LISTO

owledge, better care
professionals workir

...accent...

Hughes Syndrome

Second Edition

M. A. Khamashta (Ed.)

Hughes Syndrome
Antiphospholipid Syndrome
Second Edition

With 80 Figures

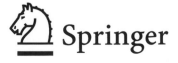 Springer

M. A. Khamashta, MD, FRCP, PhD
Deputy Head, Lupus Research Unit, St Thomas' Hospital, London, UK

Artwork marked with 📖 symbol throughout the book is original to the 1st edition (Khamashta MA. Hughes Syndrome: Antiphospholipid Syndrome. Springer-Verlag London Ltd. 2000) and is being republished in this 2nd edition.

A catalogue record for this book is available from the British Library

Library of Congress Control Number: 2005926817

ISBN-10:1-85233-873-3   Printed on acid-free paper
ISBN-13:978-1-85233-873-2

ISBN 1-85233-232-8 1st edition

First published 2000
Second edition 2006

Printed in Singapore   (EXP/KYO)

9 8 7 6 5 4 3 2 1

Springer Science+Business Media
springeronline.com

To my parents, Andrawes and Azizeh,
who have supported me throughout my life
and continue to inspire me to achieve.

Foreword to the Second Edition

The studies and discussions presented in the second edition of the *Hughes Syndrome* text had their beginning with a 1983 *British Medical Journal* publication entitled "Thrombosis, abortion, cerebral disease and the lupus anticoagulant." In the mid-20th-century, it was recognized that some patients with systemic lupus erythematosus had biological false positive serological tests for syphilis, often coincident with the presence of an anti-coagulant in plasma and the some of these patients (particularly ones with somewhat atypical of patterns of lupus) paradoxically manifested an increased incidence of procoagulant complications. Nothing much was made of these associations, however, until Graham Hughes, author of the above citation, applied his talents of astute bedside observation, knowledge of disease mechanisms, imagination, and a "bloodhound" instinct for fol-lowing relevant clues. Graham and his colleagues early-on documented vas-culopathy as basis for the diffuse (variable) pathology characteristic of the syndrome; evidence that procoagulant features were mediated by anti-phospholipid autoantibodies (aPL) followed. Over the past two decades, investigators around the world have turned their attention to the study of the Hughes syndrome. (Contributors to this text include 83 clinicians and/or scientists from 13 countries in Europe, the Americas, Near East, and Asia. They represent more than a dozen clinical subspecialties and several basic science disciplines; professionals and students in these fields will need access to this book, whether in institutional libraries or personal collections – good news for the publisher.)

Truly rational treatment and/or prevention of the Hughes syndrome will await more precise knowledge of its pathogenesis but the recognition in the 1980s that ischemic and necrotic lesions in affected organs are secondary to thrombosis rather than to inflammation played a significant role in improved management of the illness and avoidance of inappropriate therapy. Beyond anticoagulation, there is enormous potential for discovery of more specific (and potentially more effective) therapies based on better definition of the complex humoral and/or cellular events activated by aPL. For example, studies by Giradi and Salmon (described in Chapter 31) demonstrated that blockade of the complement system prevented fetal loss and thrombosis in an animal model of the Hughes syndrome, extrapolation to clinical trials of complement blockade should be forthcoming.

I would like to address the issue of terminology for this illness, herein designated the "Hughes syndrome." I have already referred to the historical role Graham Hughes played in describing the syndrome, the recognition of clinical-pathological associations, and the relationship to aPL (reviewed in more detail by Munther Khamashta in Chapter 1). This alone, in my judgment, justifies acceptance of the eponym "Hughes syndrome" rather than "antiphospholipid syndrome." There are other rationales for that recommendation: (1) the precise molecular target of aPL remains a subject of study (beta 2 glycoprotein-1 versus phospholipids), (2) in some patients the illness and presence of aPL are disassociated over time, and (3) the long-standing use of eponyms for other vasculopathies (e.g., Wegener, Churg-Strauss, Kawasaki, Henoch-Schöenlein, Behçet, Takayasu) have utility in recognizing individual clinical and pathological patterns of disease and management objectives.

Finally, I would like to draw attention to a short chapter at the end of the book, "The Future of Hughes Syndrome." In this chapter, Michael D. Lockshin summarizes recent progress in our understanding of the problem and, more importantly, identifies areas of ignorance and special opportunities for study. It is an exciting time for seeking new insights regarding the pathogenesis and management of the Hughes syndrome; this revised reference text will be an invaluable resource for anyone engaged in such inquiries.

Charles L. Christian, MD
Department of Medicine
University of Florida
Jacksonville, Florida
USA

Foreword to the First Edition

I am very happy to be asked by Dr. Munther Khamashta to write a Foreword to this first comprehensive description of the many facets of the antiphospholipid syndrome (APS). Although I have been an interested and long-time participant in studies to elucidate the nature of some human diseases associated with immunological abnormalities, I have not had a personal involvement with work on the APS. I have however watched with great fascination the evolution of this field from initial observations of clinical symptoms to studies defining the pathophysiological abnormalities.

The APS began with reports in 1983, 1984 and 1985 (see Khamashta: Hughes Syndrome, A History) on a number of clinical symptoms which appeared to have an underlying common pathogenic mechanism – vascular thrombotic episodes. These included peripheral vascular thromboses, cerebral vascular infarctions, livedo reticularis, spontaneous abortions and portal and pulmonary hypertension. A striking feature of this unfolding story was that already in 1983, suspicion was cast on the likely association of anti-cardiolipin/phospholipid antibodies with the clinical syndromes. Continuing studies on the pathophysiology have helped to fine-tune the immunological abnormalities. Most investigators believe that proteins complexed to phospholipids such as β-2–glycoprotein-1 are the primary targets of the autoantibodies but there appears to be continuing evidence that phospholipids themselves are also target antigens. The argument here may hinge on the fact that the immunogen itself might be a complex of phospholipid and protein and the humoral immune response is directed at different component parts of this complex, depending on the "immunogenicity" of different components to a genetically susceptible host. In fact, many autoantigens in lupus and other autoimmune diseases are complexes of nucleic acids and proteins, a classical example being the Sm antigens comprising complexes of small nuclear RNAs and small nuclear ribonucleoproteins.

In autoimmune diseases like lupus, we have advanced the notion that the humoral antibody responses are antigen-driven and that the antigens are self proteins rendered immunogenic due to a variety of reasons, including overexpression, ectopic localization and structural alterations of various kinds such as mutagenesis or complexing with foreign materials. An interesting aspect of the APS story is the diverse nature of clinical symptoms which involve totally different organ systems but rarely involve more than one organ system at a time. This is in contrast to lupus which is also a multi-system disease, but the individual patient often has multiple organ

Hughes Syndrome

system involvement. It is possible that the APS might fall into the following mechanistic scenario:

Different inciting agents → → → Thrombosis in different organ systems → → → antigenic modification of procoagulant phospholipid-protein → → → humoral antibody responses → → → in-situ antigen-antibody complex formation → → → inflammation, further thrombosis, recruitment of cellular immune infiltrates → → → perpetuation of repeated cycles of thrombosis, inflammation and immune responses.

The diversity of the APS could be explained on the uniqueness of the initial inciting event leading to pro-coagulation occurring in specific organ systems and thus would not have to invoke aberrant immune responses manifesting the great variety of clinical syndromes. One of the challenges in the future would be to explain or identify the different inciting agents for the different syndromes encountered.

One of the issues which has been raised is that the anti-phospholipid syndrome is a misnomer since the major target antigen appears to be the protein or the lipoprotein complex. Many investigators are inclined towards keeping the original moniker of the APS because of both historical and common usage reasons. The history of clinical medicine and bio-medical research is replete with examples where original designations have been retained in spite of subsequent studies showing that the designation was not totally correct. The important thing is that the essence of the original observations in the APS was correct.

It is rare that an investigator and his colleagues have the opportunity to open up a new field in clinical medicine and biomedical research. This has happened with the anti-phospholipid syndrome. Graham Hughes and his colleagues deserve enormous kudos for recognizing that a number of clinical syndromes shared a common feature of vascular thrombosis and for carrying this into consolidation of the clinical observations with laboratory analysis. Much clinical and basic research by many investigators worldwide have resulted from these beginnings. This volume stands as a tribute to Hughes and his colleagues.

Eng M. Tan, MD
The Scripps Research Institute
La Jolla, California 92037
USA

Prologue to the First Edition

Memory loss, migraine, strokes, accelerated atheroma, recurrent miscarriages – some of the features which make the antiphospholipid syndrome (APS) so important to patients and clinicians worldwide.

The finding that simple and reproducible assays can identify patients at risk both for venous and arterial thrombosis has opened up new avenues for treatment across many specialities.

From the early days in the late 1970's and early 1980's, I had felt strongly that the syndrome would one day outstrip lupus in frequency. Indeed my colleagues and I were often impatient at the seemingly slow acceptance of the syndrome by the medical (and obstetric) community in the early years. All that has changed. The number of papers and meetings relating to the syndrome has become a flood, and there is widespread realisation that this may, in fact be one of the most common and important auto-immune diseases.

My grateful thanks to my colleagues, mentors and friends, especially Dr Tan and Charles Christian, whose guidance I have always valued, and to Nigel Harris and Aziz Gharavi, who not only worked with me in the early days of the syndrome, but have become world leaders in APS research.

Most of all, my grateful thanks to Munther Khamashta, my colleague and friend for a decade.

His reputation in this field is truly international. It is a testimony to his personal qualities that he has been able to persuade the world leaders in APS to contribute to this volume.

Graham Hughes

Prologue to the Second Edition

"There are two 'new' diseases of the late twentieth century, AIDS and APS"
Miquel Vilardell, Dean of Medicine of the University of Barcelona

Munther Khamashta deserves plaudits for his contributions to this corner of medicine. He has not only published numerous original papers on the syndrome, notably in the field of recurrent pregnancy loss, but he has also brought together colleagues with clinical and research expertise. The first edition of his book was a triumph – an example of clinically-based research which has had a major direct impact on medical practice.

In the 5 years since the first edition, there has been a dawning realisation of the extent of the impact of the antiphospholipid syndrome in so many branches of medical practice – in Alzheimer's, in multiple sclerosis, myocardial infarction, movement disorders, leg ulcers, infertility, renal and cardiac transplantation, avascular necrosis, ischaemic fractures – and even more so with the original pillars of the syndrome – stroke, TIA, DVT, pulmonary hypertension, and recurrent pregnancy loss.

Many of us working in this field have felt frustration at the seemingly slow recognition of its importance. However, things are changing. The number of research publications, reviews and conferences is increasing. In our own clinic, the number of referrals of patients with Hughes Syndrome now promises to overtake those with lupus.

In the original description of the clinical syndrome back in 1983, I wrote.... "For those of us hardened into nihilism by years of study of various autoantibodies in SLE there is a rare sense of excitement at the implications of the associations now being reported".

Twenty-two years later, this sense of clinical excitement has not waned.

Graham Hughes
Head, Lupus Unit

Contents

Contributors

Olga Amengual, MD, PhD
Department of Medicine II,
Hokkaido University Graduate School
of Medicine, Sapporo, Japan

Paul R. J. Ames, MD
Academic Department of
Rheumatology, Leeds University
Teaching Hospitals, Leeds, UK

Mary-Carmen Amigo, MD, FACP
Department of Rheumatology,
Instituto Nacional de Cardiología
Ignacio Chávez
Mexico City, Mexico

Eduardo Anglés–Cano, MD, DSc
Institut National de la Santé et de la
Recherche Médicale, CHU Bichat-
Claude Bernard, Paris, France

Jef M. M. C. Arnout, PhD
Centre for Molecular and Vascular
Biology, Faculty of Medicine,
University of Leuven, Leuven, Belgium

Tatsuya Atsumi, MD, PhD
Department of Medicine II,
Hokkaido University Graduate School
of Medicine, Sapporo, Japan

Tiziano Barbui, MD
Division of Haematology, Ospedali
Riuniti, Bergamo, Italy

Carlos A. Battagliotti
Department of Internal Medicine and
Therapeutics, National University of
Rosario, Rosario, Argentina

H. Michael Belmont, MD
Department of Rheumatology,
Hospital for Joint Diseases, New York
University School of Medicine,
New York, NY, USA

Maria Laura Bertolaccini, MD, PhD
Lupus Research Unit, The Rayne
Institute, St Thomas' Hospital, London,
UK

Susan Bewley, MBBS, MA, MD
Department of Obstetrics, Guy's and
St. Thomas' Hospitals NHS Trust,
London, UK

Miri Blank, PhD
Department of Internal Medicine and
Center for Autoimmune Diseases,
Sheba Medical Center, Tel-Hashomer,
Ramat-Gan, Israel

Maria Orietta Borghi, PhD
Department of Internal Medicine,
IRCCS Istituto Auxologico Italiano,
University of Milan, Milan, Italy

D. Ware Branch, MD
Department Obstetrics and Gynecology,
Division of Maternal and Fetal
Medicine, University of Utah Health
Services Center, Salt Lake City, UT,
USA

Robin L. Brey, MD
Department of Medicine, University of
Texas Health Science Center,
San Antonio, TX, USA

Roberto Caporali, MD
Servizio di Reumatologia, University of
Pavia, IRCCS Policlinico S. Matteo,
Pavia, Italy

Cristina Castañon, MD
Instituto Nacional De Cardiologia I.
Chavez, Mexico City, Mexico

Ricard Cervera, MD, PhD, FRCP
Department of Autoimmune Diseases,
Hospital Clínic, Barcelona, Spain

Rolando Cimaz, MD
Paediatric Rheumatology,
Istituti Clinici di Perfezionamento,
Milano, Italy

Maria J. Cuadrado, MD, PhD
Lupus Research Unit, The Rayne
Institute, St Thomas' Hospital,
London, UK

Elena Cucurull, MD
Department of Medicine, Section of
Rheumatology, Louisiana State
University Health Sciences Center,
New Orleans, LA, USA

David P. D'Cruz, MD, FRCP
Lupus Research Unit, The Rayne
Institute, St Thomas' Hospital,
London, UK

Ronald H. W. M. Derksen, MD, PhD
Department of Rheumatology and
Clinical Immunology, University
Medical Center Utrecht, Utrecht,
Netherlands

Kieth B. Elkon, MD
Department of Medicine and
Immunology, University of
Washington, Seattle, WA,
USA

Josep Font, MD, PhD, FRCP
Department of Autoimmune Diseases,
Hospital Clínic, Barcelona, Spain

Monica Galli, MD, PhD
Division of Haematology, Ospedali
Riuniti, Bergamo, Italy

Romeo García-Torres, MD
Department of Pathology, Hospital de
Especialidades, Centro Médico La Raza
Mexico City, Mexico

Maria Gerosa, MD
Department of Internal Medicine,
IRCCS Istituto Auxologico Italiano,
University of Milan, Milan, Italy

Azzudin E. Gharavi, MD
Decreased
Department of Medicine, Morehouse
School of Medicine, Atlanta, GA, USA

Ian P. Giles, BSc, MBBS, MRCP, PhD
Centre for Rheumatology,
Department of Medicine,
University College London,
London, UK

Guillermina Girardi, PhD
Department of Medicine, Hospital for
Special Surgery, Weill Medical College
of Cornell University, New York, NY,
USA

Philip G. de Groot, PhD
Department of Haematology and
Rheumatology & Clinical Immunology,
University Medical Centre, Utrecht,
Netherlands

Beverley J. Hunt, Mb ChB, FRCP,
FRCPath, MD
Department of Clinical Haematology
and Rheumatology,
Guy's and St Thomas' Hospital Trust,
London, UK

David A. Isenberg, MD, MBBS, FRCP
Centre for Rheumatology, Department
of Medicine, University College
London, London, UK

Aharon Kessel, MD
Division of Clinical Immunology and
Allergy, Bnai Zion Medical Center,
Affiliated with Technion Faculty of
Medicine, Haifa, Israel

Munther A. Khamashta, MD, FRCP, PhD
Lupus Research Unit, The Rayne
Institute, St Thomas' Hospital,
London, UK

Kazuko Kobayashi, PhD
Department of Cell Chemistry,
Okayama University Graduate School
of Medicine and Dentistry, Okayama,
Japan

Takao Koike, MD
Department of Medicine II, Hokkaido
University Graduate School of
Medicine, Sapporo, Japan

Ilan Krause, MD
Department of Internal Medicine F,
Rabin Medical Center, Petah-Tiqva,
Israel

Lorin Lakasing, MD, MRCOG
Department of Obstetrics, Guy's and
St. Thomas' Hospitals NHS Trust,
London, UK

Michael D. Lockshin, MD
Department of Rheumatology,
Barbara Volcker Center for Women
and Rheumatic Diseases, Hospital for
Special Surgery, New York, NY, USA

Luis R. Lopez, MD
Corgenix, Inc., Westminster, CO, USA

Chary López-Pedrera, PhD
Research Unit, Reina Sofia Hospital,
Córdoba, Spain

Charles G. Mackworth-Young, MD,
FRCP
Department of Rheumatology, Charing
Cross Hospital, London, UK

Eiji Matsuura, PhD
Department of Cell Chemistry,
Okayama University Graduate School
of Medicine and Dentistry, Okayama,
Japan

Gale A. McCarty, MD, FACP, FACR
RheumEd Consulting, and Washington
Hospital Center/Georgetown University
Division of Rheumatology and
Immunology, Washington DC, USA

John A. McIntyre, PhD, FRCPath,
Dip ABHI
HLA-Vascular Biology Laboratory,
St. Francis Hospital and Health Center,
and
Department of Biology, Indiana
University-Purdue University at
Indianapolis, Indianapolis, IN, USA

Pier Luigi Meroni, MD
Department of Internal Medicine,
IRCCS Istituto Auxologico Italiano,
University of Milan, Milan, Italy

Carlomaurizio Montecucco, MD
Servizio di Reumatologia, University of
Pavia, IRCCS Policlinico S. Matteo,
Pavia, Italy

Haralampos M. Moutsopoulos, MD,
FACP, FRCP
Department of Pathophysiology,
Medical School, National University of
Athens, Athens, Greece

Neelufar Mozaffarian, MD, PhD
Department of Medicine, University of
Washington, Seattle, WA, USA

Catherine Nelson-Piercy, MBBS, MA,
FRCP
Department of Obstetrics, Guy's and
St. Thomas' Hospitals NHS Trust,
London, UK

Arianna Parisio, PhD
Department of Internal Medicine,
IRCCS Istituto Auxologico Italiano,
University of Milan, Milan, Italy

Ann L. Parke, MBBS
Department of Medicine, Division of
Rheumatic Diseases, The University of
Connecticut, School of Medicine,
Farmington, CT, USA

Debendra Pattanaik, MD
Department of Medicine, University of
Texas Health Science Center, San
Antonio, TX, USA

Michelle Petri, MD, MPH
Department of Medicine, Division of
Rheumatology, Johns Hopkins
University School of Medicine,
Baltimore, MD, USA

Silvia S. Pierangeli, PhD
Department of Microbiology,
Biochemistry and Immunology,
Morehouse School of Medicine, Atlanta,
GA, USA

Jean-Charles Piette, MD
Service de Médecine Interne, Groupe
Hospitalier Pitié-Salpetrière, Paris,
France

T. Flint Porter, MD
Obstetrics and Gynecology Diagnostic
Center, University Hospital and Clinics,
University of Utah Health Services
Center, Salt Lake City, UT, USA

Anisur Rahman, MA, BM, BCh, MRCP,
PhD
Centre for Rheumatology, Department
of Medicine, University College
London, London, UK

Jacob H. Rand, MD
Department of Pathology and Medicine,
Albert Einstein College of Medicine,
and Hematology Laboratories,
Montefiore Medical Center, Bronx, NY,
USA

Elena Raschi, PhD
Department of Internal Medicine,
IRCCS Istituto Auxologico Italiano,
University of Milan, Milan, Italy

Joan-Carles Reverter, MD, PhD
Hemotherapy and Hemostasis
Department, Hospital Clínic Barcelona,
Barcelona, Spain

Pedro A. Reyes, MD
Instituto Nacional De Cardiologia I.
Chavez, Mexico City, Mexico

Robert A. S. Roubey, MD
Division of Rheumatology, Allergy &
Immunology, Department of Medicine,
and Thurston Arthritis Research
Center, The University of North
Carolina at Chapel Hill, Chapel Hill,
NC, USA

Guillermo Ruiz-Irastorza
Service and Department of Internal
Medicine, Hospital de Cruces,
Universidad del Pais Vasco/Euskal
Herriko Unibertsitatea, Bizkaia, Spain

Jane E. Salmon, MD
Department of Medicine, Hospital for
Special Surgery, Weill Medical College
of Cornell University, New York, NY,
USA

Lisa R. Sammaritano, MD
Division of Rheumatology, Hospital for
Special Surgery, Weill Medical College
of Cornell University, New York, NY,
USA

Shirish R. Sangle, MBBS, MD
Lupus Research Unit, The Rayne
Institute, St Thomas' Hospital, London,
UK

Giovanni Sanna, MD, PhD
Department of Rheumatology,
Homerton University Hospital NHS
Foundation Trust, London, UK

Yehuda Shoenfeld, MD, FRCP
Department of Internal Medicine B and
Center for Autoimmune Diseases,
Sheba Medical Center, Tel-Hashomer,
Sackler Faculty of Medicine, Tel-Aviv
University, and Incumbent of the Laura
Schwarz-Kipp Chair for Autoimmunity,
Tel-Aviv University, Israel

Robert M. Silver, MD
Obstetrics and Gynecology Diagnostic
Center, University Hospital and Clinics,
University of Utah Health Services
Center, Salt Lake City, UT, USA

Dolors Tàssies, MD, PhD
Hemotherapy and Hemostasis
Department, Hospital Clínic Barcelona,
Barcelona, Spain

Maria G. Tektonidou, MD
Department of Pathophysiology,
Medical School, National University of
Athens, Athens, Greece

Cinzia Testoni, PhD
Department of Internal Medicine,
IRCCS Istituto Auxologico Italiano,
University of Milan, Milan, Italy

Natalia Tishkevich, MD
Department of Medicine, University of
Washington, Seattle, WA, USA

Elias Toubi, MD
Division of Clinical Immunology and
Allergy, Bnai Zion Medical Center,
Affiliated with Technion Faculty of
Medicine, Haifa, Israel

Lori B. Tucker, MD
Division of Rheumatology, British
Columbia Children's Hospital,
Vancouver, BC, Canada

Francisco Velasco, MD
Department of Haematology,
Reina Sofia Hospital, Córdoba, Spain

Jos Vermylen, MD, PhD
Centre for Molecular and Vascular
Biology, Faculty of Medicine,
University of Leuven, Leuven, Belgium

Tonia L. Vincent, MRCP, PhD
Department of Cartilage Biology,
Kennedy Institute of Rheumatology,
London, UK

Dawn R. Wagenknecht, BS, MS, CHS
(ABHI)
HLA-Vascular Biology Laboratory,
St. Francis Hospital and Health Center,
Indianapolis, IN, USA

Wendell A. Wilson, MD, FRCP
Department of Medicine, Section of
Rheumatology, Louisiana State
University Health Sciences Center,
New Orleans, LA, USA

Xiao-Xuan Wu, MD
Department of Pathology, Albert
Einstein College of Medicine,
Montefiore Medical Center, Bronx, NY,
USA

Shinsuke Yasuda, MD
Department of Medicine II, Hokkaido
University Graduate School of
Medicine, Sapporo, Japan

Section 1
Clinical Aspects

1 Hughes Syndrome: History

M. A. Khamashta

In the 21 years since Graham Hughes's detailed description of the antiphospholipid syndrome (APS), the condition has come to be regarded as one of the most common autoimmune diseases. The impact of the description has been enormous – for example, the recognition that some individuals with connective tissue diseases require anticoagulation rather than steroids or anti-inflammatory treatment has brought about a fundamental change in medical practice. In obstetrics, APS is now regarded as the most important prothrombotic cause of recurrent pregnancy loss – with pregnancy success improving from below 20% to a current live birth rate of over 80% [1].

In neurology, Hughes syndrome may be associated with up to 20% of strokes in people under 40 – a striking figure not least in terms of medical economics, let alone in potentially preventable suffering.

In vascular disease, Hughes syndrome may well provide insights into immunological factors in the pathogenesis of atheroma [2].

In short, the syndrome links immunology with thrombosis and vascular disease. The mechanisms are complex and our current knowledge will be detailed in this volume. Suffice to say that the antibodies probably bind not simply to phospholipids – nor simply to phospholipid cofactor. In view of this increasing complexity, colleagues at the Sixth APS meeting in Louvain put forward the eponym *Hughes syndrome* in honor of the physician who fully described the condition – an eponym with which most colleagues working in the field, and those contributing to this volume, are content.

Graham Hughes's description of the condition was not, as is sometimes the case, based on a single case report or a small series. It was a truly comprehensive and lifetime work, starting in the world of lupus. The 1983 description of the syndrome was the culmination of a decade of work in which careful clinical observations were combined not only with scientific studies, but also with a sharing of information. His ward rounds were and are famous for the cross-fertilization of ideas.

In 1983–1986, Dr Hughes and his team described the association of antiphospholipid antibodies (aPL) with *arterial* as well as venous thrombosis; with neurological disease, especially stroke; with pulmonary hypertension; with livedo; with occasional thrombocytopenia; and with recurrent miscarriages. More significantly, he recognized that this syndrome, which he initially named the anticardiolipin syndrome and later the primary antiphospholipid syndrome, was separable from lupus. My colleague, the late Aziz Gharavi, remembered hearing Graham forecast, at the 1985 American College of Rheumatology meeting in New Orleans, that the

3

"primary" APS would one day outstrip lupus in prevalence, and that in the world of obstetrics, anticoagulation would replace steroids in the management of recurrent fetal loss in this disease. Both forecasts are proving correct. In the early 1980s Graham Hughes's team, led initially by Drs Nigel Harris and Aziz Gharavi, and later by myself, instituted collaborative workshops and, in 1984, the first international APS meeting – a meeting which has become a regular fixture and which spawned the classification criteria [3, 4]. The following extract is, with permission, taken from Dr Hughes's own account of the description of the APS [5]:

> The description of the syndrome in 1983 came after a number of years of study of lupus, of myelopathy (especially so-called Jamaican neuropathy) and of atypical forms of connective tissue disease. We had become interested in the association of a false-positive VDRL with transverse myelopathy, and hypothesized, probably wrongly, that anticardiolipin antibodies might cross-react with neuronal phospholipids including cephalin and sphingomyelin [6]. With our large clinic population, it is relatively easy to spot subsets of disease and it soon became apparent that the presence of anticardiolipin antibodies (also the lupus anticoagulant) – hence antiphospholipid antibodies, were strongly associated with thrombosis and miscarriage. From a clinical point of view, the association with thrombosis related not merely to venous thrombosis, but – differentiating it from almost all other prothrombotic conditions – *arterial* thrombosis, especially strokes.
>
> In 1983, I was invited to present my findings to a British dermatology society meeting – the "Prosser White oration" [7]. The following extract, taken from that paper, highlights, I believe both the clinical features of the syndrome, and the recognition of a "Primary" antiphospholipid syndrome:
>
> Although many of these patients fall under the general heading of lupus, or lupus-like disease, I believe that the group is sufficiently homogeneous, and in some ways (such as the frequently negative ANA serology) sufficiently different from typical systemic lupus erythematosus (SLE) to warrant separate consideration. The manifestations of this syndrome are thrombosis (often multiple) and, frequently, spontaneous abortions (often multiple), neurological disease, thrombocytopenia and livedo reticularis. The livedo reticularis is often most florid on the knees. This may or may not be associated with mild to moderate Raynaud's phenomenon.
>
> These patients' blood pressure often fluctuates, apparently correlating with the severity of the livedo, suggesting a possible renovascular aetiology. However, this group of patients rarely has primary renal disease.
>
> The cerebral features are prominent and of three varieties: headaches – often migrainous and intractable; epilepsy (or abnormal EEGs) – often going back to early teenage. Fortunately, severe or difficult-to-control epilepsy is infrequent. Some patients have chorea. Cerebro-vascular accidents – sometimes transient and seemingly attributable to migraine, are frequently progressive.... The patients may develop transient cerebral ischaemic attacks or visual field defects, or, more significantly, progressive cerebral ischaemia.
>
> Two other features of the syndrome are a tendency to multiple spontaneous abortions and peripheral thrombosis, often with multiple leg and arm vein thrombosis. We have also seen Budd–Chiari syndrome and renal vein thrombosis in some of these patients. We have, of course, tended to group these patients under the diagnostic umbrella of systemic lupus, though an alternative label of "primary" Sjögren's syndrome covers other patients, and characteristic dry Schirmer's tests and lymphocytic infiltration of the minor salivary glands have been found in a number (though not all) of this group of patients.
>
> To my mind, however, the most striking, and often the most serious feature of the disease is the tendency to thrombosis, particularly cerebral thrombosis. So prominent has this feature been that we have some patients in their 40s and 50s who had been diagnosed as primary cerebrovascular disease or – when the labile hypertension has been observed – as hypertensive cerebrovascular disease. The finding that many of these patients may have

high titres of circulating anti-cardiolipin antibodies leads us to believe that a new line of investigation may be possible in such patients.

In the early 1980s my team then at Hammersmith, collected large numbers of patients who had the syndrome, yet did not meet the classification criteria for lupus – we called these patients "anticardiolipin syndrome" – and changed the name to the antiphospholipid syndrome when it was clear that these patients' sera were also cross-reactive with other phospholipids such as phosphatidylserine [8–10].

So, in the few years between 1983 and 1987, our description of the syndrome included recurrent fetal loss [11], livedo [7], renal thrombosis [12], strokes [13], liver thrombosis including Budd–Chiari syndrome [14], myelopathy [15], chorea [16], bowel infarction [17], thrombocytopenia [18], pulmonary hypertension [19] and dementia [20].

The clinical collaborators included Margaret Byron, Bernie Colaco, Genevieve Derue, Mee-Ling Boey, later joined by Charles Mackworth-Young, Sozos Loizou, Bupendra Patel, John Chan, Keith Elkon, Mark Walport and Ron Asherson. In the laboratory, two research fellows, Aziz Gharavi, and later Nigel Harris, spearheaded the development of immunoassays culminating in the first (*Lancet*) paper on the assay for anticardiolipin antibodies [21] which paved the way for the development of the enzyme-linked immunosorbent assay (ELISA) [22] and the widespread testing and recognition of the syndrome.

In his 1983 Prosser–White lecture, Graham Hughes emphasized his view that many of the patients did not have classic lupus, and deserved separate consideration as a syndrome [7]. His group, in the early 1980s, published a number of reports which associated aPL with the syndrome *outside* of systemic lupus. He reported aPL in Behçet's disease, idiopathic transverse myelopathy and Guillain–Barré syndrome [23], idiopathic thrombocytopenia [18], migraine, epilepsy [24], heart valve disease [25], and Addison's disease [26]. Graham Hughes's view was that this was most certainly a "distinct" syndrome which occurs in ANA-negative lupus erythematosus (LE) patients, atypical lupus patients, and, as expected, individuals with no lupus at all [7]. In 1987 his group was the first to introduce the term *antiphospholipid syndrome* and *primary antiphospholipid syndrome* [10] and 2 years later, in 1989, two large series of patients were published, one by his group [27] and another by the group in Mexico [28], which confirmed and detailed the earlier clinical descriptions.

In 1990 the next major advance, when three groups [29–31] reported that aPL required a plasma protein "cofactor" to bind cardiolipin on ELISA plates. β_2-glycoprotein I was identified as this cofactor. Since then, a number of "cofactors," including prothrombin, have been described [32]. The binding of antibodies to the antigen site is clearly complex and dependent on molecule configuration. Studies using monoclonal antibodies have, for example, suggested binding to a trimolecular site including phospholipid, protein C and cofactor [33]. It is now felt that the cumbersome term *phospholipid-cofactor syndrome* is probably wrong.

From Osler on, many observers of lupus have recognized thrombosis as a feature in some patients. Similarly, many other features, including thrombocytopenia and recurrent miscarriage, are well recognized as features of the disease. Historically, the "oldest" immunological finding in SLE is the Wasserman reaction. In 1952, Moore and Mohr recognized that their false positive (BFP-STS) syphilis tests could occur in lupus [34]. In 1957, Laurell and Nilsson [35] found that the "lupus inhibitor" was frequently associated with BFP-STS. Bowie et al [36] in clinical studies of lupus, reported thrombotic lesions in patients with a circulating anticoagulant. Beaumont et al in 1954 [37] were the first to report a patient with lupus anticoagulant and recurrent abortions. This was followed by similar observations by Nilsson et al [38] 20 years later and by Soulier and Boffa [39] 5 years after that.

This volume acknowledges the many who have worked so hard to bring recognition to the syndrome. To Nigel Harris and Aziz Gharavi – involved from the early days – to the dozens of research fellows who have trained in our laboratory, and whose names are associated with so much of the APS literature; to the late Donato Alarcon-Segovia, for his enthusiasm in endorsing the syndrome with his surveys of his own lupus patients; to Takao Koike, for providing so much to the studies of β_2-glycoprotein I; to Marie Claire Boffa, for her collaboration and organizing ability in setting up collabortive workshops; and to Yehuda Shoenfeld for contributing so much momentum, especially through his animal model studies, to our knowledge of the syndrome.

The ripples continue to spread. The world of transplantation is involved with huge implications for renal, liver, and cardiac transplantation [40], orthopaedics is embraced, not only in the predilection for avascular necrosis, but in the recent striking finding of spontaneous metatarsal and other bone fractures [41]. Internal arterial ischemia has embraced Hughes Syndrome as a possibly important cause of reno-vascular hypertension [42] and celiac axis stenosis as a "new" link to gastro-intestinal symptoms [43]. In the world of neurology the ramifications include multiple sclerosis, memory loss, migraine, and even sleep disorders [44]. In dermatology, the importance of livedo, described in Hughes' original papers, is recognized, as is the contribution to chronic leg ulcers.

This syndrome is common. Many physicians ask: "Where were all these patients before?" They were always there – in lupus clinics, in migraine clinics, in anticoagulant clinics with strokes, with multiple sclerosis, and with a gamut of vascular problems. It is also probable that many, many patients – notably those with memory loss or subtle neurological deficit – remain undiagnosed.

The description of the APS by Graham Hughes has had an impact on patients in all corners of medical practice.

References

1. `Khamashta MA, Mackworth Young C. Antiphospholipid (Hughes) syndrome – a treatable cause of recurrent pregnancy loss. Br Med J 1997;314:244.
2. Harats D, George J, Levy Y, Khamashta MA, Hughes GRV, Shoenfeld Y. Atheroma: links with antiphospholipid antibodies, Hughes syndrome and lupus. Q J Med 1999;92:57–59.
3. 8th International Symposium on Antiphospholipid Antibodies, Sapporo, Japan (1998). Lupus 7(suppl 2):1–234.
4. Wilson WA, Gharavi AE, Koike T, et al. International consensus statement on preliminary classification criteria for definite antiphospholipid syndrome. Report of an international workshop. Arthritis Rheum 1999;42:1309–1311.
5. Hughes GRV. Hughes syndrome – the syndrome behind the name (otherwise known as antiphospholipid syndrome). Isr Med Ass J 1999;1:100–103.
6. Wilson WA, Hughes GRV. Aetiology of Jamaican neuropathy. Lancet 1975;i:240.
7. Hughes GRV. Connective tissue disease and the skin. The 1983 Prosser-White oration. Clin Exp Dermatol 1984;9:535–544.
8. Hughes GRV. The anticardiolipin syndrome. Clin Exp Rheumatol 1985;3:285.
9. Harris EN, Baguley E, Asherson RA, Hughes GRV. Clinical and serological features of the antiphospholipid syndrome [abstract]. Br J Rheumatol 1987;26:19.
10. Mackworth-Young CG, David J, Loizou S, Walport MJ. Primary antiphospholipid syndrome: features in patients with raised anticardiolipin antibodies and no other disorders [abstract]. Br J Rheumatol 1987;26:94.
11. Derue GJ, Englert HJ, Harris EN, et al. Fetal loss in systemic lupus: association with anticardiolipin antibodies. J Obstet Gynaecol 1985;2:207–209.

12. Hughes GRV, Asherson RA. Formes atypiques du lupus erythemateux dissemine. In: Crosnier J, Funck-Brentano JL, Brack JF, Grungeld JP, eds. Actualites nephrologiques. Paris: Flammarion Medicine; 1984.
13. Harris EN, Gharavi AE, Asherson RA, Boey ML, Hughes GRV. Cerebral infarction in systemic lupus. Association with anticardiolipin antibodies. Clin Exp Rheumatol 1984;2:47–51.
14. Mackworth-Young CG, Gharavi AE, Boey ML, Hughes GRV. Portal and pulmonary hypertension in a case of systemic lupus erythematosus: possible relationships with clotting abnormality. Eur J Rheumatol Inflamm 1984;7:72–74.
15. Harris EN, Gharavi AE, Mackworth-Young CG, Patel BM, Derue G, Hughes GR. Lupoid sclerosis: a possible pathogenetic role for antiphospholipid antibodies. Ann Rheum Dis 1985;44:281–282.
16. Asherson RA, Hughes GRV. Antiphospholipid antibodies and chorea. J Rheumatol 1988;15:377–379.
17. Asherson RA, Morgan SH, Harris EN, Gharavi AE, Kraus T, Hughes GRV. Arterial occlusion causing large bowel infarction in SLE. Reflection of clotting diathesis. Clin Rheumatol 1986;5:102–106.
18. Harris EN, Gharavi AE, Hegde U, et al. Anticardiolipin antibodies in autoimmune thrombocytopenic purpura. Br J Haematol 1985;59:231–234.
19. Asherson RA, Mackworth-Young CG, Boey ML, et al. Pulmonary hypertension in systemic lupus erythematosus. Br Med J 1983;287:1024–1025.
20. Asherson RA, Mercy D, Philips G, et al. Recurrent stroke and multi-infarct dementia in systemic lupus erythematosus associated with antiphospholipid antibodies. Ann Rheum Dis 1987;46:605–611.
21. Harris EN, Gharavi AE, Bowie ML, et al. Anticardiolipin antibodies: detection by radioimmunoassay and association with thrombosis in SLE. Lancet 1983;ii:1211–1214.
22. Harris EN, Gharavi AE, Patel SP, et al. Evaluation of the anticardiolipin antibody test: report of a standardisation workshop held on April 4th, 1986. Clin Exp Immunol 1987;58:215–222.
23. Harris EN, Englert H, Derue G, et al. Antiphospholipid antibodies in acute Guillain–Barré syndrome. Lancet 1983;ii:1361–1362.
24. Herranz MT, Rivier G, Khamashta MA, Blaser KU, Hughes GRV. Association between antiphospholipid antibodies and epilepsy in patients with systemic lupus erythematosus. Arthritis Rheum 1994;37:568–571.
25. Khamashta MA, Cervera R, Asherson RA, et al. Association of antibodies against phospholipids with heart valve disease in systemic lupus erythematosus. Lancet 1990;335:1541–1544.
26. Asherson RA, Hughes GRV. Addison's disease and primary antiphospholipid syndrome. Lancet 1989;ii:874.
27. Asherson RA, Khamashta MA, Ordi-Ros J, et al. The "primary" antiphospholipid syndrome: major clinical and serological features. Medicine (Baltimore) 1989;68:366–374.
28. Alarcon-Segovia D, Sanchez-Guerrero J. Primary antiphospholipid syndrome. J Rheumatol 1989;16:482–488.
29. Matsuura E, Igarashi Y, Fujimoto M, Ichikawa K, Koike T. Anticardiolipin co-factor(s) and differential diagnosis of autoimmune disease. Lancet 1990;336:177–178.
30. Galli M, Comfurius P, Maassen C, et al. Anticardiolipin antibodies (ACA) are directed not to cardiolipinbut to a plasma protein co-factor. Lancet 1990;335:1544–1547.
31. McNeil HP, Simpson RJ, Chesterman CN, Krilis SA. Antiphospholipid antibodies are directed against a complex antigen that includes a lipid-binding inhibitor of coagulation: 2-glycoprotein I (apolipoprotein H). Proc Natl Acad Sci U S A 1990;87:4120–4124.
32. Roubey RAS. Auto-antibodies to phospholipid binding proteins: a new view of lupus anticoagulants and other "antiphospholipid" antibodies. Blood 1994;84:2854–2867.
33. Atsumi T, Khamashta, MA, Amengual, O et al. Binding of anticardiolipin antibodies to Protein C via β_2-glycoprotein I (β_2-GPI): a possible mechanism in the inhibitory effect of antiphospholipid antibodies on the Protein C system. Clin Exp Immunol 1998;112:325–333.
34. Moore JE, Mohr CF. Biologically false positive serological test for syphilis. Type, incidence and cause. J Am Med Ass 1952;150:467–473.
35. Laurell AB, Nilsson IM. Hypergammaglobulinaemia, circulating anticoagulant and biological false positive Wasserman reaction: a study of 2 cases. J Lab Clin Med 1957;49:694–707.
36. Bowie EJW, Thompson JH Jr, Pascuzzi CV, Owen CA. Thrombosis in systemic lupus erythematosus despite circulating anticoagulant. J Lab Clin Med 1983;62:416–430.
37. Beaumont JL. Syndrome hemorrhagique acquis du a un anticoagulant circulant. Sang 1954;25:1–15.
38. Nilsson IM, Astedt B, Hedner U, et al. Intrauterine death and circulating anticoagulant ("antithromboplastin"). Acta Med Scand 1975;197:153–159.
39. Soulier JP, Boffa MC. Avortements a repetition thromboses et anticoagulant circulant anti-thromboplastine. Nouv Press Med 1980;9:859–864.

40. McIntyre JA, Wagenknecht DR. Antiphospholipid Antibodies: risk assessment for solid organ, bone marrow, and tissue transplantation. Rheum Dis Clin N Am 2001;27:611–631.

41. Sangle SR, D'Cruz DP, Khamashta MA, Hughes GRV. Antiphospholipid antibodies, systemic lupus erythematosus and non-traumatic metatarsal fractures. Ann Rheum Dis 2004;63:1241–1243.

42. Sangle SR, D'Cruz DP, Jan W, et al. Renal artery stenosis in the antiphospholipid (Hughes) syndrome and hypertension. Ann Rheum Dis 2003;62:999–1002.

43. Sangle SR, Jan W, Lau IS, et al. Coeliac artery stenosis and antiphospholipid (Hughes) syndrome/antiphospholipid antibodies. Lupus 2005;14.

44. Hughes GRV. Migraine, memory loss, and "multiple sclerosis". Neurological features of the antiphospholipid (Hughes) syndrome. Postgrad Med J 2003;79:81–83.

2   Antiphospholipid (Hughes) Syndrome: An Overview

David P. D'Cruz

Introduction

The cardinal features of the antiphospholipid syndrome (APS), first described in 1983 by Dr Graham Hughes and his team at the Hammersmith Hospital, included recurrent arterial and venous thromboses, fetal losses, and thrombocytopenia. Although a wide variety of clinical features have been added over the last 22 years, these major features have stood the test of time. The aim of this chapter is to give a clinical overview of the spectrum of these clinical features, the assessment of aPL, and their impact on morbidity and mortality.

Demographics

APS is now recognized as a common disorder and is certainly not a "small print" disease. Its importance lies in the fact that once diagnosed, this a treatable condition. The difficulty is that for many patients diagnosis is often delayed, sometimes for years, with consequent disability, loss of livelihood, inability to start a family, or even death.

The prevalence of antiphospholipid antibodies (aPL) in otherwise healthy populations is less than 1% and up to 5% in older healthy populations. In autoimmune diseases, especially systemic lupus erythematosus (SLE), however, the prevalence is much higher. There have been several large studies of the prevalence of aPL in SLE patients. Perhaps the largest is the Euro-Lupus study that found a prevalence of 24% IgG anticardiolipin antibodies (aCL), 13% IgM aCL, and 15% lupus anticoagulant (LA) in a cohort of 1000 patients with SLE [1]. The prevalence of aPL and definite APS may increase with longer follow up, further pregnancies, and repeat testing for aPL. Thus, Perez-Vazquez et al showed that the prevalence of APS increased from 10% to 23% after 15–18 years in a large cohort of SLE patients [2]. A further study of 1000 APS patients has detailed the clinical features of the disorder [3].

Definition and Classification of APS

An international consensus statement on classification criteria for definite APS was published after a workshop in 1998 (Table 2.1) and validated [4, 5]. These

Table 2.1. Classification criteria for the antiphospholipid syndrome.

Clinical criteria

1. Vascular thrombosis:
   One or more clinical episodes of arterial, venous, or small vessel thrombosis, in any tissue or organ. Thrombosis must be confirmed by imaging or Doppler studies or histopathology, with the exception of superficial venous thrombosis. For histopathologic confirmation, thrombosis should be present without significant evidence of inflammation in the vessel wall.

2. Pregnancy morbidity
   (a) One or more unexplained deaths of a morphologically normal fetus at or beyond the 10th weeks of gestation, with normal fetal morphology documented by ultrasound or by direct examination of the fetus, or
   (b) One or more premature births of a morphologically normal neonate at or before the 34th week of gestation because of severe pre-eclampsia or eclampsia, or severe placental insufficiency or
   (c) Three more unexplained consecutive spontaneous abortions before the 10th week of gestation, with maternal anatomic, or hormonal abnormalities and paternal and maternal chromosomal causes excluded.

Laboratory criteria

1. Anticardiolipin antibody of IgG and/ or IgM isotype in blood, present in medium or high titre, on two or more occasions, at least 6 weeks apart, measured by a standard enzyme linked immunosorbent assay for β_2-glycoprotein 1-dependent anticardiolipin antibodies.
2. Lupus anticoagulant present in plasma on two or more occasions at least 6 weeks apart, detected according to the guidelines of the International Society on Thrombosis and Hemostasis.

Definite APS is considered to be present if at least one of the clinical and one of the laboratory criteria are met.

---

classification criteria were developed for use in research studies rather than as diagnostic criteria which have to date not been developed. Other well-recognized features of APS, such as thrombocytopenia, hemolytic anemia, transient ischaemic attacks, transverse myelitis, livedo reticularis, valvular heart disease, demyelinating syndromes, chorea, and migraine, were not thought to have as strong an association as the final criteria and were excluded as classification criteria, possibly resulting in lower sensitivity but higher specificity [5]. In clinical practice, however, the physician should still consider the diagnosis and commence treatment according to clinical judgment after exclusion of other causes of these clinical features.

There are numerous traps for the unwary and many other conditions can be associated with aPL but are not necessarily associated with thrombosis. Thus, aPL may occur in infections such as human immunodeficiency virus (HIV) and malignancy and may also follow exposure to certain drugs. aPL in these circumstances are not necessarily pathogenic and these conditions should therefore be considered in any differential diagnosis of APS.

Indications for aPL Testing

There is a compelling case for aPL to be tested routinely in all patients who are newly diagnosed with an autoimmune connective tissue disease, especially SLE or Sjögren's syndrome, because the prevalence of aPL in these disorders ranges between 30% and 50% [6]. The finding of aPL at disease onset may have significant consequences later in the disease course in terms of predicting morbidity and mortality [7]. In other clinical contexts, patients who suffer thrombotic events at relatively young ages should also be considered for testing. Thus, patients with strokes,

Table 2.2. Indications for the measurement of antiphospholipid antibodies.

Connective tissue disease especially SLE

Venous/arterial thrombosis before the age of 45 years
Thrombosis after trivial provocation
Association of arterial and venous thrombosis
Association of thrombosis and fetal loss
Recurrent events
Family history
Thrombosis in an unusual site: retinal vein, portal, cerebral venous sinus, renal vein
Recurrent superficial thrombophlebitis
Recurrent miscarriage
Coumarin-induced skin necrosis

myocardial infarctions, and venous thromboses under the age of 50 may be at risk of further thrombotic events if they are aPL positive. Similarly, women with pregnancy morbidity should also have aPL measured. There is a wide spectrum of aPL-related pregnancy morbidity, including miscarriage, fetal death, intra-uterine growth restriction, intra-uterine death/still birth, pregnancy-induced hypertension, pre-eclampsia, and eclampsia. There is increasing evidence though that other thrombophilic disorders may also be associated with obstetric problems [8].

The timing of measurement may be important. Some authors have suggested that aPL may be consumed during a thrombotic episode, though this remains controversial. Alternatively, due to endothelial activation and exposure of cryptic antigens, aPL may appear after the thrombotic event as an "epiphenomenon" [9]. For these reasons aPL should be measured between 6 weeks and 3 months post-thrombosis to confirm results. Steroid therapy and the development of the nephrotic syndrome may also be associated with a falsely negative result [10, 11].

A recent intriguing paper has suggested that aPL may appear many years prior to the diagnosis of an autoimmune connective tissue disease such as lupus. Moreover, aPL-positive patients appeared to be at risk of more severe lupus later in the disease course [12]. This data is in keeping with their previous findings for anti-nuclear antibodies appearing long before the onset of clinical features of SLE. These studies suggest that immune dysregulation leading to autoantibody production may precede the appearance of symptoms by many years.

What Should Be Measured?

The recommendation is that both IgG and IgM aCL isotypes should be tested as well as LA. The significance of IgA aCL antibodies remains controversial but may be more relevant in SLE populations with African ancestry in contrast to Caucasians [13, 14]. The relevance of IgA aCL is discussed in detail elsewhere in this book. Although aPL testing has been standardized, there remain major inconsistencies when standard sera are sent to various laboratories. Testing for LA is also inconsistent but there seems to be a consensus that aCL are sensitive and LA testing is more specific in the diagnosis of APS. Anti–β_2-glycoprotein I antibodies correlate well with clinical features of APS as well as with other aPL and will be discussed in detail in this book. However, most routine laboratories do not offer anti–β_2-glycoprotein I antibodies because in general there is no added value above conventional aPL testing and the assay lacks standardization.

Prevalence of aPL

General Population

The prevalence of aPL in the general population is low. Large studies have shown prevalences of between 2% and 7%. For example, in 543 blood donors under 65 years of age, Fields et al found an aCL prevalence of 2% [15]. The Antiphospholipid Antibodies in Stroke Study (APASS) Group also found a prevalence of aCL in 4.3% of 257 hospitalized non-stroke patients with a mean age 66 [16]. This was similar to the prevalence of 7.1% for at least one positive aCL in 1014 in-patients studied by Schved et al with a mean age of 66.7 years: the most frequent associations were with carcinoma or alcohol abuse [17].

Elderly

Many autoantibodies become more prevalent with increasing age and aPL is no exception. Fields found that 12% of 300 healthy individuals older than 65 years had IgG or IgM aCL antibodies and that there was an association with positive antinuclear antibodies (ANA) but not rheumatoid factor [15]. The significance of these autoantibodies remains unclear and could be related to the increasing prevalence of associated conditions in the elderly, such as malignancy and drug treatment.

Venous Thromboembolism

In patients with unselected venous thromboembolism, the prevalence of aCL varies from 3% to 17% and LA from 3% to 14%. The highest prevalence of 17% was found by Schulman et al, who tested 897 patients with venous thromboembolism as part of a treatment trial with a follow up of 4 years, in whom aCL were tested 6 months post–deep vein thrombosis (DVT). Interestingly, of 20 recurrent episodes, aCL was negative in 14 at the time of the recurrent episode [18].

Arterial Thrombosis

In the situation of stroke, Nencini et al found 18% of young patients, mean age 38 years, were positive for aPL (LA and aCL), whereas the APASS study found 9.7% of first stroke patients had a positive aCL. In myocardial infarction the prevalence of aCL is between 5% and 15% [19, 20].

Fetal Loss

There is a wide range of prevalences of aPL in otherwise healthy women who have had pregnancy morbidity, ranging from 7% to as high as 42%. The reasons for this are discussed in more detail elsewhere in this book.

Risk of Positive aPL Tests for Thrombosis and Recurrent Events

There is now abundant evidence in the literature that aPL are particularly associated with a risk of thrombosis, especially recurrent events and pregnancy morbidity. The risk appears to be higher for LA than aCL but when high titer aCL are considered, the risks are also high. For example, Kearon assessed recurrence rates in 162 patients with "idiopathic" DVT participating in a treatment trial where the hazard ratio for recurrence was 2.3 for aCL and 6.8 for LA, although only the hazard ratio for LA was significant in terms of the risk of recurrent thrombosis [21]. In a meta-analysis, Wahl examined the risk of venous thromboembolism in aPL-positive patients without autoimmune disease or previous thrombosis. The odds ratio was 11.1 for LA and 1.6 for aCL. However, that risk rose to 3.2 if higher titers of aCL were examined [22]. There were 90 DVTs in the American Physicians Health Study and aCL levels greater than the 95th percentile [greater than 33 glycophospholipid (GPL) units] had a relative risk of venous thromboembolism of 5.3 [23].

In terms of arterial disease, the American Physicians Study did not find a significant association of aCL with first stroke [23]. In a seminal paper, Nencini et al found 18% of young strokes were positive for aPL tested after a first stroke compared to 2% of controls. They also found that the recurrence rate for stroke was higher in the aPL group compared to a group of stroke patients that were negative [19].

The APASS group compared first stroke to a control population of non-stroke hospitalized patients. aCL were positive in 24 of 248 of the stroke patients compared to 11 of 257 control patients. The odds ratio for stroke in patients who were aCL positive was calculated at 2.33 [16]. The APASS group concluded that aCL were a risk factor for first ischemic stroke and the extent of association was comparable to that between stroke and hypertension [16]. Recent large studies have supported this. A Framingham cohort and offspring study of 2712 women and 2262 men found that positive aCL at baseline were an independent risk factor for future ischaemic stroke and transient ischaemic attack in women but not men [24]. However, in a surprising paper extending the APASS study, Levine et al appear to come to diametrically opposite conclusions to their earlier findings and now conclude that aPL neither predict recurrent cerebral events nor a differential response to aspirin or warfarin and say that routine testing for aPL in ischemic stroke patients is not warranted [25]. This study has, however, been heavily criticized on methodological grounds and is discussed further in the chapter on neurological complications.

Kittner reviewed a number of studies and concluded that the strength of association between aCL and stroke in patients over 50 years was comparable to hypertension with an odds ratio of 2.2. In a young population less than 50 years the odds ratio may rise to 8.3 [26]. Further information on arterial disease derives from the Helsinki heart study. In this study healthy men with a low-density lipoprotein (LDL) cholesterol greater than 5.2 mmol/L, with a mean age of 49 years, were studied for cardiac end points. In the highest quartile of aCL patients, the odds ratio for myocardial infarct was significant at 2.0. In multivariate analyses the risk was independent of other risk factors and, interestingly, aCL levels were higher in smokers [20].

In SLE, the evidence for an association between aPL and arterial and venous events as well as pregnancy morbidity is strong. The largest study to date, the Euro-

Lupus study of 1000 patients, showed a correlation between the presence of IgG aCL and thrombosis as well as fetal loss and LA correlated with thrombosis [27]. Wahl performed a meta-analysis of the risk of venous thromboembolism and examined 26 studies comprising 2249 patients. The odds ratio for LA and venous events was 6.32 and 2.17 for aCL. When recurrent venous events were examined these ratios increased to 11.6 and 3.91, respectively [28].

Mortality, Morbidity, and Damage Associated with aPL

APS has a significant impact on survival. For example, in a retrospective study of 52 patients with aCL followed over 10 years, 29% of APS patients (31 patients) had recurrent events and in the asymptomatic group (21 patients) half developed APS: mortality was 10% [29]. In another study, Jouhikainen et al compared 37 LA–positive SLE patients with 37 age- and sex-matched SLE patients without LA. During a median follow up of 22 years, 30% in the LA group died in contrast to 14% in the control group [30]. Among patients with venous thromboembolism, the mortality in Swedish patients was 15% at 4 years in those with aCL and 6% in those without antibodies ($P = 0.01$)[18]. The largest prospective study of 1000 SLE patients showed that after 10 years of follow up there were 68 deaths of whom 18 (26.5%) died from thrombosis associated with aPL [7]. The most common thrombotic events were cerebrovascular accidents (11.8%), coronary occlusions (7.4%), and pulmonary emboli (5.9%).

There is increasing evidence that thrombosis contributes to the damage accrued in patients with SLE, which in turn may contribute to morbidity as well as mortality. Two recent studies have clearly demonstrated that APS with thrombotic manifestations independently contributes to irreversible organ damage as well as mortality in lupus patients [31, 32]. Thus, Ruiz-Irastorza's study of over 200 SLE patients extending over 25 years demonstrated both higher damage scores and increased mortality in APS patients, most of whom had suffered arterial thromboses [32].

Risk Factors for Thrombosis in APS: Two Hit Hypothesis

It is clear that not all aPL-positive patients will inevitably develop clinical features of Hughes syndrome. The precise reasons for this remain unclear and suggest that additional factors are required for a first thrombotic event or pregnancy-related feature. However, previous events in the context of persistent moderate-to-high aCL levels and/or LA are the most powerful predictors of future events. Thus, in a cohort of 360 patients in the Italian aPL Registry followed prospectively for 3.9 years, with either a positive LA or aCL, 34 patients developed a thrombotic event: an incidence of 2.5%/patient-year, with a rate of 5.4%/patient-year in those with a previous thrombosis and 0.95%/patient-year in asymptomatic subjects [33]. Clearly the mere presence of aPL is not sufficient for an event. Patients with aCL greater than 40 units and previous thrombosis were important risk factors for future events. Similarly, the greater the different numbers of aPL detected in a given patient the greater the risk of thrombosis [34]. The importance of previous thrombosis as a risk factor was highlighted by the recurrence rate in our patients at St Thomas' Hospital, where those with APS and previous thrombosis had a recurrence rate of 20%/patient-year of follow-up [35]. In pregnancy, patients with a prior history of miscarriages or vascular occlusions have a significantly higher rate of adverse pregnancy outcome [33].

There are numerous other risk factors that may contribute to the development of a first thrombotic event in the presence of aPL. A recent study of 404 patients with aPL showed that at the time of the initial thrombosis, 50% of patients had had coincident risk factors for thrombosis: previous surgery and prolonged immobilization were significantly associated with venous thrombosis, and hypercholesterolemia and arterial hypertension with arterial thrombosis [36].

Virchow's observations on the three factors relevant to clot formation still hold good today: factors related to the blood (hypercoagulability), factors related to the speed of flow, and factors related to the vessel wall itself. The complex mechanisms by which aPL may affect platelets and endothelial cells to produce a procoagulant state will be discussed in detail in other chapters. However, evidence is emerging of abnormalities of the vessel wall that may be relevant to APS. Accelerated atherosclerosis is undoubtedly a feature of SLE that contributes to mortality [37]. However, studies in patients without lupus who are aPL positive have shown increased carotid intima-media thickness associated with an increased risk of arterial thrombosis [38]. Another study found a higher prevalence of an abnormal ankle–brachial index in patients with primary APS compared to healthy controls, suggesting widespread vascular abnormalities [39]. Further evidence of vessel wall abnormalities comes from data showing a higher prevalence of renal artery stenosis in association with aPL in patients with SLE. This suggests that vessels that have high velocity turbulent flow may be at increased risk of vascular abnormality in the presence of aPL [40]. Our recent unpublished data suggests a similar phenomenon with coeliac artery stenosis in aPL-positive patients. Even at the capillary level there may be abnormalities. Nailfold videocapillaroscopy in patients with primary APS showed abnormal morphology with smaller capillary diameters than controls, although these changes could not be correlated to impairment of functional parameters [41]. The authors suggested that the smaller capillary diameters resulted in lower local tissue perfusion and hypoxia, although these parameters were not directly measured. If correct though, these conditions would clearly favor a procoagulant state.

Several studies have shown that risk factors can be additive. In venous thrombosis in the young, Rosendaal found that the risk of thrombosis rose sharply with the number of risk factors and that fewer factors were required for thrombosis in older subjects [42]. Several groups have reported the additional presence of coagulation abnormalities, such as factor V Leiden, in patients with APS. Factor V Leiden and aCL can both cause the activated protein C resistance phenotype and, not surprisingly, the combination has been associated with severe thrombosis [43, 44]. Methylenetetrahydrofolate reductase $\therefore$ C 677 $\rightarrow$ T substitution (increased homocysteine) may also have an effect on age at first occlusive event [44]. Furthermore, Peddi reported the development of catastrophic APS in a patient with SLE, aCL, and antithrombin III deficiency [45].

Conditions Associated with Secondary APS

A wide spectrum of disorders has been associated with APS although primary APS, where there is no underlying disease, is common and may even exceed the

Table 2.3. Antiphospholipid antibodies in other conditions.

Autoimmune connective tissue disorders	Drugs
Systemic vasculitis	Chlorpromazine
Malignancy	Quinine/quinidine
Crohn's disease	Hydralazine
Infection	Procainamide
Syphilis/lyme	Phenytoin
Human immunodeficiency virus	Interferon-α
Hepatitis C	
Cytomegalovirus	
Mycoplasma	

prevalence of secondary APS, especially if women who only have aPL-related pregnancy morbidity are included. It has been estimated that up to half of patients with APS do not have an associated systemic disease [46]. Some conditions reported in association with aPL are listed in Table 2.3.

Thrombotic manifestations of APS are not usually seen in infection- or drug-associated aCL, although occasional reports of thrombosis in infections such as acquired immune deficiency syndrome (HIV/AIDS) and cytomegalovirus (CMV) suggests that in patients with APS, especially where there may be atypical features, an underlying infection should be considered [47, 48]. Procainamide has been shown to produce β_2-glycoprotein I–dependent antibodies that are potentially pathogenic [49].

Differences Between Primary and Secondary APS

In general, there are no significant differences in the cardinal clinical features of APS, such as arterial or venous thrombosis or pregnancy morbidity, whether the syndrome is primary or secondary to an underlying connective tissue disorder [33, 50]. Shah et al found IgM aCL more commonly in SLE than primary antiphospholipid syndrome (PAPS) but no difference in thrombotic rates [29]. Although Vianna et al found that PAPS and APS secondary to SLE had similar clinical features, heart valve disease, autoimmune hemolytic anemia, lymphopenia, neutropenia, and low C4 levels were more common in patients with SLE [50].

The distinction between PAPS and APS due to SLE can sometimes be difficult. Thrombocytopenia, anemia, renal, and central nervous system (CNS) disease may be seen in both conditions. Anti-dsDNA or antibodies to extractable nuclear antigens are not found in PAPS and their presence usually suggests SLE as a secondary cause. Piette has been a strong advocate of exclusion criteria for PAPS and these are listed in Table 2.4 [51]. In terms of genetic differences between primary and secondary APS, a recent study has suggested that there are differences in FcgammaRIIA-R/H131 polymorphisms in patients with APS secondary to SLE [52].

The number of cases reported in the literature of patients with PAPS evolving into SLE is small [53,54]. Silver et al and Mujic et al have reported the evolution in small numbers (7/71 and 3/80, respectively) but Asherson et al and Vianna et al did not find any [55,56]. The short period of follow up may have been responsible for

Table 2.4. Exclusion criteria to distinguish SLE–associated antiphospholipid syndrome from PAPS.

Malar or discoid rash

Oral, pharyngeal, or nasal ulceration
Frank arthritis
Pleurisy/pericarditis
Persistent proteinuria > 0.5 g/day, due to biopsy-proven immune-complex–related glomerulonephritis
Lymphopenia < 1000 cells/L
Antibodies to dsDNA (crithidia or radioimmunoassay), or ENA
ANA >1:320
Treatment with drugs known to produce aPL
Follow up < 5 years from the initial clinical manifestation.

the latter result (5 and 2 years, respectively) as several patients have developed the syndrome after 10 years. The presence of high titer ANA (>1:320), low complement levels, and lymphopenia may be predictive [53–56].

Seronegative APS

It is well recognized that seronegative forms of other autoimmune disorders such as rheumatoid arthritis and lupus exist and there is increasing recognition that patients with classical features of Hughes syndrome may be persistently aPL negative [57]. Clearly these patients can be difficult to diagnose though there may be several clinical clues. For example, APS is probably the only procoagualant state that can give rise to both arterial and venous thromboses as well as pregnancy morbidty, and in our experience the presence of livedo reticularis is a good marker for APS. Sometimes, aPL may appear only after prolonged follow up but in the majority of these patients there may be serological markers that are yet to be described.

Catastrophic APS

The catastrophic APS has emerged as a dramatic if rare presentation of APS with a high mortality despite expert management. The etiology of this variant of APS remains obscure although there are often factors such as recent surgery or sepsis that herald its onset. The syndrome will be described in detail in Chapter 16, although it is worth noting that immunosuppression, especially with cyclophosphamide, is relatively contraindicated and plasma exchange may be beneficial [58].

Clinical Features

Hughes syndrome, like SLE, is truly multisystem in nature and any organ or system in the body may be affected. The spectrum of clinical features associated with aPL continues to expand and will be covered extensively in the following chapters (Table 2.5). The cardinal features remain arterial and venous thrombosis, pregnancy morbidity, and thrombocytopenia. Since the last edition of this book, a number of

Table 2.5. Clinical associations.

Central Nervous System	Bone
Chorea	Avascular necrosis
Migraine	Bone marrow necrosis
Psychosis	Fractures
Epilepsy	
CVA/TIA	**Obstetric**
Hypoperfusion on SPECT scanning	Recurrent miscarriage
Sensorineural hearing loss	Pre-eclampsia
Transverse myelopathy	Growth retardation
Cognitive impairment	HELLP syndrome
Pseudotumor cerebri	
Cerebral vein/artery thrombosis	**Renal**
Retinal venous thrombosis	Glomerular thrombosis
Multiple sclerosis like syndrome	Renal artery stenosis
Renal artery thrombosis	Renal insufficiency
	Renal vein thrombosis
Gastrointestinal	
Hepatic necrosis	**Pulmonary**
Acalculous cholecystitis	Pulmonary embolism
Budd–Chiari	Pulmonary hypertension
Intestinal ischemia	ARDS
Coeliac artery stenosis	
	Endocrine
Vascular disease	Adrenal failure
Atherosclerosis	Hypopituitarism
Cardiac valvular disease	
Acute myocardial infarction	**Hematological**
Failed angioplasty	Thrombocytopenia
Diastolic dysfunction	Autoimmune hemolytic anemia
Intracardiac thrombosis	Thrombotic microangiopathy
Cardiomyopathy	
Buerger 's disease	
Skin	
Livedo reticularis	
Cutaneous ulcers	
Dego's Disease	
Splinter hemorrhages	
Superficial thrombophlebitis	
Distal cutaneous ischemia	

CVA, cerebrovascular accident; TIA, transient ischemic attack; SPECT, single positron emission computerized tomography; HELLP, hemolytic anaemia, elevated liver function tests and low platelets; ARDS, adult respiratory distress syndrome.

associations have been described, including renal artery stenosis and other renal complications. An interesting development has been the emergence of orthopedic manifestations such as rib and metatarsal fractures that follow previous descriptions of avascular necrosis. A separate chapter has been devoted to this.

Conclusion

In conclusion, the following observations can be made. aPL are present in approximately 2% to 4% of the normal population and the prevalence increases with age.

There is a high prevalence among patients with autoimmune connective tissue disorders, especially SLE. There is an association with both venous and arterial thrombosis as well as with pregnancy morbidity, but the strength of association varies amongst studies. This probably reflects different populations, study designs, and different assays and definitions used. In several studies the risk of thrombosis appears to be higher with LA and the data suggests a true association rather than epiphenomenon. In a given patient, both aCL and LA should be measured. A significant impact on long-term survival has been noted and aPL also contribute significantly to accumulated damage in diseases such as SLE. The clinical spectrum of APS features is enormous and continues to expand. It behoves us all as clinicians and health care professionals to consider an early diagnosis of Hughes syndrome, with its distinct clinical and serological features, to reduce the risk of morbidity and mortality in our patients.

References

1. Cervera R, Khamashta MA, Font J, et al. Systemic lupus erythematosus: clinical and immunologic patterns of disease expression in a cohort of 1000 patients. Medicine (Baltimore) 1993;72:113–124.
2. Perez-Vazquez ME,Villa A, Drenkard C, Cabiedes J, Alarcon-Segovia D. Influence of disease duration, continued follow up and further antiphopholipid testing on the frequency and classi fication category of antiphospholipid syndrome in a cohort of patients with SLE. J Rheumatol 1993;20:437–442.
3. Cervera R, Piette JC, Font J, et al. Antiphospholipid syndrome. Clinical and immunologic manifestations and patterns of disease expression in a cohort of 1000 patients. Arthritis Rheum 2002;46:1019–1027.
4. Wilson WA, Gharavi AE, Koike T, et al. International consensus statement on preliminary classification criteria for definite antiphospholipid syndrome. Report of an International Workshop. Arthritis Rheum 1999;42:1309–1311.
5. Lockshin MD, Sammaritano LR, Schwartzman S. Validation of the Sapporo criteria for the antiphospholipid syndrome. Arthritis Rheum 2000;43:440–443.
6. Alarcon-Segovia D, Deleze M, Oria CV, et al. Antiphospholipid antibodies and the antiphospholipid syndrome in SLE. A prospective analysis of 500 consecutive patients. Medicine 1989;68:353–365.
7. Cervera R, Khamashta MA, Font J, et al. Morbidity and mortality in systemic lupus erythematosus during a 10 year period. A comparison of early and late manifestations in a cohort of 1000 patients. Medicine (Baltimore) 2003;82:299–308.
8. Kovalevsky G, Gracia CR, Berlin JA, Sammel MD, Barnhart KT. Evaluation of the association between hereditary thrombophilias and recurrent pregnancy loss: a meta-analysis. Arch Intern Med 2004;164:558–563.
9. Drenkard C, Sanchez-Guerrero J, Alarcon-Segovia D. Fall in antiphospholipid antibody at time of thromboocclusive episodes in SLE. J Rheumatol 1989;16:614–617.
10. Perez-Vazquez ME, Cabiedes J, Cabral AR, Alarcon-Segovia D. Decrease in serum antiphospholipid antibodies upon development of the nephrotic syndrome in patients with SLE:relationship to urinary losses of IgG and other factors. Am J Med 1992;92:357–363.
11. Silveira LH, Jara LJ, Espinoza LR. Transient disappearance of serum antiphospholipid antibodies can also be due to prednisolone therapy. Clin Exp Rheumatol 1996;14:217–226.
12. McClain MT, Arbuckle MR, Heinlen LD, et al. The prevalence, onset, and clinical significance of antiphospholipid antibodies prior to diagnosis of systemic lupus erythematosus. Arthritis Rheum 2004;50:1226–1232.
13. Diri E, Curcurull E, Gharavi AE, et al. Antiphospholipid (Hughes) syndrome in African-American patients: IgA aCL and beta 2 glycoprotein 1 is the most frequent isotype. Lupus 1999;8:263–268.
14. Bertolaccini ML, Atsumi T, Amengual O, Katsumata K, Khamashta MA, Hughes GRV. IgA anticardiolipin antibody testing does not contribute to the diagnosis of antiphospholipid syndrome in patients with SLE. Lupus 1998;7(suppl 2):S184.
15. Fields R, Toubbeh H, Searles R, Bankhurst A. The prevalence of anticardiolipin antibodies in a healthy elderly population and its association with antinuclear antibodies. J Rheumatol 1989;16:623–625.

16. Antiphospholipid Antibodies in Stroke Study Group. Clinical, radiological, and pathological aspects of cerebrovascular disease associated with antiphospholipid antibodies. Stroke 1993;24(suppl 1):S1–S123.
17. Schved JF, Dupuy-Fons C, Biron C, Quere I, Janbon C. A prospective epidemiological study on the occurrence of antiphospholipid antibody: the Montpellier Antiphospholipid (MAP) Study. Haemostasis 1994;24:175–182.
18. Schulman S, Svenungsson E, Granqvist S, and the Duration of Anticoagulation Study Group. Anticardiolipin antibodies predict early recurrence of thromboembolism and death among patients with venous thromboembolism following anticoagulant therapy. Am J Med 1998;104:332–338.
19. Nencini P, Baruffi M, Abbate R, Massai G, Amaducci L, Inzitari D. Lupus anticoagulant and anti-cardiolipin antibodies in young adults with cerebral ischaemia. Stroke 1992;23:189–193.
20. Vaarala O, Puurunen M, Manttari M, et al. Anticardiolipin antibodies and risk of myocardial infarction in a prospective cohort of middle-aged men. Circulation 1995;91:23–27.
21. Kearon C, Gent M, Hirsh J, Weitz J, et al. A comparison of three months of anticoagulation with extended anticoagulation for a first episode of idiopathic venous thromboembolism. N Engl J Med 1999;340:901–907.
22. Wahl DG, Guillemin F, de Maistre E, Perret-Guillaume C, Lecompte T, Thibaut G. Meta-analysis of the risk of venous thrombosis in individuals with antiphospholipid antibodies without underlying autoimmune disease or previous thrombosis. Lupus 1998;7:15–22.
23. Ginsburg K, Liang M, Newcomer L, et al. Anticardiolipin antibodies and the risk for ischemic stroke and venous thrombosis. Ann Intern Med 1992;117:997–1002.
24. Janardhan V, Wolf PA, Kase CS, et al. Anticardiolipin antibodies and risk of ischemic stroke and transient ischemic attack. The Framingham cohort and offspring study. Stroke 2004;35:736–741.
25. Levine SR, Brey RL, Tilley BC, et al. Antiphospholipid antibodies and subsequent thrombo-occlusive events in patients with ischemic stroke. JAMA 2004;291:576–584.
26. Kittner S, Gorelick P. Antiphospholipid antibodies and stroke:an epidemiological perspective. Stroke 1992;23(suppl 1):1–19, 1–22.
27. Cervera R, Khamashta MA, Font J, et al. Morbidity and mortality in systemic lupus erythematosus during a 5 year period. A multicentre prospective study of 1000 patients. Medicine (Baltimore) 1999;78:167–175.
28. Wahl DG, Guillemin F, de Maistre E, Perret C, Lecompte T, Thibaut G. Risk for venous thrombosis related to antiphospholipid antibodies in systemic lupus crythematosus. A meta-analysis. Lupus 1997;6:467–473.
29. Shah NM, Khamashta MA, Atsumi T, Hughes GRV. Outcome of patients with anticardiolipin anti-bodies: a 10 year follow up of 52 patients. Lupus 1998;7:3–6.
30. Jouhikainen T, Stephansson E, Leirisalo-Repo M. Lupus anticoagulant as a prognostic marker in systemic lupus erythematosus. Br J Rheumatol 1993;32:568–573.
31. Soares M, Reis L, Papi JA, Cardoso CR. Rate, pattern and factors related to damage in Brazilian sys-temic lupus erythematosus patients. Lupus 2003;12:788–794.
32. Ruiz-Irastorza G, Egurbide MV, Ugalde J, Aguirre C. High impact of antiphospholipid syndrome on irreversible organ damage and survival of patients with systemic lupus erythematosus. Arch Intern Med 2004;164:77–82.
33. Finazzi G, Brancaccio V, Moia M, et al. Natural history and risk factors for thrombosis in 360 patients with antiphospholipid antibodies. A four year prospective study from the Italian Registry. Am J Med 1996;100:530–536.
34. Neville C, Rauch J, Kassis J, et al. Thromboembolic risk in patients with high titre anticardiolipin and multiple antiphospholipid antibodies. Thromb Haemost. 2003;90:108–115.
35. Khamashta M, Cuadrado M, Mujic F, Taub N, Hunt B, Hughes GRV. The management of thrombosis in the antiphospholipid–antibody syndrome. N Engl J Med 1995;332:993–997.
36. Giron-Gonzalez JA, Garcia del Rio E, Rodriguez C, Rodriguez-Martorell J, Serrano A. Antiphospholipid syndrome and asymptomatic carriers of antiphospholipid antibody: prospective analysis of 404 individuals. J Rheumatol 2004;31:1560–1567.
37. Roman MJ, Shanker BA, Davis A, et al. Prevalence and correlates of accelerated atherosclerosis in systemic lupus erythematosus. N Engl J Med 2003;349:2399–2406.
38. Medina G, Casaos D, Jara LJ, Vera-Lastra O, Fuentes M, Barile L, Salas M. Increased carotid artery intima-media thickness may be associated with stroke in primary antiphos-pholipid syndrome. Ann Rheum Dis 2003;62:607–610.
39. Baron M, D'Cruz DP, Khamashta MA, Hughes GRV. ABI in PAPS. Ann Rheum Dis 2005;64:144–???.
40. Sangle SR, D'Cruz DP, Jan W, Karim MY, Khamashta MA, Abbs IC, Hughes GR. Renal artery stenosis in the antiphospholipid (Hughes) syndrome and hypertension. Ann Rheum Dis 2003;62:999–1002.

41. Vaz JL, Dancour MA, Bottino DA, Bouskela E. Nailfold videocapillaroscopy in primary antiphospholipid syndrome (PAPS). Rheumatology (Oxford) 2004;43:1025–1027.
42. Rosendaal F. Thrombosis in the young: epidemiology and risk factors. A focus on venous thrombosis. Thromb Haemost 1997;78:1–6.
43. Brenner B, Vulfsons SL, Lanir N, Nahir M. Coexistence of familial antiphospholipid syndrome and factor V Leiden: impact on thrombotic diathesis. Br J Haematol 1996;94:166–167.
44. Ames P, Tommasino C, D 'Andrea G, Iannaccone L, Brancaccio V, Margaglione M. Thrombophilic genotypes in subjects with idiopathic antiphospholipid antibodies – prevalence and significance. Thromb Haemost 1998;79:46–49.
45. Peddi VR, Kant KS. Catastrophic secondary antiphospholipid syndrome with concomitant antithrombin III deficiency. J Am Soc Nephrol 1995;5:1882–1887.
46. Asherson RA, Khamashta MA, Ordi-Ros J, et al. The primary antiphospholipid syndrome:major clinical and serological features. Medicine 1989;68:366–374.
47. Soweid AM, Hajjar RR, Hewan-Lowe KO, Gonzalez EB. Skin necrosis indicating antiphospholipid syndrome in patient with AIDS. S Med J 1995;88:786–778.
48. Labarca J, Rabaggliati R, Radrigan F, et al. Antiphospholipid syndrome associated with cytomegalovirus infection: case report and review. Clin Infect Dis 1997;24:197–200.
49. Merrill JT, Shen C, Gugnani M, Lahita RG, Mongey AB. High prevalence of antiphospholipid antibodies in patients taking procainamide. J Rheumatol 1997;24:1083–1088.
50. Vianna JL, Khamashta MA, Ordi-Ros J, et al. Comparison of the primary and secondary antiphospholipid syndrome: a European multicenter study of 114 patients. Am J Med 1994;96:3–9.
51. Piette JC, Weschler B, Frances C, Papo T, Godeau P. Exclusion criteria for primary antiphospholipid syndrome. J Rheumatol 1993;20:1802–1804.
52. Karassa FB, Bijl M, Davies KA, et al. Role of the Fcgamma receptor IIA polymorphism in the antiphospholipid syndrome: an international meta-analysis. Arthritis Rheum 2003;48:1930–1938.
53. Seisdedos L, Munoz-Rodriguez F J, Cervera R, Font J, Ingelmo M. Primary antiphospholipid syndrome evolving into SLE. Lupus 1997;6:285–286.
54. Carbone J, Orera M, Rodriguez-Mahou M, et al. Immunological abnormalities in primary APS evolving into SLE: 6 years follow-up in women with repeated pregnancy loss. Lupus 1999;8:274-8.
55. Silver RM, Drapor MJ, Scott JR et al. Clinical consequences of antiphospholipid antibodies. An historic exhort study Obstet Gynecol 1994;83:372–77.
56. Mujic F, Cuadrado MJ, Lloyd M et al. Primary antiohospholipid syndrome evolving into SLE. J Rheumatol 1995;22:1589–1592.
57. Hughes GR, Khamashta MA. Seronegative antiphospholipid syndrome. Ann Rheum Dis 2003;62:1127.
58. Erkan D, Cervera R, Asherson RA. Catastrophic antiphospholipid syndrome: where do we stand? Arthritis Rheum 2003;48:3320–3327.

3   Epidemiology of Antiphospholipid Syndrome

Michelle Petri

This chapter will review classification criteria of the antiphospholipid syndrome (APS), the prevalence of antiphospholipid antibodies [aPL; anticardiolipin (aCL); lupus anticoagulant (LA)] in normals and in systemic lupus erythematosus (SLE), the prevalence of aPL in venous thrombosis, arterial thrombosis, and pregnancy loss, and longitudinal studies.

Classification Criteria for APS

Classification criteria for APS (Table 3.1) were developed by consensus at the Sapporo antiphospholipid meeting [1]. These criteria, for the first time, emphasized that vasculopathy (and not just thrombosis) was part of APS and broadened the pregnancy criterion to include severe pre-eclampsia. The Sapporo criteria were validated in an exercise by Lockshin et al [2]. The sensitivity was 0.71.

The Sapporo criteria were not evidence based. As part of the Taormina antiphospholipid meeting, evidenced-based criteria were prepared. These criteria required that the criterion be valid in both primary (non-SLE) and secondary (SLE) APS and be proven by more than one study (and more than one study design). The evidence-based criteria do not include pregnancy morbidity, but do include cardiac valve disease (valvular thickening and/or vegetations; Table 3.2) [3].

Table 3.1. Sapporo classification criteria for antiphospholipid syndrome.

Clinical	Laboratory*
Vascular thrombosis	IgG anticardiolipin – moderate or high
	IgM anticardiolipin – moderate or high
Pregnancy morbidity	Lupus anticoagulant
3 or more concurrent spontaneous abortions	
1 or more unexplained deaths of a normal fetus at or beyond 10th week of gestation	
1 or more premature births before 34 weeks because of severe preeclampsia or placental insufficiency	

*Present at least twice 6 weeks apart.

Table 3.2. Taormina evidence-based classification criteria for antiphospholipid syndrome.

Clinical	Laboratory
Vascular thrombosis	IgG anticardiolipin – moderate or high
	IgM anticardiolipin – moderate or high
Pregnancy	Lupus anticoagulant
3 or more early fetal losses	
1 intrauterine fetal demise	
Cardiac	
Valve thickening and/or vegetations	

Table 3.3. Prevalence of antiphospholipid antibodies in normals.

Study, year	Number of Controls	Type of controls	aCL-IgG	aCL-IgM	LA	Anti-β_2 GPI
Harris et al, 1991 [4]	1449	Pregnant women	1.8	4.3		
Infante-Rivard et al, 1991 [5]	993	Pregnant women	1.5		3.8	
Perez et al, 1991 [6]	1200	Pregnant women	1.25			
Rix et al, 1992 [7]	2856	Pregnant women			0.07	
Pattison et al, 1993 [8]	933	Pregnant women	1		1.2	
Phadke et al, 1993 [9]	504	Healthy, age-matched	4.2	5		
Juby et al, 1998 [10]	250	Healthy, young	1.2			
Bruce et al, 2000 [11]	129	Healthy				3%

Prevalence of aPL Antibodies in Normals

The prevalence of aCL in most large studies of normals has been 1% to 5%. The prevalence of the LA has been in the range of 0% to 4% (Table 3.3).

Prevalence of aPL in SLE

Representative recent studies of the prevalence of aCL, LA, and anti–β_2-glycoprotein I (anti-β_2 GPI) in SLE are compiled in Table 3.4. In general, aCL is more fre-

Table 3.4. Prevalence of antiphospholipid antibodies in systemic lupus erythematosus.

Study, year	Number of SLE	Assay	LA	aCL	Anti-β_2 GPI
Padmakumar et al, 1990 [12]	55	KCT	13%		
Mayumi et al, 1991 [13]	106	aPTT	16%		
McHugh et al, 1991 [14]	58	KCT, RVVT, TTI	22%	29%	
Wong et al, 1991 [15]	91	aPTT, RVVT, PNP, TTI	11%	44%	
Cervera et al, 1993 [16]	1000	Multiple	15%	24%	
Jones et al, 1991 [17]	200			17%	
Kutteh et al, 1993 [18]	125			25%	
Axtens et al, 1994 [19]	127			24%	
Tsutsumi et al, 1996 [20]	308			12.3%	10.1%
Bruce et al, 2000 [11]	133			13.5%	15.8%
Tubach et al, 2000 [21]	102			23.5%	18.6%

quent than LA. However, any cross-sectional study in SLE may underestimate the true frequency of aPL because disease activity and treatment lead to fluctuations over time. In the Hopkins Lupus Cohort, a longitudinal study in which aPL are measured quarterly, at 5 years of follow up the prevalence of aCL was 26% and that of the LA (by dRVVT) was 31%.

Prevalence of aPL in Venous Thrombosis

Bick and colleagues [22] found, in 100 patients with venous thrombosis, that 24% had aCL and 4% had LA. In a study of 122 consecutive venous thrombotic patients, close to 15% had LA, aPL, or anti-β_2 GPI phospholipid. The presence of the LA was strongly associated with the severity of thrombosis [23]. In 227 consecutive patients with acute deep venous thrombosis or pulmonary embolism, 31% had aPL. Anti-β_2 GPI, present in 8.4%, was associated with a higher rate of recurrent thromboembolism [24].

Prevalence of aPL in Arterial Thrombosis

The most informative studies have been the prevalence of aPL in stroke patients less than 50 years (Table 3.5). These studies suggest that about 29% of young people with a stroke have aCL.

Prospective studies have found an association of aPL with myocardial infarction in middle-aged men [31, 32]. No association of anti-β_2 GPI and coronary atherosclerosis was found in a cross-sectional study of 97 subjects [33]. A study of 60 peripheral vascular disease patients found the LA in 43% versus 0% of controls [34].

Recurrent Fetal Loss

Multiple cross-sectional studies have reported an association of aCL and/or LA with recurrent fetal loss, in a general range of 10% to 19% (Table 3.6). Anti-β_2 GPI was not associated with recurrent fetal loss in one study [45].

In terms of pregnancy morbidity, the LA was not associated with pregnancy-induced hypertension [46].

Table 3.5. Antiphospholipid antibody prevalence in young stroke patients.

Study, year	Number of patients	Assays	Frequency
Brey et al, 1990 [25]	46	LA, aCL	46%
Czlonkowska et al, 1992 [26]	49	aCL	32%
Nencini et al, 1992 [27]	44		23%
de Jong et al, 1993 [28]	44	LA, aCL	2%
Ferro et al, 1993 [29]	33	LA	18%
Tietjen et al, 1993 [30]	68	LA, aCL	43%

Table 3.6. Antiphospholipid antibody in recurrent fetal loss.

Study, year	Number of women	LA	aCL	aCL-IgG	aCL-IgM	Anti-β_2 GPI
Taylor et al, 1990 [35]	189	3%	15%			
Parazzini et al, 1991 [36]	220	7%				
Parazzini et al, 1991 [36]	99		19%			
Parke et al, 1991 [37]	81	4.9%		7.4%	4.9%	
Aoki et al, 1993 [38]	334			8%		
Bagger et al, 1993 [39]	158			4%	26%	
Toyoshima et al, 1993 [40]	148		8%			
MacLean et al, 1994 [41]	243	6.6%	8.2%			
Rai et al, 1995 [42]	500	9.6%		3.3%	2.2%	
Ogasawara et al, 1996 [43]	195	11.3%				9.7%
Kumar et al, 2002 [44]	150	10.3%				40.2%

Thrombocytopenia

In a study of 52 newly diagnosed patients with idiopathic thrombocytopenic purpura (ITP), 38% were aPL positive at diagnosis. Patients with aPL positivity were significantly more likely to have a thrombosis in the next 5 years. After 38 median months of follow up, 45% of the ITP patients with aPL had developed APS [47].

Longitudinal Studies

The Hopkins Lupus Cohort Study is a longitudinal study in which aPL (LA by dRVVT and aCL by polyclonal ELISA) are measured quarterly. SLE patients with the LA have a 50% chance of a venous thrombotic event within 10 years of diagnosis [48]. In a second SLE cohort of 139 patients, IgM aCL was negatively associated with survival. However, thromboembolic events were not a major cause of death in the cohort [49]. In a third study, 37 SLE patients with LA and 37 matched SLE patients without LA were followed for a median of 22 years. Deep venous thrombosis occurred in 54% of those with LA. Events tended to occur in the first 8 years [50].

In patients already diagnosed with APS, several studies have shown a high risk of recurrence. In a study of APS with either arterial or venous thrombotic events, the risk of thrombosis recurrence was high if anti-coagulation was not maintained [51]. In patients with APS and venous thrombosis, the risk of recurrent venous thrombosis was 50% within 2 years [52].

In patients with stroke, the odds ratio for recurrent stroke and for all events (stroke, myocardial infarction, and death) is significantly higher in those with aCL [53].

References

1. Wilson WA, Gharavi AE, Koike T, et al. International consensus statement on preliminary classification criteria for definite antiphospholipid syndrome: report of an international workshop. Arthritis Rheum 1999;42:1309–1311.

2. Lockshin MD, Sammaritano LR, Schwartzman S. Validation of the Sapporo criteria for antiphospholipid syndrome. Arthritis Rheum 2000;43:440–443.
3. Petri M, Akhtar S, Branch DW, Brey RL, Lockshin MD, Roubey RA. Evidence-based classification criteria for antiphospholipid antibody syndrome (APS) [abstract]. Arthritis Rheum 2003;48:S364.
4. Harris EN, Spinnato JA. Should anticardiolipin tests be performed in otherwise healthy pregnant women? Am J Obstet Gynecol 1991;165:1272–1277.
5. Infante RC, David M, Gauthier R, Rivard GE. Lupus anticoagulants, anticardiolipin antibodies, and fetal loss. A case-control study. N Engl J Med 1991;325:1063–1066.
6. Perez MC, Wilson WA, Brown HL, Scopelitis E. Anticardiolipin antibodies in unselected pregnant women in relationship to fetal outcome. J Perinatol 1991;11:33–36.
7. Rix P, Stentoft J, Aunsholt NA, Dueholm M, Tilma KA, Hoier-Madsen M. Lupus anticoagulant and anticardiolipin antibodies in an obstetric population. Acta Obstet Gynecol Scand 1992;71:605–609.
8. Pattison NS, Chamley LW, McKay EJ, Liggins GC, Butler WS. Antiphospholipid antibodies in pregnancy: prevalence and clinical associations. Br J Obstet Gynaecol 1993;100:909–913.
9. Phadke KV, Phillips RA, Clarke DT, Jones M, Naish P, Carson P. Anticardiolipin antibodies in ischaemic heart disease: marker or myth? Br Heart J 1993;69:391–394.
10. Juby AG, Davis P. Prevalence and disease associations of certain autoantibodies in elderly patients. Clin Invest Med 1998;21:4–11.
11. Bruce IN, Clark-Soloninka CA, Spitzer KA, Gladman DD, Urowitz MB, Laskin CA. Prevalence of antibodies to beta2-glycoprotein I in systemic lupus erythematosus and their association with antiphospholipid antibody syndrome criteria: a single center study and literature review. J Rheumatol 2000;27:2833–2837.
12. Padmakumar K, Singh RR, Rai R, Malaviya AN, Saraya AK. Lupus anticoagulants in systemic lupus erythematosus: prevalence and clinical associations. Ann Rheum Dis 1990;49:986–989.
13. Mayumi T, Nagasawa K, Inoguchi T, et al. Haemostatic factors associated with vascular thrombosis in patients with systemic lupus erythematosus and the lupus anticoagulant. Ann Rheum Dis 1991;50:543–547.
14. McHugh NJ, Moye DAH, James IE, Sampson M, Maddison PJ. Lupus anticoagulant: clinical significance in anticardiolipin positive patients with systemic lupus erythematosus. Ann Rheum Dis 1991;50:548–552.
15. Wong K-L, Liu H-W, Ho K, Chan K, Wong R. Anticardiolipin antibodies and lupus anticoagulant in Chinese patients with systemic lupus erythematosus. J Rheumatol 1991;18:1187–1192.
16. Cervera R, Khamashta MA, Font J, et al., and the European Working Party on Systemic Lupus Erythematosus. Systemic lupus erythematosus: clinical and immunologic patterns of disease expression in a cohort of 1,000 patients. Medicine (Baltimore) 1993;72:113–124.
17. Jones HW, Ireland R, Senaldi G, et al. Anticardiolipin antibodies in patients from Malaysia with systemic lupus erythematosus. Ann Rheum Dis 1991;50:173–175.
18. Kutteh WH, Lyda EC, Abraham SM, Wacholtz MC. Association of anticardiolipin antibodies and pregnancy loss in women with systemic lupus erythematosus. Fertil Steril 1993:60:449–455.
19. Axtens RS, Miller MH, Littlejohn GO, Topliss DJ, Morand EF. Single anticardiolipin measurement in the routine management of patients with systemic lupus erythematosus. J Rheumatol 1994;21:91–93.
20. Tsutsumi A, Matsuura E, Ichikawa K, et al. Antibodies to b_2-glycoprotein I and clinical manifestations in patients with systemic lupus erythematosus. Arthritis Rheum 1996;39:1466–1474.
21. Tubach F, Hayem G, Marchand J-L, et al. IgG anti-β_2-glycoprotein I antibodies in adult patients with systemic lupus erythematosus: prevalence and diagnostic value for the antiphospholipid syndrome. J Rheumatol 2000;27:1437–1443.
22. Bick RL, Jakway J, Baker WF Jr. Deep vein thrombosis: prevalence of etiologic factors and results of management in 100 consecutive patients. Semin Thromb Hemost 1992;18:267–274.
23. Eschwege V, Peynaud-Debayle E, Wolf M. Prevalence of antiphospholipid-related antibodies in unselected patients with history of venous thrombosis. Blood Coagul Fibrinolysis 1998;9:429–434.
24. Zanon E, Prandoni P, Vianello F, et al. Anti-β_2-glycoprotein I antibodies in patients with acute venous thromboembolism: prevalence and association with recurrent thromboembolism. Thromb Res 1999;96:269–274.
25. Brey RL, Hart RG, Sherman DG, Tegeler CH. Antiphospholipid antibodies and cerebral ischemia in young people. Neurology 1990;40:1190–1196.
26. Czlonkowska A, Meurer M, Palasik W, Baranska-Gieruszczak M, Mendel T, Wierzchowska E. Anticardiolipin antibodies, a disease marker for ischemic cerebrovascular events in a younger patient population? Acta Neurol Scand 1992;86:304–307.
27. Nencini P, Baruffi MC, Abbate R, Massai G, Amaducci L, Inzitari D. Lupus anticoagulant and anticardiolipin antibodies in young adults with cerebral ischemia. Stroke 1992;23:189–193.

28. de Jong AW, Hart W, Terburg M, Molenaar JL, Herbrink P, Hop WC. Cardiolipin antibodies and lupus anticoagulant in young patients with a cerebrovascular accident in the past. Neth J Med 1993;42:93–98.
29. Ferro D, Quintarelli C, Rasura M, Antonini G, Violi F. Lupus anticoagulant and the fibrinolytic system in young patients with stroke. Stroke 1993;24:368–370.
30. Tietjen GE, Levine SR, Brown E, Mascha E, Welch KMA. Factors that predict antiphospholipid immunoreactivity in young people with transient focal neurological events. Arch Neurol 1993;50:833–836.
31. Puurunen M, Manttari M, Manninen V, et al. Antibody against oxidized low-density lipoprotein predicting myocardial infarction. Arch Intern Med 1994;154:2605–2609.
32. Vaarala O, Manttari M, Manninen V, et al. Anti-cardiolipin antibodies and risk of myocardial infarction in a prospective cohort of middle-aged men. Circulation 1995;91:23–27.
33. Limaye V, Beltrame J, Cook R, Gillis D, Pile K. Evaluation of antibodies to beta2-glycoprotein 1 in the causation of coronary atherosclerosis as part of the antiphospholipid syndrome. Aust N Z J Med 1999;29:789–793.
34. Fligelstone LJ, Cachia PG, Ralis H. Lupus anticoagulant in patients with peripheral vascular disease: a prospective study. Eur J Vasc Endovasc Surg 1995;9:277–283.
35. Taylor M, Cauchi MN, Buchanan RRC. The lupus anticoagulant, anticardiolipin antibodies, and recurrent miscarriage. Am J Reprod Immunol 1990;23:33–36.
36. Parazzini F, Acaia B, Faden D, et al. Antiphospholipid antibodies and recurrent abortion. Obstet Gynecol 1991;77:854.
37. Parke AL, Wilson D, Maier D. The prevalence of antiphospholipid antibodies in women with recurrent spontaneous abortion, women with successful pregnancies, and women who have never been pregnant. Arthritis Rheum 1991;34:1231–1235.
38. Aoki K, Hayashi Y, Hirao Y, Yagami Y. Specific antiphospholipid antibodies as a predictive variable in patients with recurrent pregnancy loss. Am J Reprod Immunol 1993;29:82–87.
39. Bagger PV, Andersen V, Baslund B, et al. Anti-cardiolipin antibodies (IgG and IgA) in women with recurrent fetal loss correlate to clinical and serological characteristics of SLE. Acta Obstet Gynecol Scand 1993;72:465–469.
40. Toyoshima K, Makino T, Ozawa N, Umeuchi M, Nozawa S. Effect of anticardiolipin antibody in patients with recurrent fetal loss on thrombomodulin-dependent protein C activation. J Clin Lab Anal 1993;7:57–59.
41. MacLean MA, Cumming GP, McCall F, Walker ID, Walker JJ. The prevalence of lupus anticoagulant and anticardiolipin antibodies in women with a history of first trimester miscarriages. Br J Obstet Gynaecol 1994;101:103–106.
42. Rai RS, Regan L, Clifford K, et al. Antiphospholipid antibodies and beta 2-glycoprotein-I in 500 women with recurrent miscarriage: results of a comprehensive screening approach. Hum Reprod 1995;10:2001–2005.
43. Ogasawara M, Aoki K, Matsuura E, Sasa H, Yagami Y. Anti beta 2glycoprotein I antibodies and lupus anticoagulant in patients with recurrent pregnancy loss: prevalence and clinical significance. Lupus 1996;5:587–592.
44. Kumar KS, Jyothy A, Prakash MS, Rani HS, Reddy PP. Beta2-glycoprotein I dependent anticardiolipin antibodies and lupus anticoagulant in patients with recurrent pregnancy loss. J Postgrad Med 2002;48:5–10.
45. Maejima M, Fujii T, Okai T, Kozuma S, Shibata Y, Taketani Y. Beta2-glycoprotein I-dependent anticardiolipin antibody in early recurrent spontaneous abortion. Hum Reprod 1997;12:2140–2142.
46. Matsumoto T, Sagawa N, Ihara Y, Kobayashi F, Itoh H, Mori T. Relationship between lupus anticoagulant (LAC) and pregnancy-induced hypertension. Reprod Fertil Dev 1995;7:1569–1571.
47. Diz-Kucukkaya R, Hacihanefioglu A, Yenerel M, et al. Antiphospholipid antibodies and antiphospholipid syndrome in patients presenting with immune thrombocytopenic purpura: a prospective cohort study. Blood 2001;98:1760–1764.
48. Somers E, Magder LS, Petri M. Antiphospholipid antibodies and incidence of venous thrombosis in a cohort of patients with SLE. J Rheumatol 2002;29:2531–2536.
49. Gulko PS, Reveille JD, Koopman WJ, Burgard SL, Bartolucci AA, Alarcon GS. Anticardiolipin antibodies in systemic lupus erythematosus: clinical correlates, HLA associations, and impact on survival. J Rheumatol 1993;20:1684–1693.
50. Jouhikainen T, Stephansson E, Leirisalo-Repo M. Lupus anticoagulant as a prognostic marker in systemic lupus erythematosus. Br J Rheumatol 1993;32:568–573.
51. Rosove MH, Brewer PMC. Antiphospholipid thrombosis: clinical course after the first thrombotic event in 70 patients. Ann Intern Med 1992;117:303–308.

52. Derksen RHWM, de Groot PG, Kater L, Nieuwenhuis HK. Patients with antiphospholipid antibodies and venous thrombosis should receive long term anticoagulant treatment. Ann Rheum Dis 1993;52:689–692.
53. The Antiphospholipid Antibodies in Stroke Study Group (APASS). Anticardiolipin antibodies and the risk of recurrent thrombo-occlusive events and death. Neurology 1997;48:91–94.

4 Hemocytopenias in Antiphospholipid Syndrome

Carlomaurizio Montecucco and Roberto Caporali

Introduction

Although not included in the recently proposed preliminary criteria for the classification of the human antiphospholipid (Hughes) syndrome (APS) [1], thrombocytopenia is one of the most common laboratory abnormalities found in patients with APS [2, 3], and it is present in some animal models as well [4, 5]. Hemolytic anemia can also be found in APS although less frequently than thrombocytopenia [2, 3]. These hemocytopenias are mainly due to autoimmune mechanisms as supported by the presence of bone marrow megakaryocytes and platelet-associated immunoglobulins for thrombocytopenia and by increased reticulocytes and positive direct Coombs' test for hemolytic anemia. However, antiphospholipid antibodies (aPL) were also reported in association with thrombotic thrombocytopenia and microangiopathic hemolytic anemia.

The present chapter deals with the clinical features of aPL-associated cytopenia, either autoimmune or thrombotic/microangiopathic.

Autoimmune Thrombocytopenia

Prevalence in Primary and Secondary APS

A correlation between thrombocytopenia and aPL is well documented in spite of differences related to the criteria of patient selection and the methods employed to detect aPL. Thrombocytopenia was found in 26% of cases in a series of 319 patients with positive test for either lupus anticoagulant (LA) or anticardiolipin antibodies (aCL) collected from the Italian Registry of aPL [6]. This series included 112 patients with systemic lupus erythematosus (SLE) and 207 with primary APS (PAPS) or without any clinical syndrome. A multicenter study by Vianna et al [7] showed thrombocytopenia in 40% of patients with either PAPS or APS secondary to SLE. Recently, in a large cohort of patients with APS (either PAPS or APS secondary to SLE) from 13 European countries, thrombocytopenia was found in about 30% of cases, and was one of the most common presenting manifestation [2].

In SLE, thrombocytopenia is significantly more frequent in patients with aPL than in patients without [8, 9]; the patients with both LA and high aCL show the highest frequency of thrombocytopenia [10]. Among patients with APS, thrombocytopenia is more frequently observed in patients with SLE than in patients with PAPS [2]. In a recently published paper, McClain et al showed that the presence of aPL may precede the diagnosis of SLE and that, in these patients, thrombocytopenia was common and occurred earlier than in aPL-negative patients [11].

In pediatric APS the presence of thrombocytopenia was either confirmed [12, 13] or denied [14]. Recently, thrombocytopenia was found in 17 out of 58 (29%) of pediatric patients with APS (5 with PAPS and 12 with SLE or SLE-like disorders) [15]. In this cohort, thrombocytopenia was the most frequent APS-related manifestation observed. In SLE pediatric patients, thrombocytopenia has been reported much more frequently in patients with clinical features of APS than in other SLE patients, with or without the presence of aPL [16].

A close correlation with thrombocytopenia was reported for other markers of APS such as antimithocondrial antibodies type-M5 [17] and antibodies reacting to thromboplastin in a solid phase assay [18]. Anti-prothrombin antibodies seem to be associated with thrombocytopenia in patients with PAPS but not in patients with APS secondary to SLE [19].

On the contrary, the antibodies to oxidized low-density lipoproteins do not correlate with thrombocytopenia [20]. A strong relationship between APS features, including thrombocytopenia, and antibodies to β_2-glycoprotein I (β_2-GPI) has been reported by different groups [21, 22]. Anti-β2-GPI seems to show higher specificity but lower sensitivity for thrombocytopenia with respect to aCL or LA [23].

Many papers have addressed the relationship between aCL specific isotypes and thrombocytopenia. Most of these studies showed a stronger correlation with IgG [24, 25]; the usefulness of testing for IgA aCL and IgA anti-β2-GPI is still a matter of debate [26, 27].

Clinical Features

aPL–related thrombocytopenia is a chronic, usually mild form and is seldom associated with hemorrhagic complications. Values lower than 50×10^9 platelets/L are uncommon, although platelet count can fluctuate with time. Among the patients enrolled in the Italian Registry of aPL [6], 32 (11%) had severe thrombocytopenia and only two experienced bleeding. In a cohort of 305 patients with SLE, severe thrombocytopenia was found in 20 patients and was strongly associated with the presence of aCL [28].

It should be kept in mind that bleeding may be related to several causes other than thrombocytopenia: (a) high-intensity oral anticoagulation for thromboembolic disease; (b) hypoprothrombinemia, which has been reported in patients with LA and hemorrhagic complications; (c) acquired defects of platelet function which may be associated with aPL. Severe thrombocytopenia is likely to act as an additional risk factor for bleeding complications in these patients and it might explain a higher than expected incidence of life-threatening bleeding events in APS patients on high-intensity warfarin therapy [29].

Arterial and/or deep venous thrombosis in APS may occur despite very low platelet count; however, the frequency of aPL-associated thrombotic events may be lower when platelet count is less than 50×10^9/L [6].

aPL and Anti-platelet Antibodies

The pathogenic role for aPL in thrombocytopenia was first suggested by Harris et al [30] and is still controversial. aPL may occasionally bind to unactivated platelets [31]. However, because anionic phospholipids are concentrated in the inner leaflet of cell membrane and exposed only after platelet activation [32], aPL binding is more likely to occur following platelet activation induced by other mechanisms. Accordingly, several groups have demonstrated that aPL can bind to pre-activated platelets in a β_2-GPI dependent way, inducing further platelet activation [33]; it has also been shown that binding of dimer–β_2-GPI to platelets results in a slight activation of platelets, not enough to induce full aggregation, but enough to make them more responsive to a second agonist [22]. Moreover, purified IgG from the plasma of patients with aCL and LA were able to enhance platelet activation induced by ADP [34]. Therefore aPL may have a role in thrombocytopenia but they are not the only actor on the scene [29]. Indeed, many studies failed to detect any antiphospholipid activity in eluates from platelets of patients with aPL-related thrombocytopenia [35, 36].

Galli et al [35] found antibodies to the specific platelet membrane glycoproteins (GP) IIb/IIIa and Ib/IX in 40% of aPL-positive patients, as well as a significant correlation between these antibodies and thrombocytopenia. Anti-platelet GP antibodies are pathogenetically linked to idiopathic thrombocytopenic purpura (ITP) and the frequency found in aPL-associated thrombocytopenia (59%) was similar to that in ITP [35]. In recent years several other studies reported increased levels of specific antibodies directed to internal platelet antigens [37] or to specific membrane GP [38] in aPL-related thrombocytopenia. Godeau et al [36] showed antibodies to a large panel of platelet GP in the sera from 11 of 15 thrombocytopenic patients with APS; the same authors described a strong association between thrombocytopenia in SLE and specific anti-platelet autoantibodies, mainly directed against GPIIb/IIIa without any association with aCL antibodies [39].

The role of antibodies to platelet membrane GP is supported by the following data: (a) anti-GP are rarely found in SLE and APS with normal platelet count [37]; (b) anti-GP, but not aCL or LA, can usually be eluted from platelets of patients with aPL-associated thrombocytopenia [36, 36]; (c) anti-GP in thrombocytopenic patients do not cross-react with phospholipids or β_2-GPI [35]; (d) treatment with glucocorticoids increases platelet number and reduces anti-GP titer but not aPL titer [40]; (e) the incidence of thrombocytopenia is significantly higher in patients with APS secondary to SLE than in patients with PAPS [2].

aPL in ITP and Other Autoimmune Thrombocytopenias

Idiopathic thrombocytopenic purpura is usually associated with antiplatelet antibodies reacting to specific membrane GP. Nevertheless, higher than normal titers of aCL have been detected in 25% to 30% of ITP patients by different groups [25, 30]. Combining aCL assay and LA testing by kaolin clotting time and dilute Russel's viper venom time, Stasi and colleagues [41] were able to find either LA or aCL in 46% of ITP, and both LA and aCL in 16%.

The same anti-platelet GP antibody profile was seen in aPL-positive thrombocytopenia and classic ITP [35, 40]. Furthermore, aPL levels are neither influenced by therapy nor related to the disease activity [40]. In 149 patients with ITP [41], aPL were not associated with age, sex, platelet count, platelet-associated immunoglobulins, or severity of hemorrhages. Also, no significant difference between patients with normal and elevated aPL was found as for clinical course and response to therapy.

Recently, a prospective cohort study evaluated the prevalence and clinical significance of aPL in 82 patients with ITP [42]: 31 patients (37.8%) were aPL positive at diagnosis. After a median follow-up of 38 months, 14 of these patients (45%) developed clinical features of APS. The conclusions of this study support the fact that a persistent presence of aPL in ITP patients is an important risk factor for the development of APS. Similar results were reported in children with chronic ITP, in which the presence of anti–β_2-GPI seems able to detect those patients who are at risk for future development of SLE [15].

Even if these data are not conclusive, we believe that a careful search for other signs of APS, including direct Coombs' test (see below), should be performed in ITP patients with high-titer aCL and LA.

Heparin-induced thrombocytopenia and thrombosis (HIT) is related to specific antibodies directed to the complex of platelet factor 4 (PF4) and heparin [43]. Although pathophysiological and clinical homologies between HIT and APS have been suggested [44], the occurrence of HIT along with aPL was reported only occasionally. Lasne et al [45] showed low-titer anti- PF4/heparin antibodies and/or heparin dependent anti-platelet activity in sera from 2 of 20 patients with primary APS, and borderline values in 4 more patients. Similar results were obtained more recently by Martinuzzo and coworkers [46], who found these antibodies in some APS patients never exposed to heparin. Moreover, it was shown that antibodies from mice immunized with human anti–β_2-GPI were able to recognize not only β_2-GPI but also PF4-heparin complex [47]. The clinical relevance of this association should be further investigated.

Pseudothrombocytopenia is the phenomenon of spuriously low platelet counts due to in vitro platelet clumping in the presence of platelets antibodies and EDTA or other anticoagulants. EDTA-dependent anti-platelet antibodies are directed against membrane GP and seem to recognize cryptic antigens on the GP IIb. A positive test for aCL was reported in 56 of 88 cases of pseudothrombocytopenia [48] but the frequency of EDTA-dependent pseudothrombocytopenia in APS has not been assessed.

Autoimmune Hemolytic Anemia (AIHA)

Many different studies have noted the frequent occurrence of positive direct Coombs' test in SLE patients with LA, aCL, and anti-M5 [18, 20, 49, 50]; aPL were also associated with a positive Coombs' test occasionally found in healthy blood donors [51]. In PAPS, a positive Coombs' test was reported in 10 of 70 patients (14%) and AIHA in 3 (4%) [52].

Higher frequency was observed in APS secondary to SLE [7]. In two different series, direct Coombs' test was positive in 31% and 49.5% of aCL-positive SLE as compared with 2% and 13% of aCL-negative SLE [7, 53]. The association with AIHA is less evident probably due to its relative rareness and the mutifactorial origin of anemia in SLE; Kokori and coworkers studied 41 patients with AIHA in patients with SLE and found a strong correlation with IgG aCL, thromboses, and thrombocytopenia [54].

A significant correlation between aPL and hemolytic anemia was reported by different groups in large series of patients with SLE and related disorders [2, 55, 56]. Hemolytic anemia was reported in 9.7% of a large cohort of APS patients [2]: no differences was found between patients with PAPS or with APS secondary to SLE or SLE-like disorders. A significant association between severe haemolytic anemia and aCL was confirmed in a retrospective study including 305 SLE patients [28]. As for the specific isotypes, IgM were mainly correlated with AIHA in some studies [18, 55], even though other studies found a correlation with IgG [7, 52, 54]. Genetic and racial factors may partially account for these discrepancies.

A number of investigators found aCL in eluates from erythrocytes of patients with aCL-associated AIHA [25, 53, 57]. A direct binding of aPL to red blood cell membrane in these patients is supported by the following data: (a) aCL were not found in eluates obtained from red blood cells in aCL-negative AIHA or aCL-positive SLE without AIHA [53, 57]; (b) a correlation between serum aCL titers and hemolytic activity has been found in one case [57]; (c) anti-red blood cell binding activity present in eluates can be inhibited by absorption on phospholipid micelles [58]; (d) aCL binding activity present in eluates can be inhibited by absorption on fixed red blood cell membranes [51].

The antigen recognized on erythrocyte surface by aPL remains undefined. Cardiolipin is not present on red blood cell membrane and other negatively charged phospholipids are present only in the inner leaflet. In some patients with AIHA, IgM aCL displayed extensive cross-reactivities with different negative and neutral phospholipids, including phosphatidylcholine, that is exposed on bromelain-treated red blood cell surface [59]. Red blood cell membrane phosphatidylcholine might be a candidate target for aPL as it has been found in mice [60]. To date, however, the mechanisms underlying aPL-associated AIHA are not fully understood and we cannot exclude that other factors, such as immune complexes fixed on red blood cells, may have a role. aCL were found to be enriched in circulating immune complexes from patients with APS [61]. The presence of other anti-erythrocyte antibodies cannot be ruled out.

aPL in Idiopathic AIHA and Evans' Syndrome

IgM aCL reacting with a broad spectrum of negative and neutral phospholipids were found in 4 of 14 patients with idiopathic AIHA by Guzman et al [62]. Six of these patients also had IgG aCL, while only one of the 14 control patients with non-autoimmune hemolytic anemia had IgG aCL, and none IgM aCL. Lang et al [63] showed the presence of aPL in idiopathic AIHA as well as in AIHA associated with SLE. These authors also demonstrated that both IgG and IgM aCL titers were increased in warm-type AIHA and in cold-agglutinin disease as well. This finding is in keeping with a previous report of IgG aCL showing cold-agglutinin activity [58] and it may have clinical relevance when cardiopulmonary surgery requiring hypothermia is needed [64]. Recently, Pullarkat confirmed a high frequency of aPL in AIHA and found that aPL-positive patients showed a higher frequency of venous thromboembolism [65].

The eponymy Evans' syndrome is used to define the clinical association of autoimmune thrombocytopenic purpura with AIHA. Many of these patients have SLE or will develop SLE or SLE-like disease. Evans' syndrome was found in 5% of patients with SLE, mainly in association with high aCL levels [66], and in 10% of patients with PAPS [52]. Ten of 12 patients with SLE and Evans' syndrome studied by Delezé and colleagues [67] had positive tests for aPL. The two patients who did not have evidence of aPL were studied at the onset of SLE with active hemolysis and the authors raised the possibility of a transient seronegativity due to absorption of aPL on cell membranes [67]. In a previously published paper, we had found a positive aCL assay in 6 of 7 patients suffering from Evans' syndrome without overt SLE [25]; the only aCL-negative patient had a positive immunofluorescent assay for anti-M5 antibodies, that is, a marker of APS that do not cross-react with phospholipids and cofactors [17]. It could be of interest for readers to know that four of these patients developed overt APS in the following 10 years. Evans' syndrome associated with aPL has been described in pediatric age as well [68].

Thrombotic and Microangiopathic Hemocytopenia

Thrombotic thrombocytopenic purpura (TTP) is a rare hematologic syndrome due to an occlusive microangiopathy. It is characterized by the presence of microangiopathic schistocytic hemolytic anemia, consumption thrombocytopenia with often severe hemorragic complications, fluctuating central nervous system symptoms, fever, and, less frequently, renal impairment. Similar features can be found in other thrombotic microangiopathies such as hemolytic uremic syndrome (HUS), which is usually found in children following intestinal infections and is characterized by prominent renal involvement , and the HELLP syndrome (hemolysis, elevated liver enzymes, and low platelet count) occurring in pregnacy. Thrombocytopenia and microangiopathic hemolytic anemia are also present in disseminated intravascular coagulation (DIC).

The differential diagnosis between thrombotic microangiopathy and APS is often a clinical challenge (Table 4.1). The following points should be taken into account: (a) a minor degree of thrombocytopenia in APS could be related to increased platelet activation and consumption; (b) many clinical and laboratory features may be shared by SLE and TTP [69]; (c) TTP may develop in patients with SLE and vice versa [70]; (d) aPL may be present in some cases of TTP, HUS, and HELLP syndrome [70, 71]; (e) DIC can occur in the catastrophic APS [72]; (f) deficiency of von Willebrand factor cleaving protease (ADAMTS13) seems to be a marker of TTP [73], and simplified assays for ADAMTS13 activity are becoming available in the clinical practice [74].

aPL in TTP and Related Disorders

aPL have not been commonly detected in primary TTP, however, some definite cases of TTP were reported in patients with primary APS [75]. Thrombotic thrombocytopenic purpura may occur in SLE; traditional estimates range from 1% to 4% [69, 76], though postmortem studies may suggest higher percentages [77]. On the other hand, four cases of SLE were found among 175 TTP patients gathered by the Italian Cooperative Group for TTP [69, 78].

Table 4.1. Comparison of the main clinical and laboratory features associated with thrombocytopenia and hemolytic anemia in antiphospholipid syndrome and thrombotic microangiopathy.

	APS	CAPS	TTP	DIC
Renal involvement	+ −	+ +	+ −	+ −
CNS involvement	+ −	+ +	+ +	+ −
Multiorgan failure	+ −	+ +	+ +	+ −
Hemorrhages	− −	± −	+ −	+ +
Anti-platelet antibodies	+ −	+ −	− −	− −
Direct Coombs' test	+ −	+ −	− −	− −
Schistocytes	− −	± −	+ +	+ −
Low plasma fibrinogen	− −	± −	− −	+ +
Prolonged partial prothrombin time	+ − *	+ − *	− −	+ + [†]
Fibrin degradation products	− −	+ −	− −	+ +
Low serum complement	+ −	+ −	− − [‡]	− − [§]
Antinuclear antibodies	+ −	+ −	− − [‡]	− − [§]
Anticardiolipin antibodies	+ +	+ +	− − [‡]	− − [§]

APS = antiphospholipid syndrome; CAPS = catastrophic APS; TTP = thrombotic thrombocytopenic purpura;
DIC = disseminated intravascular coagulation.
* Negative mixing test (lupus anticoagulant);
[†] Positive mixing test;
[‡] TTP may be associated with SLE;
[§] DIC may be associated with CAPS.

In their excellent review, Musio and colleagues [70] reported on 41 cases of TTP in association with SLE. In 30 cases TTP followed SLE, in 6 TTP preceded SLE, and in 5 TTP and SLE occurred simultaneously. A positive test for aCL was found in 8 of 17 patients tested and LA in 2 of 14. Several more cases reported in recent papers were not associated with aCL and/or LA [79, 80]. Therefore, a positive aCL assay was found in about 40% of SLE with TTP, and LA in about 15%, that is, a figure similar to that expected for unselected SLE patients [49]. In a retrospective review of renal biopsies of SLE patients, 4 cases of TTP were identified and all were negative for aPL antibodies testing [81].

Two cases of chronic recurrent TTP were proven to be negative for aCL and positive for anti-phosphatidylinositol or phosphatidylserine antibodies [82]: whether other aPL may be relevant in aCL-negative TTP remains to be ascertained.

A positive assay for IgG aCL was found in 8 of 17 children with classic HUS [83]. Because this condition is triggered by intestinal infections, only further studies addressed to β_2-GPI binding will clarify the nature of these antibodies.

HELLP syndrome does usually complicate severe pre-eclampsia, that is, a disorder characterized by endothelial damage different from that induced by aPL. It seems likely that a further endothelial damage induced by aPL may switch on thrombotic microangiopathy. As a matter of fact, several cases of postpartum HUS and HELLP syndrome associated with aPL have been reported [71, 84]. A case of catastrophic APS occurring in a patient who had had HELLP syndrome 31 years before was also reported [85]. Most cases of HELLP syndrome are, however, aPL negative.

Recently clinical and laboratory features of 46 patients reported in the literature with thrombotic microangiopathic haemolytic anemia (TTP, HUS, HELLP) associated with aPL antibodies has been reported [81]. In 61% of these patients a diagnosis of PAPS was made and thrombotic microangiopathic anemia was the first clinical manifestation of APS. Even if the pathogenic role of aPL remains to be fully elucidated, these data support the need for systematic screening for aPL in all patients with clinical and laboratory features of microangiopathic hemolitic anemia.

aPL in DIC

Though DIC has been rarely found in both primary and secondary APS, a full-blown picture of DIC was observed in 14 of the 50 reviewed cases of catastrophic APS [72], as well as in one case of catastrophic APS in childhood [86]. Schistocytes were reported in 8% of cases with catastrophic APS [72]. We have described a patient with aPL and quiescent SLE who developed DIC with thrombocytopenia, severe anemia with rare schistocytes, and a clinical picture of purpura fulminans characterized by widespread cutaneous thromboses [87].

Other Hemocytopenias

Monoclonal antibodies to β_2-GPI may bind neutrophils [88] and a few studies have reported a clinical association between neutropenia and aCL in patients with SLE [55]. Leukopenia was present in 38% of patients with APS secondary to SLE or SLE-like disorders and only in 2% of patients with PAPS, suggesting that factors other than aPL (i.e., lymphocytotoxic antibodies) could play a role in the pathogenesis of this manifestation in SLE patients [2].

aPL have been reported in a number of patients suffering from hematologic malignancies [49], and hemocytopenias related to the development of non-Hodgkins lymphomas may be observed in APS [6].

Bone marrow necrosis is a rare syndrome leading to severe pancytopenia associated with poor outcome. It has been reported in patients with malignancies, severe infections, sickle cell anemia, and, more recently, APS [84, 89].

Sickle cell anemia is associated with changes in membrane lipid phase which may contribute to the generation of aPL. aPL were found in a significant though variable percentage of patients with homozygous disease [90, 91]. aPL did not correlate with the hematological and clinical features, even though APS has been reported in 1 case [92].

Patients with human immunodeficiency virus (HIV) infection may develop thrombocytopenia and show increased level of aCL. However, the presence of aCL does not seem to correlate with thrombocytopenia in these patients [25, 93, 94].

aCL with the characteristics of infection-related aPL were found in 4% to 20% of patients with chronic HCV infection [95, 96]. A trend of higher incidence of thrombocytopenia among aCL-positive patients with HCV infection was reported [97] but not confirmed by recent studies [96, 98].

References

1. Wilson WA, Gharavi AE, Koike T, et al. International consensus statement on preliminary classification criteria for definite antiphospholipid syndrome: report of an international workshop. Arthritis Rheum 1999;42:1309–1311.

2. Cervera R, Piette JC, Font J, et al. Antiphospholipid syndrome: clinical and immunologic manifestations and patterns of diseases expression in a cohort of 1,000 patients. Arthritis Rheum 2002;46:1019–1027.
3. Hughes GRV. The antiphospholipid syndrome. Ten years on. Lancet 1993;324:341–344.
4. Haj-Yahja S, Sherer Y, Blank M, et al. Anti-prothrombin antibodies cause thrombosis in an novel qualitative ex vivo animal model. Lupus 2003;12:364–369.
5. Ziporen L, Polak-Charcon S, Korczyn DA, et al. Neurological dysfunction associated with antiphospholipid syndrome: histopathological brain findings in a mouse model. Clin Dev Immunol 2004;11:67–65.
6. Finazzi G. The Italian Registry of antiphospholipid antibodies. Haematologica 1997;82:101–105.
7. Vianna JL, Khamashta MA, Ordi-Ros J, et al. Comparison of the primary and secondary antiphospholipid syndrome: a European multicenter study of 114 patients. Am J Med 1994;96:3–9.
8. Abu-Shakra M, Gladman DD, Urowitz MB, et al. Anticardiolipin antibodies in systemic lupus erythematosus: clinical and laboratory correlations. Am J Med 1995;99:624–628.
9. Font J, Cervera R, Ramos-Casals M, et al. Clusters of clinical and immunologic features in systemic lupus erythematosus : analysis of 600 patients from a single center. Semin Arthritis Rheum 2004;33:217–230.
10. Nojima J, Suehisa E, Kuratsune H, et al. High prevalence of thrombocytopenia in SLE patients with a high level of anticardiolipin antibodies combined with lupus anticoagulant. Am J Hematol 1998;58:55–60.
11. McClain MT, Arbuckle MR, Heinlen LD, et al. The prevalence, onset, and clinical significance of antiphospholipid antibodies prior to diagnosis of systemic lupus erythematosus. Arthritis Rheum 2004;50:1226–1232.
12. Briones M, Abshire T. Lupus anticoagulant in children. Curr Opin Hematol 2003;10:375–379.
13. Ravelli A, Caporali R, Di Fuccia G, et al. Anticardiolipin antibodies in pediatric systemic lupus erythematosus. Arch Pediatr Adolesc Med 1994;148:398–402.
14. Seaman DE, Londino AV Jr, Kwoh CK, et al. Antiphospholipid antibodies in pediatric Systemic Lupus Erythematosus. Pediatrics 1995;96:1040–1045.
15. Von Scheven E, Glidden DV, Elder ME. Anti-β_2-glycoprotein I antibodies in pediatric systemic lupus erythematosus and antiphospholipid syndrome. Arthritis Rheum 2002;47:414–420.
16. Campos LMA, Kiss MH, D'Amico EA, et al. Antiphospholipid antibodies and antiphospholipid syndrome in 57 children and adolescents with systemic lupus erythematosus. Lupus 2003;12:820–826.
17. La Rosa L, Covini G, Galperin C, et al. Anti-mitochondrial M5 type antibody represents one of the serological markers for anti-phospholipid syndrome distinct from anti-cardiolipin and anti β_2-glycoprotein I antibodies. Clin Exp Immunol 1998;112:144–151.
18. Font J, Lopez-Soto A, Cervera R, et al. Antibodies to thromboplastin in systemic lupus erythematosus: isotype distribution and clinical significance in a series of 92 patients. Thromb Res 1997;86:37–48.
19. Munoz-Rodriguez FJ, Reverter JC, Font J, et al. Prevalence and clinical significance of antiprothrombin antibodies in patients with systemic lupus erythematosus or with primary antiphospholipid syndrome. Haematologica 2002;632–637.
20. Hayem G, Nicaise-Roland P, Palazzo E, et al. Non-oxidized low-density-lipoprotein (OxLDL) antibodies in systemic lupus erythematosus with and without antiphospholipid syndrome. Lupus 2001;10:346–351.
21. Amengual O, Atsumi T, Khamashta MA, et al. Specificity of ELISA for antibody to beta 2-glycoprotein I in patients with antiphospholipid syndrome. Br J Rheumatol 1996;35:1239–1243.
22. De Laat HB, Derksen RHWM, De Groot PG. Beta2-GPI, the playmaker of the antiphospholipid syndrome. Clin Immunol 2004;112:161–168.
23. Sanfilippo SS, Khamashta MA, Atsumi T, et al. Antibodies to β_2-glycoprotein I: a potential marker for clinical features of antiphospholipid antibody syndrome in patients with systemic lupus erythematosus. J Rheumatol 1998;25:2131–2134.
24. Amoroso A, Mitterhofer AP, Del Porto F, et al. Antibodies to anionic phospholipids and anti-β_2-GPI: association with thrombosis and thrombocytopenia in systemic lupus erythematosus. Human Immunol 2003;64:265–273.
25. Caporali R, Longhi M, De Gennaro F, et al. Antiphospholipid antibody-associated thrombocytopenia in autoimmune dieases. Med Sci Res 1988;16:537–539.
26. Bertolaccini ML, Atsumi T, Escudero-Contreras A, et al. The value of IgA antiphospholipid testing for diagnosis of antiphospholipid (Hughes) syndrome in systemic lupus erythematosus. J Rheumatol 2001;28:2637–2643.

27. Lakos G, Kiss E, Regeczy N, et al. Isotype distribution and clinical relevance of anti-β_2-glycoprotein I antibodies: importance of IgA isotype. Clin Exp Immunol 1999;117:574–579.
28. Sultan SM, Begum S, Isenberg DA. Prevalence, patterns of disease and outcome in patients with systemic lupus erythematosus who develop severe haematological problems. Rheumatology 2003;42:230–234.
29. Galli M, Finazzi G, Barbui T. Thrombocytopenia in the antiphospholipid syndrome. Br J Haematol 1996;93:1–5.
30. Harris EN, Gharavi AE, Hedge V, et al. Anticardiolipin antibodies in autoimmune thrombocytopenic purpura. Br J Haematol 1985;59:231–234.
31. Out HJ, de Groot PG, van Vliet M, et al. Antibodies to platelets in patients with anti-phospholipid antibodies. Blood 1991;77:2655–2659.
32. Bevers EM, Smeets EF, Confurius P, et al. Physiology of membrane lipid asymmetry. Lupus 1994;3:235–240.
33. Robbins DL, Leung S, Miller-Blair DJ, et al. Effect of β_2-glycoprotein I complexes on production of thromboxane A2 by platelets from patients with antiphospholipid syndrome. J Rheumatol 1998;25:51–56.
34. Nojima J, Suehisa E, Kuratsune H, et al. Platelet activation induced by combined effects of anticardiolipin and lupus anticoagulant IgG antibodies in patients with systemic lupus erythematosus. Thromb Haemost 1999;81:436–441.
35. Galli M, Daldossi M, Barbui T. Anti-glycoprotein Ib/IX and IIb/IIIa antibodies in patients with antiphospholipid antibodies. Thromb Haemost 1994;71:571–575.
36. Godeau B, Piette JC, Fromont P, et al. Specific antiplatelet glycoprotein autoantibodies are associated with the thrombocytopenia of primary antiphospholipid syndrome. Br J Haematol 1997;98:873–879.
37. Fabris F, Steffan A, Cordiano I, et al. Specific antiplatelet autoantibodies in patients with antiphospholipid antibodies and thrombocytopenia. Eur J Haematol 1994;53:232–236.
38. Macchi L, Rispal P, Clofent-Sanchez G, et al. Anti-platelet antibodies in patients with systemic lupus erythematosus and the primary antiphospholipid antibody syndrome: their relationship with the observed thrombocytopenia. Br J Haematol 1997;98:336–341.
39. Michel M, Lee K, Piette JC, et al. Platelet autoantibodies and lupus-associated thrombocytopenia. Br J Haematol 2002;119:354–358.
40. Lipp E, vov Felten A, Sax H, et al. Antibodies against platelet glycoproteins and antiphospholipid antibodies in autoimmune thrombocytopenia. Eur J Haematol 1998;60:283–288.
41. Stasi S, Stipa E, Masi M, et al. Prevalence and clinical significance of elevated antiphospholipid antibodies in patients with idiopathic thrombocytopenic purpura. Blood 1994;84:4203–4208.
42. Diz-Kucukkaya R, Hachanefioglu A, Yenerel M, et al. Antiphospholipid antibodies and antiphospholipid syndrome in patients presenting with immune thrombocytopenic purpura : a prospective cohort study. Blood 2001;98:1760–1764.
43. Arepally G, Cines DB. Pathogenesis of heparin-induced thrombocytopenia and thrombosis. Autoimmune Rev 2002;1:125–132.
44. Arnout J. The pathogenesis of the antiphospholipid syndrome: a hypothesis based on parallelisms with heparin-induced thrombocytopenia. Thromb Haemost 1996;75:536–541.
45. Lasne D, Saffroy R, Bachelot C, et al. Test for heparin-induced thrombocytopenia in primary antiphospholipid syndrome. Br J Rheumatol 1997;97:939.
46. Martinuzzo ME, Forestiero RR, Adamczuk Y, et al. Antiplatelet factor 4-heparin antibodies in patients with antiphospholipis antibodies. Throm Res 1999;15:271–279.
47. Bourhim M, Darnige L, Legallais C, et al. Anti-β_2-GPI antibodies recognizing platelet factor-4-heparin complex in antiphospholipid syndrome in patient substantiated with mouse model. J Mol Recognit 2003;16:125–130.
48. Bizzaro N, Brandalise M. EDTA-dependent pseudothrombocytopenia. Association with antiplatelet and antiphospholipid antibodies. Am J Clin Pathol 1995;103:103–107.
49. Montecucco C, Longhi M, Caporali R, et al. Hematological abnormalities associated with anticardiolipin antibodies. Haematologica 1989;74:195–204.
50. Tincani A, Meroni PL, Brucato A, et al. Anti-phospholipid and anti-mitochondrial type M5 antibodies in systemic lupus erythematosus. Clin Exp Rheumatol 1985;3:321–326.
51. Win N, Islam SI, Peterkin MA, et al. Positive direct antiglobulin test due to antiphospholipid antibodies in normal healthy blood donors. Vox Sang 1997;72:182–184.
52. Asherson RA, Khamashta MA, Ordi-Ros J, et al. The "primary" antiphospholipid syndrome: major clinical and serological features. Medicine (Baltimore) 1989;68:366–374.
53. Hazeltine M, Rauch J, Danoff D, et al. Antiphospholipid antibodies in systemic lupus erythematosus: evidence of an association with positive Coombs' and hypocomplementemia. J Rheumatol 1998;15:80–86.

54. Kokori SIG, Ioannidis JPA, Voulgarelis M, et al. Autoimmune haemolytic anemia in patients with systemic lupus erythematosus. Am J Med 2000;108:198–204.
55. Cervera R, Font J, Lopez-Soto A, et al. Isotype distribution of anticardiolipin antibodies in Systemic Lupus Erythematosus: prospective analysis of a series of 100 patients. Ann Rheum Dis 1990;49:109–113.
56. Merkel PA, Chang Y, Pierangeli SS, et al. The prevalence and clinical associations of anticardiolipin antibodies in a large inception cohort of patients with connective tissue diseases. Am J Med 1996;101:576–583.
57. Sthoeger Z, Sthoeger D, Green L, et al. The role of anticardiolipin autoantibodies in the pathogenesis of autoimmune hemolytic anemia in systemic lupus erythematosus. J Rheumatol 1993;20:2058–2061.
58. Del Papa N, Meroni PL, Barcellini W, et al. Antiphospholipid antibodies cross-reacting with erythrocyte membranes. A case report. Clin Exp Rheumatol 1992;10:395–399.
59. Cabral AR, Cabiedes J, Alarcon-Segovia D. Hemolytic anemia related to an IgM autoantibody to phosphatidylcholine that bind in vitro to stored and to bromelain-treated human erythrocytes. J Autoimmun 1990;3:773–787.
60. Arnold LW, Haughton G. Autoantibodies to phosphatidylcholine. The murine antibromelain RBC response. Ann N Y Acad Sci 1992;651:354–359.
61. Arfors L, Lefvert AK. Enrichment of antibodies against phospholipids in circulating immune complexes (CIC) in the anti-phospholipid syndrome (APLS). Clin Exp Immunol 1997;108:47–51.
62. Guzman J, Cabral AR, Cabiedes J, et al. Antiphospholipid antibodies in patients with idiopathic autoimmune haemolytic anemia. Autoimmunity 1994;18:51–56.
63. Lang B, Straub RH, Weber S, et al. Elevated anticardiolipin antibodies in autoimmune haemolytic anaemia irrespective of underlying systemic lupus erythematosus. Lupus 1997;6:652–655.
64. Barzaghi N, Maurelli M, Emmi V, et al. Pulmonary thromboendoarterectomy in a patients with cryoagglutinins. J Cardiothorac Vasc Anesth 2000;14:447–448.
65. Pullarkat V, Ngo M, Iabal S, et al. Detection of lupus anticoagulant identifies patients with autoimmune haemolytic anaemia at increased risk for venous thromboembolism. Br J Haematol 2002;118:1166–1169.
66. Alarcon-Segovia D, Delezé M, Oria CV, et al. Antiphospholipid antibodies and the antiphospholipid syndrome in systemic lupus erythematosus. A prospective analysis of 500 consecutive patients. Medicine 1989;68:353–365.
67. Deleze M, Oria CV, Alarcon-Segovia D. Occurrence of both hemolytic anemia and thrombocytopenic purpura (Evans' syndrome) in systemic lupus erythematosus. Relationship to antiphospholipid antibodies. J Rheumatol 1998;15:611–615.
68. Avcin T, Jazbec J, Kuhar M, et al. Evans syndrome associated with antiphospholipid antibodies. J Pediatr Hematol Oncol 2003;25:755–756.
69. Porta C, Caporali R, Montecucco C. Thrombotic thrombocytopenic purpura and autoimmunity: a tale of shadow and suspects. Haematologica 1999;84:260–269.
70. Musio F, Bohen EM, Yuan CM, et al. Review of thrombotic thrombocytopenic purpura in the setting of systemic lupus erythematosus. Semin Arthritis Rheum 1998;28:1–19.
71. Huang JJ, Chen MW, Sung JM, et al. Postpartum hemolytic uremic syndrome associated with antiphospholipid antibody. Nephrol Dial Transplant 1998;13:182–186.
72. Asherson RA, Cervera R, Piette JC, et al. Catastrophic antiphospholipid syndrome. Clinical and laboratory features of 50 patients. Medicine 1988;77:195–207.
73. Tsai HM. Advances in the pathogenesis, diagnosis, and treatment of thrombotic thrombocytopenic purpura. J Am Soc Nephrol 2003;14:1072–1081.
74. Knovich MA, Craver K, Matulis MD, et al. Simplified assay for VWF cleaving protease (ADAMTS13) activity and inhibitor in plasma. Am J Hematol 2004;76:286–290.
75. Durand JM, Lefevre P, Kaplanski G, Soubeyrand J. Thrombotic microangiopathy and the antiphospholipid antibody syndrome. J Rheumatol 1991;18:1916–1918.
76. Vasoo S, Thumboo J, Fong KY. Thrombotic thrombocytopenic purpura in systemic lupus erythematosus: disease activity and the use of cytotoxic drugs. Lupus 2002;11:443–450.
77. Devinsky O, Petito CK, Alonso DR. Clinical and neuropathological findings in systemic lupus erythematosus: the role of vasculitis, heart emboli, and thrombotic thrombocytopenic purpura. Ann Neurol 1988;23:380–384.
78. Porta C, Bobbio-Pallavicini E, Centurioni R, et al. Thrombotic thrombocytopenic purpura in systemic lupus erythematosus. J Rheumatol 2002;20:1625–1626.
79. Caramaschi P, Riccetti MM, Pasini AF, et al. Systemic lupus erythematosus and thrombotic thrombocytopenic purpura. Report of three cases and review of the literature. Lupus 1988;7:37–41.
80. Jorfen M, Callejas JL, Formiga F, et al. Fulminant thrombotic thrombocytopenic purpura in systemic lupus erythematosus. Scand J Rheumatol 1998;27:76–77.

81. Espinosa G, Bucciarelli S, Cervera R, et al. Thrombotic microangiopathic haemolytic anemia and antiphospholipid antibodies. Ann Rheum Dis 2004;63:730–736.
82. Trent K, Neustater BR, Lottenberg R. Chronic thrombotic thrombocytopenic purpura and anti-phospholipid antibodies: A report of two cases. Am J Haematol 1997;54:155–159.
83. Ardiles LG, Olavarria F, Elgueta M, et al. Anticardiolipin antibodies in classic pediatric hemolytic-uremic syndrome: a possible pathogenic role. Nephron 1998;78:278–283.
84. Sinha J, Chowdhry I, Sedan S, et al. Bone marrow necrosis and refractory HELLP syndrome in a patient with catastrophic antiphospholipid syndrome. J Rheumatol 2002;29:195–197.
85. Neuwelt CM, Daikh DI, Linfoot JA, et al. Catastrophic antiphospholipid syndrome: response to repeated plasmpheresis over three years. Arthritis Rheum 1997;40:1534–1539.
86. Falcini F, Taccetti G, Ermini M, et al. Catstrophic antiphospholipid antibody syndrome in pediatric systemic lupus erythematosus. J Rheumatol 1997;24:389–392.
87. Gamba G, Montani N, Montecucco C, et al. Purpura fulminans as clinical manifestation of atypical SLE with antiphospholipid antibodies: a case report. Haematologica 1991;76:426–428.
88. Arvieux J, Jacob MC, Roussel B, et al. Neutrophil activation by anti-beta 2 glycoprotein I monoclonal antibodies via Fc gamma receptor II. J Leukoc Biol 1995;57:387–394.
89. Moore J, Ma DD, Concannon A. Non-malignant bone marrow necrosis: a report of two cases. Pathology 1998;30:318–320.
90. De Ceulaer K, Khamashta MA, Harris EN, et al. Antiphospholipid antibodies in homozygous sickle cell disease. Ann Rheum Dis 1992;51:671–672.
91. Kucuk O, Gilman-Sachs A, Beaman K, et al. Antiphospholipid antibodies in sickle cell disease. Am J Haematol 1993;42:380–383.
92. Yeghen T, Benjamin S, Boyd O, et al. Sickle cell anemia, right atrial thrombosis, and the antiphos-pholipid antibody. Am J Hematol 1995;50:46–48.
93. Hassoun A, Al-Kadhimi Z, Cervia J. HIV infection and antiphospholipid antibody: literature review and link to the antiphspholipid sindrome. AIDS Patient Care STDS 2004;18:333–340.
94. Palomo I, Alarcon M, Sepulveda C, et al. Prevalence of antiphospholipid antibodies in HIV-infected Chilean patients. J Clin Lab Anal 2003;17:209–215.
95. Cacoub P, Musset L, Amoura Z, et al. Anticardiolipin, anti-β_2-glycoprotein I, and antinucleosome antibodies in hepatitis C virus infection and mixed cryoglobulinemia. Multivirc group. J Rheumatol 1997;24:2139–2144.
96. Ordi-Ros J, Villareal J, Monegal F, et al. Anticardiolipin antibodies in patients with chronic hepatitis C virus infection: characterization in relation to antiphospholipid syndrome. Clin Diagn Lab Immunol 2000;7:241–244.
97. Leroy V, Arvieux J, Jacob MC, et al. Prevalence and significance of anticardiolipin, anti-β_2 glycopro-tein I and anti-prothrombin antibodies in chronic hepatitis C. Br J Haematol 1998;101:468–474.
98. Ramos-Casals M, Cervera R, Lagrutta M, et al. Clinical features related to antiphospholipid syn-drome in patients with chronic viral infections (hepatitis C virus/HIV infection): description of 82 cases. Clin Infect Dis 2004;38:1009–1016.

5 Cardiac Manifestations in Antiphospholipid Syndrome

Josep Font and Ricard Cervera

Introduction

Cardiac manifestations may be found in up to 40% of patients with the antiphospholipid syndrome (APS), but significant morbidity appears in less than 10% of these patients. Most of these manifestations are explicable on the basis of thrombotic lesions either on the valves or in the coronary circulation, and they may mimic other similar conditions, such as rheumatic fever or infectious endocarditis. The APS coagulopathy in these patients requires the careful and judicious use of appropriate antiaggregant and anticoagulant therapy. For this reason, the estimation of antiphospholipid antibodies (aPL) in cardiological practice assumes considerable importance.

Valvular Disease

Heart valve lesions are the most common cardiac manifestations described in patients with aPL. The introduction of two-dimensional and Doppler echocardiography revealed a high prevalence of valvular abnormalities, such as thickening, stenosis, regurgitation, and vegetations, in patients with systemic lupus erythematosus (SLE). Additionally, it appears that, since the introduction of corticosteroid therapy, valvular involvement has become more prevalent among patients with SLE due to their increased longevity [1]. In several studies, these valvular lesions have been associated with the presence of aPL [2–6]. Furthermore, valvular lesions have also been described in patients with the primary APS (PAPS) [7–9]. Although most cases are symptomless, an increasing number of papers report cases with severe valvular dysfunction resulting in cardiac failure, sometimes requiring valve replacement [2–9].

Echocardiographic Findings

Valve Dysfunction and Thickening

In 1997, Nesher et al [10] performed a meta-analysis of 13 studies on valvular involvement in SLE, as documented by Doppler-echocardiography, and they found valvulopathy in 35% of SLE patients. The mitral valve was involved most commonly, and lesions included leaflet thickening, vegetations, regurgitation, and stenosis. Most of these studies also looked at the possible relationship of valvulopathy to the presence of aPL. Although several studies documented a statistically significant association between aPL and valvulopathy [2–6], others found no significant difference in aPL-positive and aPL-negative patients [11, 12]. The meta-analysis of these studies showed that 48% of aPL-positive SLE patients had valvulopathy, compared with only 21% of aPL-negative SLE patients. Additionally, Nesher et al [10], in the analysis of studies involving patients with PAPS, found that 36% had valvulopathy.

Thickening of the valve leaflets is the most common lesion detected by echocardiography in both SLE and PAPS patients. Valve thickness increases by twofold to threefold or more compared with normal valves [7–9]. The mitral valve is involved most commonly, followed by the aortic valve. Most thickened valves develop hemodynamic abnormalities, so that thickening as the sole abnormality is uncommon. Analysis of data from multiple studies [10] show that mitral regurgitation is the most common hemodynamic dysfunction, occurring in 22% and 26% of all patients with PAPS and SLE, respectively. Aortic regurgitation is less common, occurring in 6% and 10%, respectively. Mitral and aortic stenosis are uncommon, and usually accompany valvular regurgitation. Involvement of right-sided valves is also uncommon, and probably reflects pulmonary hypertension secondary to mitral or aortic regurgitation. In many cases, two or more valves are involved.

The valvular abnormalities associated with aPL may resemble those seen in cases of rheumatic fever. However, several echocardiographic differences have been observed. In APS-related cases, valve thickening is generally diffuse, and when localized thickening is noted, it involves the leaflets' midportion or base. Chordal thickening, fusion, and calcification is rarely seen and, when present, is not prominent. In contrast, valve thickening is typically confined to the leaflets' tips in rheumatic fever, and chordal thickening, fusion, and leaflet calcification is prominent in these cases [10] (Table 5.1).

Vegetations

Early reports of the link between aPL and SLE vegetations – the so-called "Libman–Sacks endocarditis" – date back to the mid-1980s when isolated reports of the association started appearing in the literature [2, 3]. Several echocardiographic studies with larger numbers of patients confirmed that SLE patients possessing aPL have a significantly higher prevalence of vegetations, particularly on the mitral valve, than those without [4–6,13]. Information on the histological appearance of these lesions in patients with aPL derives from anecdotal reports of individual cases and systematic studies are clearly lacking.

Pathogenesis

The pathogenesis of valvular abnormalities in APS is not entirely clear. It has been postulated that in APS the aPL directly cause valvular or endothelial injury unrelated to clinical severity of the disease. Ziporen et al [1] have shown positive staining for human immunoglobulins and for complement compounds in the subendothelial ribbon-like layer along the surface of the leaflets and cups. Amital et

Table 5.1. Differential diagnosis between APS-related valve lesions, rheumatic fever and infective endocarditis.

Features	APS-related	Rheumatic fever	Infective endocarditis
Fever	+/−	+/−	+
Leucocytosis	−	−	+
C-reactive protein	−	−	+
Blood cultures/Serologies	−	−	+
aPL	+	−	−
Echocardiography	Diffuse valve thickening (if localized, it involves the leaflets' midportion or base) Chordal thickening, fusion and leaflet calcification are rare and minimal	Localized valve thickening involving the leaflets' tips. Chordal thickening, fusion and leaflet calcification are common and prominent	Mobile mass localized on the auricular surface of ventricular valves or aortic surface of aortic valve. Valve abscess and rupture are common.

+ present; − absent.

al [14] reported similar findings with the deposition of anticardiolipin antibodies (aCL) in the subendothelial layer of the valve. These findings clearly indicate that the deposition of aPL on the valves resembles the deposition of immune complexes in the dermo-epidermal junction or in the kidney basement membrane in patients with SLE.

García-Torres et al [15] hypothesized that interaction of circulating aPL with local factors in the valves may lead to endocardial damage, resulting in superficial thrombosis and subendocardial mononuclear-cell infiltration, causing fibrosis and calcification. Alternatively, the initial event could be intravalvular capillary endothelial damage caused by aPL interacting with local antigens. This can lead to intracapillary thrombosis, focal inflammation, and the development of fibrosis and scarring. Both pathways may result in valvular deformities which can be hemodinamically significant. Thus, the initial event could be binding of aPL to valvular endothelial cells, leading to local inflammatory reaction, resulting in valve deformities. This proposed mechanism may be supported by the hemodynamic and echocardiographic improvement observed in several patients following treatment with prednisone, which probably diminishes the valvular inflammatory reaction [10].

As postulated by Hojnik et al [16], the above data suggest that aPL play a pathogenetic role in the development of valvular lesions rather than being elicited by the antigens expressed in the damaged valve tissue or merely being an epiphenomenon. Thrombotic tendency may not be the only mechanism whereby aPL may mediate valve damage. At present, there is no explanation for an apparently selective vulnerability of the endocardium to the action of aPL.

Clinical Manifestations

Most cases are clinically silent and detected by either chest auscultation, echocardiography, or at autopsy. Nevertheless, 4% to 6% of all SLE and PAPS patients develop severe mitral or aortic regurgitation, and valve replacement surgery has been performed in half of these patients [10] (Fig. 5.1).

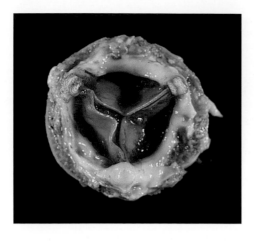

Figure 5.1. Valvular thickening and thrombosis in a prosthetic mitral valve of a patient with primary APS. 📖

Patients with severe valvular regurgitation present with symptoms of congestive heart failure such as fatigue, shortness of breath, and orthopnea. A murmur is present in most cases. It is sometimes difficult to differentiate this from valvulitis associated with rheumatic fever. However, antistreptococcal antibodies are not present, and the echocardiographic presentation is different, as previously described. Hemodynamic abnormalities and symptoms may progress over a period of several weeks or months, remain stable, or improve.

Although infective endocarditis has been described in several patients with SLE, it is a very uncommon complication of this disease. However, several SLE patients have been reported presenting with the following combination of signs and serology: (i) fever; (ii) cardiac murmurs with echocardiographic demonstration of valve vegetations; (iii) splinter hemorrhages (Fig.5.2); (iv) serological evidence of SLE activity (e.g., high titers of antibodies to dsDNA and low serum complement levels); (v) moderate-to-high elevations of aPL; and (vi) repeatedly culture-negative blood

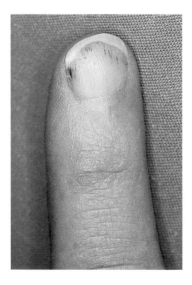

Figure 5.2. Splinter hemorrhages in a patient with valve vegetations and aPL. 📖

samples [17]. All these manifestations are explicable on the basis of SLE activity and complications associated with the APS. Interestingly, similar features were reported by our group [18] in a patient with PAPS. Three simple laboratory tests may also assist in making a differential diagnosis between true infective endocarditis and SLE activity with "pseudoinfective endocarditis" in a patient with the above combination of signs: (a) the white cell count: if low, would point to SLE activity alone, if high, to an infective etiology; (b) the C-reactive protein: SLE patients are usually unable to mount a response of this protein to disease activity alone and elevation would imply infection; and (c) the aCL level: if it is negative or low positive only, this would be in keeping with infective endocarditis, rather than clot deposition on valve alone without infection. Although it has recently been shown that patients with simple infective endocarditis, for example, on rheumatic valves, or valves congenitally abnormal, may in fact demonstrate aCL, the levels are never high positive [19]. A moderate or high positive level would also usually point towards SLE activity rather than infection (Table 5.1).

A further problem in patients with aPL and valve lesions is the development of embolic cerebrovascular complications such as transient ischemic attacks, strokes, or multi-infarct dementia. Early reports [20–22] suggested a relationship between the presence of aPL, valve disease, and ischemic cerebral events, indicating an embolic source for these episodes. Although clinical studies of embolic stroke are limited by the inability to diagnose cardiogenic stroke with certainty, the Antiphospholipid Antibodies in Stroke Study (APASS) found that one third of stroke patients who had elevated aCL levels had abnormal echocardiograms [23].

Our group has recently completed a long-term follow-up study of 61 SLE patients with serial echocardiographic evaluations and we have confirmed that the presence of high levels of IgG aCL is associated with the development of severe valvular regurgitation and with a high incidence of valvular surgery and thromboembolic events [24].

Treatment

Although most studies are retrospective and include a very small number of patients, some information on treatment of heart valve lesions in the APS is already available. Espinola-Zavaleta et al [25] performed 1-year tranesophageal echocardiographic follow up on 13 patients with PAPS receiving anticoagulant or antiplatelet therapy, most treated with aspirin (100 mg/day) and/or warfarin (international normalized ratio > 3.0). Valve lesions persisted unchanged in 6 cases (46%) but new lesions appeared in the remaining 7 (54%). The authors concluded that oral anticoagulant or antiaggregant therapy does not contribute to the disappearance of vegetations.

Nesher et al [10] described 4 patients with subacute onset of congestive heart failure secondary to severe mitral regurgitation, with leaflets thickened three- to sixfold, who had not responded to treatment with diuretics, afterload reduction, and anticoagulation, that subsequently received 40–60 mg/day prednisone and all improved: the regurgitant jet area decreased from 7.5 ± 0.8 to 1.6 ± 1.2 cm^2. Although other contributory factors (pregnancy, hypertension) were also changing, making the attribution of response to steroid therapy difficult to interpret, rapid decreased in leaflet thickness (from 14.3 ± 4 mm to 8.5 ± 3 mm) suggests that corticosteroid therapy improved the function of the valve. By contrast, Hojnik et al [16] stated, without presenting primary data, that steroid therapy is ineffective in treatment of valve disease. No systematic study on immunosuppressive or anti-inflammatory treatment of valve disease exists. In patients with SLE and recurrent systemic embolism, surgical excision of uninfected valvular vegetations may not prevent recurrence [12].

Erkan et al [26] surveyed clinicians who participated in the 9th International Congress on aPL, held in Tours, France, regarding treatment of asymptomatic patients with valve disease. Thirteen of 17 experts preferred low-dose aspirin alone, two chose no treatment, one warfarin, and one low-dose aspirin plus low-dose corticosteroid.

The careful and open discussion of these previous studies by all participants in the pre-symposium workshop on APS consensus, held in Taormina, Italy, on occasion of the 10th International Congress on aPL (29 September 2002), allowed the proposal of the following recommendations: "Since valve thickening and vegetations can serve as substrates for embolism, the Committee recommends warfarin/heparin anticoagulation for patients with valvulopathy who have had any evidence of thromboembolic disease. Prophylactic antiplatelet therapy may be appropriate for asymptomatic patients. Committee members disagreed whether corticosteroid therapy is helpful for acute valve inflammation but agree that distinguishing among reversible valve deformity, irreversible cicatricial valve deformity, and vegetations is important, as treatment implication may differ" [27].

Coronary Artery Disease

Myocardial Infarction

The incidence of myocardial infarction among women with SLE in the 35- to 44-year-old age cohort has been estimated to be 50-fold greater than that of age-matched controls [28]. Myocardial infarction in SLE is usually due to accelerated atherosclerosis – related to long-term steroid administration, hyperlipidemia, and hypertension [29] – or vasculitis [30]. To these classical mechanisms might now be added the presence of the aPL as a possible risk factor [31]. This fact was confirmed by the analysis of the Hopkins Lupus Cohort performed by Petri [32]. Currently, 9% of the cohort have had clinical evidence (myocardial infarction or angina) of coronary artery disease. To traditional coronary artery disease risk factors (prednisone therapy, hypertension, hyperlipidemia, and obesity), the list may now be extended to include age, male sex, renal insufficiency, and two "new" risk factors: homocysteine and aPL.

Many cases of myocardial infarction have been documented both in patients with APS associated with SLE and in PAPS [33]. In the "Euro-Phospholipid cohort," that includes 1000 European patients with APS, myocardial infarction was the presenting manifestation in 2.8% of the patients and it appeared during the evolution of the disease in 5.5% of the cohort [34].

In a prospective cohort of 4081 healthy middle-aged men, Vaarala et al [35] found that the presence of a high aCL level was an independent risk factor for myocardial infarction or cardiac death. The risk was estimated with logistic regression analysis using a nested case-control design with 133 patients (individuals from the cohort who developed myocardial infarction or cardiac death during the study) and 133 control subjects. Subjects with the aCL level in the highest quartile of distribution had a relative risk for myocardial infarction of 2.0 compared with the remainder of the population. This risk was independent of confounding factors, such as age, smoking, systolic blood-pressure, low-density lipoprotein (LDL), and high-density lipoprotein (HDL).

A correlation between the levels of aCL and antibodies to oxidized LDL has been described [36]. Antibodies to oxidized LDL have been considered as markers of atherosclerosis. Although aCL were associated with antibodies to oxidized LDL, the cumulative effect of these two antibodies for the risk of myocardial infarction was additive [36], suggesting that these two antibodies have, at least, partly different antibody specificities with different pathogenic pathways. The generation of antibodies to oxidized LDL probably reflects the increased oxidation of LDL in atherosclerosis. In patients with SLE, aPL have been reported to correlate with the markers of lipid peroxidation, suggesting that increased oxidative stress could be a trigger for these antibodies [37]. It is possible that part of the effect of aPL could be mediated via a cross-reacting specificity directed against oxidized LDL [38].

The prevalence of aPL in patients with myocardial infarction seems to be between 5% and 15% [38]. Elevated levels of these antibodies were initially described in young patients with myocardial infarction [39]. This finding has been confirmed by prospective studies showing that elevated levels of aCL in a non-SLE population imply an increased risk for the development of myocardial infarction [40, 41]. However, an association of aCL with coronary artery disease has been shown in several [39, 42–44] but not all studies [45, 46].

With regard to recurrent coronary events in postinfarction patients, Bili et al [47] demonstrated that elevated IgG aCL and IgM aCL at any level are independent risk factors for recurrent cardiac events. Furthermore, patients with both elevated IgG aCL and IgM aCL at any level have the highest risk. This risk was comparable to other known risk factors for recurrent coronary events: prior myocardial infarction, non–insulin-dependent diabetes, ejection fraction < 30%, and smoking. In the same study, no association was found between anti–β_2-glycoprotein I antibodies and recurrent cardiac events. Interestingly, Hamsten et al [39], in a series of 62 young survivors of myocardial infarction (under the age of 45 years), found an increase in recurrent thrombotic events in those with aPL. Specifically, in 8 out 13 patients with elevated aPL levels, recurrent cardiovascular thombotic events occurred. However, these results have not been verified by other authors [45, 46, 48]. For example, Sletnes et al [45], in the largest study of aPL in patients surviving an acute infarct, found that 13.2% of 597 patients were positive for aPL compared with 4.4% of a reference population. However, in a multivariate analysis, adjusted for major cardiovascular risk factors, aPL were not found to be an independent risk factor for mortality, reinfarction, or non-hemorrhagic stroke. These aPL might arise because of vascular injury and exposure of neoantigens and might, in fact, be different idiotypes from those pathogenic idiotypes demonstrable in patients with SLE or PAPS. The question of whether aCL can be induced in response to tissue necrosis that occurs in myocardial infarction is still unresolved [49].

Thus, general screening for aPL of all patients with myocardial infarction is not indicated. It may still be concluded that aPL are a significant factor in acute myocardial infarction in selected patients. Therefore, selective aPL estimations should be undertaken in: (i) younger patients (under 45 years of age); (ii) those with a previous history of venous or arterial thrombosis or recurrent fetal losses; and (iii) those with a family history of an autoimmune disease, especially if lupus related [50].

Unstable Angina

Although some patients with myocardial infarction and aPL presented with angina before or after the acute infarction, isolated unstable angina has been reported occasionally in patients with the APS [51]. In the "Euro-Phospholipid cohort" [34], angina was reported in 2.7% of the 1000 patients studied. Conversely, Díaz and Becker [52] found aCL in 8 out of 22 (36.4%) patients with unstable angina and Hamsted et al [39] found a high incidence of aCL in young patients with myocardial infarction. However, they were unable to identify an association between aCL positivity and either the severity of angiographic coronary disease or an adverse clinical outcome. Thus, aCL does not appear to act independently of the usual coronary risk factors or alter the morphological features of atherosclerotic coronary narrowing as determinated angiographically.

Farsi et al [53] investigated the prevalence of anti–β_2-glycoprotein I antibodies in 20 patients with unstable angina and 17 with effort angina. Positivity for anti–β_2-glycoprotein I antibodies was found in 45% of patients with unstable angina and only in 12% of patients with effort angina. In addition, both IgG and IgM levels of anti–β_2-glycoprotein I antibodies were significantly higher in patients with unstable angina compared to patients with effort angina. There was a lack of a significant difference in the prevalence of these antibodies in patients with or without a previous myocardial infarction, suggesting that anti–β_2-glycoprotein I antibodies were not induced by tissue necrosis.

Coronary Bypass Graft and Angioplasty Occlusions

There is a substantial failure rate following aortocoronary venous bypass grafting. Early graft occlusions (10%–20%) seems to be due to technical and hemodynamic factors, including the calibre of the graft and anastomosis and unsatisfactory distal run-off. Bick et al [54] disclosed that a very high percentage of young individuals (those under 50 years) who suffered acute myocardial infarction or who experienced restenosis after percutaneous transluminal coronary angioplasty (PTCA) or coronary artery bypass have aCL. In another study [55], it was found that 33% of coronary artery bypass patients suffering late graft occlusion (as determined by coronary angiography 12 months postcoronary artery bypass graft surgery) had preoperative aCL levels 2 standard deviations above control values, strongly suggesting an association between graft occlusion and aPL. Interestingly, Morton et al [56]] in a series of 83 patients who underwent coronary bypass graft surgery, found that aCL levels were elevated in those patients with late bypass graft occlusions.

Eber et al [57], in a series of 65 men with coronary artery disease treated with PTCA, have reported increased IgM aCL levels in patients with restenosis. Additionally, Chambers et al [58], described a 56-year-old woman with APS and early failure of percutaneous transluminal coronary angioplasty (PTCA) on three occasions and the patient had to be subjected to coronary artery bypass surgery. Ludia et al [59] investigated the role of aPL in restenosis after PTCA. In this study, aPL were investigated in 60 patients with ischemic heart disease before PTCA, and patients were followed up for restenosis. The aPL were found in 15/60 patients and restenosis was observed in 13/60 patients; specifically, in 7/45 (15%) aPL-negative patients and in 6/15 (40%) aPL-positive patients. In addition, restenosis occurred earlier in aPL-positive patients. Three additional APS patients with myocardial infarction were successfully managed with PTCA [60], coronary stent implantation [61], and PTCA and stenting [62], respectively. In these three cases, long-term anticoagulation was initiated immediately after the PTCA or stenting and appeared to be effective.

Intracardiac Thrombus

The endocardial surface may also be an important site for thrombus formation in patients with aPL. Primary intracardiac mural thrombi have been reported in these patients [63, 64]. It is important to stress that their presence may lead to diagnostic confusion; on occasion there may be difficulty in differentiation from a cardiac tumor, for example, atrial myxoma, using noninvasive imaging techniques.

Cardiomyopathy

Acute Cardiomyopathy

Brown et al [65] described a 22-year-old female with SLE who succumbed within 24 hours of admission with profound hypotension and peripheral circulatory collapse and who at necropsy demonstrated the presence of microthrombi in multiple organs, including the heart (cardiac "microvasculopathy"). An essentially similar patient, a male with a PAPS, who had previously suffered a myocardial infarction, transient ischemic attacks, stroke, aortic regurgitation, and who had extensive *livedo reticularis*, was described by Murphy and Leach [66]. He died suddenly and multiple platelet thrombi within the intramyocardial arteries were found at autopsy. Kattwinkel et al [67] also reported a patient with a primary APS, myocardial infarction being caused by cardiac microvasculopathy. Angiography in these patients may reveal normal coronary arteries as the disease involves the microcirculation.

Chronic Cardiomyopathy

Patients with aPL and chronic myocardial dysfunction, unexplained in the context of valve abnormalities or other obvious causes, have been documented. Leung et al [13] in a study of 75 consecutive SLE patients found that aPL were significantly associated with left ventricular (global/isolated) dysfunction. Four of 5 patients with isolated left ventricular dysfunction had positive aPL.

Conclusions

Whether the aPL are cause of these cardiac complications or simply accompany more basic underlying immunological disturbances cannot be assessed from these studies. However, serial screening of aPL in patients who develop these complications will help to assess the prevalence and usefulness of these antibodies in cardiac diseases. Until these studies become available, clinicians should consider a search for aPL in those patients with the previously reported cardiac complications in whom no other etiology could be found.

References

1. Ziporen L, Goldberg I, Arad M, et al. Libman-Sacks endocarditis in the antiphospholipid syndrome: Immunopathogenic findings in deformed heart valves. Lupus 1996;5:196–205.
2. Ford PM, Ford SE, Lillicrap DP. Association of lupus anticoagulant with severe valvular heart disease in systemic lupus erythematosus. J Rheumatol 1988;15:597–600.
3. Anderson D, Bell D, Lodge R, Grant E. Recurrent cerebral ischemia and mitral valve vegetation in a patient with lupus anticoagulant. J Rheumatol 1987;14:839–841.
4. Nihoyannopoulos P, Gomez PM, Joshi J, et al. Cardiac abnormalities in systemic lupus erythematosus. Association with raised anticardiolipin antibodies. Circulation 1990;82:369–375.
5. Khamashta MA, Cervera R, Asherson RA, et al. Association of antibodies against phospholipids with heart valve disease in systemic lupus erythematosus. Lancet 1990;335:1541–1544.
6. Cervera R, Font J, Paré C, et al. Cardiac disease in systemic lupus erythematosus: prospective study of 70 patients. Ann Rheum Dis 1992;51:156–159.
7. Cervera R, Khamashta MA, Font J, et al. High prevalence of significant heart valve lesions in patients with the 'primary' antiphospholipid syndrome. Lupus 1991;1:43–47.
8. Brenner B, Blumenfeld Z, Markiewicz W, et al. Cardiac involvement in patients with primary antiphospholipid syndrome. J Am Coll Cardiol 1991;18:931–936.
9. Galve E, Ordi J, Barquinero J, et al. Valvular heart disease in the primary antiphospholipid syndrome. Ann Intern Med 1992;116:293–298.
10. Nesher G, Ilani J, Rosenmann D, et al. Valvular dysfunction in antiphospholipid syndrome: Prevalence, clinical features, and treatment. Semin Arthritis Rheum 1997;27:27 35.
11. Metz D, Jolly D, Graciet-Richard J, et al. Prevalence of valvular involvement in systemic lupus erythematosus and association with antiphospholipid syndrome: a matched echocardiographic study. Cardiology 1994;85:129–136.
12. Roldan CA, Shively BK, Lau CC, et al. Systemic lupus erythematosus valve disease by transesophageal echocardiography and the role of antiphospholipid antibodies. J Am Coll Cardiol 1992;20:1127–1134.
13. Leung W-H, Wong K-L, Lau C-P, et al. Association between antiphospholipid antibodies and cardiac abnormalities in patients with systemic lupus erythematosus. Am J Med 1990;89:411–419.
14. Amital H, Langevitz P, Levy Y, et al. Valvular deposition of antiphospholipid antibodies in the antiphospholipid syndrome: a clue to the origin of the disease. Clin Exp Rheumatol 1999;17:99–102.
15. García-Torres R, Amigo MC, de la Rossa A, et al. Valvular heart disease in primary antiphospholipid syndrome: clinical and morphological findings. Lupus 1996;5:56–61.
16. Hojnik M, George J, Ziporen L, et al. Heart valve involvement (Libman-Sacks endocarditis) in the antiphospholipid syndrome. Circulation 1996;93:1579–1587.
17. Asherson RA, Gibson DG, Evans DW, et al. Diagnostic and therapeutic problems in two patients with antiphospholipid antibodies, heart valve lesions and transient ischaemic attacks. Ann Rheum Dis 1988;47:947–953.
18. Font J, Cervera R, Paré C, et al. Haemodynamically significant non-infective verrucous endocarditis in a patient with 'primary' antiphospholipid syndrome. Br J Rheumatol 1991;30:305–307.
19. Asherson RA, Tikly M, Staub H, et al. Infective endocarditis, rheumatoid factor, and anticardiolipin antibodies. Ann Rheum Dis 1990;49:107–108.
20. Young SM, Fisher M, Sigsbee A, et al. Cardiogenic brain embolism and lupus anticoagulant. Ann Neurol 1989;26:390–392.
21. D'Alton JG, Preston DN, Bormanis J, et al. Multiple transient ischemic attacks, lupus anticoagulant and verrucous endocarditis. Stroke 1985;16:512–514.
22. Levine SR, Kim S, Deegan MJ, et al. Ischemic stroke associated with anticardiolipin antibodies. Stroke 1987;18:1101–1106.

23. The Antiphospholipid Antibodies in Stroke Study Group. Clinical and laboratory findings in patients with antiphospholipid antibodies and cerebral ischaemia. Stroke 1990;21:1268–1273.
24. Font J, Pérez-Villa F, Cervera R, et al. Antiphospholipid antibodies and severe valvular regurgitation in patients with systemic lupus erythematosus. A long-term follow-up echocardiographic study. Arthritis Rheum 1999;42 (suppl):S366.
25. Espinola-Zavaleta N, Vargas-Barron J, Colmenares-Galvis T, et al. Echocardiographic evaluation of patients with primary antiphospholipid syndrome. Am Heart J 1999;137:973–978.
26. Erkan D, Sammaritano L, Lockshin MD. Management of the difficult aspects of antiphospholipid syndrome. In: Asherson RA, Cervera R, Piette JC, Shoenfeld Y, eds. Antiphospholipid syndrome II. Autoimmune thrombosis. Amsterdam:Elsevier; 2002:395–407.
27. Lockshin MD, Tenedios F, Petri M, et al. Cardiac disease in the antiphospholipid syndrome: recommendations for treatment. Committee consensus report. Lupus 2003;12:518–523.
28. Manzi S, Meilhan EN, Rairie J, et al. Age-specific incidence rates of myocardial infarction and angina in women with systemic lupus erythematosus comparison with the Framingham Study. Am J Epidemiol 1997;145:408–415.
29. Petri M, Lakatta C, Magder L, et al. Effect of prednisone and hydroxychloroquine on coronary artery disease risk factors in systemic lupus erythematosus: a longitudinal data analysis. Am J Med 1994;96:254–259.
30. Karrar A, Sequeira W, Block JA. Coronary artery disease in systemic lupus erythematosus: a review of the literature. Semin Arthritis Rheum 2001;30:436–443.
31. Asherson RA, Cervera R. Antiphospholipid antibodies and the heart. Lessons and pitfalls for the cardiologist. Circulation 1991;84:920–923.
32. Petri M. Detection of coronary artery disease and the role of traditional risk factors in the Hopkins Lupus Cohort. Lupus 2000;9:170–175.
33. Asherson RA, Harris EN, Gharavi AE, et al. Myocardial infarction in SLE and 'lupus-like' disease. Arthritis Rheum 1985;29:1292–1293.
34. Cervera R, Piette JC, Font J, et al. Antiphospholipid syndrome: Clinical and immunologic manifestations and patterns of disease expression in a cohort of 1,000 patients. Arthritis Rheum 2002;46:1019–1027.
35. Vaarala O, Mänttäri M, Manninen V, et al. Anti-cardiolipin antibodies and risk of myocardial infarction in a prospective cohort of middle-aged men. Circulation 1995;91:23–27.
36. Puurunen M, Manttari M, Manninen V, et al. Antibodies to oxidized low-density lipoprotein predicting myocardial infarction. Arch Intern Med 1994;154:2605–2609.
37. Iuliano L, Pratico D, Ferro D, et al. Enhanced lipid peroxidation in patients positive for antiphospholipid antibodies. Blood 1997;90:3931–3935.
38. Vaarala O. Antiphospholipid antibodies and myocardial infarction. Lupus 1998;7(suppl 2):132–134.
39. Hamsten A, Norberg R, Bjorkholm M, et al. Antibodies to cardiolipin in young survivors of myocardial infarction: an association with recurrent cardiovascular events. Lancet 1986;1:113–116.
40. Levine SR, Salowich-Palm L, Sawaya KL, et al. IgG anticardiolipin antibody titer > 40 GPL and the risk of subsequent thrombo-occlusive events and death. A prospective cohort study. Stroke 1997;28:1660–1665.
41. Adler Y, Finkelstein Y, Zandeman-Goddard G, et al. The presence of antiphospholipid antibodies in acute myocardial infarction. Lupus 1995;4:309–313.
42. Zuckerman E, Toubi E, Shiran A, et al. Anticardiolipin antibodies and acute myocardial infarction in non-systemic lupus erythematosus patients: a controlled prospective study. Am J Med 1996;171:381–386.
43. Espinosa G, Cervera R, Font J, et al. Cardiac and pulmonary manifestations in the antiphospholipid syndrome. In: Asherson RA, Cervera R, Piette JC, Shoenfeld Y, eds. The antiphospholipid syndrome II. Autoimmune thrombosis. Amsterdam: Elsevier; 2002:169–188.
44. Wu R, Nityanand S, Berglund L, et al. Antibodies against cardiolipin and oxidatively modified LDL in 50-year old men predict myocardial infarction. Arterioscler Thromb Vasc Biol 1997;17:3159–3163.
45. Sletnes KE, Smith P, Abdelnoor M, et al. Antiphospholipid antibodies after myocardial infarction and their relation to mortality, reinfarction, and non-haemorrhagic stroke. Lancet 1992;339:451–453.
46. Phadke KV, Phillips RA, Clarke DT, et al. Anticardiolipin antibodies in ischaemic heart disease: marker or myth? Br Heart J 1993;69:391–394.
47. Bili A, Moss AJ, Francis CW, et al. Anticardiolipin antibodies and recurrent coronary events. A prospective study of 1150 patients. Circulation 2000;102:1258–1263.
48. De Caterina R, D'Ascanio A, Mazzone A, et al. Prevalence of anticardiolipin antibodies in coronary artery disease. Am J Cardiol 1989;65:922–923.
49. Vaarala O. Antiphospholipid antibodies and atherosclerosis. Lupus 1996;5:442–447.

50. Baker WF Jr, Bick RL. Antiphospholipid antibodies in coronary artery disease: a review. Semin Thromb Hemost 1994;20:27–45.
51. Asherson RA, Khamashta MA, Ordi-Ros J, et al. The 'primary' antiphospholipid syndrome: Major clinical and serological features. Medicine (Baltimore) 1989;68:366–374.
52. Díaz MN, Becker RC. Anticardiolipin antibodies in patients with unstable angina. Cardiology 1994;84:380–384.
53. Farsi A, Domeneghetti MP, Fedi S, et al. High prevalence of anti-beta2-glycoprotein I antibodies in patients with ischemic heart disease. Autoimmunity 1999;30:93–98.
54. Bick RL, Ismail Y, Baker WF Jr. Coagulation abnormalities in patients with precocious coronary artery thrombosis and patients failing coronary artery bypass grafting and percutaneous transcoronary angioplasty. Semin Thromb Hemost 1993;19:411–417.
55. Gavaghan TP, Krilis SA, Daggard GE, et al. Anticardiolipin antibodies and occlusion of coronary bypass grafts. Lancet 1987;2:977–978.
56. Morton KE, Gavaghan TP, Krilis SA, et al. Coronary artery bypass graft failure: an autoimmune phenomenon? Lancet 1986;2:1353–1356.
57. Eber B, Schumacher M, Auer-Grumbach P, et al. Increased IgM anticardiolipin antibodies in patients with restenosis after percutaneous transluminal coronary angioplasty. Am J Cardiol 1992;69:1255–1258.
58. Chambers JD, Haire WD, Deligonul U. Multiple early percutaneous transluminal coronary angioplasty failures related to lupus anticoagulant. Am Heart J 1996;132:189–190.
59. Ludia C, Domenico P, Monia C, et al. Antiphospholipid antibodies: a new risk factor for restenosis after percutaneous transluminal coronary angioplasty? Autoimmunity 1998;27:141–148.
60. Takeuchi S, Obayashi T, Toyama J. Primary antiphospholipid syndrome with acute myocardial infarction recanalised by PTCA. Heart 1998;79:96–98.
61. Jankowski M, Didek D, Dubiel JS, et al. Successful coronary stent implantation in a patient with primary antiphospholipid syndrome. Blood Coagul Fibrinolysis 1998;9:753–756.
62. Umesan CV, Kapoor A, Nityanand S, et al. Recurrent acute coronary events in a patient with primary antiphospholipid syndrome: successful management with intracoronary stenting. Int J Cardiol 1999;71:99–102.
63. Lubbe WF, Asherson RA. Intracardiac thrombus in systematic lupus erythematosus associated with lupus anticoagulant. Arthritis Rheum 1988;31:1453–1454.
64. Leventhal LJ, Borofsky MA, Bergey PD, Schumacher HR Jr. Antiphospholipid antibody syndrome with right atrial thrombosis mimicking an atrial myxoma. Am J Med 1989;87:111–113.
65. Brown JH, Doherty CC, Allan DC, Morton P. Fatal cardiac due to myocardial microthrombi in systemic lupus erythematosus. Br Med J 1989;298:525.
66. Murphy JJ, Leach IA. Findings at necropsy in the heart of a patient with anticardiolipin syndrome. Br Heart J 1989;62:61–64.
67. Kattwinkel N, Villanueva AG, Labib SB, Aretz T, Walek JW, Burns DL et al. Myocardial infarction caused by cardiac microvasculopathy in a patient with the primary antiphospholipid syndrome. Ann Intern Med 1992;116:974–976.

6 Cerebral Ischemia in Antiphospholipid Syndrome

Debendra Pattanaik and Robin L. Brey

Introduction

Central nervous system (CNS) involvement is common in antiphospholipid antibody syndrome (APS). In fact neurological manifestations were only second to venous thrombosis in a recently published prospective cohort of 1000 patients with APS [1]. In addition, some of the most debilitating clinical aspects of APS are the neurological and neuropsychiatric manifestations. Clinical manifestations of APS associated with the CNS include thrombo-occlusive events, psychiatric manifestations, and a variety of other non-thrombotic neurological syndromes [2] (see Table 6.1). Nevertheless, the specific role of antiphospholipid antibodies (aPL) in the CNS remains one of the least understood aspects of this syndrome. The mechanism of neurological involvement in patients with APS is thought to be primarily thrombotic in origin. However, there are many neurological syndromes where no structural lesions are evident in imaging studies of brain, suggesting aPL-mediated mechanisms other than thrombosis may be playing a role. Several investigators have found an interaction between aPL and nervous system tissue [3, 4]. aPL may interfere with endothelial cell function and promote procoagulant activity of endothelial cells [5–8]. IgG fractions from patients with aPL also increase mononuclear cell adhesion to human umbilical vein endothelial cells [9]. The pathogenic role of aPL in the development of thrombosis is supported by animal studies [8,

Table 6.1. Neurologic syndromes associated with antiphospholipid antibodies.

Cerebrovascular ischemia	Chorea
Stroke	Transverse myelopathy
Transient ischemic attack	Guillain–Barré syndrome
Cerebral venous sinus thrombosis	Diabetic peripheral neuropathy
Ocular ischemia	Sensorineural hearing loss
Dementia	Sudden onset
Acute ischemic encephalopathy	Progressive
With Sneddon's syndrome	Transient global amnesia
Without Sneddon's syndrome	Psychiatric disorders
Atypical migrainous-like events	Orthostatic hypotension
Seizures	

10–14]. Blank and colleagues showed that bacterial peptides homologus with β_2-glycoprotein I (β_2-GPI) induce pathogenic anti–β_2-GPI along with APS manifestations in mice and proposed a mechanism of molecular mimicry in experimental APS [13]. These investigations in animal models are useful for a better understanding the pathogenic mechanisms and to test new therapies for APS.

Cerebral Ischemia

Cerebral ischemia associated with aPL is the most common arterial thrombotic manifestation [15–17]. Stroke and transient ischemic attacks (TIAs) are considered the second most common clinical manifestations of primary antiphospholipid syndrome (PAPS) after venous thrombosis [1]. The average age of onset of aPL-associated cerebral ischemia is several decades younger than the typical cerebral ischemia population [18]. Cerebral ischemic events can occur in any vascular territory (see Fig. 6.1) [19], but in general the territory of the middle cerebral artery is more affected. A link has been postulated between cervico-cranial artery dissection and APS [20]. Though infrequent, cardiac emboli may be another cause of cerebral ischemia in patients with aPL. Cerebral ischemic events are more frequent in patients with valvular heart disease. The prevalence of valvular abnormalities, particularly left sided valve lesions, is higher in systemic lupus erythematosus (SLE) patients with aPL than in those without aPL [21, 22]. A study by Khamastha and colleagues [22] showed that patients with SLE and aPL have an increased frequency of mitral valve vegetations and mitral regurgitation than aPL-negative patients (16% vs. 1.2% and 38% vs. 12%, respectively). These may represent a potential cardiac source of stroke [21–23]. In a large consecutive autopsy series, a higher incidence of

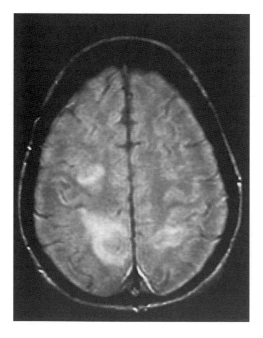

Figure 6.1. Brain magnetic resonance imaging (MRI) study showing multiple strokes in a young woman with antiphospholipid antibodies, strokes, and seizures. 📖

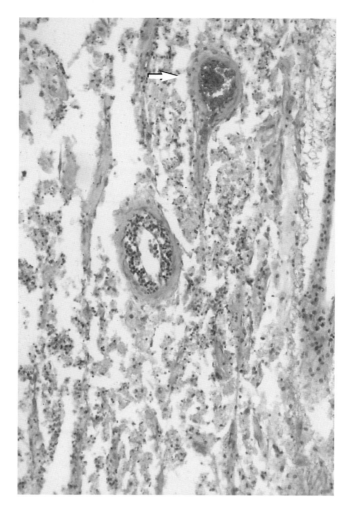

Figure 6.2. Hematoxalin and esosin–stained section of post-mortem brain tissue from a patient with aPL and the Catastrophic Antiphospholipid Antibody Syndrome. *Arrow* indicates a small cerebral blood vessel with thrombus, but no inflammation. 📖

cardiac valvular abnormalities and "bland" (non-vasculitic) thromboembolic lesions were found in patients with aPL (see Fig.6.2) [24]. Another possible source can be the heart chambers themselves or the internal carotid artery. Microthrombotic occlusive disease of multiple small vessels ("thrombotic microangiopathy") has been reported in a large number of patients with catastrophic APS [25] and in animal studies [14]. Clinical events consistent with multiple small vessel occlusion occurred in these patients within a short time period of days to weeks. Neurologic involvement is a poor prognostic factor in catastrophic APS [26].

aPL have been established as risk factors in a first ischemic stroke, but their role in recurrent stroke is less clear. Many case control and prospective studies have shown an association between different types of aPL and stroke [18, 27–38], but some have not [39–46]. All but one showed an increased risk for incident ischemic stroke in young people [45]. The presence and magnitude of the ischemic stroke risk associated with aPL in older populations is more evenly split between finding an increased risk and no increased risk. This suggests that aPL may be a more important stroke mechanism in young people. In older populations, other stroke risk factors may take on more importance. There are also methodological differences between studies, such as the type of aPL studied, sample size, and population studied, that could explain discrepant results. In addition, most of them either excluded cardio-embolic disease or did not distinguish between cardio-embolic, artery-to-artery embolic, or thrombotic mechanisms. This is an important point, because different treatment strategies may apply to these different pathophysiological mechanisms.

It is interesting that many of the larger studies find an association between aPL and incident stroke, whereas the association between aPL and recurrent stroke is weaker. This is true for two studies that reported an increased risk related to aPL for incident stroke, yet failed to find an increased risk for recurrent stroke in the same population during follow up [30, 31, 42]. The explanation for this is not clear, but as described above for the aPL-associated incident ischemic stroke in older populations, may be due to other stroke risk factors assuming more importance in risk for recurrent stroke and over-shadowing (or even negating) the recurrent stroke risk contributed by aPL in these patients, or may possibly represent a treatment effect.

Clinical and immunologic manifestations and patterns of disease expression of APS in a cohort of 1000 patients from the Euro-Phospholipid Project Group have been recently reported [1]. This project began in 1999, and employs a multi-center, consecutive, prospective design. The final cohort meets the Saporro criteria for APS [47]. There are 820 women and 180 men enrolled. PAPS was present in 53.1% of patients, APS associated with SLE in 36.2%, APS associated with "lupus-like" disease in 5.9%, and other diseases in 5.9%. At study entry, deep venous thrombosis was the most common thrombotic manifestation, occurring in 317 (31.7%) patients and stroke was the most common arterial thrombotic manifestation, occurring in 135 (13.1%) patients with myocardial infarction occurring in 28 (2.8%) patients. Additional cerebrovascular ischemic events were seen as well: transient ischemic attack in 70 (7.0%) and amaurosis fugax in 28 (2.8%) patients. While some clinical differences existed between primary and secondary APS patients, none of these included thrombotic manifestations. While follow-up information is not yet available for this extremely well-characterized cohort, invaluable information about recurrent stroke and other clinical manifestations will be forthcoming, as 10 years of follow up is planned.

In another European collaborative study, the European Working Party on SLE [17], the morbidity and mortality in patients with SLE over a 10-year period was studied in a cohort of 1000 patients. At the beginning of this study, there were 204 (20.4%) patients with anticardiolipid antibodies (aCL) IgG, 108 (10.8%) patients with aCL IgM, and 94 (9.4%) patients with lupus anticoagulant (LA) [48]. While it is not entirely clear how many of these patients had aPL positivity at follow up (and would be diagnosed as secondary APS), thromboses were the most common cause of death in the last 5 years of follow up and were always associated with APS. The most common thrombotic events in these patients were strokes (11.8%), followed by myocardial infarction (7.4%) and pulmonary embolism (5.9%). This suggests an important role for aPL and recurrent thrombosis in patients with SLE, but does not address the issue of a possibly greater increased risk in patients with secondary versus primary APS.

Another important study that evaluated the natural history and risk factors for recurrent thrombosis in patients with aPL is the Italian Registry [49]. In that study, 360 patients were studied prospectively for 4 years. Inclusion criteria were that subjects had aPL and were available for follow up. aPL assays were done clinically because of a thrombotic event, disease known to be associated with APS, or a coagulation abnormality suggesting the presence of a LA. Thirty-four patients had thrombotic events over the 4-year period, including 10 strokes (1 fatal) and 6 TIAs. Treatment was at the discretion of the attending physician. Risk factors for thrombosis in this cohort included: (1) aCL titer > 40 GPL and prior thrombotic event, and (2) aCL titer > 40 GPL units and SLE.

The Antiphospholipid Antibody and Stroke Study Group (APASS)/ Warfarin Aspirin Recurrent Stroke Study (WARSS) collaboration evaluated the recurrent stroke risk attributed to aPL in a group of nearly 2000 patients with ischemic stroke who were randomized to warfarin (international normalized ratio (INR) range, 1.2–2.8; mean INR, 2.2) versus aspirin (325 mg/day] in a double blind study [50]. Very few of these patients had a diagnosis of SLE. aCL, LA, or both at study entry did not predict recurrent stroke in either treatment group. As will be discussed further in the section below, this study included patients with low positive titers of aCL IgG, IgM, and IgA antibodies and results published thus far utilize baseline aPL values only. Thus, this study does not address the question of recurrent stroke risk in patients with APS. Another study by the APASS investigators that evaluated the risk for recurrent stroke in a multi-center, U.S. cohort of patients followed for 2 years also did not find an association between APS and recurrent stroke [32]. These patients were treated at the discretion of the attending physician.

Few prospective studies have examined the association between aPL and an initial stroke. These have been limited to aCL tested on only one occasion and therefore, patients included would not meet current criteria for APS [39, 40, 46]. Brey and colleagues performed a prospective study of the association between aCL and stroke and myocardial infarction (MI) over a 20-year period in men enrolled in the Honolulu Heart Program [36]. Only presence of β_2-GPI–dependent aCL of the IgG class was significantly associated with both incident ischemic stroke and MI. This association was attenuated in the last 5 years of follow up. The risk factor-adjusted relative odds for men with a positive versus a negative β_2-GPI–dependent aCL of the IgG class were 2.2 [95% confidence interval (CI), 1.5–3.4) at 15 years and 1.5 (95% CI, 1.0–2.3) at 20 years. For MI, the adjusted relative odds were 1.8 (95% CI, 1.2–2.6) at 15 years and 1.5 (95% CI, 1.1–2.1) at 20 years. This is the first report of a prospective association between aCL and stroke. Two other studies failed to show an association [39, 40]. Among the studies linking aCL to MI, two other prospective studies suggested the possibility of a time-dependent association between aCL and MI in men [51, 52]. In one study [51], the follow-up period was 5 years and, in the other study [51], a significant association was found only for the first 10 years of follow up, despite the fact that the second 10 years of follow up had more than double the number of events. Such weakening of the association with time could be due to changes in risk factor status during follow up, including aCL. It is unlikely that the observed associations between aCL and vascular disease are due to chance or an artifact of study design. Prospective studies of MI and stroke preclude the possibility that the antibodies were a consequence of the vascular event

but, as noted above, do not exclude the possibility that the antibodies are a consequence of pre-clinical disease or require the presence of other stroke risk factors in
order for thrombosis to occur.

Venous Sinus Thrombosis

Venous sinus thrombosis is an uncommon manifestation of APS. Deschiens and
colleagues [53] suggested that aPL may be an important factor contributing to cerebral venous sinus thrombosis (CVT) even in the presence of other potential risk
factors including the syndrome of activated protein C resistance due to Factor V
Leiden mutation. In a later study, Carhupoma and colleagues [54] reported that the
onset of CVT in patients with aPL occurs at a younger age and has more extensive
superficial and deep cerebral venous system involvement. In addition, a higher rate
of post–CVT migraine and more infarctions on brain imaging studies may possibly
be seen in patients with aPL [54].

Dementia and Other Cognitive Dysfunction

Cognitive deficits associated with primary or secondary APS can vary from mild
neurocognitive disorders to more severe vascular dementia [55]. Despite the
increased interest within the last few years, research in this area is limited and few
formal neuropsychological studies have been conducted thus far to assess the
prevalence and nature of cognitive deficits in APS. Although many studies evaluating neurocognitive deficits in patients with aPL have been anecdotal [56, 57], several
cross-sectional and prospective studies have been recently published [58–63]. There
is no specific pattern of cognitive dysfunction that has been consistently identified;
however, there are many similarities in the deficits found in aPL-positive patients
across different studies.

When cognitive dysfunction is milder, patients complain of forgetfulness, attention deficits, difficulty concentrating on tasks, and other deficits that mildly interfere with everyday function. These mild changes in the cognitive status may be the
only clinical manifestation of APS [64]. Formal neuropsychological testing may be
the most sensitive tool to measure small cognitive changes that might not be
obvious on brief bedside examinations such as the Mini Mental Status Examination
[65]. In addition, cognitive functioning assessed by these tests may provide an accurate index of the patient's general CNS status [65, 66].

There are many documented cases of neurocognitive deficits secondary to APS
that are not related to cerebrovascular disease [57, 67]. For example, Mikdashi and
Kay [56] reported 4 patients who exhibited psychomotor retardation and had the
same deficit pattern, including decreased visual attention, word retrieval problems,
executive function difficulties, and impairment of both verbal and non-verbal
memory skills. None of these patients had a history of stroke.

aPL-associated Cognitive Dysfunction: Primary APS

An association between high aCL titers and cognitive dysfunction has also been
found in patients without SLE. For example, Schmidt and colleagues found subtle

neuropsychological dysfunction in otherwise normal elderly people with increased levels of aCL IgG [67]. This correlation with aCL IgG titers was significant despite the lack of evidence of any anatomic abnormalities on magnetic resonance imaging (MRI) or correlation of aCL positivity with MRI. De Moerloose and colleagues evaluated the prevalence of aCL in 192 elderly patients [68]. The overall prevalence of aCL was 10.9% and decreased by decade in patients 70–99 years of age from 18% to 10% to 7%, whereas the prevalence of ANA positivity increased by decade from 22% to 32% to 42%. There was no association between the presence of aCL and decreased survival. In contrast, and in keeping with previous findings, Cesbron found a trend towards an increased prevalence of aCL by decade in 1042 elderly subjects between the ages of 60 and 99 years [69]. In addition, high aCL levels were associated with increased physical disability in this population independent of age, gender, visual or hearing abnormalities, Mini Mental Status Examination scores, or history of cerebrovascular or cardiovascular disease. Chapman and colleagues reported that 13 of 23 (56%) patients with APS were demented and they were significantly older than the non-demented APS group [70]. The demented patients had significantly more pathology on computed tomography (CT) scan of brain and electroencephalogram (EEG). The higher level of aPL in the demented patients suggests a direct causal relationship between autoantibodies and brain dysfunction.

aPL-associated Cognitive Dysfunction: Secondary APS

aPL positivity has been associated with several different patterns of cognitive dysfunction in patients with secondary APS, depending on the study. Verbal memory deficits, decreased psychomotor speed, and decreased overall productivity have been significantly correlated to elevated aPL levels [59–62]. Denburg and colleagues found LA-positive patients to score significantly lower than LA-negative patients on measures of verbal memory, cognitive flexibility, and psychomotor speed [59]. In addition, the cognitive deficits were noted even in patients who had no past or present clinical neuropsychiatric event, suggesting a specific association between the antibodies and cognitive functioning. Several recent studies have also reported cognitive dysfunction with increased IgG aCL titers [60, 62]. Menon and colleagues reported that SLE patients with consistently elevated IgG aCL levels over a period of 2 to 3 years performed significantly worse than SLE patients with occasionally elevated or never elevated titers on a variety of neuropsychological tests [62]. These results were not observed with anti-DNA antibody titers or C3 levels. Attention and concentration, as well as psychomotor speed, were the domains most affected. Hanly and colleagues followed 51 female SLE patients over a 5-year period and found that persistent aCL IgG elevations were associated with decreased psychomotor speed, while persistent aCL IgA elevations were correlated with problems with executive functioning and reasoning abilities [59]. They also found no association between cognitive deficits and anti-DNA antibodies.

Sneddon's Syndrome and Other aPL-associated Dementia

Recurrent stroke in patients with livedo reticularis (Sneddon's syndrome) has been associated with aPL [71]. The frequency of aPL in patients with Sneddon's syndrome has ranged from 0% to 85% [71–73]. This syndrome is also frequently accompanied by dementia, most likely on the basis of multiple infarctions.

Sneddon's original patients all had focal neurological deficits, which he considered to be "limited and benign," leaving little residual disability [74]. Subsequent descriptions of the syndrome have revealed a spectrum of clinical neurological manifestations. Zelger and colleagues described three stages of neurological involvement: (1) "prodromal" symptoms such as dizziness or headaches preceding focal neurological deficits by years; (2) recurrent focal neurological deficits due to recurrent cerebral ischemia, also lasting years; and (3) progressive cognitive impairment leading to severe dementia [72]. Tourbah and colleagues correlated the MRI abnormalities found in 26 patients with Sneddon's syndrome with disability, presence of cardiovascular risk factors, cardiac valvular abnormalities on ECHO, and titer of aPL [73]. Disability (defined by memory disturbance or ability to perform activities of daily living) was found in 50% of the patients. Severe disability, which was consistent with dementia, was present in over half of the patients with disability. Systemic hypertension was present in 65%, cardiac valvular abnormalities in 61%, and aPL in 42% of patients with no correlation found between any of these and MRI abnormalities. The presence of disability was correlated with increasing severity of MRI lesions.

An aPL-associated dementia without the other features of Sneddon's syndrome has also been described. In many patients this appears to be due to multiple cerebral infarctions [75]. In addition, the catastrophic APS can present with an acute organic brain syndrome characterized by fulminant encephalopathy [76]. Asherson reported that in a group sample of 50 patients with catastrophic APS over 50% had CNS involvement [25].

Neuroimaging Studies

Brain MRI studies in patients with APS (primary or secondary) have revealed small foci of high signal in subcortical white matter scattered throughout the brain [77–79]. This type of pattern is seen in many other disease processes and is, as such, non-specific. The correlation between MRI lesions in patients with aPL and clinical nervous system symptoms is reported to be high by some investigators [77–79] and not by others [67, 80].

Toubi and colleagues [79] found aPL immunoreactivity in 53/96 (55%) SLE patients with CNS manifestations as compared to 20/100 (20%) of SLE patients without them. In this study, 53 patients with CNS manifestations underwent MRI imaging and 33 showed high-intensity lesions that were interpreted as "suggestive of vasculopathy." MRI abnormalities were seen more frequently in patients with as compared to those without aPL immunoreactivity. Some of these patients with MRI abnormalities had seizures or psychiatric disturbances and not stroke. This suggests that in some cases, aPL-associated neurologic manifestations may be due to an aPL–brain phospholipid interaction whereas in other the underlying pathogenic feature may be thrombotic. Although useful in demonstrating structural lesions such as infarcts and hemorrhages in the brains of patients with focal lesions, imaging techniques are poorly correlated with diffuse or global dysfunction. For example, the status of aCL titers in a group of 233 normal elderly participants was found to have no influence in the MRI results [67]. Using brain MRI and PET imaging, neuropsychological testing, a neurological examination, and serum testing for aPL antibodies and antineuronal antibodies, Sailer and colleagues [80] studied 35 SLE patients whose disease was inactive. Twenty patients had neurological deficits, 3 had psychiatric symptoms, and 10 had cognitive impairment. No differences in global glucose utilization by PET imaging were seen between SLE patients with as compared to those without neurological or cognitive abnormalities. On MRI imaging, the number and size of the white matter lesions correlated with the presence of neurological deficit, but were unrelated to the severity of cognitive impairment. Large lesions (8 mm or greater) were associated with high aCL IgG levels. In a study evaluating the association between neuropsychological abnormalities and aPL in an elderly population, no association between aCL and MRI lesions was found, supporting Sailer's findings in the group with cognitive impairment only [67].

Hachulla and colleagues performed brain MRI in patients with primary and secondary APS [81]. Both cerebral atrophy and white matter lesions were more common in both groups in comparison with control subjects. The number and volume of white matter lesions were increased in patients with primary and secondary APS who also had neurological symptoms. Only a weak correlation was found between the presence of LA and cerebral atrophy.

Treatment

Primary Prevention

There are no data that address the use of any specific treatment strategies for primary prevention of aPL-associated stroke. Several ongoing studies are likely to provide some data addressing this issue over the next few years. An ongoing study in the United Kingdom is randomizing SLE patients with aPL and adverse pregnancy outcomes to receive low-dose aspirin (75 mg/day) or low-intensity warfarin [2]. The aforementioned Euro-Phospholipid Project Group will also have some information that will shed light on the issue of primary prevention, although in that study patients are not randomized to a specific treatment [17]. Some information in this regard may already be available in the Euro-Lupus data set. Finally, the APSCORE registry in the United States (Robert Roubey, University of North Carolina, Principal Investigator) is enrolling subjects with primary APS, secondary APS, and aPL-positive patients not meeting Sapporo criteria [47]. Thus, the issue of true primary prevention (aPL positive at a moderate-to-high titer on at least two occasions at least 6 weeks apart but without clinical manifestations) can potentially be prospectively evaluated.

Secondary Prevention

Treatment such as platelet antiaggregant and anticoagulant therapy for secondary stroke prevention have both been used in APS and in cerebrovascular disease associated with aPL immunoreactivity [49, 82–84]. Two groups have retrospective data to suggest that high-intensity warfarin treatment (vs. low- or moderate-intensity warfarin or aspirin treatment) is associated with better outcomes in selected cohorts with various types of thrombotic events [82, 83]. Patients reported on in these studies did not have repeat aPL testing and would not fulfill current criteria for APS.

Crowther and colleagues recently reported the results of the first randomized, double-blind, controlled trial of two different intensities of warfarin treatment on the prevention of recurrent thrombotic events in patients with APS [84]. There were 114 patients enrolled in the study and followed for an average of 2.7 years. The average INR values in the moderate and high-intensity groups were 2.3 and 3.3, respectively. Recurrent thrombosis occurred in 2/58 (3.4%) patients assigned to moderate-intensity warfarin and in 6/56 (10.7%) patients assigned to receive high-intensity warfarin. In the moderate-intensity group, recurrent events included MI and deep venous thrombosis. The INR values at the time of recurrent thrombosis in this group were 1.6 and 2.8. In the high-intensity group, recurrent events included 3 deep venous thromboses, 1 pulmonary embolism, 1 MI, and 1 stroke. The INR values for these patients at the time of recurrent thrombosis were 3.1, 1.0, 0.9, 1.0, 3.9, and 1 patient had stopped warfarin 137 days before the recurrent event. Thirteen patients in the moderate and 21 patients in the high-intensity group discontinued warfarin prematurely. Thus, 22.4% of the low-intensity group and 37.5% of the high-intensity group either had thrombosis on therapy or complications leading to the need for discontinuation of warfarin. The most common reasons for stopping warfarin included withdrawal of consent, thrombotic event, and bleeding. There was no difference in major bleeding rates between the two groups. These results suggest that high-intensity warfarin treatment is *not* more effective than moderate-intensity treatment in preventing recurrent thrombotic events in patients with APS. The study did not specifically address the end-point of stroke.

The APASS Group recently completed the first prospective study of the role of aPL in recurrent ischemic stroke in collaboration with the WARSS group [50]. This controlled and blinded study was initiated in 1993 and compared the risk of recurrent stroke and other thrombo-embolic disease over a 2-year follow-up period in patients with ischemic stroke who were randomized to either aspirin therapy (325 mg/day) or warfarin therapy at a dose to maintain the INR between 1.4 and 2.8. The suggested target INR was 2.2. This study was not designed to be a treatment trial, but rather collected additional laboratory data from subjects enrolled in WARSS. The purpose of the study was to collect information about recurrent stroke rates in aPL-positive versus aPL-negative patients controlling for treatment. Exclusion criteria for WARSS included indication for warfarin therapy (e.g., atrial fibrillation), contraindication for warfarin therapy, and high-grade carotid stenosis suggesting the need for carotid endarterectomy. There were 882 patients randomized to warfarin and 890 patients randomized to aspirin who participated in APASS. The primary analysis assessed the impact of baseline aPL positivity within each WARSS treatment group separately, after risk factor adjustment (because these aPL+ vs. aPL– comparisons were not randomized). No increased risk of thrombotic event was associated with the baseline aPL in either the warfarin-treated patients (RR 0.97; 95% CI, 0.74–1.27; $P = 0.82$), or the aspirin-treated patients (RR 0.96; 95% CI, 0.71–1.29; $P = 0.77$). The overall event rate was 22.2% among aPL-positive subjects and 21.8% among those who were aPL negative. There was no treatment by aPL interaction ($P = 0.96$). Patients with baseline positivity for both LA and aCL antibodies tended to have a higher event rate (31.7%) than patients who were negative on both antibodies (24.0%; RR 1.36; (95% CI, 0.97–1.92; $P = 0.07$). Classification by Regression Tree (CART) analyses failed to identify a specific LA test or aCL isotype or titer that was associated with an increased risk of thrombotic event. There was no difference in major bleeding complications between treatment groups. Thus, it appears that for patients with a positive aPL determination at a single time point at the time of ischemic stroke (including low titers of aCL and/or IgA aCL) who do not have either atrial fibrillation or high-grade carotid stenosis, aspirin and warfarin therapy at an INR of approximately 2.0 are equivalent regarding stroke recurrence and major bleeding complications.

There are some important limitations that must be kept in mind when applying these data to individual patients. First, the analyses that are currently available from the WARSS/APASS data do not address the issue of whether or not meeting the proposed criteria for the diagnosis of definite APS is an important factor in stroke recurrence or therapeutic response. A pre-specified analysis explored the relationship between aPL levels at study entry (and not APS status) and outcome. Second, both the INR and the aspirin dose selected for this study were based on treatment recommendations for secondary prevention of ischemic stroke in patients without aPL at the time the study was undertaken nearly 10 years ago. That is, a high INR-producing dose of warfarin was not used. The average INR was, however, nearly identical to the average dose of warfarin used in the moderate-intensity group in the study of Crowther and colleagues [84]. This dose was found to be equally effective to high-intensity warfarin treatment in preventing recurrent thrombotic events. A lower dose of aspirin (60–81 mg) may have theoretical advantages over the dose used in WARSS, however, new attention is being paid to the issue of aspirin resistence in stroke treatment. It may be that aspirin dose, like warfarin dose, will provide optimal efficacy if the dose is tailored to the individual patient.

It remains possible, although unproven, that high-intensity doses of warfarin can better prevent recurrence in some patients with aPL-associated ischemic stroke, particularly in patients with APS. Any benefit of high-intensity doses of warfarin may be negated by a higher rate of major bleeding complications, although this was not found to be the case in the study of Crowther and colleagues [84]. Ruiz-Irastorza and colleagues also addressed this question in an analysis of 66 patients with APS (58% of them with a previous stroke) on high-intensity warfarin therapy and found a major bleeding rate of 6 cases to 100 patient-years, with no cases of fatal bleeding and only 1 case of intracranial (subdural) hematomas [85]. In all cases, bleeding was associated with a clear precipitating factor. Interestingly, this group also found a high rate of thrombotic recurrences despite anticoagulant therapy, primarily in the same vascular territory as the original thrombotic episode (9.1 cases per 100 patient-years). In all but 1 case patients were documented to have an INR lower than 3.0 at the time of recurrent thrombosis, suggesting that in some patients with persistent medium-high titers of aCL and/or LA oral anticoagulation to high-intensity target range may be needed to prevent recurrent thrombotic events. Alternatively, antiplatelet therapy may benefit these patients, as well.

Derksen and colleagues recently described the course and outcome of 8 patients with ischemic stroke as the first thrombotic manifestation of APS who received low-dose aspirin as treatment for secondary prevention [86]. During 8.9 years of follow up, 2 patients had a recurrent stroke, for a recurrent stroke rate of 3.5/100 patient-years on aspirin. Although this is a very small series of patients, the recurrent stroke rate with aspirin treatment is actually lower than in the patients on high-intensity warfarin described by Ruiz-Irastorza and colleagues [85].

Thus, the issue of optimal treatment in preventing recurrent stroke in patients with aPL/APS remains an open question. It is possible that subgroups with different recurrence risks and for whom specific treatments are optimal will be identified in the coming years.

References

1. Cervera R, Piette J, Font J, et al. Antiphospholipid syndrome clinical and immunologic manifestations and patterns of disease expression in a cohort of 1000 patients Arthritis Rheum 2002;46:1019–1027.
2. Sanna G, Bertolaccini ML, Cuadrado MJ, Khamashta MA, Hughes GRV. Central nervous system involvement in the antiphospholipid (Hughes) syndrome. Rheumatology (Oxford) 2003;42:200–213.
3. Sun KH, Liu WT, Tsai CY, et al. Inhibition of astrocyte proliferation and binding to brain tissue of anticardiolipin antibodies purified from lupus serum [abstract]. Ann Rheum Dis 1992;51:707.
4. Khalili A, Cooper RC. A study of immune responses to myelin and cardiolipin in patients with systemic lupus erythematosus (SLE). Clin Exp Immunol. 1991;8:365–372.
5. Oosting JD, Derksen RH, Blokzijl L, Sixma JJ, de Groot PG. Antiphospholipid antibody positive sera enhance endothelial cell procoagulant activity – studies in a thrombosis model. Thromb Haemost 1992;68:278–284.
6. Del Papa N, Guidali L, Sala A, et al. Endothelial cells as target for antiphospholipid antibodies. Arthritis Rheum 1997;40:551–561.
7. Del Papa N, Raschi ER, Catelli L, et al. Endothelial cells as a target for antiphospholipid antibodies: role of anti-beta-2-glycoprotein 1 antibodies. Am J Reprod Immunol 1997;38:212–217.
8. Pierangeli SS, Harris EN. Probing antiphospholipid-mediated thrombosis: the interplay between anticardiolipin antibodies and endothelial cells. Lupus 2003;12:539–545.
9. Simantov R, LaSala JM, Lo SK, et al. Activation of cultured vascular endothelial cells by antiphospholipid antibodies. J Clin Invest 1995;96:2211–2219.
10. Kent M, Vogt E, Rote NS. Monoclonal antiphosatidylserine antibodies react directly with feline and murine central nervous system. J Rheumatol 1997;24:1725–1733.
11. Kent MN, Alvarez FJ, Ng AK, Rote NS. Ultrastructural localization of monoclonal antiphospholipid antibody binding to rat brain. Exp Neurol 2000;163:173–179.
12. Ziporen L, Shoenfeld Y, Levy Y, Korczyn AD. Neurological dysfunction and hyperactive behavior associated with antiphospholipid antibodies. A mouse model. J Clin Invest 1997;100:613–619.
13. Blank M, Krause I, Fridkin M, et al. Bacterial induction of autoantibodies to beta2-glycoprotein-I accounts for the infectious etiology of antiphospholipid syndrome. J Clin Invest 2002;109:797–804.
14. Ziporen L, Polak-Charcon S, Korczyn DA, et al. Neurological dysfunction associated with antiphospholipid syndrome: histopathological brain findings of thrombotic changes in a mouse model. Clin Dev Immunol 2004;11:67–75.
15. Connor P, Hunt BJ. Cerebral haemostasis and antiphospholipid antibodies. Lupus 2003;12:929–934.
16. Brey RL, Chapman J, Levine SR, et al. Stroke and the antiphospholipid syndrome: consensus meeting Taormina 2002. Lupus 2003;12:508–513.
17. Cervera R, Khamashta MA, Font J, et al. Morbidity and mortality in Systemic Lupus Erythematosus during a 10-year period: a comparison of early and late manifestations in a cohort of 1,000 patients. Medicine (Baltimore) 2003;82:299–308.
18. Levine SR, Brey RL, Sawaya KL, et al. Recurrent stroke and thrombo-occlusive events in the antiphospholipid syndrome. Ann Neurol 1995;38:119–124.
19. Coull BM, Levine SR, Brey RL. The role of antiphospholipid antibodies and stroke. Neurol Clin 1992;10:125–143.
20. Sibilia J, Hercelin D, Gottenberg JE, et al. Cervico-cranial artery dissection and antiphospholipid syndrome: is there a link? Am J Med 2004;116:138–139.
21. Ford SE, Lillicrap DM, Brunet D, Ford PM. Thrombotic endocarditis and lupus anticoagulant, a pathogenetic possibility for idiopathic rheumatic type valvular heart disease. Arch Pathol Lab Med 1989;113:350–353.
22. Khamashta MA, Cervera R, Asherson RA, et al. Association of antibodies against phospholipids with valvular heart disease in patients with systemic lupus erythematosus. Lancet 1990;335:1541–1544.
23. Badui E, Solorio S, Martinez E, et al. The heart in the primary antiphospholipid syndrome. Arch Med Res 1995;26:115–120.
24. Nesher G, Ilany J, Rosenmann D, Abraham AS. Valvular dysfunction in antiphospholipid syndrome: prevalence, clinical features and treatment. Semin Arthritis Rheum 1997;27:27–35.

25. Asherson RA. The catastrophic antiphospholipid syndrome. A review of the clinical features, possible pathogenesis and treatment. Lupus 1998;7(suppl 2):55–62.
26. Olguin-Ortega L, Jara LJ, Becerra M, et al. Neurological involvement as a poor prognostic factor in catastrophic antiphospholipid syndrome: autopsy findings in 12 cases. Lupus 2003;12:93–98.
27. Brey RL, Hart RG, Sherman DG, Tegeler CT. Antiphospholipid antibodies and cerebral ischemia in young people. Neurology 1990;40:1190–1196.
28. Levine SR, Deegan MJ, Futrell N, Welch KMA. Cerebrovascular and neurologic disease associated with antiphospholipid antibodies: 48 cases. Neurology 1990;40:1181–1189.
29. Nencini P, Baruffi MC, Abbate R, Massai G, Amaducci L, Inzitari D. Lupus anticoagulant and anticardiolipin antibodies in young adults with cerebral ischemia. Stroke 1992;23:189–193.
30. Antiphospholipid Antibodies in Stroke Study (APASS) Group. Anticardiolipin antibodies are an independent risk factor for first ischemic stroke. Neurology 1993;43:2069–2073.
31. Heinzlef O, Abuaf N, Cohen A, et al. Recurrent stroke and vascular events in elderly patients with anticardiolipin antibodies: a prospective study. J Neurol 2001;248:373–379.
32. Antiphospholipid Antibody in Stroke Study Group (APASS). Anticardiolipin antibodies and the risk of recurrent thrombo-occlusive events and death. Neurology 1997;48:91–94.
33. Toschi V, Motta A, Castelli C, Paracchini ML, Zerbi D, Gibelli A. High prevalence of antiphosphatidylinositol antibodies in young patients with cerebral ischemia of undetermined cause. Stroke 1998;29:1759–1764.
34. Tuhrim S, Rand JH, Wu X, et al. Elevated anticardiolipin antibody titer is an independent risk factor for stroke in a multiethnic population independent of isotype or degree of positivity. Stroke 1999;30:1561–1565.
35. Tuhrim S, Rand JH, Wu X, et al . Antiphosphatidyl serine antibodies are independently associated with ischemic stroke. Neurology 1999;53:1523–1527.
36. Brey RL, Abbott RD, Curb JD, et al. beta(2)-Glycoprotein 1-dependent anticardiolipin antibodies and risk of ischemic stroke and myocardial infarction: the Honolulu Heart Program. Stroke 2001;2:1701–1706.
37. Singh K, Gaiha M, Shome DK, Gupta VK, Anuradha S. The association of antiphospholipid antibodies with ischemic stroke and myocardial infarction in young and their correlation: a preliminary study. J Assoc Physicians India 2001;49:537–529.
38. Brey RL, Stallworth CL, McGlasson DL, et al. Antiphospholipid antibodies and stroke in young women. Stroke 2002;33:2396–2400.
39. Ginsburg KS, Liang MH, Newcomer L, et al. Anticardiolipin antibodies and the risk for ischemic stroke and venous thrombosis. Ann Intern Med 1992;117:997–1002.
40. Muir KW, Squire IB, Alwan W, Lees KR. Anticardiolipin antibodies in an unselected stroke population. Lancet 1994;344:452–456.
41. Metz LM, Edworthy S, Mydlarski R, Fritzler MJ. The frequency of phospholipid antibodies in an unselected stroke population. Can J Neurol Sci 1998;25:64–69.
42. Zielinska J, Ryglewicz D, Wierzchoska E, Lechowicz W, Hier DB, Czlonkiwska A. Anticardiolipin antibodies are an indepdendent risk factor for ischemic stroke. Neurol Res 1999;21:653–657.
43. Tanne D, D'Olhaberriague L, Schultz LR, Salowich_Palm L, Sawaya KL, Levine SR. Anticardiolipin antibodies and their associations with cerebrovascular risk factors. Neurology 1999;52:1368–1373.
44. Ahmed E, Stegmayr B, Trifunovid J, et al. Anticardiolipin antibodies are not an independent risk factor for stroke: an incident case-referent study nested within the MONICA and Västerbotten cohort project. Stroke 2000;31:1289.
45. Blohorn A, Guegan-Massardier E, Triquenot A, et al. Antiphospholipid antibodies in the acute phase of cerebral ischemia in young adults: a descriptive study of 139 patients. Cerebrovasc Dis 2002;13:156–162.
46. Tanne D, D'Olhaberriague L, Trivedi AM, Salowich-Palm L, Schyltz LR, Levine SR. Anticardiolipin antibodies and mortality in patients with ischemic stroke: a prospective follow-up study. Neuroepidemiology 2002;21:93–99.
47. Wilson A, Gharavi AE, Koike T, et al. International consensus statement on preliminary classification criteria for definite antiphospholipid syndrom. Artheritis Rheum 1999;42:1309–1311.
48. Cervera R, Khamashta MA, Font J, et al. Morbidity and mortality in Systemic Lupus Erythematosus during a 5-year period: a multicenter prospective study of 1,000 patients. Medicine (Baltimore) 1999;78:167–175.
49. Finazzi G, Brancaccio V, Moia M, et al. Natural history and risk factors for thrombosis in 360 patients with antiphospholipid antibodies: a four-year prospective study from the Italian registry. Am J Med 1996;100:530–536.

50. Levine SR, Brey RL, Tilley BC, et al. Antiphospholipid antibodies and subsequent thrombo-occlusive events in patients with ischemic stroke. JAMA 2004;291:576–584.
51. Sletnes KE, Smith P, Abdolnoor M, Arnosen H, Wisloff F. Antiphospholipid antibodies after myocardial infarction and their relation to mortality, reinfarction, and non-harmorrhagic stroke. Lancet 1992;339:451–453.
52. Wu R, Nityanand S, Berlund L, Lithell H, Holm G, Lefvert AK. Antibodies against cardiolipin and oxidatively modified LDL in 50-year-old men predict myocardial infarction. Aterioscler Thromb Vasc Bio 1997;17:3159–3163.
53. Deschiens MA, Conrad J, Horellou MH, et al. Coagulations studies, factor V Leiden, and anticardiolipin antibodies in 40 cases of cerebral venous sinus thrombosis. Stroke 1996;27:1724–1730.
54. Carhuapoma JR, Mitsias P, Levine SR. Cerebral venous thrombosis and anticardiolipin antibodies. Neurology 1997;28:2363–2369.
55. Coull BM, Goodnight, SH. Antiphospholipid antibodies, prethrombotic states, and stroke. Stroke 1990;21:1370–1374.
56. Mikdashi JA, Kay GG. Neurocognitive deficits in Antiphopholipid syndrome [abstract]. Neurology 1996;46:A359.
57. Van Horn G, Arnett FC, Dimachkie MM. Reversible dementia and chorea in a young woman with the lupus anticoagulant. Neurology 1996;46:1566–1603.
58. Klemp P, Cooper RC, Strauss FJ, et al. Anticardiolipin antibodies in ischemic heart disease. Clin Exp Immunol 1988;89:411–419.
59. Denburg SD, Carbotte, RM, Ginsberg, JS, Denburg, J. The relationship of antiphospholipid antibodies to cognitive function in patients with systemic lupus erythematosus. J Intern Neuropsychol Soc 1997;3:377–386.
60. Hanly JG, Hong C, Smith S, Fisk JD. A prospective analysis of cognitive function and anticardiolipin antibodies in systemic lupus erythematosus. Arthritis Rheum 1999;42:728–734.
61. Long AA, Denburg SD, Carbotte RM, Singal DP, Denburg JA. Serum lymphocytotoxic antibodies and neurocognitive function in systemic lupus erythematosus. Ann Rheum Dis 1990;49:249–253.
62. Menon S, Jameson-Shortall E, Newman SP, Hall-Craggs MR, Chinn R, Isenberg DA. A longitudinal study of anticardiolipin antibody levels and cognitive functioning in systemic lupus erythematosus. Arthritis Rheum 1999;42:735–741.
63. McLaurin EY, Holliday SL, Williams P, Brey RL. Predictors of cognitive dysfunction in patients with systemic lupus erythematosus. Neurology 2004. In press.
64. Denburg SD, Carbotte, RM, Denburg, JA. Cognition and mood in systemic lupus erythematosus. Ann N Y Acad Sci 1997;823:45–59.
65. Lezak MD. Neuropsychological assessment, 3rd ed. New York: Oxford University Press; 1998:18.
66. Spreen O, Strauss E. A compendium of neuropsychological tests: administration, norms, and commentary. New York: Oxford University Press; Chap. 8.
67. Schmidt R, Auer-Grumbach P, Fazekas F, Offenbacher H, Kapeller P. Anticardiolipin antibodies in normal subjects. Neuropsychological correlates and MRI findings. Stroke 1995;26:749–754.
68. de Moerloose P, Boehlen F, Reber G. Prevalence of anticardiolipin and antinuclear antibodies in an elderly hospitalized population and mortality after a 6-year follow-up. Age Ageing 1997;26:319–320.
69. Cesbron J-Y, Amouyel Ph, Masy E. Anticardiolipin antibodies and physical disability in the elderly. Ann Intern Med 1997;126:1003.
70. Chapman J, Abu-Katash M, Inzelberg R, et al. Prevalence and clinical features of dementia associated with the antiphospholipid syndrome and circulating anticoagulants. J Neurol Sci 2002; 203–204:81–84.
71. Kalashnikova LA, Nasonov EL, Kushekbaeva AE, Gracheva LA . Anticardiolipin antibodies in Sneddon's syndrome. Neurology 1990;40:464–467.
72. Zelger B, Sepp N, Stockhammer G, et al. Sneddon's syndrome: a long term follow-up of 21 patients. Arch Dermatol 1993;129:437–444.
73. Tourbah A, Peitte JC, Iba-Zizen MT, Lyon-Caen O, Godeau P, Frances C. The natural course of cerebral lesions in Sneddon syndrome. Arch Neurol 1997;54:53–60.
74. Sneddon IB. Cerebral vascular lesions in livedo reticularis. Br J Dermatol 1965;77:180–185.
75. Coull BM, Bourdette DN, Goodnight SH, Briley DP, Hart R. Multiple cerebral infarctions and dementia associated with anticardiolipin antibodies. Stroke 1987;18:1107–1112.
76. Chinnery PF, Shaw PI, Ince PG, Jackson GH, Bishop RI. Fulminant encephalopathy due to the catastrophic primary antiphospholipid syndrome. J Neurol Neurosurg Psych 1997;62:300–301.
77. Molad Y, Sidi Y, Gornish M, et al. Lupus anticoagulant: correlation with magnetic resonance imaging of brain lesions. J Rheumatol 1992;19:556–561.

78. Provenzale JM, Heinz ER, Ortel TL, Macik BG, Charles LA, Alberts MJ. Antiphospholipid antibodies in patients without systemic lupus erythematosus: neuroradiologic findings. Radiology 1994;192:531–537.
79. Toubi E, Khamashta MA, Panarra A, Hughes GRV. Association of antiphospholipid antibodies with central nervous system disease in systemic lupus erythematosus. Am J Med 1995;99:397–401.
80. Sailer M, Burchert W, Ehrenheim C, et al. Positron emission tomography and magnetic resonance imaging for cerebral involvement in patients with systemic lupus erythematosus. J Neurol 1997;244:186–193.
81. Hachulla E, Michon-Pasturel U, Leys D, et al. Cerebral magnetic imaging in patients with or without antiphospholipid antibodies. Lupus 1998;7:124–131.
82. Rosove MH, Brewer PMC. Antiphospholipid thrombosis: clinical course after the first thrombotic event in 70 patients. Ann Intern Med 1992;117:303–308.
83. Khamashta MA, Cuadrado MJ, Mujic F, Taub NA, Hunt BJ, Hughes GRV. The management of thrombosis in the antiphospholipid antibody syndrome. N Engl J Med 1995;332:993–997.
84. Crowther MA, Ginsberg JS, Julian J, et al. A comparison of two intensities of warfarin for the prevention of recurrent thrombosis in patients with the antiphospholipid antibody syndrome. N Engl J Med 2003;349:1133–1138.
85. Ruiz-Irastorza G, Khamashta KA, Hunt BJ, Escuedero A, Cuadrado MJ, Hughes GRV. Bleeding and recurrent thrombosis in definite antiphospholipid syndrome: an analysis of a series of 66 patients treated with oral anticoagulation to a target international normalized ratio of 3.5. Arch Intern Med 2002;162:1164–1169.
86. Derksen RHWM, de Groot PG, Kappelle LJ. Low dose aspirin after ischemic stroke associated with antiphospholipid syndrome. Neurology 2003;61:111–114.

7 Cerebral Disease Other than Stroke and Transient Ischemic Attack in Antiphospholipid Syndrome

Giovanni Sanna

Central nervous system (CNS) involvement is one of the most prominent clinical manifestations of antiphospholipid (Hughes) syndrome (APS) and includes arterial and venous thrombotic events, psychiatric features, and a variety of other non-thrombotic neurological syndromes.

In 1983, Hughes, in his original description of the syndrome, highlighted the importance of cerebral disease in patients with APS [1]. In the early 1980s, his group reported the presence of antiphospholipid antibodies (aPL) in association with cerebrovascular accidents, intractable headache or migraine, epilepsy, chorea, idiopathic transverse myelitis, Guillain-Barré syndrome, and dementia [2–5].

The full impact of APS on neurology is now becoming increasingly recognized [6]. The range of neurological features of APS is comprehensive and includes focal symptoms attributable to lesions in a specific area of the brain as well as diffuse or global dysfunction [7–10]. Table 7.1 summarizes the wide spectrum of CNS manifestations that have been reported in association with aPL.

Although the mechanism of neurological involvement in APS is thought to be thrombotic in origin and cerebral ischemia is the most common manifestation [9], a number of other neuropsychiatric manifestations, including chronic headache, dementia, cognitive dysfunction, psychosis, depression, transverse myelitis, multiple sclerosis-like disease, chorea, and seizures have been associated with the presence of aPL [4, 6, 10–14]. Many of these manifestations cannot be explained solely by hypercoagulability and it is possible that some of them (e.g., cognitive dysfunction, seizures, chorea) may have more complex causes.

It is not completely understood why the CNS is particularly vulnerable in patients with APS.

There is an increasing body of evidence which supports the hypothesis that aPL may also have more direct effects on the brain [11]. It has been shown that aPL bind neurons, glial cells, and myelin and disrupt their function [15, 16]. aPL also interfere with endothelial cell function and promote the procoagulant activity of endothelial cells [17–20]. Lai and Lan [21] found high levels of IgG anticardiolipin antibodies (aCL) in cerebrospinal fluid of systemic lupus erythematosus (SLE) patients with CNS involvement, including headache, acute psychosis, and cognitive impairment, suggesting that aPL may also produce direct neurologic tissue damage

Table 7.1. Neuropsychiatric manifestations associated with the presence of antiphospholipid antibodies.

Cerebrovascular disease
    Transient ischemic attacks
    Ischemic stroke
    Acute ischemic encephalopathy
    Cerebral venous thrombosis
Seizures
Headache
Chorea
Multiple sclerosis–like syndrome
Transverse myelitis
Idiopathic intracranial hypertension
Other neurological syndromes
    Sensorineural hearing loss
    Guillain-Barré syndrome
    Transient global amnesia
    Ocular syndromes
    Dystonia–Parkinsonism
    Progressive supranuclear palsy
Cognitive dysfunction
Dementia
Other psychiatric disorders
    Depression
    Psychosis

through immune-mediated mechanisms. Animal models are providing important insights in some of the underlying mechanisms for CNS dysfunction in APS [22–24].

In this chapter we will attempt to highlight the broad spectrum of the neuropsychiatric manifestations that have been reported in association with aPL with a particular emphasis on those without a well-defined underlying thrombotic mechanism. Cerebrovascular disease will be described in another chapter of this book.

Seizures

A number of studies – mainly in SLE patients – have confirmed the original observation of Mackworth-Young and Hughes in 1985 [25] of the association between aPL and seizures [14, 26–32].

Herranz et al [27] found that moderate-to-high titers of IgG aCL were associated with seizures in SLE patients, suggesting an important role for these antibodies in the aetiopathogenesis of this manifestation. Liou et al [29] confirmed the association between epilepsy and aCL in 252 SLE patients recruited in a prospective study, where the odds ratio of developing seizure for those patients who had a high level of aCL was 3.7 when compared with those without a detectable level of aCL.

Our most recent experience confirmed a strong association between the presence of aPL and seizures in a series of 323 SLE patients [32]. We found that the prevalence of aCL was higher in patients with seizures than in those without. The association of seizures with aCL remained significant after excluding 47 patients with cerebrovascular accidents. We also showed that IgG and IgM aCL were both independently associated with cerebrovascular accidents and seizures by multivariate analysis.

The increased prevalence of autoantibodies in patients with epilepsy has also been attributed to the use of antiepileptic drugs [33, 34]. However, recent studies showed no association between the presence of autoantibodies, including aPL, and antiepileptic medication in patients with epilepsy [30, 35–37].

Verrot et al [30] studied 163 consecutive patients with epilepsy with no clinical signs of SLE or APS and found that aCL were present in 20% of the patients, independently of the type of epilepsy, the antiepileptic treatment, or the age or sex of the patients.

Peltola et al [35] found no association between the presence of aPL and antiepileptic medications. They found that the prevalence of aPL was greater in patients with epilepsy – including newly diagnosed seizure – confirming the association between aPL and seizure disorder.

In accordance with these reports, a recent paper from Ranua et al [37] showed that the use of antiepileptic medication does not have an effect on the presence of aPL or other autoantibodies. They found an association between the presence of aCL and long duration of partial epilepsy, as well as an association between the presence of these antibodies and poor seizure control despite antiepileptic treatment, supporting the hypothesis that an immune dysregulation may play a role at least in certain types of epilepsy.

Different forms of seizures are seen in association with aPL and all ages may be affected [6, 36, 38]. A recent paper from the Euro-Phospholipid Project Group reported seizures in 7% of 1000 patients with APS [9], but this figure is probably an underestimate.

Shoenfeld et al [14] recently reported epilepsy in 8.6% of 538 patients with APS. Epilepsy was more prevalent among patients with APS secondary to SLE (13.7%) when compared to those with primary APS (6%). They also found that patients with epilepsy had a higher prevalence of focal ischemic events, suggesting that in many cases seizures may be the expression of an underlying ischemic event occurring as a result of hypercoagulability. However, this explains only part of the increased occurrence of epilepsy in APS and the pathogenetic mechanism underlying the association of this manifestation with aPL remain uncertain.

There may be a primary immunological basis for seizures in APS. In fact there is increasing evidence supporting the hypothesis of a direct interaction of aPL with neuronal tissue as a possible alternative mechanism to hypercoagulability [7, 11, 39, 40].

aCL obtained from patients with SLE who had seizures have been shown to reduce a gamma-aminobutyric acid (GABA) receptor-mediated chloride current in snail neurons [39], suggesting the there is a direct and reversible mechanism through which aPL might lower the seizure threshold.

Also, aPL have been demonstrated to bind directly to ependyma amd myelin of fixed cat [41] and rat brain [42]. The recent finding that aPL depolarize brain nerve terminals [40] has provided further evidence that these antibodies may play a role in the pathogenesis of seizures in APS.

Headache

One of the most prominent features in patients with APS is headache. This symptom, a common complaint of APS patients in clinical practice, can vary from classic intermittent migraine to almost continuous incapacitating headache.

The association of migraine and aPL is controversial, with widely varying results from different series [43]. Many authors have reported association with LA or aCL [44, 45] and others no association at all [46].

The difficulty in demonstrating a true association between aCL positivity and migraine stems in part from the high prevalence of migraine in the normal population and the relatively low prevalence of aCL positivity in otherwise healthy individuals. One of the major problems is also that headaches, often non-migrainous, have been loosely termed "migraine," and these headaches may precede or accompany transient ischemic attacks (TIAs) or cerebrovascular accident (CVA) [47]. aPL have been also detected in patients with transient neurologic symptoms including migraine aura. Therefore, the controversy may be in part due to the inherent difficulty in distinguishing the transient focal neurologic events of migraine from TIA.

The available data suggest an association between the migraine-like phenomena and aPL, but not between migraine headache and aPL. In 1989, Shuaib et al [48] described migraine as an early prominent symptom in 6 patients with aPL, but Tietjen [49] pointed out that the role of these antibodies in the pathogenesis of migraine was poorly understood, calling for prospective, controlled studies to elucidate the actual role of aPL in migraine.

Montalban et al [50] carried out a prospective study in 103 consecutive patients with SLE, including a control group of 58 patients with migraine not associated with SLE. Although they found a high frequency of headache in SLE patients, they failed to find an association between the presence of aCL and migraine. No migraine control patients were found to have aCL.

Tietjen et al [51] assessed the frequency of aCL in migraine in a large prospective study that evaluated adults patients and normal controls under 60 years of age. The authors studied a group of 645 patients with transient focal neurological events, including 518 with migraine with aura, another group of 497 individuals with migraine without aura, and the 366 healthy controls. The frequency of aCL did not differ significantly between groups.

Verrotti et al [52] studied the prevalence of aCL in children with migraine. In this study, 40 patients were divided into two groups according to the type of migraine: group I included 22 cases suffering from migraine with and without aura; group II consisted of 18 children having migraine with prolonged aura or migrainous infarction, also called complicated migraine. Two groups of children were studied as controls: a group of 35 children with juvenile chronic arthritis and a group of 40 healthy sex- and age-matched children who did not suffer from migraine or any other neurological disease. No statistically significant differences were found in levels of aCL between group I and II and controls. The authors concluded that, in children with migraine, aCL are not more frequent than in healthy controls, suggesting that aCL are not implicated in the pathogenesis of migraine.

To date prospective studies using appropriate control groups failed to demonstrate association between aPL and migraine in SLE patients and higher prevalence of aPL in migraine sufferers.

Our recent study in 323 SLE patients showed that although the prevalence of headache in SLE was similar to that reported for the general population, aPL, in particular IgG aCL, were more significantly prevalent in the group of patients with headache compared with those without [32]. However, we failed to demonstrate an association of aPL with a particular subtype of headache or with migraine.

Recent anecdotal reports described a dramatic clinical improvement in patients with APS and chronic severe headache after commencing anticoagulation to prevent recurrences of thrombosis [53–55].

However, a double-blind crossover trial comparing low-molecular-weight heparin with placebo in patients with aPL and chronic incapacitating headache, not responsive to conventional treatment, did not show any beneficial effect [56].

Cognitive Dysfunction

Cognitive dysfunction varies from global dysfunction in the context of multi-infarct dementia to subtle cognitive deficits in otherwise asymptomatic patients with aPL. One of the most common complaints in these patients is of poor memory, difficulty in concentrating, or difficulty in keeping their attention for a long time, indicating a probable preclinical phase of neurological involvement.

In the largest published series of APS to date a prevalence of 2% was reported for multi-infarct dementia but no data were provided on other different type of cognitive impairment [9]. Less severe forms of cognitive impairment are considered common in APS patients, but the exact prevalence is unknown. The estimated prevalence of cognitive dysfunction in SLE patients range from 17% to 59% [57].

The recognition of subtle forms of cognitive dysfunction has been greatly facilitated by the application of formal neuropsychological assessment, mainly in patients with SLE. The relationship of cognitive dysfunction with aPL, detected by the presence of lupus anticoagulant (LA) or aCL, has been investigated in cross-sectional [58, 59] and prospective/longitudinal studies [60, 61]. These studies showed that aPL may play a primary role in the pathogenesis of cognitive impairment and that the application of neuropsychological testing is useful in detecting an early neuropsychiatric involvement in patients with SLE.

A cross-sectional study of 70 patients with SLE [58] showed that delayed recognition memory performance was poorer in patients with elevated aCL levels. Denburg et al [59] evaluated the relationship between aPL positivity (expressed as the LA) and cognitive dysfunction in patients with SLE in a cross-sectional study. LA-positive patients were 2 to 3 times more likely than were LA-negative patients to be designated as cognitively impaired by the application of specific psychometric tests, with lower performance on tasks of verbal memory, cognitive flexibility, and psychomotor speed. These deficits occurred independently of clinically overt neuropsychiatric manifestations. The authors speculated that LA positivity is associated with subclinical nervous system compromise, possibly on the basis of ongoing LA-related microthrombotic events or vasculopathy.

Menon et al [61] determined the relationship between persistently raised aCL levels and neuropsychological performance in 45 patients with SLE. They found that levels of IgG aCL that were persistently elevated over a 2- to 3-year period (as opposed to never or occasionally elevated) were associated with significantly poorer performance in cognitive function. Tasks requiring speed of attention and concentration appeared to be particularly affected in these patients.

Hanly et al [60] analysed prospectively the association between changes in cognitive function and aCL over a period of 5 years in SLE patients using standardized tests of cognitive function. Their results showed that patients with persistent IgG aCL positivity had a reduction in psychomotor speed, and patients with persistent IgA aCL positivity had a reduction in conceptual reasoning and executive ability, suggesting that IgG and IgA aCL may be responsible for long-term subtle deterioration in cognitive function in patients with SLE. An important finding of this study was that the observed changes in cognitive performance were not associated with persistent elevation of the level of anti-dsDNA antibodies, showing that they can occur independently of generalized SLE disease activity and supporting the hypothesis that aPL play a primary role in the etiology of these manifestations.

Whether these cognitive deficits result from recurrent cerebral ischemia or whether there is other underlying mechanisms is not clear. An increasing evidence for a direct pathogenic role of aPL in causing cognitive and behavioral impairments has been recently provided from animal model of APS [24, 40].

Clinical implications of these findings are that, although the current evidence does not support the introduction of aggressive anticoagulation as a strategy to prevent subclinical cognitive impairment, there may be a role for more benign therapies such as low-dose aspirin or antimalarials. On the other hand, anecdotal reports of improvement of these symptoms after anticoagulation therapy commenced for other reasons in APS patients [55], may provide some support for the theory that arterial thrombosis and/or ischemia represent the primary cause of this type of CNS dysfunction, supporting the utility of further longitudinal case-control trials to answer the question of whether an anticoagulation treatment with low targeted international normalized ratio (INR) could be superior to aspirin in these patients.

Long-term prospective studies are also required to determine if the risk of cognitive impairment in patients with persistently elevated aPL levels is cumulative over time. If this is confirmed, the next step will be to identify effective therapies with an acceptable benefit/toxicity ratio.

Dementia

A chronic multifocal disease, defined as a recurrent or progressive neurological deterioration attributable to cerebrovascular disease, can produce multi-infarct dementia. Asherson et al [5] first described this manifestation in 1987. They went on to describe in 1989 [62] the clinical and serologic features of 35 patients with aPL and cerebrovascular disease. Strokes were often multiple and were followed by multi-infarct dementia in 9 patients. This dementia, generally associated with a loss of cognitive functions and impairment of skills, concentration, memory dysfunction, language impairment, and judgemental defects, does not present with peculiar characteristics. It cannot be differentiated from other kinds of dementia, such as in Alzheimer's disease, senile dementia, or metabolic/toxic conditions involving the brain. Many other authors have since reported this complication in patients with recurrent strokes [63–65].

Westermann et al [66] described brain biopsy findings from a patient with multi-infarct dementia and APS. Microscopic examination showed luminal occlusion by thrombi, and marked endothelial hyperplasia of small meningeal and cortical arterioles, suggesting that the pathogenesis of this cerebral vasculopathy is non-inflammatory and is associated with reactive endothelial hyperplasia and thrombosis of small arterioles.

Hilker et al [67] reported on a 55-year-old man suffering from progressive dementia and primary APS (PAPS), in whom cerebral glucose metabolism and blood flow were examined by positron emission tomography (PET). Cerebral atrophy and a moderate number of white matter hyperintensities were detected on magnetic resonance imaging (MRI), whereas the PET scans showed a considerable diffuse impairment of cortical glucose metabolism combined with a reduced cerebral perfusion in the arterial border zones. These findings indicate that PAPS-associated vascular dementia is accompanied by a cortical neuronal loss, presumably caused by a small-vessel disease with immune-mediated intravascular thrombosis.

Mosek et al [68] examined the relationship of aPL to dementia in the elderly in a case-controlled study. They found that 5 of the 87 demented patients (6%), but none of the 69 controls, had significantly elevated aCL IgG levels (above 20 GPL). All the patients with high aCL IgG levels were diagnosed clinically as having dementia of the Alzheimer type, except for 1 who had mixed dementia, and none had features of an immune-mediated disease. This study showed that a small but significant number of patients with dementia have high levels of aPL. The role of the aPL in these patients, with apparently diffuse brain disease, is currently unknown.

Chapman et al [69] recently confirmed the association of APS with dementia in a hospital-based study. They found that 13 out of 23 patients (56%) with PAPS were demented, with higher levels of aPL and significantly older when compared with the non-demented APS patients. The authors suggested that the length of exposure to aPL may play an important role – as well the presence of high levels of aPL – in determining the development of dementia.

Other Psychiatric Disorders

To date there have been surprisingly few studies detailing the psychiatric manifestations of APS. Mood disorder and psychosis may be present in patients with APS, although both the frequency and the pathophysiological relationship to APS remain controversial [13].

It should always be kept in mind that corticosteroid treatment may itself induce psychosis and negative effects on cognition and mood, particularly in patients with long-term treatment and/or treated with high doses corticosteroids [70]. Nevertheless, these effects have also been seen in healthy volunteers [71]. This in particular applies to patients with SLE and secondary APS.

It remains unclear whether the presence of aPL may represent an adverse response to neuroleptic treatment. However, Schwartz et al [72] found no association between the presence of aCL or LA and neuroleptic treatment in 34 patients with acute psychosis, suggesting that the presence of aPL may be primarily associated with psychosis.

However, we recently found no association between the presence of aPL and psychiatric disorder in 323 patients with SLE [32].

Animal studies recently showed a propensity to hyperactivity and exploratory behavior in induced animal models of APS [23, 73, 74], suggesting a possible association between human hyperactive behavior and aPL [11]. However, a recent study showed no significant difference in the level of aPL between children diagnosed with attention deficit/hyperactivity disorder when compared to the control group [75].

Chorea

A strong relationship between aPL and chorea has been reported in retrospective studies. Chorea is a rare manifestation, occurring in 1% to 3% of SLE and APS patients [9]. This type of movement disorder has been documented in pregnancy and as a complication of oral contraceptives [76]. Its association with aPL alone [77], or, more commonly, with SLE has been infrequently reported [78, 79]. It seems that chorea is more frequent in patients with PAPS than in those with SLE.

Because chorea in SLE is often unilateral, acute in onset, and is often followed by other CNS manifestations, a vascular pathogenesis is probable in these patients. A similar mechanism may also be present in patients who demonstrate the disorder subsequent to taking oral contraceptives. It is also possible that increased dopaminergic activity within the corpus striatum, a mechanism postulated to occur particularly in patients taking compounds such as d-amphetamine and levodopa, may also play some role [80].

It has been postulated that aPL can cause chorea by an antigen/antibodies mechanism binding phospholipid in the basal ganglia [81].

Cervera et al [82] reviewed the clinical, radiologic, and immunologic characteristics of 50 patients with chorea and the APS. Fifty-eight percent of patients had defined SLE, 12% "lupus-like" syndrome, and 30% had PAPS. Twelve percent of patients developed chorea soon after they started taking estrogen-containing oral contraceptives, 6% developed chorea gravidarum, and 2% of patients developed chorea shortly after delivery. Most patients (66%) had only 1 episode of chorea. Chorea was bilateral in 55% of patients. Computed tomography and MRI scans reported cerebral infarcts in 35% of patients. The chorea in these patients responded to a variety of medications, for example, steroids, haloperidol, antiaggregants, anticoagulants, or a combination of therapy, usually prescribed in the presence of other manifestations of APS or SLE. Many patients responded well to haloperidol and to the discontinuation of oral contraceptives if this was the precipitating factor.

Multiple Sclerosis–like Syndrome

Clinical syndromes mimicking multiple sclerosis (MS), mainly in its relapsing–remitting pattern, are reported to occur in association with aPL [83–85]. Differential diagnosis may be difficult and some APS patients can be misdiagnosed as having MS.

In 1994, Scott et al [83] reported 4 patients presenting with multiple neurological manifestations, including vertigo, aphasia, unilateral visual loss, diplopia, or hemiparesis, in different combinations over several years, with variable degrees of recovery after the episodes. All had white-matter lesions and all had received the clinical diagnosis of MS. IgG aCL were positive at medium-to-high levels in the 4 patients, and LA was also found in 3 of them. In addition, all but 1 patient had previous clinical manifestations suggestive of APS, such as venous thrombosis, recurrent miscarriages, and thrombocytopenia.

More recent studies showed a controversial relationship between MS and the presence of aPL.

Tourbah et al [86] found that patients with MS with autoimmune features, including those with titers of antinuclear antibodies (ANA) of 1:100 or less and/or aPL, were not different than others with MS regarding age of onset, presenting symptoms and signs, neurological examination findings, or disease course. The authors found that patients with an MS-like illness and aPL were so similar to patients with MS that in their opinion they should not be excluded from clinical trials.

In 1998, Karussis et al [87] screened a population of 70 classic and 100 non-classic MS patients, labeling as non-classic those with features unusual for MS. They found a strikingly significant proportion of aCL-positive patients in the non-classic MS group. Most of the positive patients in the non-classic MS group had a similar clinical manifestation pattern, such as progressive myelopathy, spinocerebellar syndrome, or neuromyelitis optica. They concluded that a clinical subset of patients with probable or definite diagnosis of MS but with consistently elevated levels of aCL show a slower progression and some atypical features for MS, such as persistent headaches and absence of oligoclonal bands in the cerebrospinal fluid. Therefore, in patients with MS showing such clinical features, aCL testing is recommended. They speculated that these antibodies may be involved in the pathogenesis of the neurological symptoms, and therefore, management should include antiplatelet or even anticoagulant agents.

Recently, Cuadrado et al [85] analyzed the clinical, laboratory, and imaging findings of MS-like expression in a cohort of patients with APS in an attempt to identify parameters that might differentiate the two entities. These authors studied 27 patients with a previous diagnosis of probable or definite MS made by a neurologist, all of them referred because of symptoms suggesting an underlying connective tissue disease, uncommon findings for MS on MRI, atypical evolution of MS, or aPL positivity. MRI was performed in every patient and compared with MRI of 25 definite MS patients who did not have aPL. In the past medical history, 8 patients with PAPS and 6 with APS secondary to SLE had had symptoms related to these conditions. Neurological symptoms and the results of physical examination of the patients were not different from those common in MS patients. Laboratory findings and MRI studies were not useful tools to distinguish APS from MS. Most of the patients with PAPS showed a good response to oral anticoagulant treatment. In patients with secondary APS, the outcome was poorer. The authors concluded that APS and MS can be difficult to distinguish. A careful medical history, a previous history of thrombosis and/or fetal loss, and the response to anticoagulant therapy might be helpful in the differential diagnosis. They recommended testing for aPL in all patients with MS.

Roussel et al [88] studied the prevalence of serum aPL, aCL, and anti–β_2 glycoprotein I (anti–β_2-GPI), in 89 patients affected with possible, probable, or definite MS and no clinical evidence of associated autoimmune disorder. About one third of the patients had aPL, either aCL, anti–β_2-GPI, or both. Because of the known high frequency of aCL in ischemic stroke they also studied sera from a series of such patients, and the frequency of both aCL and anti–β_2-GPI was higher in MS than in ischemic stroke. No correlation was found between aPL and the category of MS, its clinical course or clinical symptoms, nor atypical lesions by MRI. They concluded that aCL and anti–β_2-GPI are neither rare in MS nor associated with a specific clinical form of the disease and therefore they cannot be used as a diagnosis exclusion criteria.

Sastre-Garriga et al [89] recently studied 296 randomly selected patients with MS and 51 healthy controls; aCL, anti–β_2-GPI, or antiprothrombin were found in 6 patients. No predominance of any kind of clinical manifestation and no cardinal manifestation of primary APS were found in these patients. They concluded that aCL tests should be performed only when a suspicion of APS is raised and atypical clinical presentation for MS is found, but not in unselected cases. In this case the different results can be justified on the basis of different population selection criteria and differences in laboratory techniques.

We believe that some APS patients can be misdiagnosed as having MS, making this a crucial point for the therapeutic approach [6]. A careful interview of the patient, a past medical history of thrombotic events, and pregnancy morbidity in female patients may be useful in the differential diagnosis, favoring APS. The abruptness of onset and resolution of symptoms, especially in regard to visual symptoms (i.e., amaurosis fugax), and atypical neurological features for MS such as headache or epilepsy, strongly suggest APS rather than MS. We think that if not all, at least a subgroup of patients with "non-classic" MS should be tested for aPL.

Transverse Myelitis

Harris et al [4] described in 1985 the case of a 45-year-old woman who developed transverse myelitis in the context of a lupus-like illness. Antibodies to cardiolipin of the IgM class were detected in high titers in the serum. The authors speculated that these aCL may have played a part in the pathogenesis of this peculiar neurologic manifestations in this patient.

Subsequently, many other authors confirmed the association between aPL and transverse myelitis. The prevalence of aPL had been shown to be higher in SLE patients with transverse myelitis compared with SLE patients in general [46].

Lavalle et al [90] reported a strong association between transverse myelitis in SLE and the presence of aPL. They found 10 of 12 patients with transverse myelitis and SLE as having aCL, and in the other 2 patients they found evidence of venereal disease research laboratory (VDRL) positivity and prolonged activated partial thromboplastin time (aPTT). Both IgG and IgM aCL were detected in 8/10 patients.

Kovacs et al [91] evaluated 14 patients with SLE and transverse myelitis and 91 additional cases published in the literature. Forty-three percent of their patients and 64% of the patients reported in the literature were aPL positive.

More recent studies provided good supporting evidence for a role for aPL in the development of transverse myelitis. Sherer et al [92] described 4 patients out of a cohort of 100 aPL-positive patients who had transverse myelitis, and, more recently, D'Cruz et al [93] described a series of 15 patients with transverse myelitis as the presenting manifestation of SLE or lupus-like disease. They found a strong association with aPL, with 11 of 15 patients positive (73%). In 2 patients, however, aPL did not become detectable until long after presentation. The high prevalence of aPL in these patients and the good functional outcome in those patients who had combination of anticoagulation with immunosuppression provides further evidence of a possible pathogenic role for these antibodies in the development of transverse myelitis.

Idiopathic Intracranial Hypertension

Idiopathic intracranial hypertension, also known as pseudotumor cerebri, is the term used to describe the occurrence of raised intracranial pressure which is not due to mass lesions, obstruction of cerebrospinal fluid flow, or focal structural abnormalities, in alert and oriented patients. The term *idiopathic* requires the exclusion of intracranial venous sinus thrombosis. Idiopathic intracranial hypertension can be the presenting symptom of APS. The association of idiopathic intracranial hypertension with aPL has been only acknowledged recently [94]. However, its true incidence is still unknown. Sussman et al [95] reported on 11 out of 38 patients (29%) with aPL and idiopathic intracranial hypertension. However, only 4 had aCL without other prothrombotic risk factors or evidence of sinus thrombosis.

Leker et al [96] found aCL in 6 out of 14 patients (43%) with idiopathic intracranial hypertension. They did not find differences in clinical, laboratory, or radiological findings to distinguish between patients with idiopathic intracranial hypertension with and without aCL.

Kesler et al [97], in a retrospective study, confirmed the association between idiopathic intracranial hypertension and aCL, although they found a lower frequency of aCL in their patients. Three out of 37 patients (8.1%) were shown to be aCL positive, with a prevalence lower than that reported in the two previously published studies.

Sensorineural Hearing Loss

A link between sensorineural hearing loss and autoimmune disease has been postulated by many authors who described the association of sensorineural hearing loss with aPL in several reports [98–100].

Hisashi et al [98] described the occurrence of sensorineural hearing loss in an young woman diagnosed with SLE. Serologic tests for syphilis were false-positive and IgG aCL were positive. The authors postulated the association of sudden profound sensorineural hearing loss with aCL in patients with autoimmune diseases.

Casoli et al [99] described a 55-year-old woman with a 6-year history of Sjögren syndrome who presented IgG and IgM aCL and developed a sudden onset of sensorineural hearing loss associated with vertigo.

Toubi at al [101] studied 30 patients, 11 suffering from sudden deafness and 19 from progressive sensorineural hearing loss, and 20 matched healthy controls. They found that 27% of patients had low-moderate titers of aCL, while none of the control group presented aCL. The authors concluded that aPL may play an important role in the pathogenesis of this disability, speculating about the possibility of anticoagulant therapy for these patients.

Naarendorp et al [102] described 6 patients with SLE or a lupus-like syndrome who developed sudden sensorineural hearing loss and had elevated serum levels of aCL or LA. They concluded that acute onset of sensorineural hearing loss in presence of aPL may be a manifestation of APS, and that anticoagulation treatment was to be recommended for these patients.

Guillain-Barré Syndrome

Guillain-Barré syndrome is a transient neurological disorder characterized by an inflammatory demyelination of peripheral nerves. Although the pathogenesis of this disorder has not been elucidated, there is increasing evidence pointing to an autoimmune etiology. This demyelinating neuropathy, also uncommon in SLE patients, was associated with aPL in the original descriptions of the Hughes syndrome [2].

Gilburd et al [103] studied the reactivity of Guillain-Barré syndrome sera with various phospholipids which are known to be important constituents of myelin, and serve as autoantigens in other autoimmune conditions, demonstrating that some Guillain-Barré syndrome patients produce autoantibodies to various phospholipid and nuclear antigens. However, these autoantibodies are probably produced as a result of the myelin damage rather than cause the demyelination.

Transient Global Amnesia

Transient global amnesia, a syndrome of sudden unexplained short-term memory loss in association with aPL, was reported by Montalban et al [104]. Some regard this disturbance as migrainous in origin, but other mechanisms such as epileptic seizure have been advocated as involved in its pathogenesis [105].

Ocular Syndromes

Amaurosis fugax suggests cerebral ischemia, and is one of the most common ocular manifestations in APS. Other visual disturbances have been associated with the presence of aPL. Ischemic optic neuropathy is less frequently described in APS [106] when compared with SLE patients [107, 108]. Giorgi et al [108] reported on 6 SLE patients with optic neuropathy, one of them also diagnosed with APS. This patient had monolateral optic neuropathy, whereas the other 5 SLE patients had bilateral optic nerve disease. These authors considered the monolateral occurrence of optic neuropathy as a focal neurological disease due to a thrombotic event involving the ciliary vasculature. Conversely, bilateral optic nerve damage in SLE was considered to be due to different immunological mechanisms, such as vasculitis.

Vaso-occlusive retinopathy has also been described in the presence of aPL [109]. This is a rare but severe form of retinopathy characterised by microthrombosis and often associated with other CNS manifestations [110].

Dystonia–Parkinsonism

There are only a few anecdotal reports of Parkinsonism in association with APS [111, 112]. Milanov et al [112] recently reported on the combination of dystonia with parkinsonian-like symptoms as presenting clinical manifestation of APS in a 60-year-old man who had ischemic lesions in the basal ganglia on MRI and positive aPL. It has been suggested that anticoagulation should be considered in patients with aPL and dystonia–Parkinsonism in order to prevent further deterioration in case of lack of clinical improvement with levodopa, bromocriptine, and anticholinergics [113].

Progressive Supranuclear Palsy

There are recent anecdotal reports of progressive supranuclear palsy in association with aPL [114, 115]. Aleem et al [114] reported the case of young man with recurrent stroke presenting as pseudobulbar palsy, and, more recently, Reiblat et al [115] reported on a 53-year-old male who presented with severe headache, progressive dementia, and ataxia, and developed features of progressive supranuclear palsy (downgaze palsy, disproportionate axial predominance of rigidity, and no response to l-dopa treatment). Interestingly he also had livedo reticularis, thrombocytopenia, increased titers of aCL, and a positive LA. Brain MRI showed presence of cortical and subcortical infarcts. The authors suggested that progressive supranuclear palsy might be part of the neurological manifestations of APS.

Small High-density Lesions on Brain MRI

Brain MRI in aPL patients with ischemic stroke typically shows cortical abnormalities consistent with large vessel occlusion. However small high-density lesion on the brain MRI are frequently found in patients with aPL and, in our experience, also in SLE patients with or without overt neuropsychiatric manifestations [116]. The significance of these lesions is not completely understood. They are often defined as consistent with the presence of small vessel disease by the neuroradiologists. It has been suggested that they may be due to multiple small infarcts [117]. There is also evidence that the presence of similar lesions is associated with a higher risk for stroke [118], dementia, and cognitive decline in the elderly population [119]. The finding of white matter hyperintensities on the brain MRI may represent a diagnostic and therapeutic dilemma especially when recognized in young patients. In our experience, subclinical cognitive disorders, usually undetected in the absence of a formal neuropsychological assessment, are frequent in these patients. In a recent study we also found that small high-density lesions on the brain MRI were associated with the presence of LA [32], supporting the hypothesis of an underlying ischemic/thrombotic mechanism for these lesions.

References

1. Hughes GRV. Thrombosis, abortion, cerebral disease and the lupus anticoagulant. BMJ 1983;287:1088–1089.
2. Harris EN, Englert H, Derue G, Hughes GRV, Gharavi A. Antiphospholipid antibodies in acute Guillain-Barré syndrome. Lancet 1983;ii:1361–1362.
3. Hughes GRV. The Prosser-White oration 1983. Connective tissue disease and the skin. Clin Exp Dermatol 1984;9:535–544.

4. Harris EN, Gharavi AE, Mackworth-Young CG, Patel BM, Derue G, Hughes GRV. Lupoid sclerosis: a possible pathogenetic role for antiphospholipid antibodies. Ann Rheum Dis 1985;44:281–283.
5. Asherson R, Mercey D, Phillips G, et al. Recurrent stroke and multi-infarct dementia in systemic lupus erythematosus: association with antiphospholipid antibodies. Ann Rheum Dis 1987;46:605–611.
6. Hughes GR. Migraine, memory loss, and "multiple sclerosis." Neurological features of the antiphospholipid (Hughes') syndrome. Postgrad Med J 2003;79:81–83.
7. Levine SR, Deegan MJ, Futrell N, Welch KM. Cerebrovascular and neurologic disease associated with antiphospholipid antibodies: 48 cases. Neurology 1990;40:1181–1189.
8. Brey RL, Escalante A. Neurological manifestations of antiphospholipid antibody syndrome. Lupus 1998;7(suppl 2):S67–S74.
9. Cervera R, Piette JC, Font J, et al. Antiphospholipid syndrome: clinical and immunologic manifestations and patterns of disease expression in a cohort of 1,000 patients. Arthritis Rheum 2002;46:1019–1027.
10. Sanna G, Bertolaccini ML, Cuadrado MJ, Khamashta MA, Hughes, GR. Central nervous system involvement in the antiphospholipid (Hughes) syndrome. Rheumatology (Oxford) 2003; 42:200–213.
11. Katzav A, Chapman J, Shoenfeld Y. CNS dysfunction in the antiphospholipid syndrome. Lupus 2003;12:903–907.
12. Sastre-Garriga J, Montalban X. APS and the brain. Lupus 2003;12:877–882.
13. Chapman J, Rand JH, Brey RL, et al. Non-stroke neurological syndromes associated with antiphospholipid antibodies: evaluation of clinical and experimental studies. Lupus 2003;12:514–517.
14. Shoenfeld Y, Lev S, Blatt I, et al. Features associated with epilepsy in the antiphospholipid syndrome. J Rheumatol 2004;31:1344–1348.
15. Sun KH, Liu WT, Tsai CY, et al. Inhibition of astrocyte proliferation and binding to brain tissue of anticardiolipin antibodies purified from lupus serum. Ann Rheum Dis 1992;51:707–712.
16. Khalili A, Cooper RC. A study of immune responses to myelin and cardiolipin in patients with systemic lupus erythematosus (SLE). Clin Exp Immunol 1991;85:365–372.
17. Oosting JD, Derksen RH, Blokzijl L, Sixma JJ, de Groot PG. Antiphospholipid antibody positive sera enhance endothelial cell procoagulant activity – studies in a thrombosis model. Thromb Haemost 1992;68:278–284.
18. Simantov R, LaSala JM, Lo SK, et al. Activation of cultured vascular endothelial cells by antiphospholipid antibodies. J Clin Invest 1995;96:2211–2219.
19. Del Papa N, Guidali L, Sala A, et al. Endothelial cells as target for antiphospholipid antibodies. Human polyclonal and monoclonal anti-beta 2-glycoprotein I antibodies react in vitro with endothelial cells through adherent beta 2-glycoprotein I and induce endothelial activation. Arthritis Rheum 1997;40:551–561.
20. Meroni P, Tincani A, Sepp N, et al. Endothelium and the brain in CNS lupus. Lupus 2003;12:919–928.
21. Lai NS, Lan JL. Evaluation of cerebrospinal anticardiolipin antibodies in lupus patients with neuropsychiatric manifestations. Lupus 2000;9:353–357.
22. Blank M, Krause I, Fridkin M, et al. Bacterial induction of autoantibodies to beta2-glycoprotein-I accounts for the infectious etiology of antiphospholipid syndrome. J Clin Invest 2002;109:797–804.
23. Shrot S, Katzav A, Korczyn AD, et al. Behavioral and cognitive deficits occur only after prolonged exposure of mice to antiphospholipid antibodies. Lupus 2002;11:736–743.
24. Shoenfeld Y, Nahum A, Korczyn AD, et al. Neuronal-binding antibodies from patients with antiphospholipid syndrome induce cognitive deficits following intrathecal passive transfer. Lupus 2003;12:436–442.
25. Mackworth-Young CG, Hughes GRV. Epilepsy: an early symptom of systemic lupus erythematosus. J Neurol Neurosurg Psychiatry 1985;48:185.
26. Inzelberg R, Korczyn AD. Lupus anticoagulant and the late onset seizures. Acta Neurol Scand 1989;79:114–118.
27. Herranz MT, Rivier G, Khamashta MA, Blaser KU, Hughes GR. Association between antiphospholipid antibodies and epilepsy in patients with systemic lupus erythematosus. Arthritis Rheum 1994;37:568–571.
28. Toubi E, Khamashta MA, Panarra A, Hughes GR. Association of antiphospholipid antibodies with central nervous system disease in systemic lupus erythematosus. Am J Med 1995;99:397–401.
29. Liou HH, Wang CR, Chen CJ, et al. Elevated levels of anticardiolipin antibodies and epilepsy in lupus patients. Lupus 1996;5:307–312.

30. Verrot D, San-Marco M, Dravet C, et al. Prevalence and signification of antinuclear and anticardi-olipin antibodies in patients with epilepsy. Am J Med 1997;103:33–37.
31. Shrivastava A, Dwivedi S, Aggarwal A, Misra R. Anti-cardiolipin and anti-beta2 glycoprotein I anti-bodies in Indian patients with systemic lupus erythematosus: association with the presence of seizures. Lupus 2001;10:45–50.
32. Sanna G, Bertolaccini ML, Cuadrado MJ, et al. Neuropsychiatric manifestations in systemic lupus erythematosus: prevalence and association with antiphospholipid antibodies. J Rheumatol 2003;30:985–992.
33. Jain KK. Systemic lupus erythematosus (SLE)-like syndromes associated with carbamazepine therapy. Drug Saf 1991;6:350–360.
34. Echaniz-Laguna A, Thiriaux A, Ruolt-Olivesi I, Marescaux C, Hirsch E. Lupus anticoagulant induced by the combination of valproate and lamotrigine. Epilepsia 1999;40:1661–1663.
35. Peltola JT, Haapala A, Isojarvi JI, et al. Antiphospholipid and antinuclear antibodies in patients with epilepsy or new-onset seizure disorders. Am J Med 2000;109:712–717.
36. Eriksson K, Peltola J, Keranen T, Haapala AM, Koivikko M. High prevalence of antiphospholipid antibodies in children with epilepsy: a controlled study of 50 cases. Epilepsy Res 2001;46:129–137.
37. Ranua J, Luoma K, Peltola J, et al. Anticardiolipin and antinuclear antibodies in epilepsy–a popula-tion-based cross-sectional study. Epilepsy Res 2004;58:13–18.
38. Gibbs JW 3rd, Husain AM. Epilepsy associated with lupus anticoagulant. Seizure 2002;11:207–209.
39. Liou HH, Wang CR, Chou HC, et al. Anticardiolipin antisera from lupus patients with seizures reduce a GABA receptor-mediated chloride current in snail neurons. Life Sci 1994;54:1119–1125.
40. Chapman J, Cohen-Armon M, Shoenfeld Y, Korczyn AD. Antiphospholipid antibodies permeabi-lize and depolarize brain synaptoneurosomes. Lupus 1999;8:127–133.
41. Kent M, Alvarez F, Vogt E, Fyffe R, Ng AK, Rote N. Monoclonal antiphosphatidylserine antibodies react directly with feline and murine central nervous system. J Rheumatol 1997;24:1725–1733.
42. Kent MN, Alvarez FJ, Ng AK, Rote NS. Ultrastructural localization of monoclonal antiphospho-lipid antibody binding to rat brain. Exp Neurol 2000;163:173–179.
43. Cuadrado MJ, Sanna G. Headache and systemic lupus erythematosus. Lupus 2003;12:943–946.
44. Levine SR, Joseph R, G, DA, Welch KM. Migraine and the lupus anticoagulant. Case reports and review of the literature. Cephalalgia 1987;7:93–99.
45. Hogan MJ, Brunet DG, Ford PM, Lillicrap D. Lupus anticoagulant, antiphospholipid antibodies and migraine. Can J Neurol Sci 1988;15:420–425.
46. Alarcon-Segovia D, Deleze M, Oria CV, et al. Antiphospholipid antibodies and the antiphospho lipid syndrome in systemic lupus erythematosus. A prospective analysis of 500 consecutive patients. Medicine (Baltimore) 1989;68:353–365.
47. Tzourio C, Kittner SJ, Bousser MG, Alperovitch A. Migraine and stroke in young women. Cephalalgia 2000;20:190–199.
48. Shuaib A, Barklay L, Lee MA, Suchowersky O. Migraine and anti-phospholipid antibodies. Headache 1989;29:42–45.
49. Tietjen GE. Migraine and antiphospholipid antibodies. Cephalalgia 1992;12:69–74.
50. Montalban J, Cervera R, Font J, et al. Lack of association between anticardiolipin antibodies and migraine in systemic lupus erythematosus. Neurology 1992;42:681–682.
51. Tietjen GE, Day M, Norris L, et al. Role of anticardiolipin antibodies in young persons with migraine and transient focal neurologic events: a prospective study. Neurology 1998;50:1433–1440.
52. Verrotti A, Cieri F, Pelliccia P, Morgese G, Chiarelli F. Lack of association between antiphospho-lipid antibodies and migraine in children. Int J Clin Lab Res 2000;30:109–111.
53. Cuadrado MJ, Khamashta MA, Hughes GRV. Migraine and stroke in young women. Q J Med 2000;93:317–318.
54. Cuadrado MJ, Khamashta MA, Hughes GR. Sticky blood and headache. Lupus 2001;10:392–393.
55. Hughes G, Cuadrado M, Khamashta M, Sanna G. Headache and memory loss: rapid response to heparin in the antiphospholipid syndrome. Lupus 2001;10:778.
56. Cuadrado MJ, Sanna G, Sharief M, Khamashta MA, Hughes GR. Double blind, crossover, ran-domised trial comparing low molecular weight heparin versus placebo in the treatment of chronic headache in patients with antiphospholipid antibodies [abstract]. Arthritis Rheum 2003;48:S364.
57. Denburg S, Denburg J. Cognitive dysfunction and antiphospholipid antibodies in systemic lupus erythematosus. Lupus 2003;12:883–890.
58. Hanly JG, Walsh NM, Fisk JD, et al. Cognitive impairment and autoantibodies in systemic lupus erythematosus. Br J Rheumatol 1993;32:291–296.
59. Denburg SD, Carbotte RM, Ginsberg JS, Denburg JA. The relationship of antiphospholipid antibod-ies to cognitive function in patients with systemic lupus erythematosus. J Int Neuropsychol Soc 1997;3:377–386.

60. Hanly JG, Hong C, Smith S, and Fisk JD. A prospective analysis of cognitive function and anticardiolipin antibodies in systemic lupus erythematosus. Arthritis Rheum 1999;728–734.

61. Menon S, Jameson-Shortall E, Newman SP, Hall-Craggs MR, Chinn R, Isenberg DA. A longitudinal study of anticardiolipin antibody levels and cognitive functioning in systemic lupus erythematosus. Arthritis Rheum 1999;42:735–741.

62. Asherson RA, Khamashta MA, Gil A, et al. Cerebrovascular disease and antiphospholipid antibodies in systemic lupus erythematosus, lupus-like disease, and the primary antiphospholipid syndrome. Am J Med 1989;86:391–399.

63. Kushner M, Simonian N. Lupus anticoagulants, anticardiolipin antibodies, and cerebral ischemia. Stroke 1989;20:225–229.

64. Montalban J, Fernandez J, Arderiu A, et al. Multi-infarct dementia associated with antiphospholipid antibodies. Presentation of 2 cases. Med Clin (Barc) 1989;93:424–426.

65. Kurita A, Hasunuma T, Mochio S, Shimada T, Isogai Y, Kurahashi T. A young case with multi-infarct dementia associated with lupus anticoagulant. Intern Med 1994;33:373–375.

66. Westerman EM, Miles JM, Backonja M, Sundstrom WR. Neuropathologic findings in multi-infarct dementia associated with anticardiolipin antibody. Evidence for endothelial injury as the primary event. Arthritis Rheum 1992;35:1038–1041.

67. Hilker R, Thiel A, Geisen C, Rudolf J. Cerebral blood flow and glucose metabolism in multi-infarct-dementia related to primary antiphospholipid antibody syndrome. Lupus 2000;9:311–316.

68. Mosek A, Yust I, Treves TA, Vardinon N, Korczyn AD, Chapman J. Dementia and antiphospholipid antibodies. Dement Geriatr Cogn Disord 2000;11:36–38.

69. Chapman J, Abu-Katash M, Inzelberg R, et al. Prevalence and clinical features of dementia associated with the antiphospholipid syndrome and circulating anticoagulants. J Neurol Sci 2002;203–204:81–84.

70. Wolkowitz OM, Reus VI, Canick J, Levin B, and Lupien S. Glucocorticoid medication, memory and steroid psychosis in medical illness. Ann N Y Acad Sci 1997;823:81–96.

71. Wolkowitz OM, Reus VI, Weingartner H, et al. Cognitive effects of corticosteroids. Am J Psychiatry 1990;147:1297–1303.

72. Schwartz M, Rochas M, Weller B, et al. High association of anticardiolipin antibodies with psychosis. J Clin Psychiatry 1998;59:20–23.

73. Ziporen L, Shoenfeld Y, Levy Y, Korczyn AD. Neurological dysfunction and hyperactive behavior associated with antiphospholipid antibodies. A mouse model. J Clin Invest 1997;100:613–619.

74. Katzav A, Pick CG, Korczyn AD, et al. Hyperactivity in a mouse model of the antiphospholipid syndrome. Lupus 2001;10:496–499.

75. Bujanover S, Levy Y, Katz M, Leitner Y, Vinograd I, Shoenfeld Y. Lack of association between antiphospholipid antibodies (APLA) and Attention Deficit/Hyperactivity Disorder (ADHD) in children. Clin Dev Immunol 2003;10:105–109.

76. Fernando SJ. An attack of chorea complicating oral contraceptive therapy. Practitioner 1966;197:210–211.

77. Agrawal BL, Foa RP. Collagen vascular disease appearing as chorea gravidarum. Arch Neurol 1982;39:192–193.

78. Herd JK, Medhi M, Uzendoski DM, Saldivar VA. Chorea associated with systemic lupus erythematosus: report of two cases and review of the literature. Pediatrics 1978;61:308–315.

79. Watanabe T, Onda H. Hemichorea with antiphospholipid antibodies in a patient with lupus nephritis. Pediatr Nephrol 2004;19:451–453.

80. Klawans HL, Weiner WJ. The pharmacology of choreatic movement disorders. Prog Neurobiol 1976;6:49–80.

81. Asherson RA, Hughes GRV. Antiphospholipid antibodies and chorea. J Rheumatol 1988; 15:377–379.

82. Cervera R, Asherson RA, Font J, et al. Chorea in the antiphospholipid syndrome. Clinical, radiologic, and immunologic characteristics of 50 patients from our clinics and the recent literature. Medicine (Baltimore) 1997;76:203–212.

83. Scott TF, Hess D, and Brillman J. Antiphospholipid antibody syndrome mimicking multiple sclerosis clinically and by magnetic resonance imaging. Arch Intern Med 1994;154:917–920.

84. Ijdo J, Conti-Kelly AM, Greco P, et al. Anti-phospholipid antibodies in patients with multiple sclerosis and MS-like illnesses: MS or APS? Lupus 1999;8:109–115.

85. Cuadrado MJ, Khamashta MA, Ballesteros A, Godfrey T, Simon MJ, Hughes GRV. Can neurologic manifestations of Hughes (antiphospholipid) syndrome be distinguished from multiple sclerosis? Analysis of 27 patients and review of the literature. Medicine (Baltimore) 2000;79:57–68.

86. Tourbah A, Clapin A, Gout O, et al. Systemic autoimmune features and multiple sclerosis: a 5-year follow-up study. Arch Neurol 1998;55:517–521.

87. Karussis D, Leker RR, Ashkenazi A, Abramsky O. A subgroup of multiple sclerosis patients with anticardiolipin antibodies and unusual clinical manifestations: do they represent a new nosological entity? Ann Neurol 1998;44:629–634.
88. Roussel V, Yi F, Jauberteau MO, et al. Prevalence and clinical significance of anti-phospholipid antibodies in multiple sclerosis: a study of 89 patients. J Autoimmun 2000;14:259–265.
89. Sastre-Garriga J, Reverter JC, Font J, Tintore M, Espinosa G, Montalban X. Anticardiolipin antibodies are not a useful screening tool in a nonselected large group of patients with multiple sclerosis. Ann Neurol 2001;49:408–411.
90. Lavalle C, Pizarro S, Drenkard C, Sanchez-Guerrero J, Alarcon-Segovia D. Transverse myelitis: a manifestation of systemic lupus erythematosus strongly associated with antiphospholipid antibodies. J Rheumatol 1990;17:34–37.
91. Kovacs B, Lafferty TL, Brent LH, DeHoratius RJ. Transverse myelopathy in systemic lupus erythematosus: an analysis of 14 cases and review of the literature. Ann Rheum Dis 2000;59:120–124.
92. Sherer Y, Hassin S, Shoenfeld Y, et al. Transverse myelitis in patients with antiphospholipid antibodies–the importance of early diagnosis and treatment. Clin Rheumatol 2002;21:207–210.
93. D'Cruz D, Mellor-Pita S, Joven B, et al. Transverse myelitis as the first manifestation of systemic lupus erythematosus or lupus-like disease: good functional outcome and relevance of antiphospholipid antibodies. J Rheumatol 2004;31:280–285.
94. Orefice G, De Joanna G, Coppola M, Brancaccio V, Ames PR. Benign intracranial hypertension: a non-thrombotic complication of the primary antiphospholipid syndrome? Lupus 1995;4:324–326.
95. Sussman J, Leach M, Greaves M, Malia R, Davies-Jones GA. Potentially prothrombotic abnormalities of coagulation in benign intracranial hypertension. J Neurol Neurosurg Psychiatry 1997;62:229–233.
96. Leker RR, Steiner I. Anticardiolipin antibodies are frequently present in patients with idiopathic intracranial hypertension. Arch Neurol 1998;55:817–820.
97. Kesler A, Ellis MH, Reshef T, Kott E, Gadoth N. Idiopathic intracranial hypertension and anticardiolipin antibodies. J Neurol Neurosurg Psychiatry 2000;68:379–380.
98. Hisashi K, Komune S, Taira T, Uemura T, Sadoshima S, Tsuda, H. Anticardiolipin antibody-induced sudden profound sensorineural hearing loss. Am J Otolaryngol 1993;14:275–277.
99. Casoli P, Tumiati B. Cogan's syndrome: a new possible complication of antiphospholipid antibodies? Clin Rheumatol 1995;14:197–198.
100. Tumiati B, Casoli P. Sudden sensorineural hearing loss and anticardiolipin antibody. Am J Otolaryngol 1995;16:220.
101. Toubi E, Ben-David J, Kessel A, Podoshin L, Golan TD. Autoimmune aberration in sudden sensorineural hearing loss: association with anti-cardiolipin antibodies. Lupus 1997;6:540–542.
102. Naarendorp M, Spiera H. Sudden sensorineural hearing loss in patients with systemic lupus erythematosus or lupus-like syndromes and antiphospholipid antibodies. J Rheumatol 1998;25:589–592.
103. Gilburd B, Stein M, Tomer Y, et al. Autoantibodies to phospholipids and brain extract in patients with the Guillain-Barre syndrome: cross-reactive or pathogenic? Autoimmunity 1993;16:23–27.
104. Montalban J, Arboix A, Staub H, et al. Transient global amnesia and antiphospholipid syndrome. Clin Exp Rheumatol 1989;7:85–87.
105. Brey RL, Gharavi AE, Lockshin MD. Neurologic complications of antiphospholipid antibodies. Rheum Dis Clin North Am 1993;19:833–850.
106. Frohman L, Turbin R, Bielory L, Wolansky L, Lambert WC, Cook S. Autoimmune optic neuropathy with anticardiolipin antibody mimicking multiple sclerosis in a child. Am J Ophthalmol 2003;136:358–360.
107. Reino S, Munoz-Rodriguez FJ, Cervera R, Espinosa G, Font J, Ingelmo M. Optic neuropathy in the "primary" antiphospholipid syndrome: report of a case and review of the literature. Clin Rheumatol 1997;16:629–631.
108. Giorgi D, Gabrieli CB, Bonomo L. The clinical-ophtalmological spectrum of antiphospholipid syndrome. Ocular Immunol Inflamm 1998;6:269–273.
109. Wiechens B, Schroder JO, Potzsch B, Rochels R. Primary antiphospholipid antibody syndrome and retinal occlusive vasculopathy. Am J Ophthalmol 1997;123:848–850.
110. Au A, O'Day J. Review of severe vaso-occlusive retinopathy in systemic lupus erythematosus and the antiphospholipid syndrome: associations, visual outcomes, complications and treatment. Clin Exp Ophthalmol 2004;32:87–100.
111. Milanov IG, Rashkov R, Baleva M, Georgiev D. Antiphospholipid syndrome and parkinsonism. Clin Exp Rheumatol 1998;16:623–624.
112. Milanov I, Bogdanova D. Antiphospholipid syndrome and dystonia-parkinsonism. A case report. Parkinsonism Relat Disord 2001;7:139–141.

113. Adhiyaman V, Meara RJ, Bhowmick BK. Antiphospholipid syndrome and dystonia-parkinsonism: need for anticoagulation. Parkinsonism Relat Disord 2002;8:215.
114. Aleem MA, Govindaraj K, Senthil VJ, Kanagaraj V, Jayapal V. Primary antiphopholipid syndrome presenting as pseudobulbar palsy in a young male. J Assoc Physicians India 2001;49:1036–1038.
115. Reiblat T, Polishchuk I, Dorodnikov E, et al. Primary antiphospholipid antibody syndrome masquerading as progressive supranuclear palsy. Lupus 2003;12:67–69.
116. Sanna G, Piga M, Terryberry JW, et al. Central nervous system involvement in systemic lupus erythematosus: cerebral imaging and serological profile in patients with and without overt neuropsychiatric manifestations. Lupus 2000;9:573–583.
117. Stimmler MM, Coletti PM, Quismorio FPJ. Magnetic resonance imaging of the brain in neuropsychiatric systemic lupus erythematosus. Semin Arthritis Rheum 1993;22:335–349.
118. Vermeer SE, Hollander M, van Dijk EJ, Hofman A, Koudstaal PJ, Breteler MM. Silent brain infarcts and white matter lesions increase stroke risk in the general population: the Rotterdam Scan Study. Stroke 2003;34:1126–1129.
119. Vermeer SE, Prins ND, den Heijer T, Hofman A, Koudstaal PJ, Breteler MM. Silent brain infarcts and the risk of dementia and cognitive decline. N Engl J Med 2003;348:1215–1222.

8   Skin Manifestations of Antiphospholipid Syndrome

Carlos A. Battagliotti

Several skin manifestations have been described in patients with antiphospholipid syndrome (APS) (Table 8.1) [1–3]. The most frequent skin lesions are livedo reticularis and skin ulcers.

Vascular occlusion is generally the first and most frequent manifestation observed in patients with antiphospholipid antibodies (aPL), accounting for 41% of the cases. Forty percent of these patients present with other multisystem thrombotic phenomena during the course of the disease, underscoring the significance of skin lesions as a diagnostic marker and predictor of systemic involvement.

In spite of the association of skin lesions with different isotypes of immunoglobulins, the presence of IgA anticardiolipin antibodies (aCL) has been reported as an independent predictive factor for skin lesions (skin ulcers, chilblain lupus, and vasculitis) [4].

Livedo Reticularis

Livedo reticularis is the most common skin manifestation in patients with APS, characterized by a dark purple reticular pattern usually involving the upper and lower limbs [3, 5].

The skin normally receives its blood supply through a vascular system arranged in the form of cones with their base towards the skin surface. Each cone is supplied by an arteriole. The pattern of livedo reticularis corresponds to areas of anastomo-

Table 8.1. The skin and antiphospholipid syndrome.

- Livedo reticularis
- Sneddon's syndrome
- Skin ulcers
- Necrotizing vasculitis
- Livedoid vasculitis
- Cutaneous gangrene
- Super cial thrombophlebitis
- Pseudovasculitic lesions: Nodules, papules, pustules, palmar–plantar erythema
- Subungual bleeding
- Anetoderma

Table 8.2. Livedo reticularis and associated diseases. 📖

- Antiphospholipid syndrome
- Systemic lupus erythematosus (with or without aPL)
- Systemic vasculitis (polyarteritis nodosa, cryoglobulinemia)
- Pseudovasculitic syndromes (cholesterol embolization)
- Overlapping syndromes
- Scleroderma
- Infectious diseases (syphilis, tuberculosis)

sis between the two cones where diminished blood flow is associated with the dilatation of venules and capillaries. Therefore, the alteration in arterial blood flow caused by the livedo may result from:

- Blood inflow obstruction
- Blood hyperviscosity
- Blood outflow obstruction

Livedo may be observed in normal subjects, especially women, after exposure to cold, displaying a symmetrical and regular mottled pattern. However, the relationship with a large number of pathological conditions (Table 8.2) is very important. A detailed examination of the features of the reticular pattern, including location, extension, symmetry, and regularity, and the presence of associated skin lesions will contribute to the differential diagnosis [3, 6–8].

The pattern of involvement associated with APS is generally disseminated, with incomplete circular segments, non-infiltrated, persistent, or irregular with wide ramifications (livedo racemosa). Some patients present a fine, regular, and complete network (Fig. 8.1).

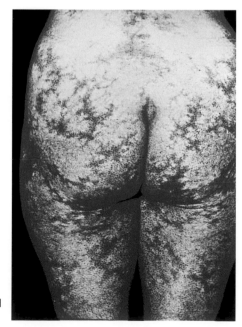

Figure 8.1. Livedo reticularis of the gluteal region and both thighs of a patient with SLE and APS. 📖

In a recent study, the presence of livedo reticularis was associated with arterial but no venous events, suggesting that livedo reticularis could be consider as a marker of the arterial APS subset [9].

Sneddon's Syndrome

In 1965, Sneddon described the association between livedo reticularis and stroke [10]. Later on, the presence of aPL in some of the patients that carry the syndrome suggests that a subset of patients might have APS [11–13].

Although there are differences in the terminology used for the Sneddon syndrome livedo, its features are very clear. The skin lesions are extensive, patchy, persistent, and do not disappear with skin heating. Usually, this is the pattern observed in patients with a prior condition that accounts for the vascular lesion (secondary Sneddon's syndrome), such as autoimmune or thrombophilic diseases.

Beyond the initial description, there are numerous reports of cardiac and renal involvement and development of hypertension, as well as gynecological and obstetrical complications [14, 15]. There are no laboratory tests that contribute to a definite diagnosis; however, 35% of patients with Sneddon's syndrome have anti-endothelial cell antibody as opposed to patients with stroke and no livedo reticularis. Prognosis is variable, mainly depending on the extension and progression of brain lesions that might lead to a severe and definite mental deterioration.

The pathological study of livedo reticularis shows endothelitis and obliterating endarteritis without necrotizing vasculitis [13]. In some cases the characteristics of APS overlap so that in all patients affected with livedo reticularis with non-inflammatory small vessel thrombosis in their biopsy, the measurement of aPL is mandatory.

Skin Ulcers

Lower limb ulcers are one of the most frequent skin manifestations in patients with APS [2]. They have been observed in 20% to 30% of patients. The prevalence of skin ulcers is very high when associated with aCL in systemic lupus erythematosus (SLE) [3, 5].

Although characteristics are variable, ulcers are painful, small (0.5–3.0 cm in diameter), with stellate, oval, or irregular borders surrounded by a purple-brownish and recurrent purple halo. They are generally located in the ankles, legs, and feet. Healing is difficult; when accomplished it results in a white scar with a pigmented halo [16, 17] (Fig. 8.2).

Giant ulcers and cases resembling gangrenous pyoderma have been reported [18–20], although in the latter case, the characteristic undercut of the borders of pyoderma are absent. Post-phlebitic ulcers are seldom seen though an increased prevalence of aPL has been described in elderly patients with venous ulcers (Figs. 8.2 and 8.3).

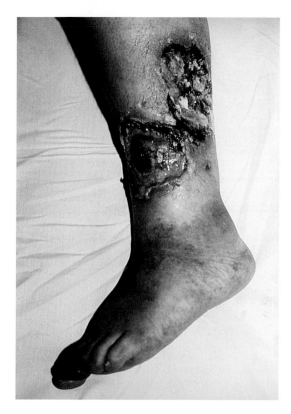

Figure 8.2. Patient with primary APS that presents necrotic ulcers on the leg and necrosis of the toes. 📖

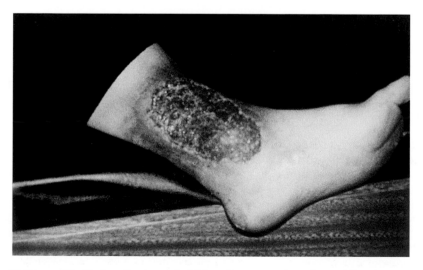

Figure 8.3. Primary APS with giant skin ulcer on the left leg refractory to anticoagulant and fibrinolytic treatment. 📖

Necrotizing Vasculitis and Livedoid Vasculitis

Generally, no inflammatory changes are observed in the biopsies taken from skin lesions of patients suffering from APS. The association with vasculitis might reflect the coexistence of two diseases, most commonly SLE.

In 1967, Bard and Winkelmann described a group of patients with chronic and recurrent livedoid-like lesions circumscribed to the lower limbs and with histological images of hyalinizing segmentary vasculitis of the dermis vessels related to thrombotic occlusion and lymphocytic infiltration [21]. This disorder was termed *livedoid vasculitis* or *segmentary hyalinizing vasculitis*. These cases presented with livedo lesions, purpura with a trend towards ulceration that became covered with dark crusts, and inflammatory borders. After weeks or months they healed, forming porcelain-white star-like scars, atrophic with telangiectasis and hyperpigmented borders. These latter lesions have been termed *white atrophy* and some authors consider it as a disorder per se. The term was coined by Milian in 1929, who attributed its formation to a previous ulceration with a probable syphilitic or tuberculous etiology. There is consensus in that there are different stages in the evolution of the same process that leads to livedoid vasculitis. Other authors believe that "white atrophy" is the end stage of different disorders that result in a stellate porcelain-like star [22–24].

Livedoid vasculitis predominates in young women with characteristic lesions on the lower limbs; it recurs with seasonal exacerbations. Its presentation might be primary or idiopathic. However, it is sometimes related to SLE, Sjögren's syndrome, APS, polyarteritis nodosa, rheumatoid arthritis, scleroderma, Raynaud's phenomenon, cryoglobulinemia, macroglobulinemia, venous vascular pathology, and diabetes [23, 25].

Controversy exists as to the pathogenesis but possible suggested mechanisms include imbalance of the coagulation and fibrinolysis system and alteration of platelet function.

Skin lesions typically found are erythematosus plaques, petechial purpura, livedo, painful ulcers of different sizes, white atrophy, telangiectases, and hyperpigmentation. In some patients, direct immunofluorescence of skin vessels reveals IgG, IgM, IgA, fibrin, and, to a lesser degree, deposits of complement [26].

Histological characteristics of livedoid vasculitis overlap with the vascular changes seen in the APS. Segmental hyalinization and non-inflammatory occlusion of the dermal arterioles leading to skin ulceration is observed.

Cutaneous Gangrene and Necrosis

Digital gangrene is a well-recognized manifestation in patients with APS [2, 3, 27]. The process starts with erythematosus macules, cyanosis, or pseudocellulitis ending in necrosis. In patients with SLE or other autoimmune diseases, aPL quite often coexists with other pathogenic factors such as cryoglobulins, antiendothelial cell antibodies, or hepatitis viruses. Patients who are smokers, hypertensive, or are on oral contraceptives have an increased risk of necrosis (Figs 8.4, 8.5, and 8.6). Angiographic images show occlusion or severe stenosis of middle- and large-size vessels.

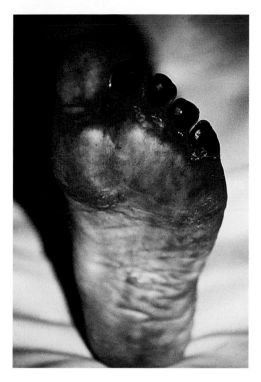

Figure 8.4. Evolution to gangrene with distal necrosis of the left foot toes in the patient carrier of primary APS shown in Figure 8.3. 📖

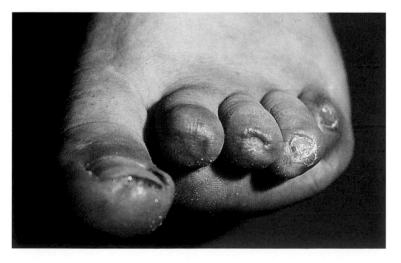

Figure 8.5. Cure by spontaneous amputation of the left foot toes affected with gangrene in a patient with primary APS. 📖

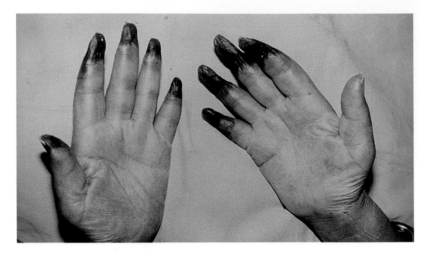

Figure 8.6. Digital necrosis with gangrene of the fingers of a patient with SLE and APS. 📖

Some patients (3%) develop extensive superficial skin necrosis generally involving the limbs, head, and buttocks [28]. The onset is sudden, with an extensive and painful purpuric lesion followed by a necrotic plaque with purpuric and active edges and bullous lesions. The thrombozing microangiitis seen in examined tissues is characteristic [2, 29].

Superficial Thrombophlebitis

Thrombotic episodes in the deep veins of the lower limbs are common. Similar mechanisms might lead to the involvement of the superficial venous territory [3].

Pseudo-vasculitic Lesions: Nodules, Papules, Pustules, Palmo–Plantar Erythema

A wide variety of skin lesions might be included under the term pseudo-vasculitic, erythematosus macules, painful nodules, and purpura, among others. APS accounts for the microthrombosis observed in skin vessels [3, 30] (Figs. 8.7 and 8.8).

Subungual Hemorrhages

Chipe-like subungual hemorrhages are longitudinally distributed, small reddish-to-black linear lesions, which persist after ungual compression. They are not exclusively associated with the APS because ungual trauma can be seen in healthy subjects as well as patients with infectious endocarditis. They are caused by thrombotic or embolic phenomena. It is worth pointing out that the presence of these

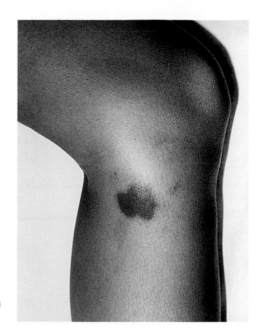

Figure 8.7. SLE along with APS presenting with papuloerythematosus skin lesion (irregular borders) on the lower limb. 📖

lesions in several fingers is related to an underlying pathological process [3, 5]. Their sudden onset on multiple fingers is usually concomitant to other thrombotic event [31, 32].

Anetoderma

Anetoderma is a rare elastolytic disorder characterized by a limited area of slack skin associated with loss of substance on examination and a loss of elastic tissue in the histopathology [33]. Although its cause is unknown, an immunological mechanism has been suggested as playing an important role in this elatolytic disease. Some reports suggest that anetoderma may be the presenting sign of autoimmune disorders [34, 35], particularly in those with aPL [25, 35].

What Do Skin Lesion Biopsies of Patients with APS Show?

The main histopathological picture is non-inflammatory thrombosis in small- and medium-sized arteries and/or veins of the dermis and hypodermis [3, 36]. A pattern that might be associated or be the only one observed is that of obliterating endarterial occlusion, characterized by narrowing of the vessel lumen with endothelial cell proliferation and fibrohyalinization of the vessel wall. The absence of vasculitis is characteristic. Lymphocytic or lymphoplasmocytic infiltrating isolates might be

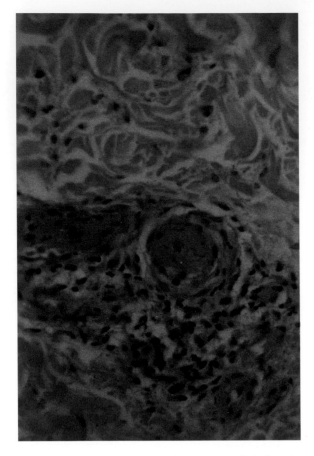

Figure 8.8. Biopsy of skin with non-inflammatory vascular thrombosis (venular) of a patient with SLE and APS. 📖

observed. Based on skin involvement, the following histopathologic pattern is observed [36]:

- Gangrenous lesion
    Vascular thrombosis
    Dermal hemorrhage
    Obliterating endarteritis
    Epidermal necrosis
- Ulcerous lesion
    Vascular thrombosis
    Capillary proliferation
    Obliterating endarteritis
    Dermal hemorrhage
    Deposit of hemosiderin

- Livedo reticularis
    Center of the reticular pattern (apparently normal skin):
        Normal biopsy
        Obliterating endarteritis in deep arterioles of the dermis or hypodermis
    Tissue of the reticulate (involved segment of the skin):
        Hyperplasia of dermal vessels

Wherever the site of biopsy in livedo reticularis, thrombosis is rare except in the case of catastrophic APS or in the presence of ulcers and necrosis.

Association of Skin Lesions with Different Organ Involvement

It should be remembered that 41% of patients with APS begin their disease with skin manifestations and that 40% of patients will develop multisystem thrombotic phenomena during the course of the disease. The association of livedo reticularis with cerebrovascular involvement has already been pointed out (Sneddon's syndrome). The presence of multiple subungual hemorrhages might coincide with thrombotic events of other organs such as the brain, skin, adrenal glands, kidney, etc.

Entities Associated with APS

Different pathologic entities have been described to occur in association with APS. It should be underscored that patients affected with inflammatory bowel disease (ulcerative colitis, Crohn's disease) are susceptible to thrombosis during the active stage of the disease in relation to aPL. Up to 10% of patients will develop ischemic lesions of the central nervous system and embolic events, including peripheral necrosis [37, 38]. Skin lesions observed in this life-threatening syndrome are livedo reticularis, acrocyanosis, extensive skin necrosis, palmar erythema, and gangrene [39].

Treatment

It is hard to predict if the patient who only has a skin lesion will later develop an extra cutaneous thrombotic event. However, it is worth remembering that 40% of patients that begin with skin lesions will eventually undergo systemic involvement. Hence, it is important to consider extensive skin necrosis and digital ischemia as major thrombotic events; in these cases, patients should receive long-term anticoagulant treatment [40–42]. The approach to minor skin manifestations is less clear. It is yet to be defined whether platelet antiaggregation is enough or whether it will be necessary to attempt the use of more aggressive treatments.

Alternative treatments should be developed for patients resistant to standard approaches [43]. Thrombolytic agents in low dose have been proposed in patients with skin lesions where the thrombotic events account for the clinical picture (i.e., livedoid vasculitis). Thrombolytic agents not only accomplish the patency of involved arteries but also play a significant role by increasing microcirculation.

Some patients have been treated with streptokinase or urokinase with or without heparin with varying degree of responses. The intravenous infusion of recombinant tissue plasminogen activator at a dose of 20 mg/day diluted in saline solution during 8 hours for 10 days resulted in the healing of ulcer lesions [44]. Unwanted effects such as bleeding that might threaten the patient's life should be considered. This therapeutic modality should be selected when all the other alternatives have failed. It is critical to test coagulation status prior to and during infusion; treatment should be withdrawn as soon as minimum bleeding is noticed [44, 45].

Although anecdotal, the efficacy of sildenafil, a phosphodiesterase inhibitor, in the treatment of non-healing ulcers has also been reported [46].

Conclusion

aPL are strongly related to thrombotic events. It is the most common acquired coagulation defect among the ones accountable for procoagulant states.

Skin involvement might be the first manifestation of APS (41%) and over one third of these patients will develop multisystem thrombotic events during the course of the disease. Therefore, a close monitoring of these patients is warranted.

References

1. Battagliotti CA. Sindrome de anticuerpos antifosfolipidicos. In: Battagliotti CA, Greca A, et al, eds. Temas relacionados de terapeutica clinica. Rosario: UNR Editora; 1996:328–334.
2. Alegre VA, Gastineau DA, Winkelmann RK. Skin lesions associated with circulating lupus anticoagulant. Br J Dermatol 1989;120:419–429.
3. Gibson GE, Su WP, Pittelkow MR. Antiphospholipid syndrome and the skin. J Am Acad Dermatol 1997;36:970–982.
4. Tajima C, Suzuki Y, Mizushima Y, Ichikawa Y. Clinical significance of immunoglobulin A antiphospholipid antibodies: possible association with skin manifestations and small vessel vasculitis. J Rheumatol 1998;25:1730–1736.
5. Eng AM. Cutaneous expressions of antiphospholipid syndromes. Semin Thromb Hemost 1994;20:71–78.
6. Naldi L, Locati F, Marchesi L, et al. Cutaneous manifestations associated with antiphospholipid antibodies in patients with suspected primary antiphospholipid syndrome: a case-control study. Ann Rheum Dis 1993;52:219–222.
7. Asherson RA, Mayou SC, Merry P, Black MM, Hughes GR. The spectrum of livedo reticularis and anticardiolipin antibodies. Br J Dermatol 1989;120:215–221.
8. Weinstein C, Miller MH, Axtens R, Buchanan R, Littlejohn GO. Livedo reticularis associated with increased titers of anticardiolipin antibodies in systemic lupus erythematosus. Arch Dermatol 1987;123:596–600.
9. Niang S, Frances C, Barete S, et al. Dermatologic manifestations of the antiphospholipid syndrome [abstract]. Arthritis Rheum 2003;48:S879.
10. Sneddon IB. Cerebro-vascular lesions and livedo reticularis. Br J Dermatol 1965;77:180–185.
11. Martinez Hernandez PL, Lopez Guzman A, Espinosa Arranz E, Monereo Alonso A, Arnalich Fernandez F. Sindrome de Sneddon: valor diagnostico de los anticuerpos antifosfolipidicos. Rev Clin Esp 1991;189:272–274.
12. Tourbah A, Piette JC, Iba-Zizen MT, Lyon-Caen O, Godeau P, Frances C. The natural course of cerebral lesions in Sneddon syndrome. Arch Neurol 1997;54:53–60.
13. Stephens CJ. Sneddon's syndrome. Clin Exp Rheumatol 1992;10:489–492.

14. Macario F, Macario MC, Ferro A, Goncalves F, Campos M, Marques A. Sneddon's syndrome: a vascular systemic disease with kidney involvement? Nephron 1997;75:94–97.
15. Ohtani H, Imai H, Yasuda T, et al. A combination of livedo racemosa, occlusion of cerebral blood vessels, and nephropathy: kidney involvement in Sneddon's syndrome. Am J Kidney Dis 1995;26:511–515.
16. Grattan CE, Burton JL. Antiphospholipid syndrome and cutaneous vasoocclusive disorders. Semin Dermatol 1991;10:152–159.
17. Reyes E, Alarcon-Segovia D. Leg ulcers in the primary antiphospholipid syndrome. Report of a case with a peculiar proliferative small vessel vasculopathy. Clin Exp Rheumatol 1991;9:63–66.
18. Grob JJ, Bonerandi JJ. Cutaneous manifestations associated with the presence of the lupus anticoagulant. A report of two cases and a review of the literature. J Am Acad Dermatol 1986;15:211–219.
19. Schmid MH, Hary C, Marstaller B, Konz B, Wendtner CM. Pyoderma gangrenosum associated with the secondary antiphospholipid syndrome. Eur J Dermatol 1998;8:45–47.
20. Chacek S, MacGregor-Gooch J, Halabe-Cherem J, Nellen-Hummel H, Quinones-Galvan A. Pyoderma gangrenosum and extensive caval thrombosis associated with the antiphospholipid syndrome – a case report. Angiology 1998;49:157–160.
21. Bard JW, Winkelmann RK. Livedo vasculitis. Segmental hyalinizing vasculitis of the dermis. Arch Dermatol 1967;96:489–499.
22. Leroux B, Baron E, Garrido G, Alonso A, Bergero A, Fernandez-Bussy R. Vasculitis livedoide: nuestra experiencia. Dermatol Argent 1998;2:121–126.
23. Winkelmann RK, Schroeter AL, Kierland RR, Ryan TM. Clinical studies of livedoid vasculitis: (segmental hyalinizing vasculitis). Mayo Clin Proc 1974;49:746–750.
24. Kern AB. Atrophie blanche. Report of two patients treated with aspirin and dipyridamole. J Am Acad Dermatol 1982;6:1048–1053.
25. Stephansson EA, Niemi KM, Jouhikainen T, Vaarala O, Palosuo T. Lupus anticoagulant and the skin. A longterm follow-up study of SLE patients with special reference to histopathological findings. Acta Derm Venereol 1991;71:416–422.
26. Hassan ML, Di Fabio NA, Martinez Aquino E, Schroh R, Kien C, Magnin PH. Vasculitis livedoide. Estudio clinico, histopatologico y laboratorial de 10 casos. Rev Arg Dermatol 1987;68:311–319.
27. Hughes GR. The Prosser-White oration 1983. Connective tissue disease and the skin. Clin Exp Dermatol 1984;9:535–544.
28. Paira S, Roverano S, Zunino A, Oliva ME, Bertolaccini ML. Extensive cutaneous necrosis associated with anticardiolipin antibodies. J Rheumatol 1999;26:1197–1200.
29. Dodd HJ, Sarkany I, O'Shaughnessy D. Widespread cutaneous necrosis associated with the lupus anticoagulant. Clin Exp Dermatol 1985;10:581–586.
30. Asherson RA, Jacobelli S, Rosenberg H, McKee P, Hughes GR. Skin nodules and macules resembling vasculitis in the antiphospholipid syndrome – a report of two cases. Clin Exp Dermatol 1992;17:266–269.
31. Frances C, Piette JC, Saada V, et al. Multiple subungual splinter hemorrhages in the antiphospholipid syndrome: a report of five cases and review of the literature. Lupus 1994;3:123–128.
32. Frances C, Piette JC. Antiphospholipid antibody syndrome (Hughes' syndrome). Dermatol Ther 2001;14:117–125.
33. Hodak E, Feuerman H, Molad Y, Monselise Y, David M. Primary anetoderma: a cutaneous sign of antiphospholipid antibodies. Lupus 2003;12:564–568.
34. Disdier P, Harle JR, Andrac L, et al. Primary anetoderma associated with the antiphospholipid syndrome. J Am Acad Dermatol 1994;30:133–134.
35. Stephansson EA, Niemi KM. Antiphospholipid antibodies and anetoderma: are they associated? Dermatology 1995;191:204–209.
36. Alegre VA, Winkelmann RK. Histopathologic and immunofluorescence study of skin lesions associated with circulating lupus anticoagulant. J Am Acad Dermatol 1988;19:117–124.
37. Martinovic Z, Perisic K, Pejnovic N, Lukacevic S, Rabrenovic L, Petrovic M. Antiphospholipid antibodies in inflammatory bowel diseases. Vojnosanit Pregl 1998;55:47–49.
38. Mevorach D, Goldberg Y, Gomori JM, Rachmilewitz D. Antiphospholipid syndrome manifested by ischemic stroke in a patient with Crohn's disease. J Clin Gastroenterol 1996;22:141–143.
39. Asherson RA, Cervera R, Piette JC, et al. Catastrophic antiphospholipid syndrome. Clinical and laboratory features of 50 patients. Medicine (Baltimore) 1998;77:195–207.
40. Lockshin MD. Which patients with antiphospholipid antibody should be treated and how? Rheum Dis Clin North Am 1993;19:235–247.
41. Derksen RH, de Groot PG, Kater L, Nieuwenhuis HK. Patients with antiphospholipid antibodies and venous thrombosis should receive long term anticoagulant treatment. Ann Rheum Dis 1993;52:689–692.

42. Khamashta MA, Cuadrado MJ, Mujic F, Taub NA, Hunt BJ, Hughes GR. The management of thrombosis in the antiphospholipid-antibody syndrome. N Engl J Med 1995;332:993–997.
43. Curwin J, Jang IK, Fuster V. Expanded use of thrombolytic therapy. Mayo Clin Proc 1992;67:1004–1005.
44. Gertner E, Lie JT. Systemic therapy with fibrinolytic agents and heparin for recalcitrant nonhealing cutaneous ulcer in the antiphospholipid syndrome. J Rheumatol 1994;21:2159–2161.
45. Klein KL, Pittelkow MR. Tissue plasminogen activator for treatment of livedoid vasculitis. Mayo Clin Proc 1992;67:923–933.
46. Gertner E. Treatment with sildenafil for the healing of refractory skin ulcerations in the antiphospholipid syndrome. Lupus 2003;12:133–135.

9 Kidney Disease in Antiphospholipid Syndrome

Mary-Carmen Amigo and Romeo García-Torres

Even though the kidney is a major target organ in antiphospholipid syndrome (APS), until recently the renal manifestations associated with antiphospholipid antibodies (aPL) have received scarce attention. This can be explained because APS was first described in patients with systemic lupus erythematosus (SLE) and such research studies were focused on the immune-complex–mediated glomerulonephritis rather than renal vascular lesions that could be secondary. In addition, because of the frequent occurrence of thrombocytopenia and systemic hypertension, renal biopsy in APS patients would often be considered a high-risk procedure to be discouraged if not formally contraindicated [1].

Nevertheless, knowledge about renal vascular involvement in APS has slowly acquired a critical mass and it is now clear that large vessels, both arterial and venous, as well as the intraparenchymatous arteries and microvasculature may all be affected, with the clinical consequences shown in Table 9.1.

Renal Artery Lesions

Large- and medium-size vessel occlusion has been associated with APS in the context of SLE as well as in its primary form [2, 3].

Table 9.1. Renal vascular involvement in antiphospholipid syndrome.

Vascular lesion	Clinical consequences
Renal artery lesions: (trunk or main branches) Thrombosis/occlusion/stenosis?	Renovascular hypertension (severe) Renal infarcts (silent, painful, hematuria)
Glomerular capillary thrombosis leading to glomerular sclerosis (studied mainly in SLE)	Increased likelihood of renal insufficiency
Renal thrombotic microangiopathy (glomerular capillaries, afferent arterioles, and interlobular arteries) with/without focal or difuse necrosis (cortical necrosis)	Systemic hypertension (usually severe) Renal failure (mild to end stage), Proteinuria (mild to nephrotic range) Cortical atrophy
Renal vein thrombosis (unilateral or bilateral)	Renal failure (if bilateral compromise)

Renal artery occlusion/stenosis has been reported in patients with positive assays for aPL. Some of these patients had autoimmune rheumatic conditions, mainly SLE, while others had the primary APS (PAPS).

An early observation by Ostuni et al [4] described a 13 year-old girl with SLE and severe systemic hypertension. Bilateral renal artery stenosis/thrombosis resulted in a poorly perfused kidney and cortical irregularities were present in the contralateral kidney. Hernández et al [5] reported on a young woman with sudden, severe hypertension and a renal infarction who, 14 years later, developed SLE. Asherson et al [6] described a young man with PAPS, arterial hypertension, and a right renal artery stenosis with renal infarction which was thought to be caused by thrombotic occlusion. Ames et al [7] reported an instance of bilateral renal artery occlusion in a patient with PAPS and an unclear systemic disease. Of major interest is a paper by Rossi et al [8] reporting 2 cases of renovascular hypertension with renal artery stenosis and suggesting a pathogenetic link between renal artery stenosis, thrombosis, fibromuscular dysplasia, and aPL. Similar considerations were independently made by Mandreoli and coworkers [9, 10]. Particularly interesting is a report by Poux et al [11] on an athletic 35- year-old man with PAPS who suddenly developed arterial hypertension and a left renal infarction. Angiographic studies revealed complete thrombosis of the aorta below the renal arteries plus an extensive colateral circulation arising from the superior mesenteric artery. More recently, several cases of renal artery stenosis, mainly in young patients with PAPS, have been reported. These consistent findings confirm that this syndrome may be a significant cause of renal artery stenosis [12–14].

In the presence of aPL, renal infarctions result from partial or total, transient or permanent occlusion of renal arteries [4, 5, 8, 9, 15, 16]. Such occlusion may be caused by diverse mechanisms such as in situ thrombosis/stenosis of a renal artery or an embolic event originating on a verrucous cardiac valve. In still other cases the cause of a renal infarction was not found [17].

Clinically, severe systemic hypertension, pain in the renal area, hematuria, and renal failure are common forms of presentation of major vessel involvement in PAPS. As commented by Hughes et al [18], arterial hypertension may be labile in early disease. Occasionally, a silent infarct is fortuitously discovered on computed tomography (CT). It cannot be overemphasized that in cases of renal artery stenosis of unknown origin, APS must be excluded. Renal scintigraphy and selective renal angiography are useful procedures to confirm diagnosis and determine the extent of damage.

Successful treatment with antihypertensive drugs [8, 15], aspirin [16], anticoagulant therapy [4, 7, 9, 15] as well as transluminal angioplasty [6, 12, 13] has been reported. Nephrectomy, with subsequent normalization of blood pressure and secondary aldosteronism, was performed in 1 patient because the kidney was seriously and irreversibly damaged [14]. However, adverse outcomes may occur [5]. The sooner an arterial lesion causing arterial hypertension is relieved, the likelier a successful outcome.

Glomerular Capillary Thrombosis

Hyaline thrombi have been described in patients with active, usually proliferative lupus nephritis. The prevalence and significance of this finding have been carefully studied by Kant et al [19] and Glueck et al [20]. They found an overall rate of capillary thrombosis of near 50% in cases of proliferative glomerulonephritis, including 78% in patients with detectable lupus anticoagulant (LA) and only 38% in those without. The presence of glomerular thrombi in the initial biopsy was a strong predictor of glomerular sclerosis. Other studies have not shown an association between aPL and prognosis in lupus nephritis [21–23]. However, Moroni et al recently documented the impact of aPL in 111 patients with lupus nephritis followed up for a mean of 173 ± 100 months. A strong association between aPL and the development of chronic renal insufficiency in the long term was found. With multivariate analysis, aPL positivity, high plasma creatinine level at presentation, and chronicity index were independent predictors of chronic renal function deterioration [24]. With these data, one should keep in mind that the detection of aPL in patients with lupus nephritis is useful not only to identify patients at risk for vascular and obstetric manifestations, but also for their potential deleterious impact on renal outcome.

Intra-renal Vascular Lesions

Thrombotic Microangiopathy

The association of the distinctive lesion known as thrombotic microangiopathy (TMA) with aPL was initially described in patients with SLE [25–27]. In another clinical setting, Kincaid-Smith and coworkers [28] showed acute or healed TMA in 22 biopsies obtained in 12 patients with LA and pregnancy-related renal failure. Subsequently, isolated cases of TMA in patients with PAPS were reported [29, 30]. In 1992, at a time in which some still doubted about the very existence of primary

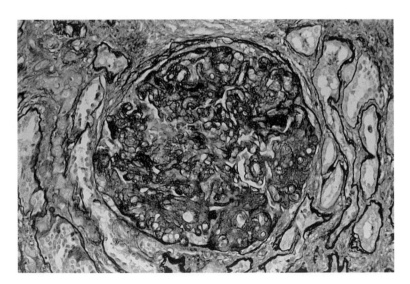

Figure 9.1. Severe and advanced glomerular thrombotic microangiopathy. Capillary lumina are occluded by severe mesangiolysis and deposition of heterogeneous subendothelial material, leading to a segmental "double contour" aspect (PAS).

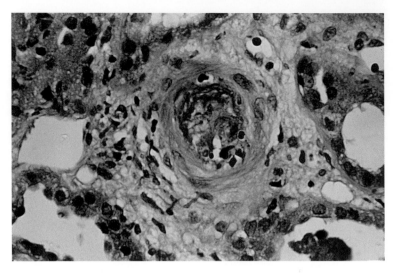

Figure 9.2. A small arteriole with a recent, almost occlusive, partially laminated thrombus. Some complete and fragmented white and red cells are seen (hematoxylin/eosin).

PAPS, we had the opportunity to study 5 patients who had renal disease and arterial hypertension among 20 consecutive patients with PAPS [31]. Mild renal failure was present in 3 patients while 2 had end-stage renal failure requiring hemodyalisis. Proteinuria in the mild-to-nephrotic range was also present. Biopsy findings in all 5

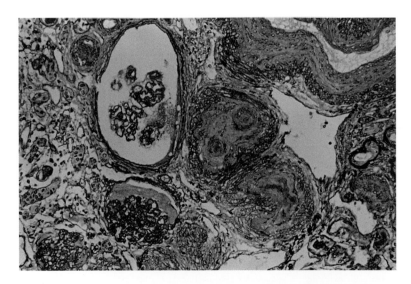

Figure 9.3. Chronic cortical lesions. There are obsolescent sclerotic glomeruli and a hypoperfused glomerulus with a wide Bowman´s space and retracted capillaries. On one of its sides there is a small arteriole with a recanalized thrombus and two lumina. On the other side there are two completely occluded arterioles showing thrombosis, recanalization, and refibrosis. A tortuous arteriole with slightly cellular subendothelial fibrosis is also seen (PAS).

patients were consistent with TMA . Some biopsies showed diffuse damage while others had only focal parenchymatous lesions. Microangiopathy involved both the vascular tree and the glomerular tufts (Fig. 9.1).

Recent and recanalized thrombi were observed (Figs. 9.2 and 9.3), as if acute lesions were superimposed on the chronic, healed damage (Table 9.2). Ultra-estructural studies showed electron lucent subendothelial deposits and ischemic obsolescence of glomeruli in absence of histologic and immunohistochemical findings suggestive of SLE. We concluded that in PAPS, depending on the degree and extension of damage, patients could have isolated hypertension, severe proteinuria, and renal failure including cortical necrosis. In chronic cases, fibrosis and focal atrophy could be found as well as arterial and arteriolar fibromuscular hyperplasia [Figs. 9.4 and 9.5).

Subsequent isolated cases or small series have confirmed our findings [32–34]. Recently, it has been emphasized that APS should be considered in the differential diagnosis of systemic hypertension and that APS-related TMA may cause isolated hypertension without significant renal impairment [35]. TMA is the characteristic histologic lesion of the microvasculature in PAPS-related nephropathy. A noninflammatory vasculopathy with or without thrombosis (the "APS vasculopathy") is a common finding in larger vessels. Of course, TMA is not pathognomonic of PAPS, as there is a wide range of conditions that present the same histological appearance (Table 9.3). Nochy et al [36] have confirmed our initial observations on glomerular and interlobular arteriolar lesions, and, in addition, have emphasized the common presence of focal cortical atrophy (Fig. 9.6).

Finally, other types of renal involvement, including membranous glomerulonephritis, IgA nephropathy, pauci-immune crescentic glomerulonephritis, glomerulonephritis with isolated C3 mesangial deposits, focal segmental glomeru-

Table 9.2. Primary antiphospholipid syndrome–associated nephropathy: main histologic features. 📖

Acute lesions	Chronic lesions
Glomerular	Glomerular
Mesangial expansion	Basement membrane thickening
Mesangiolysis	Cellular vanishing
Glomerular capillary collapse	Glomerular tuft retraction
Basement membrane wrinkling	Bowman's space widening
"Double contours" with mesangial interposition	Ischemic obsolescence
Translucent subendothelial deposits	Segmental or global glomerular sclerosis
Intracapillary thrombi	
Thrombotic/hemorrhagic infarction	
Arterioles	Arterioles
Recent occlusive thrombi	Mural organized thrombi
Laminar thrombi	Recanalizing occlusive thrombi
Endothelial edema/degeneration	Microaneurisms
Subendothelial mucoid edema	Plexiform lesions
Necrosis	Subendothelial fibrosis
	Concentric and muscular hyperplasia
	Myofibroblastic proliferation
	Diffuse fibrosis
⬇	
TMA with/without focal necrosis	Ischaemic atrophy

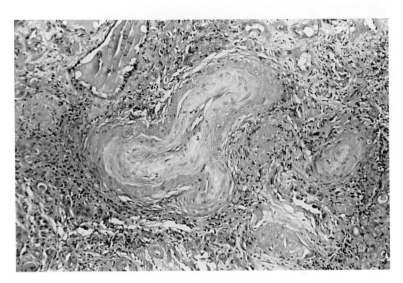

Figure 9.4. Typical histology of an interlobular arteriole which is almost occluded by a slightly cellular mucoid material. The lumen is distorted and the muscular media is partially destroyed and fibrotic. There is interstitial fibrosis with a moderate inflammatory infiltration. A dilated tubule containing hyaline material is seen (Masson). 📖

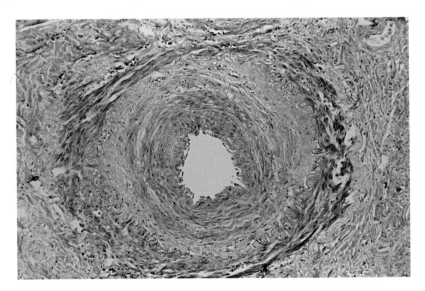

Figure 9.5. Chronic stage of an intraparenchymatous renal artery. Slight medial hyperplasia, fractures of the internal elastica, severe subendothelial fibrosis, myofibroblastic proliferation, and a drastic reduction of the lumen (Masson). 📖

losclerosis and, vasculitis, associated with aPL or with APS, but without SLE, have been published [37–39]. It is unclear, however, whether in addition to thrombosis, other mechanisms could also contribute to the pathogenesis of APS nephropathy. There is evidence that aCL recognize β_2-glycoprotein I (β_2-GPI) on the endothelial

Table 9.3. Some conditions that associate with TMA. 📖

Thrombotic thrombocytopenic purpura
Haemolytic uraemic syndrome
Post-partum renal failure
Pre-eclampsia/eclampsia
Scleroderma
Malignant arterial hypertension
Oral contraceptives
Renal transplantation / allograft rejection
Cyclosporine A toxicity
Chemotherapy

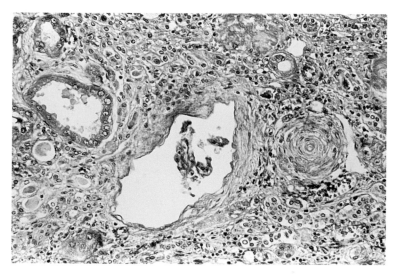

Figure 9.6. Focal cortical atrophy. There are ischemic glomeruli, an arteriole with "onion skin" hyperplasia of the media, and a "pin point" lumen, generalized tubular atrophy with early dilation in one, and interstitial fibrosis (Masson). 📖

cell membrane, leading to increased expression of adhesion molecules and increased adhesion of monocytes on endothelial cell surface [40]. These events could perhaps explain the inflammation found in some of these uncommon cases.

Cortical Renal Ischemia

Occlusion of small isolated parenchymatous renal vessels gives rise to small foci of cortical necrosis. These are generally asymptomatic; however, if they are multiple or generalized they may lead to patchy or diffuse cortical necrosis as described in the catastrophic APS [41]. These cases feature oligo/anuria, severe hypertension, and frequently have a fatal outcome. Some patients eventually recover, leaving a variable degree of renal impairment expressing cortical ischemia. Isolated cases and series of patients with cortical renal ischemia and aPL have been published [17, 35, 42, 43]. One of the first reported cases [42] was a 27-year-old man with coronary occlusion, arterial hypertension, thrombophlebitis, atrial thrombus, and positive aPL. An abdominal CT scan revealed cortex hypodensity in both kidneys. Renal biopsy showed diffuse interstitial fibrosis, mononuclear infiltration, sclerotic and ischemic glomeruli, and negative immunofluorescence studies. These findings suggested cortical sclerosis and atrophy as sequelae from old cortical necrosis. In this patient, aside from arterial hypertension, there were no additional clinical evidences of renal damage.

Cacoub's series of 5 cases [17] included patients with sudden presentation of malignant hypertension. While large renal vessels were patent on angiography, renal biopsy revealed glomerular ischemia, interstitial fibrosis, tubular atrophy, and vascular sclerosis with thrombosis. There was no vasculitis and immunofluorescence studies were negative. Four of these patients did well and 1 died, probably as a result of a catastrophic syndrome.

Pérez et al [43] reported on a man with PAPS and multi-organ arterial and venous thrombosis, seemingly a catastrophic syndrome. This patient had a 2-cm renal cortical infarction and multiple petechiae in the renal cortex. At autopsy, an organizing interlobular vein thrombus plus microthrombi in the microvasculature of the medulla were found. This case illustrates medium- and small-vessel thrombosis affecting the intra- and extra-renal vasculature.

From the above observations, it may be concluded that cortical renal ischemia (Fig. 9.6) is a well-defined clinico-pathologic entity in patients with APS. The lesion may recover ad integrum or it may leave a variable impairment of renal function.

An additional presentation of renal cortical ischemia was described by Leaker et al [44]. This is an insidious, slowly progressive nephropathy that causes renal failure in the long term. Clinically, patients have arterial hypertension, mild proteinuria, and a slowly progressive renal failure.

In a recent multicenter study, Nochy et al [36] reported 16 patients with PAPS followed for at least 5 years, all of whom had renal biopsy. In all patients there were small vessel vaso-occlussive lesions and focal cortical atrophy was present in 10.

Renal Vein Thrombosis

The main renal vein, as well as minor veins, may thrombose in APS. Asherson [45] first described the association between aPL and renal vein thrombosis in 2 cases of SLE with proliferative nephritis and nephrotic syndrome. An interesting study by Glueck et al [20] demonstrated renal vein thrombosis in 3 of 18 SLE patients with LA, compared with none in the 59 LA-negative patients without. Liano et al [46] described a man with SLE, LA, and end-stage renal disease who received a renal transplant. Nineteen months after transplantation, thrombosis of the graft's renal vein occurred and autopsy showed membranous glomerulonephritis.

Isolated cases of renal vein thrombosis have been reported in patients with PAPS [47], including 1 case with bilateral renal vein thrombosis in the postpartum period [48].

End-stage Renal Disease (ESRD)

A poorly studied issue is the occasional presence of aPL in patients with ESRD [49]. The information at hand about this interesting finding is incomplete and little more can be said about it. Similar considerations apply to the high titers of aCL and positive LA found in patients undergoing hemodialysis, a setting in which vascular access thrombosis is very common [50]. Recently, in a study of 97 hemodialysis patients, Brunet et al [51] found a prevalence of 31% of aPL (LA in 16.5% and aCL in 15.5%). The presence of aPL was independent of age, time on dialysis, gender, type of dialytic membrane used, drugs used, or presence of hepatitis B or C. There was a higher prevalence of aPL when the cause of the ESRD could not be determined. Analyzing the association between vascular access thrombosis and aPL, they found a striking correlation with the presence of LA (62% vs. 26%; $P = 0.01$) but not with aCL.

Renal Transplantation

Very few studies have addressed the impact of aPL on renal transplantation.

Reports of aPL-related morbidity among SLE transplant patients are limited by the relatively small number of subjects available for study at any given center.

In the UCSF study, 15.4% of allograft failures were attributed to aPL-associated events [52].

Radhakrishna et al [53] in a retrospective study of SLE, compared 8 patients with aCL to 5 patients without, transplanted during the same period. Thrombotic episodes occurred in 3 patients in the aCL-positive group but none in the aCL-negative group. Neither of the 2 groups differ in the number of rejection episodes, rate of graft loss, or renal function at follow up. The authors concluded that patients with SLE and aCL can be successfully transplanted.

Findings have been quite different in PAPS. Mondragón-Ramírez et al [54] reported 2 cases of PAPS with renal TMA who underwent renal transplantation and in whom, despite intensive anticoagulant therapy, the disease relapsed in the graft. Massive thrombosis in the graft in 1 case [Figs. 9.7 and 9.8) and TMA in the other suggested recurrence of the disease. We postulated that the surgical procedure plus endothelial damage, a common feature of allograft rejection, may act synergistically in amplifying the hypercoagulable state. Both patients also had thrombosis in the vascular access used for hemodialysis as has been reported by others [49, 50].

In an interesting report by Knight et al [55], a woman with aCL lost a renal allograft in the immediate postoperative period due to renal artery thrombosis. Six months later she underwent successful re-transplantation under full anticoagulation despite the presence of postoperative bleeding.

Vaidya et al [56] confirmed that patients with APS are at high risk for post-transplant renal thrombosis. Within a group of 78 patients who received renal transplant, 6 had APS. Each of these 6 patients thrombosed their renal allografts within a week of the transplant. In contrast, the remaining 72 patients were all doing well 1 year post-transplant. More recently, isolated cases as well as retrospective and prospective studies have addressed the impact of aPL on renal transplantation. In 1999, a retrospective study in 96 patients with ESRD quantified the negative impact of aPL on renal transplantation [57]. In another multicenter study, 502 ESRD patients awaiting renal transplantation were screened for APS. The potential risks associated with APS were assessed, and strategies for therapeutic intervention were reviewed. The conclusion of this study was that patients with APS are at high risk of

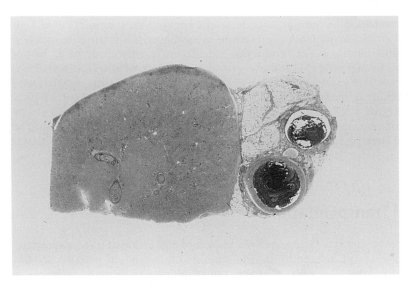

Figure 9.7. Fragment of the transplanted kidney in a female patient with PAPS. The whole vascular tree (from the intraparenchymatous vessels to the main intrarenal artery and vein) shows recent thrombotic occlusion (hematoxilin/eosin). 📖

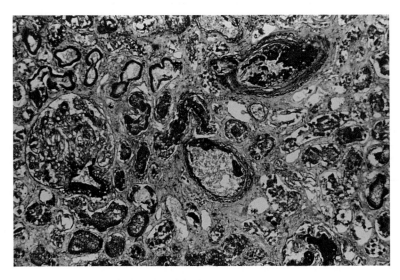

Figure 9.8. This micrograph belongs to the same kidney shown in Figure 7. There is generalized thrombosis of the microvasculature including glomerular capillaries, afferent arterioles, and interlobular arteries. Generalized necrosis without inflammatory cell infiltration is also observed (Masson). 📖

post-transplant renal thrombosis and that anticoagulant therapy could prevent this complication [58]. Interestingly, the same group of investigators reported their experience with 9 APS renal-transplant patients. Seven patients were treated with coumadin, whereas 2 were treated with heparin. Of the 2 patients treated with heparin, 1 had early allograft loss, whereas the other patient is doing well at 5 years post-transplant. Of the 7 patients treated with coumadin, 2 are doing well, 2 had early allograft loss, and the remaining 3 patients returned to dialysis after they were taken off the coumadin because of bleeding complications. The conclusions of this study are that anticoagulation therapy is beneficial to some but not all APS renal-transplant patients and, in addition, bleeding complications are a serious side effect in this setting [59]. With these data, one should question which patients with APS should be transplanted and which therapeutic intervention(s) could be used to avoid a catastrophic outcome.

Concluding Comments

In agreement with Nochy et al [36], we believe the TMA to be the characteristic nephropathy of PAPS. The lesion may have an abrupt or an insidious onset and may vary in severity and exent. All vascular structures of the kidney may be affected including glomeruli, arterioles, and parenchymatous arteries. Acute lesions as they heal give way to reparative fibrosis and focal atrophy. They are worsened by recurrent acute damage. In other cases, the lesion is insidious and slowly progressive, causing similar focal reparative fibrosis and tissue atrophy, arterial hypertension, and in some instances ESRD.

In patients with PAPS, renal involvement is probably underestimated. Hopefully, current knowledge of renal disease in APS will soon permeate all branches of internal medicine making possible an appropriate diagnosis.

References

1. Piette JC, Cacoub P, Wechsler B. Renal manifestations of the antiphospholipid syndrome. Semin Arthritis Rheum 1994;23:357–366.
2. Harris EN, Gharavi AE, Boey C, Mackworth-Young CG, Loizou Z, Hughes GR. Anticardiolipin antibodies: detection by radioimmunoassay and association with thrombosis in systemic lupus erythematosus. Lancet 1983;ii:1211–1214.
3. Alarcón-Segovia D, Cardiel MH, Reyes E. Antiphospholipid arterial vasculopathy. J Rheumatol 1989;16:762–767.
4. Ostuni PA, Lazzarin P, Pengo V, Ruffarti A, Schiavon F, Gambari P. Renal artey thrombosis and hypertension in a 13 year-old girl with antiphospholipid syndrome. Ann Rheum Dis 1990;49:184–187.
5. Hernández D, Domínguez ML, Díaz F, et al. Renal infarction in a severely hypertensive patient with lupus erythematosus and antiphospholipid antibodies. Nephron 1996;72:298–301.
6. Asherson RA, Noble GE, Hughes GRV. Hypertension, renal artery stenosis and "primary "antiphospholipid syndrome. J Rheumatol 1991;18:1413–1415.
7. Ames PRJ, Cianciaruso B, Vellizzi V, et al. Bilateral renal artery occlusion in a patient with primary antiphospholipid antibody syndrome: thrombosis, vasculitis or both? J Rheumatol 1992;19:1802–1806.
8. Rossi E, Sani C, Zini M, Casoli MC, Restori G. Anticardiolipin antibodies and renovascular hypertension. Ann Rheum Dis 1992;51:1180–1181.
9. Mandreoli M, Zuccala A, Zucchelli P. Fibromuscular dysplasia of the renal arteries associated with antiphospholipid auotantibodies: two case reports. Am J Kidney Dis 1992;20:500–503.
10. Mandreoli M, Zucchelli P. Renal vascular disease in patients with primary antiphospholipid antibodies. Nephrol Dial Transplant 1993;8:1277–1280.
11. Poux JM, Boudet R, Lacroix P, et al. Renal infarction and thrombosis of the infrarenal aorta in a 35 year-old man with primary antiphospholipid syndrome. Am J Kidney Dis 1996;27:721–725.

12. Godfrey T, Khamashta MA, Hughes GRV, Abbs I. Antiphospholipid syndrome and renal artery stenosis. Q J Med 2000;93:127–129.
13. Aizawa K, Nakamura T, Sumino H, et al. Renovascular hypertension observed in a patient with antiphospholipid-antibody syndrome. Jpn Circ J 2000;64:541–543.
14. Riccialdelli L, Arnaldi G, Giacchetti G, Pantanetti P, Mantero F. Hypertensin due to renal artery occlusion in a patient with antiphospholipid syndrome Am J Hypertens 2001;14:62–65.
15. Sonpal GM, Sharma A, Miller A.Primary antiphospholipid antibody syndrome, renal infarction and hypertension. J Rheumatol 1993;20:1221–1223.
16. Peribasekar S, Chawla K, Rosner F, Depestre M. Complete recovery from renal infarcts in a patient with mixed connective tissue disease. Am J Kidney Dis 1995;26:649–653.
17. Cacoub P, Wechsler B, Piette JC, et al. Malignant hypertension in antiphospholipid syndrome without overt lupus nephritis. Clin Exp Rheumatol 1993;11:479–485.
18. Hughes GRV, Harris EN, Gharavi AE. The anticardiolipin syndrome. J Rheumatol 1987;13:486–489.
19. Kant KS, PollaK VE, Weiss MA, Glueck HI, Miller MA, Hess EV. Glomerular thrombosis in systemic lupus erythematosus: Prevalence and significance. Medicine (Baltimore) 1981;60:71–86.
20. Glueck HI, Kant KS, Weiss MA, Pollak VE, Miller MA, Coots M. Thrombosis in systemic lupus erythematosus. Relation to the presence of circulating anticoagulants. Arch Intern Med 1985;145:1389–1395.
21. Leaker B, Cairley KF, Dowling J, Kincaid-Smith P. Lupus nephritis: clinical and pathological correlation. Q J Med 1987;238:163–179.
22. Cervera R, Khamashta MA, Font J, et al. Systemic lupus erythematosus: clinical and immunologic patterns of disease expression in a cohort of 1,000 patients. Medicine (Baltimore) 1993;72:113–124.
23. Miranda JM, García-Torres R, Jara LJ, Medina F, Cervera H, Fraga A. Renal biopsy in systemic lupus erythematosus: significance of glomerular thrombosis. Analysis of 108 cases. Lupus 1994;3:25–29.
24. Moroni G, Ventura D, Riva P, et al. Antiphospholipid antibodies are associated with an increased risk for chronic renal insufficiency in patients with lupus nephritis. Am J Kidney Dis 2004;43:28–36.
25. Bhathena DB, Sobel BJ, Migdal SD. Non-inflammatory renal microangiopathy of systemic lupus erythematosus. ("lupus vaculitis"). Am J Nephrol 1981;1:144–159.
26. Baldwin DS, Gluck MC, Lowenstein J, Gallo GR. Lupus nephritis: clinical course as related to morphological forms and their transitions. Am J Med 1997;62:12–30.
27. Kleinknecht D, Bobrie G, Meyer O, Noel LH, Callard P, Ramdane M. Recurrent thrombosis and renal vascular disease in patients with a lupus anticoagulant. Nephrol Dial Transplant 1989;4:854–858.
28. Kincaid-Smith P, Fairley KF, Kloss M. Lupus anticoagulant associated with renal thrombotic microangiopathy and pregnancy-related renal failure. Q J Med 1988;69:795–815.
29. Becquemont L, Thervet E, Rondeau E, Lacave R, Mougenot B, Sraer JD. Systemic and renal fibrinolytic activity in a patient with anticardiolipin syndrome and renal thrombotic microangiopathy. Am J Nephrol 1990;10:254–258.
30. D'Agati V, Kunis C, Williams G, Appel GB. Anti-cardiolipin antibody and renal disease: a report of three cases. J Am Soc Nephrol 1990;1:777–784.
31. Amigo MC, García-Torres R, Robles M, Bochiccio T, Reyes PA. Renal involvement in Primary Antiphospholipid Syndrome. J Rheumatol 1992;19:1181–1185.
32. Hughson MD, Nadasdy T, McCarty GA, Sholer C, Min K-W, Silva F. Renal thrombotic microangiopathy in patients with systemic lupus erythematosus and the antiphospholipid syndrome. Am J Kidney Dis 1992;20:150–158.
33. Lacueva J, Enríquez R, Cabezuelo JB, Arenas MD, Teruel A, González C. Acute renal failure as first clinical manifestation of the primary antiphospholipid syndrome. Nephron 1993;64:479–480.
34. Domrongkitchaiporn S, Cameron EC, Jetha N, Kassen BO, Sutton RAL. Renal microangiopathy in the primary antiphospholipid syndrome: a case report with literature review. Nephron 1994;68:128–132.
35. Karim MY, Alba P, Tungekar MF, et al. Hypertension as the presenting feature of the antiphospholipid syndrome. Lupus 2002;11:253–256.
36. Nochy D, Daugas E, Droz D, et al. The intrarenal vascular lesions associated with Primary Antiphospholipid Syndrome. J Am Soc Nephrol 1999;10:507–518.
37. Wilkowski M, Arroyo R, McCabe K. Glomerulonephritis in a patient with anticardiolipin antibody. Am J Kidney Dis 1990;15:184–186.
38. Almeshari K, Alfurayh O, Akhtar M. Primary antiphospholipid syndrome and self-limited renal vasculitis during pregnancy: case report and review of the literature. Am J Kidney Dis 1994;24:505–508.
39. Fakhouri F, Noel LH, Zuber J, et al. The expanding spectrum of renal diseases associated with antiphospholipid syndrome. Am J Kidney Dis 2003;41:1205–1211.

40. Branch DW, Rodgers GM. Induction of endothelial cell tissue factor activity by sera from patiens with antiphospholipid syndrome: a possible mechanism for thrombosis. Am J Obstet Gynecol 1993;168:206–210.
41. Asherson RA. The catastrophic antiphospholipid syndrome. J Rheumatol 1992;19:508–512.
42. Ramdane M, Gryman R, Bacques P, Callard P, Kleinknecht D. Ischémie rénale corticale, thrombose auriculaire droite et occlusion coronaire au cours d'un syndrome des anticorps antiphospholipides. Néphrologie 1989;10:189–193.
43. Pérez RE, McClendon JR, Lie JT. Primary antiphospholipid syndrome with multiorgan arterial and venous thromboses. J Rheumatol 1992;19:1289–1292.
44. Leaker B, Mc Gregor AO, Griffiths M, Snaiyh A, Neild GH, Isenber D. Insidious loss of renal function in patients with anticardiolipin antibodies and absence of overt nephritis. Br J Haematol 1991;30:422–425.
45. Asherson RA, Lanham JG, Hull RG, Boey ML, Gharavi AE, Hughes GR. Renal vein thrombosis in systemic lupus associated with the lupus anticoagulant. Clin Exp Rheumatol 1984;2:47–51.
46. Liano F, Mampaso F, García Martín F. Allograft membranous glomerulonephritis and renal vein thrombosis in a patient with a lupus anticoagulant factor. Nephrol Dial Transplant 1998;3:684–689.
47. Morgan RJ, Feneley CL. Renal vein thrombosis caused by primary antiphospholipid syndrome. Br J Urol 1994;74:807–808.
48. Asherson RA, Buchanan N, Baguley E, Hughes GRV. Postpartum bilateral renal vein thrombosis in the primary antiphospholipid syndrome. J Rheumatol 1993;20:874–876.
49. García-Martín F, De Arriba G, Carrascosa T, et al. Anticardiolipin antibodies and lupus anticoagulant in end stage renal disease. Nephrol Dial Transplant 1991;6:543–547.
50. Nied Prieto L, Suki NW. Frequent hemodyalisis graft thrombosis: association with antiphospholipid antibodies. Am J Kidney Dis 1994;23:587–590.
51. Brunet P, Aillaud MF, SanMarco M, et al. Antiphospholipids in hemodialysis patients: relationship between lupus anticoagulant and thrombosis. Kidney Int 1995;48:794–800.
52. Stone J, Amend W, Criswell L. Outcome of renal transplantation in SLE: 97 cyclosporine –era patients and matched controls. Arthritis Rheum 1997;27:17–26.
53. Radhakrishna J, Williams GS, Appel GB, Cohen DJ. Renal transplantation in anticardiolipin antibody-positive lupus erythematosus patients. Am J Kidney Dis 1994;23:286–289.
54. Mondragón-Ramírez G, Bochicchio T, García-Torres R, et al. Recurrent renal thrombotic angiopathy after kidney transplantation in two patients with primary antiphospholipid syndrome (PAPS). Clin Transplantation 1994;8:93–96.
55. Knight RJ, Schanzer H, Rand JH, Burrows L. Renal allograft thrombosis associated with the antiphospholipid antibody syndrome. Transplantation 1995;60:614–615.
56. Vaidya S, Wang CC, Gugliuzza C, Fish JC. Relative risk of post-transplant renal thrombosis in patients with antiphospholipid antibodies. Clin Transplant 1998;12:439–444.
57. Stone J, Amend W, Criswell L. Antiphospholipid antibody syndrome in renal transplantation: ocurrence of clinical events in 96 consecutive patients with systemic lupus erythematosus. Am J Kidney Dis 1999;34:1040–1047.
58. Vaidya S, Sellers R, Kimball P. Frequency, potential risk and therapeutic intervention in end-stage renal disease patients with antiphospholipid antibody syndrome: a multicenter study. Transplantation 2000;69:1348–1352.
59. Vaidya S, Gugliuzza K, Daller J. Efficacy of anticoagulation therapy in end-satge renal disease patients with antiphospholipid antibody syndrome. Transplantation 2004;77:1046–1049.

10 Systemic Hypertension in Antiphospholipid Syndrome

Shirish R. Sangle and David P. D'Cruz

Introduction

In the original description of antiphospholipid syndrome (APS), Hughes described a correlation between hypertension and livedo reticularis [1]. Although hypertension is a recognized and common feature, the literature on hypertension in APS is surprisingly scanty. The information so far aggregated is mainly based on the renal/reno-vascular pathology and associated hypertension in the patients with APS/antiphospholipid antibody (aPL). Indeed, it was suggested that the hypertension seen in these patients is exclusively renal in origin. Recent studies, however, do not support this concept as the only explanation for hypertension. In this chapter we have outlined the possible mechanisms of hypertension in the patients with aPL.

Prevalence of Hypertension in APS and aPL

APS is classified as a primary disorder, primary APS (PAPS), and secondary APS in association mostly with systemic lupus erythematosus (SLE). Nasssanov et al described a prevalence of hypertension up to 50% in her series of 28 primary APS patients [2]. To our knowledge there are no previous studies on the prevalence of hypertension in primary or secondary APS and /or aPL-positive patients. In our cohort of 600 patients with aPL, 173 (29%) had definite hypertension requiring therapy. The prevalence of hypertension in primary APS or aPL-positive patients was significantly high (44%) as compared to 27 % of secondary APS/aPL-positive patients. Our patients with APS/aPL were relatively young (median age, 46 years) and, in contrast with essential hypertension which is more common in Afro-Caribbean population, most of our patients (greater than 90%) were Caucasian women [3]. Other risk factors like diabetes and obesity/overweight were present in less than 10% of these hypertensive patients.

Aetio-pathogenesis

Renal and reno-vascular pathology remains the major cause of hypertension in APS. Thrombotic microangiopathy (TMA) affecting the kidney has been described

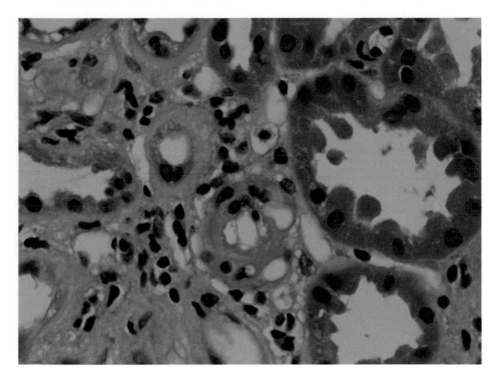

Figure 10.1. Renal thrombotic micro-angiopathy seen in a patient with APS and hypertension.

in both primary and secondary APS [4] and is reviewed in detail in elsewhere in this book. The renal impairment due to TMA ranges from mild to end-stage renal failure and mild-to-nephrotic range proteinuria is also not uncommon. Nochy et al described renal hypertension as a feature of APS in his patients with TMA [5]. The severity of hypertension varies from mild labile to severe accelerated hypertension. Hughes suggested that the labile hypertension seen in these patients fluctuates with the severity of livedo reticularis [1]. Malignant or accelerated hypertension is also not uncommonly observed in patients with TMA without any evidence of lupus nephritis (see Fig. 10.1) [6]. Previously, anecdotal reports of renal artery stenosis and hypertension in APS/aPL were reported and it is now an established fact that renal artery stenosis is more frequently seen in APS patients with uncontrolled hypertension compared to young aPL-negative hypertensives and healthy controls. The renal artery stenosis seen in these patients appears to be unique to this syndrome and is completely different from that seen in atherosclerotic disease and fibro-muscular dysplasia (see Fig. 10.2) [7]. Although the precise mechanisms are not clear, the renal artery occlusion may be secondary to thrombosis or possibly embolization from the cardiac valves. There is also a possibility that endothelin activation leading to smooth muscle hyperplasia and/or accelerated atherosclerosis are also pathogenic in renal artery stenosis. It may lead to renal infarcts and acute renal shut down has also been reported [8–10]. Obviously in patients with SLE, lupus nephritis may be an additional factor in the development of hypertension in patients with secondary APS.

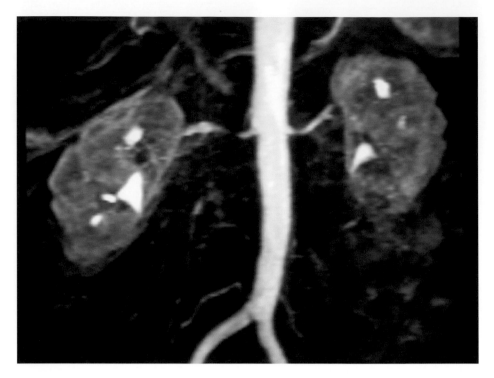

Figure 10.2. Magnetic resonance angiogram showing renal artery stenosis in a patient with APS and hypertension.

Interestingly, in our cohort of hypertensive APS patients approximately one third (66/173) had renal involvement either in the form of TMA, renal artery stenosis, and/or lupus nephritis. Other non-renal risk factors like obesity, patients receiving high-dose corticosteroids (prednisolone >7.5 mg/day), diabetes mellitus, and hyperlipidaemia were less than 10% of the patients [3]. This suggests that there are other non-renal factors responsible for developing hypertension in these relatively young patients.

There is an established link between accelerated atherosclerosis and aPL [11]. aPL interacts with oxidized low-density lipoprotein (LDL) and monocytes triggering the atherosclerotic process (12–14). Atsumi et al has demonstrated that endothelin levels are raised in arterial occlusion in patients with APS [15]. Our preliminary studies have shown that inflammatory markers, such as fasting insulin and high sensitivity C-reactive protein, are elevated in hypertensive APS patients in comparison to non-hypertensive APS and healthy controls. This data supports the idea that accelerated atherosclerosis may be a major factor in the development of hypertension in APS patients [16].

Livedo reticularis is a term used to explain the violaceous discoloration of the skin. Sneddon described the relationship between livedo reticularis and cerebrovascular accidents [17]. In addition, pregnancy morbidity, arterial and venous occlusions, and low platelets were also noticed in increased frequency in patients with livedo and aPL [18]. In our cohort, 80% of hypertensive patients were found to have livedo reticularis. Although the precise mechanisms are not clear, it is likely that the livedo may have a role in the development of hypertension.

Therapy

APS is a pro-thrombotic condition. Thrombotic insult to the kidneys in the form of TMA and renal artery stenosis are important causes of hypertension in patients with APS. This brings up the issue of anticoagulation in the patients with hypertension having renal involvement. Remondino et al described re-canalization of renal arteries in a hypertensive patient with bilateral renal artery stenosis with APS. At the end of 2 years on anticoagulation, she did not require hypotensive drugs to control the blood pressure [19]. Our preliminary studies indicate anticoagulation [target international normalized ratio (INR) 3.0–4.5] in patients with renal artery stenosis gives better control of blood pressure and may improve renal function [20]. Although there are no published data on the effect of anticoagulation in TMA, as with renal artery stenosis, we suggest that anticoagulation may be helpful in these patients.

In summary, hypertension in APS/aPL-positive patients may develop at a relatively young age and is more common in Caucasian women. The presence of aPL appears to be a distinct parameter associated with hypertension which may vary from mild labile hypertension to severe malignant hypertension. Hypertension seen in these patients is multi-factorial. Although renal pathology, renal artery stenosis, and/or TMA, are prominent etiological factors, the majority of the patients did not have any obvious renal pathology. The role of livedo reticularis certainly needs to be explored. Preliminary studies suggest anticoagulation may have a role in the management of hypertensive APS patients with renal artery stenosis.

References

1. Hughes G. Connective tissue diseases and the skin. The 1983 Prosser–White Oration. Clin Exp Dermatol 1984;9:535–544.
2. Nassonov EL, Karpov IuA, Alekberova ZS, et al. Arterial hypertension and the antiphospholipid syndrome Ter Arkh 1996;68:37–40.
3. Sangle S, D'Cruz D, Khamashta MA, Hughes GRV. Prevalence of hypertension in patients with Prevalence of hypertension in 600 patients with antiphospholipid syndrome. Arthritis Rheum 2003;48:S360.
4. Amigo MC, Garcia-Torres R, Robles M, Bochicchio T, Reyes PA. Renal involvement in primary antiphospholipid syndrome. J Rheumatol 1992;19:1181–1185.
5. Nochy D, Dougas E, Droz D, et al. The intra-renal vascular lesions associated with primary antiphospholipid syndrome. J Am Soc Nephrol 1999;10:507–518.
6. Cacoub P, Wechsler B, Piette JC, et al. Malignant hypertension in antiphospholipid syndrome without overt lupus nephritis. Clin Exp Rheumatol 1993;11:479–485.
7. Sangle S, D'Cruz D, Jan W, et al. Renal artery stenosis in antiphospholipid syndrome and hypertension. Ann Rheum Dis 2003;62:999–1002.
8. Ostuni PA, Lazzarin P, Pengo V, et al. Renal artery thrombosis and hypertension in a 13 year old girl with antiphospholipid syndrome. Ann Rheum Dis 1990;49:184–187.
9. Hernandez D, Domingues MI, Diaz F, et al. Renal infarction in a severely hypertensive patient with lupus erythematosus and antiphospholipid antibodies. Nephron 1996;72:298–301.
10. Rysava R, Zabka J, Peregrin JH, et al. Acute renal failure due to bilateral renal artery thrombosis associated with primary antiphospholipid syndrome. Nephrol Dial Transplant 1998;13:2645–2647.

11. George J, Shoenfeld Y. The antiphospholipid "Hughes syndrome" syndrome: a cross roads of autoimmunity and atherosclerosis. Lupus 1997;6:559–560.
12. Harats D, George J, Levy Y, Khamashta MA, Hughes GR, Shoenfeld Y. Atheroma: links with antiphospholipid antibodies, Hughes syndrome and lupus. QJM 1999;92:57–59.
13. Vaarala O, Alfthan G, Jauhiainen M, Leirisalo-Repo M, Aho KND, Palosuo T. Cross reaction between antibodies to oxidized low-density lipoprotein and to cardiolipin in systemic lupus erythematosus. Lancet 1993;ii:923–925.
14. Hasunuma Y, Matsura E, Makita Z, Katahira T, Nishi S, Koike T. Involvement of ß2 glycoprotein I and anticardiolipin antibodies in oxidatively modified low density lipoprotein uptake by macrophages. Clin Exp Immunol 1997;107:569–574.
15. Atsumi T, Khamashta MA, Haworth RS, et al. Arterial disease and thrombosis in the antiphospholipid syndrome, a pathogenic role for Endothelin 1. Arthritis Rheum 1998;41:800–807.
16. Horwood N, Sangle S, D'Cruz D, Khamashta M, Abbs I, Hughes GRV. Peripheral arterial disease in antiphospholipid syndrome and renal artery stenosis. Rheumatology 2004;43:104.
17. Sneddon IB. Cerebrovascular lesions and livedo reticularis. Br J Dermatol 1965;77:180–185.
18. Englert H, Loizou S, Derue G, Walport M, Hughes GRV. Clinical and immunological features of livedo reticularis in lupus: a case-control study. Am J Med 1989;87:408–410.
19. Remondino GI, Mysler E, Pissano MN, et al. A reversible bilateral renal artery stenosis in association with antiphospholipid syndrome. Lupus 2000;9:65–67.
20. Sangle S, D'Cruz D, Khamashta MA, Hughes GRV. Renal artery stenosis in hypertensive patients with antiphospholipid syndrome: the effects of anticoagulation. Arthritis Rheum 2003;43:S359.

11 Pulmonary Hypertension and Antiphospholipid Antibodies

Jean-Charles Piette and Beverley J. Hunt

Pulmonary hypertension (PH) is defined as a mean pulmonary artery pressure greater than 25 mm Hg [1, 2]. After many years of debate, it is now agreed that PH can be classified according to three features: anatomical localization of vascular disorder, presence or not of any associated disease, and severity, with the magnitude of reduction of cardiac output as the best predictor survival [1] (Table 11.1). The term *primary pulmonary hypertension* (PPH) has been used extensively in literature, leading to some confusion. PPH usually means that diverse mechanisms have been ruled out, especially chronic causes of hypoxia, left ventricular failure, and repeated pulmonary embolism, and that plexogenic arteriopathy can be found on histological lung examination. PPH is a rare but life-threatening condition, whose pathophysiology has remained mysterious for a while. Advances have suggested the importance of diverse factors, such as: imbalance in vasoactive agents, that is, deficiency of nitric oxide and prostacyclin synthase versus overexpression of endothelin-1; vascular endothelial growth factor (VEGF) expression; K+ channel anomalies; genetic susceptibility; and, last but not least, clonal expansion of endothelial cells in primary but not secondary PH [2–6]. Though PPH frequently remains "unexplained," several comorbid conditions have been identified as possible etiologies, with human immunodeficiency virus (HIV) infection, prior use of anorectic agents, and connective tissue diseases (CTD) as leaders [2, 7] (Table 11.1). Whatever the "cause," severe PH may be complicated by (a) superimposed in situ

Table 11.1. Classification of pulmonary hypertension.

Arterial pulmonary hypertension (changes in precapillary arteries)
"Primary" arterial PH
Secondary arterial PH (scleroderma, MCTD and other CTD, congenital heart disease, portal hypertension, HIV, anorectic agents, cocaine, etc.)
Postcapillary pulmonary hypertension (changes in pulmonary veins)
Left-sided heart failure
Rarely: pulmonary veno-occlusive disease, pulmonary hemangiomatosis, chronic Sclerosing mediastinitis, congenital pulmonary vein anomaly
Proximal pulmonary artery involvement
Mainly: chronic thromboembolic PH
Rarely: metastatic neoplasm, parasites, miscellaneous emboli
Extrinsic vascular compression
Secondary to all chronic causes of hypoxia

thromboses affecting distal pulmonary arteries [8] and, (b) the development of plexogenic lesions, both thought to occur as a consequence of chronic endothelial injury [1, 6]. More recently, infection with human herpes virus 8 has been implicated as having a pathogenic role in the development of plexiform lesions in PPH, for a study showed the presence of the virus in plexiform lesions [9].

Mutations in the bone morphogenic protein receptor type 2 (BMPR2) have now been linked to familiar cases of PPH [10]. BMPR2 is an interesting protein to be implicated so strongly in the pathogenesis of the disease. It is a cell surface receptor belonging to the superfamily of receptors for ligands of the transforming growth factors (TGF) β family. How might the BMPR2 mutations account for the disease? PPH [10] is a disease of vascular remodeling per excellence and BMPs 2 and 7 have been shown to inhibit vascular smooth muscle cell proliferation and to induce apoptosis in some cell types in culture. It is thus tempting to suggest that PPH arises out of an impairment of control of cellular proliferation. The molecular defects in common non-familial PPH are unknown. Recent studies suggest that these forms of PPH are linked by defects in the signaling pathways involving angiopoietin-1 TIE2, BMPR1A, and BMPR2 [11], fitting in with the hypothesis that there may be impaired cellular proliferation in PPH.

This chapter will give a brief overview of PH within antiphospholipid syndrome (APS), question the possible role of antiphospholipid antibodies (aPL) in the pathophysiology of "unexplained" PPH and thromboembolic pulmonary hypertension, and then discuss practical aspects of the management.

Pulmonary Hypertension and APS

APS mainly occurs either in association with systemic lupus erythematosus (SLE), or as a primary disorder named primary APS [12]. Within these two subsets, the prevalence of PH has been estimated 1.8% and 3.5%, respectively, in a multicenter study [13]. In two other large studies performed on SLE patients, the prevalence of PH was 2% [14] and 5% [15]. Within APS, PH may result from various causes listed in Table 11.2 [16, 17].

Table 11.2. Pulmonary hypertension within APS. 📖

APS related
    Pulmonary embolism (acute/chronic)
    Left-sided heart failure
    Heart valve dysfunction
    Myocardial infarction
    Myocardiopathy
    "Primary" pulmonary hypertension (?)
    Miscellaneous (rare)
    Portal hypertension
    Pulmonary veno-occlusive disease

Not directly APS-related
    Chest disorder leading to chronic hypoxia
    Mainly fibrosing alveolitis
    Coincidental

Pulmonary embolism is assumed to be the leading cause of PH in APS. Due to the frequent mixing of the terms pulmonary embolism with deep venous thrombosis in articles, its frequency cannot be precisely determined, but it ranged from 17% to 33% in three non-purely obstetrical APS series [13, 18, 19], and seemed to be similar in SLE-related and in primary APS: 21% versus 24%, respectively [13]. Although "catastrophic" APS is characterized by widespread microvascular involvement, 8 of 50 patients had multiple pulmonary emboli in a recent series [20]. Pulmonary embolism approximately occurs in one third of APS patients with deep venous thrombosis [21]. It may originate from nearly all sites, including inferior vena cava and/or renal vein thrombosis [22], tricuspid valve vegetations [23], or right-sided intracardiac thrombosis [24, 25]. The latter site underlines the need to systematically perform an echocardiography in all patients with APS and pulmonary embolism. The presence of anticardiolipin antibodies (aCL) has been shown to be associated with the further occurrence of deep venous thrombosis/pulmonary embolism in a cohort of healthy males [26]. Among patients with a first episode of "idiopathic" venous thromboembolism, the presence of aCL [27] or of a lupus anticoagulant (LA) [28] was significantly associated with recurrences. Permanent PH may be found in patients with SLE-related or primary APS and pulmonary embolism [15, 29–31], sometimes as the presenting manifestation [32], but its occurrence has not yet been quantified by prospective studies. It is probably higher than the estimated 0.1% prevalence seen after acute pulmonary embolism in the general population [30]. Fatalities may result from embolic recurrences [19, 29, 33], and pulmonary embolism was responsible for 4% of 222 deaths in a collaborative study on SLE [34].

The diverse causes of left-sided heart failure leading to PH being discussed in another part of this book will be briefly summarized. Heart valve dysfunction is a frequent feature of SLE-related and primary APS [35–37]. It mainly affects the mitral, then the aortic valve, and features as valve incompetence or incompetence plus stenosis, rarely as stenosis alone. Echocardiogram usually shows diffuse valve thickening and rigidity, whereas nodular masses are less frequent. These valve lesions may lead over years to significant hemodynamic intolerance [38], and though frank improvement has been reported in some cases under steroid treatment [39], surgical replacement or repair may be necessary [38, 40]. Despite the recent finding of subendothelial aCL deposits [37], the pathophysiology of these valve lesions remains poorly understood. Myocardial infarction is a well-established manifestation of the APS [41], and the presence of antiphospholipid antibodies (aPL) must be looked for, especially when it occurs in patients aged less than 50 years. Diffuse myocardiopathy thought to result from distal microthromboses may occur, especially within "catastrophic" APS [20, 42, 43]. Myocardial dysfunction may also be the consequence of systemic hypertension resulting from thrombosis affecting renal vessels.

Other mechanisms leading to PH, such as portal hypertension [44] or pulmonary veno-occlusive disease [45], are occasionally encountered within APS.

There has been increased interest recently in chronic thromboembolic pulmonary hypertension (CTPH), for it was considered a relatively rare complication of pulmonary embolism but was associated with considerable morbidity and mortality. A paper by Pengo et al has suggested that it is in fact a relatively common, serious complication of pulmonary embolism, with cumulative incidences of symptomatic chronic thromboembolic pulmonary hypertension being 1% (95%

confidence interval (CI), 0.0–2.4) at 6 months, 3.1% (95% CI, 0.7–5.5) at 1 year, and 3.8% (95% CI, 1.1–6.5) at 2 years. The risks were greatest for those with more than one episode of pulmonary embolism, younger age, a larger perfusion defect, and idiopathic pulmonary embolism at presentation [46]. In patients with CTPH, thromboemboli do not resolve, but rather form endothelialized, fibrotic obstructions of the pulmonary vascular bed, including the major branches. aPL are detected in 30% of such patients [47]. Making an accurate diagnosis of CTPH requires collaboration among experienced cardiologists, respiratory physicians, cardiothoracic surgeons, and intensive care physicians. There are about 20 CTPH centers worldwide, where these patients are treated surgically. Jamieson pioneered the original technique from San Diego, where they have now treated 2000 patients surgically [48]. Pulmonary thromboendarterectomy is a classical bilateral endarterectomy in which the thrombus and adjacent medial layer are carefully dissected with dedicated surgical instruments. This is now the procedure of choice for CTPH, if available, although the perioperative mortality is not inconsiderable. It can result in an improvement of symptoms and reduction in pulmonary artery pressure that is unprecedented, including vasodilators, lung transplantation, balloon atrial septostomy, and balloon pulmonary angioplasty. One author's experience (BJH) with a patient with PAPS who underwent this operation, reduced the pulmonary artery pressure from over 100 mm Hg to normal levels and a change from constant dyspnoea and right heart failure to normality.

"Primary" Pulmonary Hypertension and aPL

Data concerning the "heart of the topic" remain scarce. PH is known for years to occur in association with CTD, mainly mixed connective tissue disease (MCTD) and scleroderma, especially in the Calcinosis, Raynaud's, esophageal dysmotility, sclerodactyly, telangiectasia (CREST) variety [2]. Within this setting, PH may complicate the course of chronic interstitial lung disease leading to pulmonary fibrosis, or occur in its absence, then featuring as "primary" PH. aCL are frequently found in these diverse CTD [49], but interestingly it has been recently shown that the only autoantibodies that were specifically associated with PH-related deaths in a long-term study of patients with MCTD were IgG aCL [50]. None of these aCL-positive patients had thromboembolic manifestations. However, in this study, pulmonary involvement was statistically associated with PH, though the 4 autopsied patients had little or no interstitial fibrosis [50].

Concerning SLE, the relationship between PH and aPL was first suspected as early as 1983 [51]. The same group reported in 1990 an extended study on 24 patients with PH, of whom 22 had SLE [15]. Two had thromboembolic PH and 1 with SLE–scleroderma overlap had pulmonary fibrosis. In the others, PH was said to resemble PPH, that is, "with clear lung fields and no overt clinical evidence of pulmonary thromboembolism," and it was prudently suggested that the higher than expected prevalence of aPL (68%) observed in the whole group might be relevant to the pathogenesis of SLE-related PH [15]. Raynaud's phenomenon was also highly prevalent among these 24 patients. However, due to the absence of systematically performed pulmonary angiograms/nuclear perfusion scans, this study carries several limitations concerning the classification of PH as "primary" in most of patients. Subsequent data came from the Mexican group directed by Alarcon-Segovia. In a prospective analysis of 500 consecutive patients with SLE, these authors reported that PH was statistically associated with the presence of IgA aCL above 2 standard deviations (SD), whereas results were neither significant for higher IgA titers nor for IgG, IgM, or any aCL isotype [52]. An extended study performed on 667 SLE patients confirmed the association of PH with aPL, but the criteria used were not precisely defined [14]. Subsequently, Alarcon-Segovia proposed to delete PH and transverse myelitis from criteria for "definite" APS, due to their rare occurrence [53]. Sturfelt et al also found an increased frequency of aCL in SLE patients with mild HT [54]. On the other hand, Petri et al found no association between aPL and PH in a short series of 60 patients with SLE [55], and Miyata et al were unable to correlate aCL titer and the mean pulmonary artery pressure in 10 SLE patients, whereas a significant correlation was present in 12 patients with MCTD [56]. PH has also been reported in patients with aPL and either Sjögren syndrome [57] or anticentromere antibodies [58], but in both cases, it was probably due to thromboembolism.

Several cases of PPH complicating primary APS have been described or mentioned [18, 59–62]. Despite the anatomical demonstration of plexogenic lesions [59], the diagnosis of PPH has been debated in the patient reported by Luchi et al, due to the coexistence of a large thrombus in the right main pulmonary artery [30]. In a multicenter study of 70 patients with primary APS, PH was present in 2, thromboembolic in 1 and suggestive of PPH in the other, to compare with 18 patients in the series who had pulmonary embolism [18].

The alternative way to investigate the potential role of aPL in PPH is to study aPL prevalence in large series of consecutive patients with "unexplained" PPH. Similar studies have shown that diverse autoantibodies, namely antinuclear [62] and anti-Ku antibodies [63] are frequently found in this setting. In the group of 30 patients with idiopathic (without SLE) PPH studied by Asherson et al, 4 had aPL, that is, LA in 2 and low IgG aCL in 3 [15]. None of the 31 patients with PPH reported by Isern et al had aCL above mean + 5 SD [63]. Martinuzzo et al recently studied 54 consecutive patients with PH: 23 with primary PH, 20 with secondary PH (mainly congenital heart diseases, CTD, or pulmonary disorders), and 11 with CTph [64]. The latter group was characterized by a strikingly higher prevalence of LA and IgG antibodies directed to cardiolipin, β_2-glycoprotein I, and prothrombin, whereas both primary and secondary PH patients usually had negative or low-positive tests. Similarly, in a recent study, high aPL were much more prevalent in thromboembolic PH compared to PPH [65]. Among 216 patients referred for a possible surgical treatment of CTph, Auger et al found positive LA in 10.6%, of whom none had SLE, but aCL were not determined [66]. Conversely, Karmochkine et al reported the presence of aPL in 4 of 9 patients with "unexplained" PPH, but also in 7 of 29 patients with precapillary PH secondary to diverse causes, whereas the 8 patients with postcapillary PH were all aPL negative [67]. This raises the central question of the true nature of aPL, that is, cause or consequence? Keeping in mind that all forms of severe PH may be complicated by superimposed in situ thromboses [8], a risk exists to categorize as Definite APS [68] some patients with PH due to other causes. This theoretical risk is illustrated by the example of PH associated with HIV infection, given that aCL of questionable pathogenic significance are frequently present in this condition [69].

Finally, the possible role of aPL in the pathophysiology of "unexplained" PPH remains unclear to date. Consideration of the mechanisms potentially involved are therefore highly speculative. It seems unlikely that the "classical" thrombogenic properties of aPL are initially involved in the diffuse process leading to PPH. Other explanations could imply a role for activated platelets or for an interaction between aPL and endothelial cells of pulmonary arteries, leading to vascular remodeling. Similar mechanisms may also be proposed to explain the development of aPL-associated heart valve thickening. The occurrence of these peculiar lesions in some but not all patients might result from a double heterogeneity, that is, that of aPL and of endothelial cells. In vitro studies using aPL from patients with distinct vascular manifestations and focusing on the interaction of aPL with endothelial cells originated from various sites might help to solve this question. Another point that deserves comment is the possible implication of endothelin-1, a peptide known to induce a strong vasoconstriction and to stimulate the proliferation of vascular muscle cells. High levels of endothelin-1 have been found on the one hand in both plasma and lung tissue of patients with PPH [70], and on the other hand, in plasma of APS patients with systemic arterial thrombosis [71]. It would then be interesting to study plasma endothelin-1 levels of patients with "unexplained" PPH, according to the presence, or not, of aPL. Beside aPL but in keeping with endothelin-1, anti-endothelial cell antibodies might also be involved in the pathogenesis of SLE-associated non-thromboembolic PH [72, 73].

Practical Management

Evaluation includes careful personal and familial history, complete physical examination, electrocardiogram, chest X-ray, transesophageal echocardiogram, pulmonary function tests with arterial blood gas tension and additional sleep studies when sleep apnea may be suspected, routine blood tests, liver function tests, complete autoantibody screening including aPL determination, HIV serology, and either pulmonary angiogram or helicoidal chest computerized tomography scan that should be preferred to ventilation–perfusion isotopic scan. It should be emphasized that CTph may masquerade as PPH until appropriate imaging studies, as attested by our experience of several patients referred for severe PPH and possible heart–lung transplantation, who in fact had thromboembolic PH. Within the peculiar setting of aPL-related manifestations, the need to look for malignancies needs to be underlined. Indeed, cancer may present not only as recurrent venous thromboembolic events [74] sometimes associated with aPL [75–77], but can also masquerade as PPH; the correct diagnosis of pulmonary tumor microembolism being only made at necropsy [78]. In this respect, de novo occurrence of aPL-related events should be regarded cautiously in patients aged 60 or more [79].

Treatment options are conditioned by the mechanism and cause of PH. However, chronic anticoagulation is needed in all cases, at least to prevent the development of superimposed thrombosis [3], and this seems especially true for patients with aPL.

When PH results from chronic thromboembolism, inferior vena cava filter may be recommended [66], and successful thromboenarterectomy has been performed in some patients with very severe disease [30, 31, 66]. Within this setting, Auger et al have reported a high incidence of thrombocytopenia induced by unfractionated heparin in LA-positive patients [66].

Concerning aPL-related PPH, given the absence of definite management guidelines, the following regimens are those used in "unexplained" or CTD-associated PPH. Beside chronic anticoagulation and oxygen administration, patients are given vasodilators according to the results of acute drug testing. Calcium channel blockers may be sufficient in moderate forms, whereas continuous intravenous prostacyclin infusion using a pump is needed in severe cases, where it frequently provides a substantial benefit but may require sustained upward dosage adjustment [3, 60, 80]. The initiation of this complex and costly procedure is restricted to experienced centers. Monthly cyclophosphamide infusions have been claimed to be beneficial in a few reports of CTD-associated PPH [81, 82]. Diverse surgical procedures are discussed in advanced forms refractory to medical regimens. Atrial septectomy is used by several teams [3]. Transplantation, either double-lung, single lung, or heart–lung, may cure the disease [3, 15], but mortality remains high and donors scarce.

A better understanding of PPH pathophysiology and the development of new drugs are both needed to improve the prognosis of this rare disorder.

References

1. Gosney JR. Pulmonary hypertension. In: Halliday, Hunt, Poston, Schachter, eds. An introduction to vascular biology. Cambridge: Cambridge University Press; 1998:100–111.
2. Galie N, Manes A, Uguccioni L, et al. Primary pulmonary hypertension: insights into pathogenesis from epidemiology. Chest 1998;114(suppl 3):184S–194S.
3. Haworth SG. Primary pulmonary hypertension. J R Coll Physicians Lond 1998;32:187–190.
4. Lee SD, Shroyer KR, Markham NE, Cool CD, Voelkel NF, Tuder RM. Monoclonal endothelial cell proliferation is present in primary but not secondary pulmonary hypertension. J Clin Invest 1998;101:927–934.
5. Mecham RP. Conference summary: biology and pathobiology of the lung circulation. Chest 1998;114(suppl 3):106S–111S.
6. Voelkel NF, Cool C, Lee SD, Wright L, Geraci MW, Tuder RM. Primary pulmonary hypertension between inflammation and cancer. Chest 1998;114(suppl 3):225S–230S.
7. Fishman AP. Etiology and pathogenesis of primary pulmonary hypertension: a perspective. Chest 1998;114(suppl 3):242S–247S.
8. Chaouat A, Weitzenblum E, Higenbottam T. The role of thrombosis in severe pulmonary hypertension. Eur Respir J 1996;9:356–363.
9. Cool CD, Rai PR, Yeager ME, et al. Expression of human herpsevirus 8 in primary pulmonary hypertension. N Engl J Med 2003;349:1113–1122.
10. The International PPH Consortium. Heterozygous germline mutations in BMPR2, encoding a TGF-β receptor, cause familia primary pulmonary hypertension. Nat Genet 2000;26:81–84.
11. Du L, Sullivan CC, Chu D, et al. Signaling molecules in nonfamilial pulmonary hypertension. N Engl J Med 2003;348:500–509.
12. Piette JC. 1996 diagnostic and classification criteria for the antiphospholipid/cofactors syndrome: a "mission impossible"? Lupus 1996;5:354–363.
13. Vianna JL, Khamashta MA, Ordi-Ros J, et al. Comparison of the primary and secondary antiphospholipid syndrome: a European multicenter study of 114 patients. Am J Med 1994;96:3–9.
14. Alarcon-Segovia D, Perez-Vazquez ME, Villa AR, Drenkard C, Cabiedes J. Preliminary classification criteria for the antiphospholipid syndrome within systemic lupus erythematosus. Semin Arthritis Rheum 1992;21:275–286.
15. Asherson RA, Higenbottam TW, Dinh Xuan AT, Khamashta MA, Hughes GRV. Pulmonary hypertension in a lupus clinic: experience with twenty-four patients. J Rheumatol 1990;17:1292–1298.
16. Koike T, Tsutsumi A. Pulmonary hypertension and the antiphospholipid syndrome. Intern Med 1995;34:938.
17. Kunieda T. Antiphospholipid syndrome and pulmonary hypertension. Intern Med 1996;35:842–843.
18. Asherson RA, Khamashta MA, Ordi-Ros J, et al. The "primary" antiphospholipid syndrome: major clinical and serological features. Medicine (Baltimore) 1989;68:366–374.

19. Font J, Lopez-Soto A, Cervera R, et al. The "primary" antiphospholipid syndrome: antiphospholipid antibody pattern and clinical features of a series of 23 patients. Autoimmunity 1991;9:69–75.
20. Asherson RA, Cervera R, Piette JC, et al. "Catastrophic" antiphospholipid syndrome: clinical and laboratory features of 50 patients. Medicine (Baltimore) 1998;77:195–207.
21. Cervera R, Garcia-Carrasco M, Asherson RA. Pulmonary manifestations in the antiphospholipid syndrome. In: Asherson RA, Cervera R, Piette JC, Shoenfeld Y, eds. The antiphospholipid syndrome. Boca Raton: CRC Press; 1996:161–167.
22. Mintz G, Acevedo-Vazquez E, Guttierrez-Espinosa G, Avelar-Garnica F. Renal vein thrombosis and inferior vena cava thrombosis in systemic lupus erythematosus. Arthritis Rheum 1984;27:539–544.
23. Brucato A, Baudo F, Barberis M, et al. Pulmonary hypertension secondary to thrombosis of the pulmonary vessels in a patient with the primary antiphospholipid syndrome. J Rheumatol 1994;21:942–944.
24. Day SM, Rosenzweig BP, Kronzon I. Transesophageal echocardiographic diagnosis of right atrial thrombi associated with the antiphospholipid syndrome. J Am Soc Echocardiogr 1995;8:937–940.
25. O'Hickey S, Skinner C, Beattie J. Life-threatening right ventricular thrombosis in association with phospholipid antibodies. Br Heart J 1993;70:279–281.
26. Ginsburg KS, Liang MH, Newcomer L, et al. Anticardiolipin antibodies and the risk for ischemic stroke and venous thrombosis. Ann Intern Med 1992;117:997–1002.
27. Schulman S, Svenungsson E, Granqvist S, and the Duration of Anticoagulation Study Group. Anticardiolipin antibodies predict early recurrence of thromboembolism and death among patients with venous thromboembolism following anticoagulant therapy. Am J Med 1998;104:332–338.
28. Kearon C, Gent M, Hirsh J, et al. A Comparison of three months of anticoagulation with extended anticoagulation for a first episode of idiopathic venous thromboembolism. N Engl J Med 1999;340:901–907.
29. Anderson NE, Ali MR. The lupus anticoagulant, pulmonary thromboembolism, and fatal pulmonary hypertension. Ann Rheum Dis 1984;43:760–763.
30. Sandoval J, Amigo MC, Barragan R, et al. Primary antiphospholipid syndrome presenting as chronic thromboembolic pulmonary hypertension. Treatment with thromboendarterectomy. J Rheumatol 1996;23:772–775.
31. Ando M, Takamoto S, Okita Y, et al. Operation for chronic pulmonary thromboembolism accompanied by thrombophilia in 8 patients. Ann Thorac Surg 1998;66:1919–1924.
32. Miyashita Y, Koike H, Misawa A, Shimizu H, Yoshida K, Yasutomi T. Asymptomatic pulmonary hypertension complicated with antiphospholipid syndrome case. Intern Med 1996;35:912–915.
33. Jeffrey PJ, Asherson RA, Rees PJ. Recurrent deep vein thrombosis, thromboembolic pulmonary hypertension and the "primary" antiphospholipid syndrome. Clin Exp Rheumatol 1989;7:567–569.
34. Rosner S, Ginzler EM, Diamond HS, et al. A multicenter study of outcome in systemic lupus erythematosus. II. Causes of death. Arthritis Rheum 1982;25:612–617.
35. Khamashta MA, Cervera R, Asherson RA, et al. Association of antibodies against phospholipids with heart valve disease in systemic lupus erythematosus. Lancet 1990;335:1541–1544.
36. Cervera R, Khamashta MA, Font J, et al. High prevalence of significant heart valve lesions in patients with the "primary" antiphospholipid syndrome. Lupus 1991;1:43–47.
37. Hojnik M, George J, Ziporen L, Shoenfeld Y. Heart valve involvement (Libman–Sacks endocarditis) in the antiphospholipid syndrome. Circulation 1996;93:1579–1587.
38. Roldan CA, Shively BK, Crawford MH. An echocardiographic study of valvular heart disease associated with systemic lupus erythematosus. N Engl J Med 1996;335:1424–1430.
39. Nesher G, Ilany J, Rosenmann D, Abraham AS. Valvular dysfunction in antiphospholipid syndrome: prevalence, clinical features, and treatment. Semin Arthritis Rheum 1997;27:27–35.
40. Piette JC, Amoura Z, Papo T. Valvular heart disease and systemic lupus erythematosus [letter]. N Engl J Med 1997;336:1324.
41. Asherson RA, Khamashta MA, Baguley E, Oakley CM, Rowell NR, Hughes GRV. Myocardial infarction and antiphospholipid antibodies in SLE and related disorders. Q J Med 1989;73:1103–1115.
42. Kattwinkel N, Villanueva AG, Labib SB, et al. Myocardial infarction caused by cardiac microvasculopathy in a patient with the primary antiphospholipid syndrome. Ann Intern Med 1992;116:974–976.
43. Nihoyannopoulos P, Gomez PM, Joshi J, Loizou S, Walport MJ, Oakley CM. Cardiac abnormalities in systemic lupus erythematosus: association with raised anticardiolipin antibodies. Circulation 1990;82:369–375.
44. De Clerck LS, Michielsen PP, Ramael MR, et al. Portal and pulmonary vessel thrombosis associated with systemic lupus erythematosus and anticardiolipin antibodies. J Rheumatol 1991;18:1919–1921.

45. Hussein A, Trowitzsch E, Brockmann M. Pulmonary veno-occlusive disease, antiphospholipid antibody and pulmonary hypertension in an adolescent. Klin Padiatr 1999;211:92–95.
46. Pengo V, Lensing AWA, Prins MH, et al. Incidence of chronic thromboembolic pulmonary hypertension after pulmonary embolism. N Engl J Med 2004;350:2257–2264.
47. Fedullo PF, Auger WR, Kerr KM, Rubin LJ. Chronic thromboembolic pulmonary hypertension. N Engl J Med 2001;345:1465–1472.
48. Jamieson SW, Kapelanski DP, Sakakibara N, et al. Pulmonary endarterectomy: experience and lessons learned in 1,500 cases. Ann Thorac Surg 2003;76:1457–1464.
49. Merkel PA, Chang YC, Pierangeli SS, Convery K, Harris EN, Polisson RP. The prevalence and clinical associations of anticardiolipin antibodies in a large inception cohort of patients with connective tissue diseases. Am J Med 1996;101:576–583.
50. Burdt MA, Hoffman RW, Deutscher SL, Wang GS, Johnson JC, Sharp GC. Long-term outcome in mixed connective tissue disease: longitudinal clinical and serologic findings. Arthritis Rheum 1999;42:899–909.
51. Asherson RA, Mackworth-Young CG, Boey ML, et al. Pulmonary hypertension in systemic lupus erythematosus. Br Med J 1983;287:1024–1025.
52. Alarcon-Segovia D, Deleze M, Oria CV, et al. Antiphospholipid antibodies and the antiphospholipid syndrome in systemic lupus erythematosus. A prospective analysis of 500 consecutive patients. Medicine (Baltimore) 1989;68:353–365.
53. Alarcon-Segovia D. Clinical manifestations of the antiphospholipid syndrome. J Rheumatol 1992;19:1778–1781.
54. Sturfelt G, Eskilsson J, Nived O, Truedsson L, Valind S. Cardiovascular disease in systemic lupus erythematosus. A study of 75 patients from a defined population. Medicine (Baltimore) 1992;71:216–223.
55. Petri M, Rheinschmidt M, Whiting-O'Keefe Q, Hellmann D, Corash L. The frequency of lupus anticoagulant in systemic lupus erythematosus. A study of sixty consecutive patients by activated partial thromboplastin time, Russell viper venom time, and anticardiolipin antibody level. Ann Intern Med 1987;106:524–531.
56. Miyata M, Suzuki K, Sakuma F, et al. Anticardiolipin antibodies are associated with pulmonary hypertension in patients with mixed connective tissue disease or systemic lupus erythematosus. Int Arch Allergy Immunol 1993;100:351–354.
57. Biyajima S, Osada T, Daidoji H, et al. Pulmonary hypertension and antiphospholipid antibody in a patient with Sjögren's syndrome. Intern Med 1994;33:768–772.
58. Tilley S, Newman J, Thomas A. Antiphospholipid and anticentromere antibodies occurring together in a patient with pulmonary hypertension. Tenn Med 1996;89:166–168.
59. Luchi ME, Asherson RA, Lahita RG. Primary idiopathic pulmonary hypertension complicated by pulmonary arterial thrombosis. Association with antiphospholipid antibodies. Arthritis Rheum 1992;35:700–705.
60. De la Mata J, Gomez-Sanchez MA, Aranzana M, Gomez-Reino JJ. Long-term iloprost infusion therapy for severe pulmonary hypertension in patients with connective tissue diseases. Arthritis Rheum 1994;37:1528–1533.
61. Nagai H, Yasuma K, Katsuki T, et al. Primary antiphospholipid syndrome and pulmonary hypertension with prolonged survival. A case report. Angiology 1997;48:183–187.
62. Rich S, Kieras K, Hart K, Groves BM, Stobo JD, Brundage BH. Antinuclear antibodies in primary pulmonary hypertension. J Am Coll Cardiol 1986;8:1307–1311.
63. Isern RA, Yaneva M, Weiner E, et al. Autoantibodies in patients with primary pulmonary hypertension: association with anti-Ku. Am J Med 1992;93:307–312.
64. Martinuzzo ME, Pombo G, Forastiero RR, Cerrato GS, Colorio CC, Carreras LO. Lupus anticoagulant, high levels of anticardiolipin, and anti-beta2-glycoprotein I antibodies are associated with chronic thromboembolic pulmonary hypertension. J Rheumatol 1998;25:1313–1319.
65. Wolf M, Boyer-Neumann C, Parent F, et al. Thrombotic risk factors in pulmonary hypertension. Eur Respir J 2000;15:395–399.
66. Auger WR, Permpikul P, Moser KM. Lupus anticoagulant, heparin use, and thrombocytopenia in patients with chronic thromboembolic pulmonary hypertension: a preliminary report. Am J Med 1995;99:392–396.
67. Karmochkine M, Cacoub P, Dorent R, et al. High prevalence of antiphospholipid antibodies in precapillary pulmonary hypertension. J Rheumatol 1996;23:286–290.
68. Wilson WA, Gharavi AE, Koike T, et al. International consensus statement on preliminary classification criteria for definite antiphospholipid syndrome: report of an international workshop. Arthritis Rheum 1999;42:1309–1311.

69. Opravil M, Pechere M, Speich R, et al. HIV-associated primary pulmonary hypertension. A case control study. Swiss HIV Cohort Study. Am J Respir Crit Care Med 1997;155:990–995.

70. Cacoub P, Dorent R, Nataf P, et al. Endothelin-1 in the lungs of patients with pulmonary hypertension. Cardiovasc Res 1997;33:196–200.

71. Atsumi T, Khamashta MA, Haworth RS, et al. Arterial disease and thrombosis in the antiphospholipid syndrome: a pathogenic role for endothelin 1. Arthritis Rheum 1998;41:800–807.

72. Yoshio T, Masuyama J, Sumiya M, Minota S, Kano S. Antiendothelial cell antibodies and their relation to pulmonary hypertension in systemic lupus erythematosus. J Rheumatol 1994;21:2058–2063.

73. Yoshio T, Masuyama J, Mimori A, Takeda A, Minota S, Kano S. Endothelin-1 release from cultured endothelial cells induced by sera from patients with systemic lupus erythematosus. Ann Rheum Dis 1995;54:361–365.

74. Prandoni P, Lensing A, Büller HR, et al. Deep-vein thrombosis and the incidence of subsequent symptomatic cancer. N Engl J Med 1992;327:1128–1133.

75. Zuckerman E, Toubi E, Golan TD, et al. Increased thromboembolic incidence in anti-cardiolipin-positive patients with malignancy. Br J Cancer 1995;72:447–451.

76. Ruffatti A, Aversa S, Del Ross T, Tonetto S, Fiorentino M, Todesco S. Antiphospholipid antibody syndrome associated with ovarian cancer. A new paraneoplastic syndrome? J Rheumatol 1994;21:2162–2163.

77. Papagiannis A, Cooper A, Banks J. Pulmonary embolism and lupus anticoagulant in a woman with renal cell carcinoma. J Urol 1994;152:941–942.

78. Hibbert M, Braude S. Tumour microembolism presenting as "primary pulmonary hypertension". Thorax 1997;52:1016–1017.

79. Piette JC, Cacoub P. Antiphospholipid syndrome in the elderly: caution [editorial]. Circulation 1998;97:2195–2196.

80. Humbert M, Sanchez O, Fartoukh M, Jagot JL, Sitbon O, Simonneau G. Treatment of severe pulmonary hypertension secondary to connective tissue diseases with continuous IV epoprostenol (prostacyclin). Chest 1998;114:80S–82S.

81. Groen H, Bootsma H, Postma DS, Kallenberg CGM. Primary pulmonary hypertension in a patient with systemic lupus erythematosus: partial improvement with cyclophosphamide. J Rheumatol 1993;20:1055–1057.

82. Tam LS, Li EK. Successful treatment with immunosuppression, anticoagulation and vasodilator therapy of pulmonary hypertension in SLE associated with secondary antiphospholipid syndrome. Lupus 1998;7:495–497.

12   Osteoarticular Manifestations of Antiphospholipid Syndrome

Maria G. Tektonidou and Haralampos M. Moutsopoulos

Antiphospholipid syndrome (APS) is a multi-system disorder characterized by arterial or venous thrombosis, pregnancy morbidity, and the presence of aPL, namely anticardiolipin antibodies (aCL) and lupus anticoagulant (LA). The syndrome is classified as primary or as secondary when it occurs in the context of other autoimmune disorders, especially systemic lupus erythematosus (SLE). A plethora of clinical manifestations have been associated with APS, some well recognized and others less widely known. Osteoarticular manifestations have not been commonly reported in clinical studies with APS patients, probably because of their uncertain association with the syndrome. Arthralgias represent the most well-defined osteoarticular features of primary and secondary APS, whereas arthritis is mainly described in SLE-related APS. Osteonecrosis has been documented in association with antiphospholipid antibodies (aPL) in SLE patients with or without APS, but usually in the presence of steroid treatment. The existence of osteonecrosis in patients with primary APS (PAPS), in the absence of steroid administration, suggests an association between this disorder and APS.

Osteonecrosis

Osteonecrosis, also known as avascular necrosis or aseptic necrosis, is a disease in which cell death occurs in the components of bone as a result of interruption of the blood supply. It is a multi-factorial disorder associated with various traumatic and non-traumatic conditions and clinical entities (Table 12.1). If the etiology of osteonecrosis can not be identified, the disease is classified as idiopathic. Despite new developments in its diagnosis and treatment, the pathogenetic mechanisms of osteonecrosis remain partially elucidated. The most predominant hypotheses include the presence of mechanical vascular interruption (caused by trauma, fractures), injury to or pressure on a vessel wall (associated with vasculitis, infection, radiation, Gaucher disease), vascular embolism (by fat, nitrogen bubbles, sickle cells), and thrombosis [1].

Osteonecrosis has been associated with autoimmune diseases, including rheumatoid arthritis, systemic sclerosis, systemic vasculitis, and, especially, SLE [2–4]. Small vessel vasculitis or thrombotic microvasculopathy associated with aPL have been suggested as the pathogenetic mechanisms in these disorders.

Table 12.1. Etiologic factors associated with osteonecrosis.

Trauma	Connective tissue diseases
Hematologic disorders	Systemic lupus erythematosus
Sickle cell disease	Antiphospholipid syndrome
Thalassemias	Rheumatoid arthritis
Disseminated intravascular coagulation	Systemic vasculitis
Polycythemia	Systemic sclerosis
Hemophilia	Cytotoxic agents
Clotting disorders	Vincristine
Inherited thrombophilic factors	Vinblastine
Protein C deficiency	Cisplatin
Protein S deficiency	Bleomycine
Antithrombin III deficiency	Methotrexate
Factor V Leiden	Cyclophosphamide
Homocysteinemia	5-fluorouracil
Dysfibrinogenemia	Infections
Tissue plasminogen activator decrease	Human immunodeficiency virus
Plasminogen activator inhibitor increase	Meningococcemia
Acquired thrombophilic factors	Metabolic conditions
APL	Gaucher disease
Nephrotic syndrome	Hyperparathyroidism
Smoking	Hyperlipidemia
Alcohol	Hemodialysis
Pregnancy	Renal transplantation
Estrogens	Diabetes
Obesity	Gout
Diabetes mellitus	Gastrointestinal diseases
Cushing syndrome	Pancreatitis
Corticosteroids	Inflammatory bowel disease
Malignancies	Others
Hepatic failure	Radiation therapy
Hyperlipidemia	Legg-Calve-Perthes disease
	Dysbaric osteonecrosis
	Fabry disease

APL and Osteonecrosis

Ischemia has been postulated as the predominant mechanism resulting in osteonecrosis since the first description of the disease [5]. In 1974, Jones et al suggested that intravascular coagulation with fibrin thrombosis, activated by several factors, is the likely final pathway leading to bone necrosis [6]. The above hypothesis has gained support by numerous studies reporting diverse coagulation abnormalities in the patients with osteonecrosis. Idiopathic osteonecrosis of the femoral head in adults and Legg-Calve-Perthes disease in children has been associated with several thrombophilic factors including protein C, S, or antithrombin III deficiency, activated protein C resistance, factor V Leiden, homocysteinemia, and aPL, as well as with abnormal fibrinolysis [7–11].

aPL are associated with vessel thromboses of all sizes and at multiple organ sites [12–14]. Thus, these antibodies may play an important role in osteonecrosis development, promoting thrombotic vasculopathy in the intraosseous microcirculation. In some patients with non-traumatic osteonecrosis, histopathologic examinations have revealed thrombosis of terminal arteries in the subchondral areas [15].

However, histologic studies of the bone necrotic areas in patients with idiopathic osteonecrosis or in patients with autoimmune disorders are limited.

The presence of aPL has been described in several cases with idiopathic osteonecrosis of the jaw and femoral head. In a study by Glueck et al, 43 of the 55 patients with idiopathic osteonecrosis had one or more tests positive for thrombophilia and/or hypofibrinolysis; 8 out of those patients (33%) were aCL positive [16]. aPL were also detected in 3 of 16 patients with Kienbock's disease (3 patients had aCL and 2 had LA) [17]. Gruppo et al found abnormal serum aCL titers in 18 (33%) of 55 patients with idiopathic alveolar osteonecrosis of the jaw [18]. Korompilias et al noted an increased prevalence of medium and high aCL titres (37.5%) among 40 patients with non-traumatic hip osteonecrosis (7 with idiopathic osteonecrosis). No difference was found in the frequency of aCL between patients with idiopathic osteonecrosis and those with known risk factors for osteonecrosis (28.5% vs. 39.4%; $P = 0.4$) [19]. Jones et al examined 40 patients with osteonecrosis who had several etiologic associations (SLE, steroid treatment, heavy alcohol or tobacco), and 5 patients with idiopathic osteonecrosis [20]. They found that 37 (82%) of the above 45 patients had at least one coagulation factor abnormality versus 30% of controls ($P < 0.0001$). Four (80%) of the 5 patients with idiopathic osteonecrosis had abnormal IgG aCL levels (> 22 GPL). The high frequency of aPL in all the above studies with idiopathic osteonecrosis suggests an important role for these antibodies in the pathogenesis of the osteonecrotic lesions.

In addition, an association between osteonecrosis and aPL has been observed in patients with human immunodeficiency virus (HIV) infection, in the absence of known risk factors for osteonecrosis. In 1991, Solomon et al published a series of 8 HIV-infected patients with osteonecrosis and they noted that all of 5 patients tested for aCL were positive [21]. Additional cases of osteonecrosis in association with aCL have been subsequently reported [22–25]. Olive and coworkers reported 4 cases with hip osteonecrosis in a cohort of 1920 patients with HIV syndrome; three of them (75%) had positive aCL [26]. Another study undertaken by Brown et al found a prevalence of 50% of aCL in a group of 6 patients with osteonecrosis and underlying HIV infection [27]. Recently, Calza et al described 7 HIV-infected persons with femoral head involvement. Among them, only 4 patients were on antiretroviral therapy, 1 had moderate hypertriglyceridemia, and 3 were aCL positive [28]. In another recent study, 339 asymptomatic HIV-infected adults were examined prospectively by magnetic resonance imaging (MRI) for osteonecrosis of the hip. Fifteen (4.4%) of 339 participants had osteonecrosis, while 14 (93%) of the above 15 patients had detectable levels of aCL [29].

However, the overall significance of these antibodies in the development of osteonecrosis in HIV-infected patients remains unknown. Some authors suggested that the high frequency of aCL in patients with HIV with osteonecrosis should be interpreted with caution because these antibodies have been detected at high frequency in many studies with HIV-infected patients [30, 31]. The reported prevalence for IgG aCL in HIV varied from 0% to 90%. Moreover, there have been several cases of osteonecrosis occurring in HIV individuals with negative aPL [32–34]. HIV itself and hypertriglyceridemia secondary to protease inhibitor treatment have also been implicated in the pathogenesis of osteonecrosis [35]. Nevertheless, the first cases of osteonecrosis in HIV patients were reported before protease inhibitors became available [22, 32]. Hence, the presence of aPL may be an added risk factor for the development of osteonecrosis in HIV-infected patients, but more studies are required in larger groups of patients.

SLE and osteonecrosis

Osteonecrosis is a well-known complication in patients with SLE, contributing to significant morbidity. The reported prevalence of osteonecrosis in SLE varies from 5% to 40% in different studies including symptomatic and asymptomatic patients [36–39]. It was first documented in 1960 by Dubois and Cozen, who suggested that SLE itself or vasculitis are the main causes of osteonecrosis [40]. Since then, a number of pathogenetic factors have been analyzed. Corticosteroid treatment has long been recognized as a major predisposing factor for osteonecrosis in SLE [41–44]. The duration of steroid therapy, the total cumulative dosage, and the highest daily dosage have been independently involved [6, 36, 45]. However, the role of corticosteroids was not confirmed by other authors [40, 46, 47] who suggested additional risk factors such as fat emboli [45], hyperlipidemia [7], leukopenia [47], young age at the disease onset [38, 48], and Raynaud's phenomenon [44, 49]. Gladman et al demonstrated that corticosteroid treatment, the presence of arthritis, and the use of cytotoxic drugs were independent risk factors for the development of osteonecrosis in SLE patients [50]. Another study showed that patients with osteonecrosis had higher frequency of Cushingoid body habitus, thrombophlebitis, vasculitis, cigarette smoking, and preeclampsia [51]. An association with SLE activity, hypertension, and lupus nephritis has also been proposed by some authors [46, 52], but not by others [48, 53]. aPL have been strongly implicated in the pathogenesis of osteonecrosis.

The association between osteonecrosis and aPL in patients with SLE was first described in 1985 by Asherson et al [54]. One year later, Lavilla et al reported 2 other SLE patients with osteonecrosis and positive aCL [55]. Nagasawa et al noted that SLE features such as Raynaud's phenomenon, hyperlipidemia, nephrotic syndrome, hypertension, and disease activity were not related to osteonecrosis in a study with 111 SLE patients. On the other hand, the percentage of patients who had LA was found to be greater in those with osteonecrosis than in those without [56]. Mok et al [57] showed also an increased risk for osteonecrosis in SLE patients who were positive for LA ($P = 0.02$). Abeles et al described a higher prevalence of aCL in SLE patients with osteonecrosis in comparison with those without osteonecrosis (35% vs. 4%; $P = 0.008$). In 1993, Asherson and coworkers found that 27 (73%) of 37 patients with SLE with symptomatic osteonecrosis had positive aPL [51]. In 1997, Mont et al documented an association between osteonecrosis and IgG aCL levels. In a European multi-center study including 1000 patients with primary and secondary APS, the prevalence of symptomatic osteonecrosis was 2.4% [13]. With regards to patients with catastrophic APS, Egan et al described a 25-year-old woman presenting with multiple sites of thrombosis and multiple sites of osteonecrosis [59]. In a series of 80 patients with catastrophic APS, symptomatic osteonecrosis was found in 7% of cases [60].

All the above studies stressed the importance of aPL in predisposition to osteonecrosis. However, some authors consider that aCL do not play a determinant role in the pathogenesis of osteonecrosis suggesting other risk factors. Alarcon-Segovia et al failed to detect any association between osteonecrosis and aCL in a study including 500 consecutive SLE patients [61]. In 1995, in the Hopkins Lupus

Cohort, daily corticosteroid dosage, Raynaud's phenomenon, and vasculitis were considered important risk factors for osteonecrosis, while LA and aCL were not [62]. Pistiner et al reported the presence of osteonecrosis in 26 (5.3 %) of 488 studied SLE patients and noticed a lack of correlation between osteonecrosis and aCL [63]. In the study by Migliaresi and coworkers, osteonecrosis occurred in 7 (10%) of 69 unselected SLE patients and was related to continuous high-dose steroid treatment but not to detectable aCL levels [64]. Mok et al reported that no relationship could be found between aCL or LA and the development of osteonecrosis in a cohort of 265 SLE patients receiving long-term follow up from 1978 to 1998 [65]. In another series of 280 SLE patients followed for 10 years, no increased frequency of aPL, Raynaud's phenomenon, leukopenia, or SLE activity was found in the patients with osteonecrosis (N = 7) compared to those without osteonecrosis [53]. In a study undertaken by Cozen and Wallace, 26 (5%) of 488 patients with SLE developed asymptomatic osteonecrosis; no association with aCL or thromboembolic disease was observed [33]. Houssiau and associates examined prospectively by MRI the prevalence of osteonecrosis in a group of 40 SLE patients. The prevalence of osteonecrosis was 37.5% and its presence was correlated strongly with corticosteroid treatment but not with aCL status [66].

Therefore, no definite conclusions regarding the association between osteonecrosis and aPL could be deduced from the above studies. This could be explained in several ways. In almost all the previous publications, osteonecrosis has been described in patients who had received corticosteroid therapy, which is one of the major predisposing factors for bone necrosis. Most of these studies were retrospective and examined only symptomatic patients. However, it is well known that osteonecrosis can be entirely asymptomatic, especially in the early stage of disease. The diagnosis of osteonecrosis has been made using mainly plain radiographs which can identify advanced disease but can not detect early stage osteonecrosis [67, 68]. In addition, the diagnostic method for aCL measurement, the upper limit of normal, and the aCL serum levels (low, medium, or high titers) have not been reported in all the above studies. It has not been clearly reported also if the aPL were detected positive once or on more occasions. In addition, in some studies the measurement of aPL was done in samples drawn at the time of osteonecrosis while in others at the time of first observation or during the follow-up period.

PAPS and Osteonecrosis

Corticosteroid treatment is widely used in the patients with SLE or SLE-related APS, but rather rarely in the patients with PAPS. The existence of osteonecrosis in PAPS patients in the absence of steroid use was first documented by Asherson et al, suggesting an association between osteonecrosis and APS. They found that 2 out of 70 studied patients with PAPS had symptomatic osteonecrosis, and that it was the initial manifestation of the syndrome in one of them [69]. Alijotas et al reported the presence of aPL in 3 of 16 patients with Kienbocks disease; 1 had a history of deep vein thrombosis and recurrent abortions in association with positive aCL and LA [17]. Vela et al described a patient with PAPS who suffered a previous deep vein thrombosis and who subsequently developed osteonecrosis of the hip [70]. Similarly, a patient who had a history of hemiplegic migraine, cerebrovascular infarcts, and osteonecrosis of the left hip and the right knee has been reported [71].

Dubost documented a case with fatal PAPS and multiple bone necrotic areas [72]. In a retrospective study, Weber and associates analyzed the data from 108 APS patients followed from 1987 to 1996. They reported that symptomatic osteonecrosis was found in 7 (10%) of 69 patients with secondary APS but in none of 22 patients with PAPS [73].

Until recently, no prospective studies examining the prevalence of osteonecrosis in symptomatic and asymptomatic patients with PAPS were found in the literature. In a prospective study from our department, we evaluated the prevalence of osteonecrosis in patients with PAPS who were asymptomatic for osteonecrosis and had not taken corticosteroids [74]. Thirty patients with PAPS who had never received corticosteroids, 19 patients with SLE (with and without aCL) who had not previously received steroids and 30 healthy individuals, were examined prospectively by MRI of the femoral heads. Established MRI criteria were used for a diagnosis of early, intermediate, and advanced osteonecrosis. In positive cases, radiographs and dynamic scintigraphy were also performed. Asymptomatic osteonecrosis was found in 6 (20%) of the 30 patients with PAPS: 3 of them had intermediate bilateral osteonecrosis with the characteristic double-line sign on MRI (Fig. 12.1) and the other 3 patients had early osteonecrosis findings (Fig.12.2). No cases with advanced osteonecrosis were observed. Hip and pelvis radiography and dynamic scintigraphy were negative in all of 6 patients. None of the SLE patients (with and without aCL) and none of the healthy controls had documented osteonecrosis. In the osteonecrosis-positive cases, follow-up MRI 6 months after the initial examination revealed no changes. One of the 3 patients

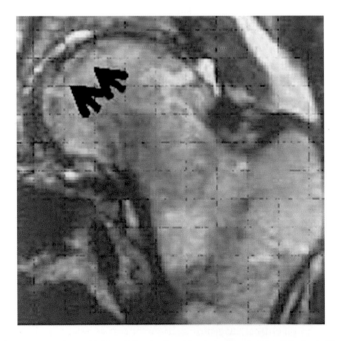

Figure 12.1. Early osteonecrosis on this T_2-weighted spin echo magnetic resonance is indicated by the low intensity band in the subchondral zone of the femoral head (*band sign*) – a feature that is characteristic of osteonecrosis. Asymptomatic patient with primary antiphospholipid syndrome.

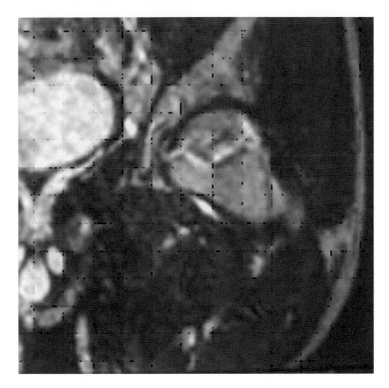

Figure 12.2. Osteonecrosis indicated by the presence of the double line sign (*arrow*) seen on T$_2$-weighted spin echo image.

with intermediate osteonecrosis suffered from knee pain 3 months after the initial examination, and an additional MRI showed avascular necrosis (AVN) of both knees. Osteonecrosis was found to be more prevalent in younger patients and in patients with livedo reticularis. No associations with other clinical characteristics (venous or arterial thrombosis, thrombocytopenia, abortions, Raynaud's phenomenon), aCL titer, presence of LA or anti–β$_2$-glycoprotein I antibodies could be identified.

The increased incidence of osteonecrosis in PAPS patients in the absence of other predisposing factors confirms the association between osteonecrosis and aPL, and suggests that osteonecrosis may represent an additional clinical feature of APS. Furthermore, all the above findings raise the possibility that a proportion of young patients with osteonecrosis with positive aPL, in the absence of other risk factors, may have a form of PAPS.

Clinical Manifestations and Diagnosis of Osteonecrosis

Osteonecrosis can be entirely asymptomatic or it can be associated with pain and/or limitation of the movement in the affected joints. The most susceptible sites for osteonecrosis are the bones with single blood terminal supply such as the femoral head, the talus, the humerus head, or the carpal bones. The femoral head appears to be the most vulnerable site for the development of osteonecrosis. Atypical sites of osteonecrosis have also been described in patients with APS [75]. Involvement of multiple bones may occur, especially in patients with SLE [76], and the condition may be often bilateral as it was shown in our study [73].

Given the unpredictable natural history of osteonecrosis, it is conceivable that early diagnosis is crucial in selecting the appropriate treatment options [77, 78]. Radiographic findings in early stages are unremarkable. In advanced disease, flattening, subchondral radiolucent lines (crescent sign) and collapse may be present. MRI is recognized as the most sensitive tool for the early recognition of osteonecrosis, having more than 95% overall sensitivity. It is significantly more sensitive than radiographs, radionuclide bone scan, or computerized tomography [79, 80]. MRI findings in early osteonecrosis include the presence of a decreased signal intensity band or rim in the subchondral zone on both T_1- and T_2-weighted images (band sign). The characteristic appearance of osteonecrosis, the double-line sign occurs later in the disease process. The double-line sign is seen on T_2-weighted images as a high signal intensity line in an inner zone combined with low-signal intensity in an outer zone. Advanced osteonecrosis is characterized by the combination of the above findings plus collapse and joint congruity. MRI imaging detects also the bone marrow edema, which can be associated with early osteonecrosis. Van de Berg et al showed that lack of accompanying subchondral changes on T_2-weighted or contrast-enhanced T_1-weighted images had 100% positive predictive value for a transient phenomenon [81].

Treatment of Osteonecrosis

Treatment strategies primarily depend on the location, size, and stage of the lesion. Conservative therapy, used in early stages, includes non-steroidal agents or other analgesics for pain relief, steroid tapering, weight-bearing avoidance, bed rest, or even immobilization for some cases. However, conservative therapies usually fall to inhibit the progression of osteonecrosis. It has been well documented that without specific treatment, approximately 70% to 80% of hips with clinically established osteonecrosis have radiologic and clinical progression leading to the femoral head collapse [82]. Thus, various prophylactic surgical procedures have been proposed in order to suppress the evolution of further degenerative changes. The goals of these procedures are the reduction of intramedullary pressure, removal of the necrotic area from the weight-bearing zone, and restoration of the blood supply in the necrotic area. The surgical treatment of choice in early stages, especially in young active patients, is core decompression with or without bone grafting [83]. Osteotomy has also been used with variable success [84]. Total joint arthroplasty is recommended for the late stage which is characterized by necrotic subchondral bone, articular cartilage collapse, and secondary osteoarthrosis (19).

Because of the ambiguity concerning the pathogenesis of osteonecrosis, the treatment of this disabling disorder has not focused on mechanisms of the disease process, but rather on the management of the end-stage bone changes. However, in patients with osteonecrosis and positive aPL the use of anticoagulants might provide an effective therapy. This hypothesis should be investigated in large, prospective studies.

Arthralgias and Arthritis in APS

Arthralgias are rather common in PAPS and SLE-related APS [13, 73, 86]. In 1989, Mackworth-Young et al described the clinical and serological features of 20 patients with PAPS and they found that 3 (15 %) of them had recurrent attacks of arthralgias [87]. In the largest cohort of APS patients with 1000 cases, the presence of arthralgias was documented in 271 (38.7%) patients with a similar distribution among primary and secondary APS [13]. Weber et al reported that arthralgias or arthritis was documented in 83% of SLE-related APS patients and in 41% of PAPS patients [73]. They also noticed that it was difficult to distinguish frank and sustained arthritis from arthralgias on the basis of patient history, because most patients reported their articular symptoms as arthralgias.

The existence of arthritis in APS has been almost exclusively reported in patients with APS secondary to SLE or in lupus-like syndrome [69, 86]. In a retrospective study, Asherson et al observed that arthritis as well as other characteristic features of SLE (serositis, vasculitic rash, renal disease) were absent in PAPS [69]. In 1992, Piette et al suggested that the American Rheumatism Association criteria for SLE were of limited value in classifying patients with APS into primary or SLE-related APS. One year later, the same authors proposed a set of empirical exclusion criteria to distinguish PAPS from SLE-related APS [88]. According to these criteria the presence of frank arthritis excluded the diagnosis of PAPS. However, in a letter to the editor, Querel et al reported 8 patients with PAPS who suffered from non-erosive polyarthritis [89]. They noted though that 3 patients had lupus-like syndrome before or after the diagnosis of PAPS. Replying to the above letter, Piette and Asherson suggested that patients with persistent "true" APS should be distinguished from those who progressively develop clinical and serologic abnormalities associated with SLE, including arthritis [90]. In a cohort of 1000 APS individuals, episodes of arthritis were observed in 56% of the patients with SLE-related APS compared to only 3% of patients with PAPS [13]. According to the above, it seems that arthritis is a rare manifestation of well-defined PAPS.

The management of arthralgias/arthritis includes the use of nonsteroidal antinflammatory agents or other analgesics but they should be used with caution in cases receiving chronic coumarin treatment. In SLE-related APS, treatment with hydroxychloroquine or corticosteroids can also be used according to the severity of the articular symptoms and lupus activity. Besides its effect on arthralgias or arthritis, the role of hydroxychloroquine on thrombosis and lipids should also be stressed in patients with PAPS and SLE-related APS [91].

Conclusion

Diverse conditions associated with thrombotic lesions either in large vessels or in the microvasculature may be part of the APS clinical spectrum. Besides the classic clinical manifestations, including arterial and venous thrombosis or recurrent fetal loss, a number of other clinical conditions characterized as microangiopathic syndromes have been associated with APS. These syndromes can affect several organs including skin, brain, heart, and kidneys. Osteonecrosis may be another distinct clinical feature of APS associated with arterial or venous microthrombosis. Clinicians should be aware of the possible association between APS and osteonecrosis because early diagnosis may lead to early and proper management of this disabling disease. Patients with persistent symptoms originating from sites most susceptible to osteonecrosis should undergo MRI evaluation. A systematic screening for aPL in all cases with diagnosed osteonecrosis in the absence of precipitating factors should also be considered.

References

1. Mankin HJ. Nontraumatic necrosis of bone (osteonecrosis). N Engl J Med 1992;326:1473–1479.
2. Zabinski SJ, Sculco TP, Dicarlo EF, et al. Osteonecrosis in the rheumatoid femoral head. J Rheumatol 1998;25:1674–1680.
3. Chang HK, Choi YJ, Baek SK, et al. Osteonecrosis and bone infarction in association with Behcet's disease: report of two cases. Clin Exp Rheumatol 2001;19(suppl 24):S51–S4.
4. Wilde AH, Mankin HJ, Rodman GP. Avascular necrosis of the femoral head in scleroderma. Arthritis Rheum 1970;13:445–447.
5. Phemister DB. Fractures of the neck of the femur, dislocation of hip and obscure vascular disturbances producing aseptic necrosis of the head of the femur. Surg Gynec Obstet 1934;59:415.
6. Jones JP Jr, Sakovich L, Anderson CE. Experimentally produced osteonecrosis as a result of fat embolism. In: Beckman EL, Elliott DH, Smith EM, eds. Dysbarism-related osteonecrosis. HEW Publ (NIOSH) 75-153. Washington DC: U.S Government Printing Office; 1974:117–132.
7. Boettcher WG, Bonfiglio M, Hamilton HH, et al. Nontraumatic necrosis of the femoral head. Relation of altered hemostasis to etiology. J Bone Joint Surg Am 1970;52:312–313.
8. Glueck CJ, Freiberg R, Tracy T, et al. Thrombophilia and hypofibrinolysis. Pathophysiologies of osteonecrosis. Clin Orthop 1997;334:43–56.
9. Glueck CJ, Glueck HI, Greenfield D, et al. Protein C and S deficiency, thrombophilia and hypofibrinolysis: pathophysiologic causes of Legg Perthes disease. Pediat Res 1994;35:383–388.
10. Van Veldhuizen PJ, Neff J, Murphey M, et al. Decreased fibrinolytic potential in patients with idiopathic avascular necrosis and transient osteoporosis of the hip. Am J Hematol 1993;44:243–248.
11. Glueck CJ, Crawford A, Roy D, et al. Association of antithrombotic factor deficiencies and hypofibrinolysis with Legg-Perthes disease. J Bone Joint Surg 1996;78:3–13.
12. Hughes GR. The antiphospholipid syndrome: ten years on. Lancet 1993;342:341–344.
13. Cervera R, Piette JC, Font J, et al. Antiphospholipid syndrome: clinical and immunological manifestations and patterns of disease expression in a cohort of 1000 patients. Arthritis Rheum 2002;46:1019–1027.
14. Tektonidou MG, Ioannidis JP, Boki KA, et al. Prognostic factors and clustering of serious clinical outcomes in antiphospholipid syndrome. QJM 2000;93:523–530.
15. Jones JP Jr. Intravascular coagulation and osteonecrosis. Clin Orthop 1992;277:41–53.
16. Glueck CJ, McMahon RE, Bouquot JE, et al. The pathophysiology of idiopathic osteonecrosis of the jaws: thrombophilia and hypofibrinolysis [abstract]. J Invest Med 1995;43(suppl 2):234.
17. Alijotas J, Argemi M, Barquinero J. Kienbock's disease and aPL. Clin Exp Rheumatol 1990; 8:297–298.
18. Gruppo R, Glueck CJ, McMahon RE. The pathophysiology of alveolar osteonecrosis of the jaw: anticardiolipin antibodies, thrombophilia and hypofibrinolysis. J Lab Clin Med 1996;127:481–488.
19. Korompilias AV, Gilkeson GS, Ortel TL, et al. Anticardiolipin antibodies and osteonecrosis of the femoral head. Clin Orthop 1997;345:174–180.
20. Jones LC, Mont MA, Le TB, et al. Procoagulants and osteonecrosis. J Rheumatol 2003;30:783–791.
21. Solomon G, Brancato L, Winchester R. An approach to the human immunodeficiency virus positive patient with a spondyloarthropathic disease. Rheum Dis Clin North Am 1991;17:43–58.
22. Chevalier X, Larget-Pier B, Hernigou P, et al. Avascular necrosis of the femoral head in HIV-infected patients. J Bone Joint Surg Br 1993;75:160.
23. Belmonte MA, Garcia-Portales R, Domenech I, et al. Avascular necrosis of bone in human immunodeficiency virus infection and aPL. J Rheumatol 1993;20:1425–1428.
24. Molina JF, Citera G, Rosler D. Coexistence of human immunodeficiency virus infection and systemic lupus erythematosus. J Rheumatol 1995;22:347–350.

25. Koeger AC, Banneville B, Gerster JC, et al. Avascular osteonecrosis in HIV-infected patients: 10 cases [abstract 277]. Arthritis Rheum 1995;38(Suppl):S119.
26. Olive A, Queralt C, Sierra G, et al. Osteonecrosis and HIV-infection: 4 more cases. J Rheumatol 1998;25:1243–1244.
27. Brown P, Crane L. Avascular necrosis of bone in patients with human immunodeficiency virus infection: report of 6 cases and review of the literature. Clin Infect Dis 2001;32:1221–1226.
28. Calza L, Manfredi R, Chiodo F. Osteonecrosis in HIV-infected patients and its correlation with highly active antiretroviral therapy (HAART). Presse Med 2003;32:595–598.
29. Miller KD, Masur H, Jones E, et al. High prevalence of osteonecrosis of the femoral head in HIV-infected adults. Ann Intern Med 2002;137:17–25.
30. Stimmler MM, Quismorio FP, McGehee WG, et al. Anticardiolipin antibodies in acquired immunodeficiency syndrome. Arch Intern Med 1989;149:1833–1835.
31. Coll Daroca J, Gutierrez-Cebollada J, Yazbeck H, et al. Anticardiolipin antibodies and acquired immunodeficiency syndrome: prognostic marker or association with HIV infection. Infection 1992;20:140–142.
32. Gerster JC, Camus JP, Chave JP, et al. Multiple site avascular necrosis in HIV infected patients. J Rheumatol 1991;18:300–302.
33. Llauger J, Palmer J, Roson N, et al. Osteonecrosis of the knee in an HIV-infected patient. AJR Am J Roentgenol 1998;171:987–988.
34. Johns DG, Gill MJ. Avascular necrosis in HIV infection. AIDS 1999;13:1997–1998.
35. Monier P, McKown K, Bronze MS. Osteonecrosis complicating highly active antiretroviral therapy in patients infected with human immunodeficiency virus. Clin Infect Dis 2000;31:1488–1492.
36. Goldie I, Tibblin G, Scheller S. Systemic lupus erythematosus and aseptic bone necrosis. Acta Med Scand 1967;182:55–63.
37. Hurley RM, Steinberg RH, Patriquin H, et al. Avascular necrosis of the femoral head in childhood systemic lupus erythematosus. Can Med Assoc J 1974;111:781–784.
38. Kalla AA, Learmonth ID, Klemp P. Early treatment of avascular necrosis in systemic lupus erythematosus. Ann Rheum Dis 1986;45:649–652.
39. Gladman DD, Chaudhry-Ahluwalia V, Ibanez D, et al. Outcomes of symptomatic osteonecrosis in 95 patients with systemic lupus erythematosus. J Rheumatol 2001;28:2226–2269.
40. Dubois EL, Cozen L. Avascular (aseptic) bone necrosis associated with systemic lupus erythematosus. JAMA 1960;174:966–971.
41. Fisher DE, Bickel WH. Corticosteroid-induced avascular necrosis. A clinical study of seventy-seven patients. J Bone Joint Surg Am 1971;53:859–873.
42. Felson DT, Anderson JJ. Across-study evaluation of association between steroid dose and bolus steroids and avascular necrosis of bone. Lancet 1987;i:902–906.
43. Abeles M, Urman JD, Rothfield NF. Aseptic necrosis of bone in systemic lupus erythematosus. Relation to corticosteroid therapy. Arch Intern Med 1978;138:750–754.
44. Zizic TM, Marcoux C, Hungerford DS, et al. Corticosteroid therapy associated with ischemic necrosis of bone in systemic lupus erythematosus. Am J Med 1985;79:596–604.
45. Jones JP Jr, Engelman EP, Steinbach HL, et al. Fat embolization as a possible mechanism producing avascular necrosis [abstract]. Arthritis Rheum 1965;8:449.
46. Nilsen KH. Systemic lupus erythematosus and avascular bone necrosis. N Z Med J 1977;85:472–475.
47. Klipper AR, Stevens MB, Zizic TM, et al. Ischemic necrosis of bone in systemic lupus erythematosus. Medicine (Baltimore) 1976;55:251–257.
48. Smith FE, Sweet DE, Brunner CM, et al. Avascular necrosis in SLE. An apparent predilection for young patients. Ann Rheum Dis 1976;35:227–232.
49. Hungerford DS. Pathogenetic considerations in ischaemic necrosis of bone. Can J Surg 1981;24:583–587.
50. Gladman DD, Urowitz MB, Chaudry-Ahluwalia C, et al. Predictive factors for symptomatic osteonecrosis in patients with systemic lupus erythematosus. J Rheumatol 2001;28:761–765.
51. Mont MA, Glueck CJ, Pacheco IH, et al. Risk factors for osteonecrosis in systemic lupus erythematosus. J Rheumatol 1997;24:654–662.
52. Cozen L, Wallace DJ. Avascular necrosis in systemic lupus erythematosus: clinical associations and a 47-year perspective. Am J Orthop 1998;27:352–354.
53. Rascu A, Manger K, Kraetsch HG, et al. Osteonecrosis in systemic lupus erythematosus, steroid induced or a lupus-dependent manifestation? Lupus 1996;5:323–327.
54. Asherson RA, Jungers P, Liote F, et al. Ischaemic necrosis of bone associated with the "lupus anticoagulant" and antibodies to cardiolipin [abstract]. In: Proceedings of the XVIth International Congress of Rheumatology, Sydney (Australia), 1985:373.

55. Lavilla P, Gil A, Khamashta MA, et al. Avascular necrosis of the bone and systemic lupus erythematosus. Rev Clin Esp 1987;181:289–290.
56. Nagasawa K, Ishi Y, Mayumi T, et al. Avascular necrosis of bone in systemic lupus erythematosus: possible role of haemostatic abnormalities. Ann Rheum Dis 1989;48:672–676.
57. Mok CC, Lau CS, Wong RW. Risk factors for avascular bone necrosis in systemic lupus erythematosus. Br J Rheumatol 1998;37:895–900.
58. Asherson RA, Liote F, Page B, et al. Avascular necrosis of bone and aPL in systemic lupus erythematosus. J Rheumatol 1993;20:284–288.
59. Egan RM, Munn RK. Catastrophic antiphospholipid antibody syndrome presenting with multiple thromboses and sites of avascular necrosis. J Rheumatol 1994;21:2376–2379.
60. Asherson RA, Cervera R, Piette JC, et al. Catastrophic antiphospholipid syndrome: clues to the pathogenesis from a series of 80 patients. Medicine (Baltimore) 2001;80:355–377.
61. Alarcon-Segovia D, Deleze M, Oria CV, et al. APL and the antiphospholipid syndrome in systemic lupus erythematosus. A prospective analysis of 500 consecutive patients. Medicine (Baltimore) 1989;68:353–365.
62. Petri M. Muscosceletal complications of systemic lupus erythematosus in the Hopkins Lupus Cohort: an update. Arthritis Care Res 1995;8:137–145.
63. Pistiner M, Wallace DJ, Nessim S, et al. Lupus erythematosus in the 1980s: a survey of 570 patients. Sem Arthritis Rheum 1991;21:55–64.
64. Migliaresi S, Picillo U, Ambrosone L, et al. Avascular osteonecrosis in patients with SLE: relation to corticosteroid therapy and anticardiolipin antibodies. Lupus 1994;3:37–41.
65. Mok MY, Farewell VT, Isenberg DA. Risk factors for avascular necrosis of bone in patients with systemic lupus erythematosus: is there a role for aPL? Ann Rheum Dis 2000;59:462–467.
66. Houssiau FA, N' Zeusseu Toukap A, Depresseux G, et al. Magnetic resonance imaging-detected avascular osteonecrosis in systemic lupus erythematosus: lack of correlation with antiphospholid antibodies. Br J Rheumatol 1998;37:448–453.
67. Mitchell DG, Rao VM, Dalinka MK, et al. Femoral head avascular necrosis: correlation of MR imaging, radiographic staging, radionuclide imaging, and clinical findings. Radiology 1987;162:709–715.
68. Fordyce MJ, Solomon L. Early detection of avascular necrosis of the femoral head by MRI. J Bone Joint Surg Br 1993;75:365–367.
69. Asherson RA, Khamashta MA, Ordi-Ros J, et al. The 'primary' antiphospholipid syndrome: major clinical and serological features. Medicine (Baltimore) 1989;68:366–374.
70. Vela P, Battle E, Salas E, et al. Primary antiphospholipid syndrome and osteonecrosis. Clin Exp Rheumatol 1991;9:545–546.
71. Seleznick MJ, Silveira LH, Espinosa LR. Avascular necrosis associated with anticardiolipin antibodies. J Rheumatol 1991;18:1416–1417.
72. Dubost JJ, Kemeny JL, Soubrier M, et al. Primary antiphospholipid syndrome of fatal course and osteoarticular cytosteatonecrosis. Rev Med Interne 1994;15:535–540.
73. Weber M, Hayem G, de Bandt M, et al. Classification of an intermediate group of patients with antiphospholipid syndrome and lupus-like disease: primary or secondary antiphospholipid syndrome? J Rheumatol 1999;26:2131–2136.
74. Tektonidou MG, Malagari K, Vlachoyiannopoulos PG, et al. Asymptomatic avascular necrosis in patients with primary antiphospholipid syndrome in the absence of corticosteroid use: a prospective study by magnetic resonance imaging. Arthritis Rheum 2003;48:732–736.
75. Mok MY, Isenberg DA. Avascular necrosis of a single vertebral body, an atypical site of disease in secondary APLS. Ann Rheum Dis 2000;59:494–495.
76. Fishel B, Caspi D, Eventov I, et al. Multiple osteonecrotic lesions in systemic lupus erythematosus. J Rheumatol 1987;14:601–604.
77. Assouline-Dayan Y, Chang C, Greenspan A, et al. Pathogenesis and natural history of osteonecrosis. Semin Arthritis Rheum 2002;32:94–124.
78. Ohzono K, Saito M, Takaoka K, et al. Natural history of nontraumatic avascular necrosis of the femoral head. J Bone Joint Surg Br 1991;73:68–72.
79. Tervonen O, Mueller DM, Matteson EL, et al. Clinically occult avascular necrosis of the hip: prevalence in an asymptomatic population at risk. Radiology 1992;182:845–847.
80. Coleman BG, Kressel HY, Dalinka MK, et al. Radiographically negative avascular necrosis: detection with MR imaging. Radiology 1998;168:525–528.
81. Vande Berg BC, Malghem JJ, Lecouvet FE, et al. Idiopathic bone marrow edema lesions of the femoral head: predictive value of MR Imaging findings. Radiology 1999;212:527–535.

82. Merle d'Aubigne R, Postel M, Mazabraud A, et al. Idiopathic necrosis of femoral head in adults. J Bon Joint Surg Br 1965;47:612–633.
83. Mont MA, Carbone JJ, Fairbank AC. Core decompression versus nonoperative management for osteonecrosis of the hip. Clin Orthop 1996;324:169–178.
84. D'Souza SR, Sadiq S, New AM, et al. Proximal femoral osteotomy as the primary operation for young adults who have osteoarthritis of the hip. J Bone Joint Surg Am 1998;80:1428–1438.
85. Cornell CN, Salvati EA, Pelicci PM. Long term follow-up of total hip replacement in patients with osteonecrosis. Orthop Clin North Am 1985;16:757–769.
86. Vianna JL, Khamashta MA, Ordi-Ros J, et al. Comparison of the primary and secondary antiphospholipid syndrome: a European multicenter study of 114 patients. Am J Med 1994;96:3–9.
87. Mackworth-Young CG, Loizou S, Walport MJ. Primary antiphospholipid syndrome: features of patients with raised anticardiolipin antibodies and no other disorder. Ann Rheum Dis 1989;48:362–367.
88. Piette JC, Whechsler B, Frances C, et al. Exclusion criteria for primary antiphospholipid syndrome. J Rheumatol 1993;20:1802–1804.
89. Queyrel V, Hachulla E, Cardon T. Arthritis in primary antiphospholipid syndrome? J Rheumatol 1996;23:1305.
90. Piette JC, Asherson RA. Arthritis in primary antiphospholipid syndrome? Reply. J Rheumatol 1996;23:1305–1306.
91. Edwards MH, Pierangeli S, Liu X, et al. Hydroxychloroquine reverses thrombogenic properties of aPL in mice. Circulation 1997;96:4380–4384.
92. Arruda VR, Belangero WD, Ozelo MC, et al. Inherited risk factors for thrombophilia among children with Legg-Calve-Perthes disease. J Pediatr Orthop 1999;19:84–87.

13   The Ear and Antiphospholipid Syndrome

Elias Toubi and Aharon Kessel

Introduction

Evidence now exists that inner-ear pathology is frequently associated with immune dysfunction, including the presence of anticardiolipin antibodies (aCL) in the sera of these patients.

The pathogenesis of sensorineural hearing loss (SNHL) is still considered idiopathic, in most cases. Sudden deafness, severe hearing loss of acute onset, is usually unilateral but may also occur bilaterally as well. Patients with progressive SNHL, develop bilateral progressive hearing loss over the course of a few days to 1–2 months, although as many as 20% initially present a unilateral loss. Both disabilities occur in previously healthy subjects, with an equal preponderance among males and females.

In addition to auditory symptoms, these patients may also present vestibular complaints, such as true vertigo, lightheadedness, or ataxia. Tinnitus and aural pressure are also frequent symptoms, and may occur in one half and one third of all patients, respectively.

The potential role of autoimmunity in the pathogenesis of hearing loss was first reported by McCabe in 1979 [1], who described a pattern of bilateral SNHL characterized by rapid progression over days to months. This was based on the finding of a positive lymphocyte migration inhibition assay to cochlear antigens and the steroid responsiveness of the hearing loss in such patients. Additional support includes the following: both cellular and humoral elements of the immune system can normally be identified in inner-ear tissue; animal models demonstrate inner-ear damage after immunization with inner-ear tissue extracts; and such an injury is transferable with sensitized T cells; human SNHL can occur in the context of systemic immunological disease; and SNHL can be treated by immunosuppressive therapy [2–5]. However, the definite proof of an autoimmune etiology is still lacking because in most studies the exact nature of the immunizing antigenic epitope(s) has not yet been identified.

The Association of SNHL with Autoimmune Disease

During the last decade many reports described the association of SNHL with various autoimmune disorders such as: systemic lupus erythematosus (SLE), Sjögren syndrome, chronic ulcerative colitis, rheumatoid arthritis, polyarthritis nodosa, polymyositis, Hashimoto's thyroiditis, and Cogan's syndrome [6–9]. The beneficial effect of immunosuppressive therapy observed in some of these patients supports the immune-mediated etiology. It was stressed that immediate treatment with corticosteroids or other immunosuppressive agents is essential because delay may lead to irreversible hearing loss [10]. The benefit of plasmapheresis in patients with suspected immune-mediated hearing loss was evaluated: improved hearing was observed in 8/16 (50%) patients and only 25% of the patients required additional immunosuppressive maintenance therapy [11]. In 1986, Bowman et al [12], prospectively tested the hearing status of 30 patients hospitalized during SLE flares and observed an 8% incidence of substantial, previously undetected hearing loss. In the same year, Caldarelli et al [13] reported profound SNHL of the right ear in a 51-year-old woman, followed 3 weeks later by a similar finding in her left ear. This was concomitant with symptoms of her newly diagnosed SLE. In 1992, Kobayashi et al [14], described bilateral SNHL in a 32-year-old woman that improved dramatically after plasmapheresis, 2 years before the diagnosis of SLE was established. They suggested that circulating immune complexes or antiphospholipid antibodies (aPL) might play a pathological role in the hearing impairment in SLE patients. In 1995, Kataoka et al [15] documented another case of intermittent bilateral SNHL in conjunction with SLE.

In the same year, Andonopoulos et al [16] reported an association between SNHL and SLE, without correlation to SLE disease activity, concluding that factors other than inflammation may be involved in the pathogenesis of this disorder. Later, Sperling et al found that out of 84 SLE patients, 31% were reported to suffer from aural symptoms, such as tinnitus and hearing loss, suggesting that these findings are also related to the immune complex nature of the disease [17].

In yet another study, the symptoms of SNHL were observed in 38% of 37 unselected systemic sclerosis (SSc) patients, suggesting that SSc may be included among the autoimmune diseases which may cause audiovestibular disturbances [18]. The association between Behcet's disease and SNHL was also reported in 1 patient who had fluctuating hearing loss, tinnitus, and dizziness, proposing a causative relationship between autoimmune vasculitis and endolymphatic hydrops [19].

Animal Models for Immune-mediated SNHL

To aid in the investigation of SNHL, several animal models were introduced. In 1983, Yoo et al [20] immunized rats with native bovine type II collagen, a major structural element of the inner ear, and induced SNHL in these animals. Ruckenstein et al [21] proposed the MRL-lpr/lpr mouse strain as a potential model of autoimmune inner-ear pathology (a strain known to develop an SLE-like disease at the age of 4–5 months) in which the authors observed cochlear pathology in 6/11 animals of this age. Based on the above, Iwai et al [22] demonstrated in severe combined immunodeficient (SCID) mice, infused with MRL-lpr/lpr spleen cells, the induction of cochlear damage which normally would not have developed in such animals. In a recent study, Billings [23] described a mouse model of CD4+ T cell–mediated autoimmune SNHL induced by immunization with peptides from the inner ear–specific proteins cochlin and β-tectorin. However, it is not yet clear how accurately this model reflects events occurring in the spontaneous idiopathic disease.

Immunological Profile in Sensorineural Hearing Disorders

Laboratory studies of peripheral blood lymphocytes from patients suffering from SNHL and serological assays of antigen-specific immune responses to sonicated inner-ear antigen preparations have provided evidence that the disease may have an autoimmune etiology. The two tests most commonly used are the lymphocyte transformation test and the Western blot immune assay [24].

In 1993, Mayot et al [25] reported in 57 individuals with SD (n = 17; group 1) and progressive SNHL (n = 40; group 2) an abnormality of the T-cell subgroups in peripheral blood. The reduced presence of CD3+ and CD4+ cells was observed in group 1, and there was marked decrease of CD8+ cells for both groups. In addition, antinuclear and antithyroid antibodies were frequently detected in the sera of group 2 patients (75%), whereas anticochlear and anticartilage antibodies were present in both groups with a similar frequency (71%). Boulassel et al [26] used two-dimensional gel electrophoresis and immunoblot analysis to define, at the molecular level, the inner-ear auto-antigens recognized by auto-antibodies in the sera of patients suffering from inner-ear diseases. Forty-four percent of the patients' sera had antibodies for several inner-ear proteins, of which the 30, 42, and 68 kDa proteins were found to be the most reactive. The 30 and 42 kDa inner-ear proteins were found to be the major peripheral myelin protein P0 and the beta-actin protein, respectively.

A study by Shin et al [27] using a Western blot immune assay suggested that approximately 40% of patients with rapidly progressive SNHL have antibodies to 68 kDa (heat-shock protein-70; hsp-70) inner-ear antigen. Such immunoblot testing provides 58% sensitivity and 98% specificity for hsp-70 antibodies.

In a different study, sera from patients with various inner-ear diseases, especially Meniere's disease, were investigated by a Western blot against guinea pig inner-ear proteins. Out of 45 patients, 24 (53%) with various inner-ear diseases had antibodies against inner-ear proteins compared with 0/10 in control subjects without inner-ear diseases. Of the 10 proteins that showed a positive reaction with the patient's sera, the 28-kDa band was unique in that it appeared only in the membranous fraction of the inner-ear proteins and was highly positive (28%) in reaction with Meniere's disease patient's sera. These results suggest that the antibody to the 28-kDa protein may be a candidate for detecting autoimmune inner-ear disease [28].

In another study, 16/18 SLE patients had antibodies to guinea pig inner-ear antigens (detected by immunobloting), whereas none were detected in the sera of the 11 normal subjects. This suggested that the inner ear might be one of the targets involved in SLE [29]. In this regard immunological abnormalities were demonstrated in 25/50 patients with SNHL; high immunoglobulin titers were observed in 18/50. Six patients were seropositive for antinuclear antibody and rheumatoid factor, whereas 2/50 revealed high anti-DNA titers [30]. In addition, abnormal low serum complement levels were detected in 6 cases. In summary, based on all of the above facts, sensorineural hearing loss is associated with immunological dysregulation.

Sensorineural Hearing Loss and APS

Because the internal auditory artery is an end artery, disturbed circulation of the inner ear has long been suggested as the cause of sudden SNHL. In 1994, de Kleyn postulated a central vascular lesion in many SNHL cases [31]. Later, some authors have attributed these symptoms to a deficient homeostasis, often in conjunction with additional risk factors for vascular disease, such as arteriosclerosis and high blood viscosity. Others have postulated a viral cause, having a detrimental effect on the rheologic properties of blood.

Primary APS and SNHL

Because microthrombosis associated with aPL is known to affect either dermal or retinal vasculature, a similar involvement of the cochlear vessels could be envisioned, causing sudden SNHL.

In 1996, Hisashi et al [32] reported 3 female patients with sudden SNHL having elevated levels of aCL in their sera: 1/3 had IgM aCL and 2/3 had IgG aCL. Corticosteroid therapy was effective only in the first patient, whereas in another case, hearing loss improved only after adding prostaglandin E and ticlopidine to the corticosteroids. The author concluded that corticosteroids as well as prostaglandin E and ticlopidine therapy might be effective in patients with SNHL with aCL.

In 1997 we reported our results on the presence of aCL in the sera of patients with SNHL [33]. Low-to-moderate positive aCL to one or both IgG/IgM isotypes (range, 18–35 units) were found in 8/30 (27%) patients, whereas none were detected in healthy controls ($P < 0.02$). Another study supported the notion that primary APS is associated with the development of SNHL. In the sera of 55 patients with SD and 80 with progressive SNHL, aCL was present in 49% and 50% of these patients, respectively [34]. The conclusions from these studies were missing as the requirement for a true positive aCL test is based on at least two consecutive seropositive aCL results that were not performed in these studies. It is also important to note that anti–β_2-glycoprotein I (anti–β_2-GPI) antibodies were not analyzed in these patients. Recently, in an extended study we assessed 51 patients (31 women and 20 men) who met the diagnostic criteria of SNHL. We found low to moderately positive titers of aCL in 16 patients (31%) compared with 2 (6%) in the healthy controls ($P = 0.004$). Six patients (12%, all aCL positive) were also positive for anti–β_2-GPI. Three months later positive aCL persisted in 7 (14%) patients, four of whom were also positive for anti–β_2-GPI [35]. This is consistent with the knowledge that anti–β_2-GPI antibodies are more specifically associated with thromboembolism [36].

Tests for antibodies to CMV, EBV, and HCV were found negative in all aCL-positive patients. This "positiveness" for aCL together with anti–β_2-GPI further supports the assumption of an association between SNHL and aPL in some patients, whereas in others it is of a transient character. Although a transient increase in aCL is not considered pathogenic, it is possible that in some cases the increase in antibody titer is capable of inducing transient vascular damage and, hence, microthrombosis. The pathogenic effect of aCL/anti–β_2-GPI induced by viral or bacterial peptides is the subject of many recent investigations. It is generally believed that aCL induced by infection (such as EBV or CMV) are independent of β_2-GPI , and do not appear to be pathogenic. Some reports suggest, however, that certain infections may induce β_2-GPI–dependent aCL as well as clinical features of

APS. This finding strongly suggests that viral antigens can induce aCL and some-times anti–β_2-GPI positivity in humans, and that these antibodies cross-react with the self-phospholipids and consequently are potentially pathogenic [37, 38].

Secondary APS and Progressive SNHL

In the past SNHL has been reported to be one of the symptoms complicating autoimmune diseases, but only recently its association with aCL seropositive data was reported. In 1993, Hisashi et al [39] reported on the occurrence of SNHL in a patient with SLE who was also seropositive for IgG aCL. In 1995, Casoli and Tumiati [40] reported, in a 55-year-old woman with Sjögren syndrome and aCL, seropositiv-ity of IgG and IgM isotypes. She developed a sudden SNHL in association with vertigo, suggesting the presence of atypical Cogan's syndrome.

In a different study [41], 30 women suffering from Sjögren syndrome were evalu-ated for audiovestibular disorders, in comparison with 40 healthy age-matched female controls. In 14/30 patients (46%), SNHL was found, compared to only one control subject (2.5%). Nine of the above 14 patients (64%) tested seropositive for aCL compared with 3/40 controls. This study suggested that SNHL in Sjögren syn-drome is correlated with the presence of aCL .

Naaredrop and Spiera [42] also reported 6 patients who developed sudden deafness in association with moderate-to-high levels of aCL and/or a positive lupus anticoagulant test.

Many studies evaluated the association between autoimmune SNHL and various viral infections, such as parvovirus B19, measles, mumps, and influenza, suggesting that these viruses may bc of possible etiology in this inner-ear disease [43, 44]. On the other hand, the finding of positive aCL is also frequently related to such viruses, but without clear evidence that aCL may be the cause of recurrent thrombosis. However, some studies reported on the association between thrombosis and infec-tious induced aPL [45].

Therefore, it is important to analyze the possible relationship between SNHL, aCL, and various viral infections. If such a positive association can be established, the use of anticoagulant therapy should be its logical consequence [46].

Closing Comments

The etiology of SNHL remains idiopathic in most cases, despite many attempts to relate this condition to infectious diseases, immune-mediated vascular disorders, or microthrombosis [47]. In some reports, SNHL was shown to be associated with the presence of various auto-antibodies and/or the dysregulation of cellular immu-nity. Reports by the authors and by others describe an association between SNHL and aCL [35], raising the speculation that this disorder is microthrombotic in origin. The persistence of aCL over time and the coexistence of anti–β_2-GPI in some patients further support this assumption. In the absence of histological or imaging tool to demonstrate microthrombosis in the inner ear of patients with SNHL and APS, the next rational step is the assessment of the use of anticoagulant therapy in such patients.

References

1. McCabe BF. Autoimmune sensorineural hearing loss. Ann Otol 1979;88:585–589.
2. Hughes GB, Kinney SE, Hamid MA, Barna BP, Calabrese LH. Autoimmune vestibular dysfunction. Laryngoscope 1984;95:758–766.
3. Harris JP. Experimental autoimmune sensorineural hearing loss. Laryngoscope 1987;97:63–76.
4. Chen CY, Halpin C, Rauch SD. Oral steroid treatment of sudden sensorineural hearing loss: a ten year retrospective analysis. Otol Neurotol 2003;24:728–733.
5. Solares CA, Edling AE, Johnson JM, et al. Murine autoimmune hearing loss mediated by CD4+ T cells specific for inner ear peptides. J Clin Invest 2004;113:1210–1217.
6. Peeva E, Barland P. Sensorineural hearing loss in conjunction with aortic insufficiency in systemic lupus erythematosus. Scand J Rheumatol 2001;30:45–47.
7. Kumar BN, Walsh RM, Wilson PS, Carlin WV. Sensorineural hearing loss and ulcerative colitis. J Laryngol Otol 1997;111:277–278.
8. Raut VV, Cullen J, Cathers G. Hearing loss in rheumatoid arthritis. J Otolaryngol 2001;30:289–294.
9. Lunardi C, Bason C, Leandri M, et al. . Autoantibodies to inner ear and endothelial antigens in Cogan's syndrome. Lancet 2002;360:915–921.
10. Saracaydin A, Katircioglu S, Karatay MC. Azathioprine in combination with steroids in the treatment of autoimmune inner-ear disease. J Intern Med Res 1993;21:192–196.
11. Luetje CM, Berliner KI. Plasmapheresis in autoimmune ear disease: long-term follow-up. Am J Otol 1997;18:572–576.
12. Bowman CA, Linthicum FH Jr, Nelson RA, Mikami K, Quismorio F. Sensorineural hearing loss associated with systemic lupus erythematosus. Otolaryngol Head Neck Surg 1986;94:197–204.
13. Caldarelli DD, Rejowaski JE, Corey JP. Sensorineural hearing loss in lupus erythematosus. Am J Otol 1986;7:210–213.
14. Kobayashi S, Fujishiro N, Sugiyama K. Systemic lupus erythematosus with sensorineural hearing loss and improvement after plasmapheresis using the double filtration method. Intern Med 1992;31:778–781.
15. Kataoka H, Takeda T, Nakatani H, Saito H. sensorineural hearing loss of suspected autoimmune ethiology: a report of three cases. Auris Nasus Larynx 1995;22:53–58.
16. Andonopoulos AP, Naxakis S, Goumas P, Lygatsikas C. Sensorineural hearing loss disorders in systemic lupus erythematosus. A controlled study. Clin Exp Rheumatol 1995;13:137–141.
17. Sperling NM, Tehrani K, Liebling A, Ginzler E. Aural symptoms and hearing loss in patients with lupus. Otolaryngol Head Neck Surg 1998;118:762–765.
18. Berrettini S, Ferri C, Pitaro N, et al. Audiovestibular involvment in systemic sclerosis. ORL J Otorhinolaryngol Relat Spec 1994;56:195–198.
19. Igarashi Y, Watanabe Y, Aso S. Case of Behcet's disease with otologic symptoms. ORL J Otorhinolaryngol Relat Spec 1994;56:295–298.
20. Yoo TJ, Tomoda K, Stuat JM, Cremer MA, Towens AS, Kang AH. Type II collagen-induced autoimmune SNHL and vestibular dysfunction in rats. Ann Otol Rhinol Laryngol 1983;92:267–271.
21. Rukemstein MJ, Mount RJ, Harrison RV. The MRL-*lpr/lpr* mouse: a potential model of autoimmune inner-ear disease. Acta Oto Laryngologica 1993;113:160–165.
22. Iwai H, Tomoda K, Hosaka N, et al. Induction of immune-mediated hearing loss in SCID mice by injection of MRL/lpr mouse spleen cells. Hearing Res 1998;117:173–177.
23. Billings P. Experimental autoimmune hearing loss. J Clin Invest 2004;113:1114–1117.
24. Hughes GB, Moscicki R, Barna BP, San Martin JE. Laboratory diagnosis of immune inner ear disease. Am J Otol 1994;15:198–202.
25. Mayot D, Bene MC, Dron K, Perrin C, Faure GC. Immunologic alterations in patients with sensorineural hearing disorders. Clin Immunol Immunopathol 1993;68:41–45.
26. Boulassel MR, Deggouj N, Tomasi JP, Gersdorff M. Inner ear autoantibodies and their targets in patients with autoimmune inner ear diseases. Acta Otolaryngol 2001;121:28–34.
27. Shin S, Billings P, Keithley EM, Harris PJ. Comparison of anti-heat shock protein-70 (anti hsp-70) and anti 68-kDa inner-ear protein in the sera of patients with Menieres disease. Laryngoscope 1997;107:222–227.
28. Suzuki M, Krug MS, Cheng KC, Yazawa Y, Bernstein J, Yoo TJ. Antibodies against inner-ear proteins in the sera of patients with inner-ear diseases. ORL J Otorhinolaryngol Relat Spec 1997;59:10–17.
29. Xiao H, Wang J. Western blot analysis of serum autoantibodies against inner-ear antigens in patients with systemic lupus erythematosus. Chung Hau Erh Pi Yen Hou Ko Chin 1995;30:236–238.

30. Takahashi M, Sakata A, Unno T, Hokunan K, Shigyo H. Immunological abnormalities in patients with etiology unknown sensorineural hearing loss. Nipon Jibiinkoka Gakkai Kaiho 1998;101:1260–1265.
31. de Kleyn A. Sudden complete or partial loss of function of the octavus-system in apparently normal persons. Acta Otolaryngol 1994;32:407–429.
32. Hisashi K, Komune S, Komiyama S, Nakamura K. Sudden sensorineural hearing loss associated with cardiolipin antibody. Nippon Jibiinkoka Gakkai Kaiho1996;99:1157–1161.
33. Toubi E, Ben-David J, Kessel A, Podoshin L, Golan TD. Autoimmune aberration in sudden sensorineural hearing loss: association with anti-cardiolipin antibodies. Lupus 1997;6:540–542.
34. Heller U, Becker EW, Zenner HP, Berg PA. Incedence and clinical relevance to phospholipids, serotonin and gangiloside in patients with sudden deafness and progressive inner-ear hearing loss. HNO 1998;46:583–586.
35. Toubi E, Ben-David J, Kessel A, Halas K, Sabo E, Luntz M. Immune-mediated disorders associated with idiopathic sudden sensorineural hearing loss. Ann Otol Rhinol Laryngol 2004;113:445–449.
36. Amengual O, Atsumi T, Khamashta MA, Hughes GRV. Specificity of ELISA for antibody to b2 glycoprotein 1 in patients with antiphospholipid syndrome. Br J Rheumatol 1996;35:1239–1243.
37. Fairweather D, Kaya Z, Shellam GR, Lawson CM, Rose NR. From infection to autoimmunity. J Autoimmun 2001;16:175–186.
38. Miller SD, Olson JK, Croxford JL. Multiple pathways to induction of virus-induced autoimmune demyelination: lessons from theiler's virus. J Autoimmun 2001;16:21–227.
39. Hisashi K, Komune S, Taira T, Uemura T, Sadoshima S, Tsuda H. Anticardiolipin antibody-induced sudden profound sensorineural hearing loss. Am J Otolaryngol 1993;14:275–277.
40. Casoli P, Tumiati B. Cogan's syndrome: a new possible complication of antiphospholipid antibodies? Clin Rheumatol 1995;14:197–198.
41. Tumiata B, Casoli P, Parmeggiani A. Hearing loss in sjogren syndrome. Ann Intern Med 1997;15:450–453.
42. Naarendrop M, Spiera H. Sudden sensorineural hearing loss in patients with systemic lupus erythematosus or lupus-like syndrome and antiphospholipid antibodies. J Rheumatol 1998;25:589–592.
43. Cotter CS, Singleton GT, Corman LC. Immune-mediated inner ear disease and parvovirus B19. Laryngoscope 1994;104:1235–1239.
44. Garcia Berrocal JRG, Ramirez-Camacho R, Portero F, Vargas JA. Role of viral and Mycoplasma pneumoniae infection in idiopathic sudden sensorineural hearing loss. Acta Otolaryngol 2000;120:835–839.
45. Uthman IW, Gharavi AE. Viral infections and antiphospholipid antibodies. Semin Arthritis Rheum 2002;31:256–263.
46. Yue WL, Li P, Qi PY, Li HJ, Zhou H. Role of low-molecular-weight heparins in the treatment of sudden hearing loss. Am J Otolaryngol 2003;24:328–333.
47. Koc A, Sanisoglu O. Sudden sensorineural hearing loss: literature survey on recent studies. J Otolaryngol 2003;32:308–313.

14 The Eye in Primary Antiphospholipid Syndrome

Cristina Castañon and Pedro A. Reyes

Clinical associations of antiphospholipid antibodies (aPL) include venous and arterial thrombosis, recurrent fetal loss, blood cytopenias, thrombocytopenia, and multi-organ compromise [1–13]. Vessel occlusion is a hallmark of this association; it may occur within the context of several diseases, mainly autoimmune disorders such as systemic lupus erythematosus (SLE), or it may be present without any recognizible disease, the so-called primary antiphospholipid syndrome or Hughes syndrome [14].

In the past there were isolated reports describing the eye involved in the primary antiphospholipid syndrome (APS) and serious ocular damage, like optic neuritis and ocular vaso-occlusive disease in patients with Hughes syndrome [15–17]. This association was challenged by Merry et al [18] based on the absence of aPL in a group of patients with ocular vaso-occlusive disease. However, Asherson et al [19] found that the presence of ocular vaso-occlusive disease in patients with SLE was definitely related to the presence of antiphospholipid autoantibodies and several studies agree on a high prevalence of vasculopathic eye disease in subjects with Hughes syndrome [20–25]. Maybe the different appreciation reflects both a selection bias (the presence of ocular disease was the inclusion criterion in some studies) and a low prevalence of Hughes syndrome among patients with ocular vaso-occlusive disease of miscellaneous origin.

At present, some cases or some series [26–48] which describe ocular findings in the presence of aPL, or associated to other diseases, are added to our clinical observations, and confirm that the eye is frequently affected. Also, they confirm that the damage is predominant in the posterior segment, as retinal or choroidal vaso-occlusive diseases, which can be arterial, venous, or both. A higher number of studied cases has made it possible to identify, in the literature, a more frecuently anterior segment damages. Anterior and posterior scleritis, related to aPL, were also reported. However, in our APS ocular disease experience, we have not seen yet this manifestation. Besides this, there is nothing new to be added to our clinical study at present.

Clinical Study

We performed and reported a cross-sectional ophthalmology study [49] on 28 consecutive patients (18 women, 10 men; median ages, 30.5 and 40 years, respectively)

Table 14.1. Primary antiphospholipid syndrome: clinical and laboratory findings.   📖

Clinical findings	No.	Laboratory findings	No.
Ocular disease	24/28	IgG aCL	28/28[a]
Recurrent fetal loss	8/10[b]	PTT > 10	14/17
Venous thrombosis	16/28	False-positive results of VDLR	11/28
Arterial occlusion	10/28[d]	Lupus anticoagulant	4/9[b]
Migraine	11/28	Cytopenia	10/28[c]
Livedo reticularis	7/28	FANA (low titer)	3/28
Leg ulcers	3/28		
Chorea	1/28		

PTT = partial thromboplastin time; FANA = fluorescent antinuclear antibodies.
[a]More than 5 SD above the mean value.
[b]Subjects at risk or those in whom the test was done.
[c]Thrombocytopenia, 9; leukopenia, 1.
[d]Seven of these 10 patients had brain infarction demonstrated by computed tomography.

with APS, all of them were seen at the Instituto Nacional de Cardiología Ignacio Chávez from 1987 to 1996. Irrespective of visual symptoms, 27 patients were evaluated prospectively by the ophthalmologist in an equivalent search effort. One patient had visual symptoms, and primary antiphospholipid antibody syndrome (PAPS) was subsequently identified. The diagnosis was based on proposed clinical criteria [5]. SLE was ruled out clinically and serologically over a 48-month follow up. Anticardiolipin antibodies (aCL) were detected by enzyme-linked immunosorbent assay according to Gharavi et al [50], with some modifications by the authors [51]. Test for serum lipid profile, fluorescent antinuclear antibodies, rheumatoid factors, syphilis (VDRL, fluorescent treponemal absorbed antibody), and a clotting profile were performed in every patient using standard laboratory techniques.

The eye examination included a survey of ocular symptoms; tests for visual acuity, ocular movements, and intraocular pressure; and slit-lamp biomicroscopy to evaluate the anterior segment and the fundus. Twenty-four patients agreed to a standard retinal fluorangiography [52].

All patients (Table 14.1) had high titer [>5 standard deviations (SD) above the mean] IgG aCL in at least two determinations. No other non–organ-specific antibodies nor lipid abnormalities were detected. In 14 out of 17 patients, a prolonged phospholipid-dependent clotting assay (PTT) was identified. In the remaining 11 patients, the test was not performed because the patients were receiving anticoagulant drugs. A false-positive VDRL test was present in 11 patients. Nine patients had thrombocytopenia, 1 more case had persistent leukopenia. Four out of 9 patients at risk in whom the test was done presented a positive lupus anticoagulant (LA) test.

Ocular Findings

As shown in Table 14.2, 19 (68%) patients had visual symptoms. Transient visual disturbance (transient blurred vision or amaurosis fugax) was present in 16 eyes (8 patients), decreased vision in 7 (4 patients), transient diplopia in 8 (4 patients), and transient field loss associated with headache and photopsy in 8 (4 patients). Visual acuity with or without correction was 20/20 to 20/ 40 in 46 eyes, 20/60 to 20/100 in 3

Table 14.2. Ocular vaso-occlusive disease in primary antiphospholipid syndrome.

Case no.	1	2	3	4	5	6	7	8	9	10	11	12	13	14	15	16	17	18	19	20	21	22	23	24	25	26	27	28	Total no. eyes
Ocular findings visual symptoms (18/28)																													
Decreased vision	R/L											L	R/L											R/L					7
Transient blurring						R/L	R/L	R/L											R/L	R/L	R/L				R/L	R/L			16
Transient diplopia			R/L						R/L											R/L					R/L				8
Transient field loss										R/L							R/L									R/L	R/L		8
Photopsy																	R/L	R/L										R/L	6
Ocular findings anterior segment (9/28)																													
Conjunctival telangiectases									R/L					R/L	R/L				R/L	R/L					R/L				12
Conjunctival microaneurysms									R/L					R/L	R/L				R/L	R/L					R/L				12
Simple episcleritis				R/L																									2
Limbal keratitis																R													1
Corneal opacity									R																				1
Ocular findings eye fundi (24/28)																													
Vitreous hemorrhage	R												R/L																3
Preretinal hemorrhage														R/L															2
Swelling optic disc						R						L	R											R					4
Venous tortuosity			R/L		R/L	R/L	R/L	R/L	R/L	R/L	R/L	R/L	R/L	R/L	R/L	R/L	R/L		R/L			R/L	R/L		R/L		R/L		38
Vascular sheathing			R/L*					L*	L*			L					R/L			R/L*				L		R			10
Rarefacción y Rectificación																		R/L											
Pigment abnormalities			R/L						L	R/L		R													R/L			R	9
Flame-shaped hemorrhages									L		R/L	R	L		R/L														7
Cotton-wool spots						R							R																2
Microaneurysms									L		L		L											L					4
Macular serous detachment									L																				1
IRMAs								L																					1
Peripheral druscen					R/L																						R/L		4

R = right eye; L = left eye; IRMAs = intraretinal microvascular abnormalities.
*Peripheral vessels.

eyes, and 20/400 or worse in 7 eyes (4 patients). All patients had normal intraocular pressures (12–18 mm Hg), except for a case with cerebrovascular disease and 20 mm Hg intraocular pressure in both eyes who had an inferior temporal quadrantanopia, due to an obstruction of a branch of retinal artery.

Anterior segment abnormalities were mild and relatively uncommon: conjunctival telangiectases or microaneurysms were present in 12 eyes (6 patients), simple episcleritis in 2 (1 patient), and limbal keratitis in 1. The latter two abnormalities resolved with local corticosteroid treatment. One patient had a monocular posttraumatic superficial corneal opacity since childhood.

Posterior segment abnormalities were found in 24 patients (86%; Table 14.2). Tortuosity of first-order venous vessels or peripheral terminals in 38 eyes (19 patients) was the most common finding. Swelling of the optic disc was found in 4 eyes (cases 1, 12, 13, and 24). Vitreous hemorrhage occurred in 3 eyes (cases 1, 12, and 24; Fig. 14.1); vitreous bands adherent to the optic disc subsequently developed in 2 of these eyes (case 12, 24) after the hemorrhage. One of these (case 1) fully recovered under treatment. Serous detachment at the macula with preretinal hemorrhage was observed in one eye (case 13) . Other patient, had segmental dilatation of capillary vessels, microaneurysms, and intraretinal microvascular abnormalities in 1 eye (case 8). There were cotton-wool spots in two eyes (cases 1 and 13), flame-shaped hemorrhages in 8 eyes (cases 1, 8, 9, 12, 13, and 24), microaneurysms in 3 eyes (cases 8, 9, and 14); sheathing of first-order veins in 2 eyes (case 1), arterial sheathing in 1 additional patient (case 25). Equatorial and peripheral hypopigmentation was noted in 2 eyes (case 3), and reticular pigment clumps around the temporal vascular arcade of both eyes, associated with widespread areas of atrophy, were seen in case 10. Two eyes (case 26) presented grayish lines extended radially on temporal retina from optic disc, with an hypertrophic scar in the temporal aspect of the macula in the right eye. One eye had minor irregular clumps of pigment near superior temporal vessels (case 28).

Retinal fluorescein angiography was performed in 24 patients (Table 14.3) and it was abnormal in 18 eyes (12 patients, 50%). Although in general the procedure

Table 14.3. Ocular vaso-occlusive disease in primary antiphospholipid syndrome*

Case no.		1	3	8	9	10	12	13	20	24	25	26	28	Total no. eyes
Abnormalities	12/24													
Vitreous	Hemorrhage	R					L			L				3
Choroidal	Blocked fluorescence					R/L		L				R	R	5
	Window defects		R/L		L	R/L						R/L		7
Vascular	Tortuosity	R/L	R/L	R/L	R/L		R/L	R/L		L	L			14
	Microaneurysms			R/L	L			R/L						5
	Capilar ectasis	R/L	L					R/L		L				6
	Leakage	R/L	L						L	L				5
	Noncapillary perfusion	R/L		L	L		L	L		R/L	L			9
	Obstruction*	R/L		L	L			L		R/L	L	R		9
	Neoformation			L										1
Retinal	Hemorrhages	R/L		L	L			R/L						6
	Cotton-wool spots	R						R						2
Optic disc	Leakage	R						R		R				3

R = right; L = left.
*Ocular findings, retinal fluorescein angiography (12/24).

confirmed the funduscopic findings, it showed unsuspected occlusion of the peri-macular arteriole in 1 eye (case 9), focal late hiperfluorescence, and leakage of retinal capillaries superior in 1 eye (case 20), and pigment epithelial window defects considered to be secondary to choriocapillary vessels obstruction in 2 eyes (case 3). In case 10, early hyperfluorescence of atrophic areas around pigment clumps created a window effect, which was interpreted as reticular degeneration of the pigmentary epithelium. Two eyes (case 26) showed fluorescence in the arterial phase which persisted after the dye had disappeared from retinal veins; these angioid streaks did occur in absence of systemic evidence of pseudoxanthoma elasticum. This patient also had vessel occlusion inferior to macula and hipertrophic scar in right eye. Case 24 had hyperfluorescence and poor arterial filling because of retinal central artery occlusion in right eye with vitreous hemorrhage and vaso-occlusive retinopathy in left eye.

A generalized vaso-occlusive retinopathy with fluorescein leakage and areas of hypoperfusion was noted in 5 eyes (cases 1, 12, and 25). In another patient, a macular serous detachment was present (case 13). Of particular interest were the angiographic findings in one eye (case 8), including focal occlusion of temporal arterioles and venules near the macula, areas of capillary hypoperfusion, fluorescein leakage, and retinal neovascularization. Emergency photocoagulation treatment was used on this patient; 4 years later the recurrence on these vessels required further treatment.

Follow Up

Six patients were lost: 2 died and 4 left the hospital. Ophtalmologic follow up from 5 to 9 years has been completed in 8 patients, 11 more were followed from 1 to 3 years, and 3 for less than a year. All cases were treated with chronic anticoagulants, with international normalization radio (INR) between 2 and 3, as well as chronic low dosage of acetilsalycilic acid, except case 19, who had an associated clotting defect, von Willebrand disease, which prevent the use of anticlotting measures.

Most patients recovered and stay visually asymptomatic for long periods, up to 9 years. Some of them required photocoagulation therapy, usually once, but one of them required a second treatment. A patient (case 13) with extensive bilateral arterial and venous ocular obstruction developed a neovascular glaucoma and right-eye ptisis bulbi in a 2-year period; the left eye conserved a corrected 20/50 vision

Table 14.4. Retinal vascular obstruction 12/56 eyes.   📖

Case No.	CRA	RA branch	CRV
1	–	–	R/L
8	–	–	L
9	–	L	–
12	–	–	L
13	R	–	R/L
24	R	–	L
25	–	L	–
26	–	L	–

CRA = central retinal artery; RA branch = retinal artery branch; CRV = central retinal vein.

without further problems. Another patient (case 18) developed retinal microa-neurysms and hemorrhages in both eyes which disappeared in a year.

In summary, ocular vaso-occlusive disease is a common finding in APS; it is easy to identify this complication by systematic eye exam. Prompt recognition and anticlotting therapy limits organ damage and usually achieve sustained improvement.

Discussion

Since the first edition of this book was published in 2000, growing evidence has confirmed eye morbidity as part of the clinical expression of PAPS. Authors from all over the world have made contributions, case reports, case series, and case-control studies describing many different forms of eye vasocclusive disease in PAPS patients and some forms of inflammatory disease which may be linked to focal ischaemia due to arterial or venous occlusions.

The posterior pole, mainly venous or arterial retinal vessels, are the most commonly affected vessels; venous engorgement and tortuosity, occluded central vein and arterial involvement with sheathered vessels appearing as white lines in funduscopy, hemorrhage due to wall damage, and abnormalities in fluorangiography are frequent findings in one or both eyes in these patients. Sometimes central nervous system damage in specific nuclei manifested as eye abnormalities such as oculomotor nerve palsy.

Vitreous hemorrhage and choroidal vessel involvement has been described, in one case, as the first manifestation of eye compromise in PAPS.

Occasionally an inherited defect on clotting mechanisms, such as Leiden or pro-thrombin G20210A mutations, homocysteine levels, or abnormal S or C proteins, coincides with aPL; however, in most cases the antibody alone is the culprit of the eye disease. All these pathogenic mechanisms may explain eye symptoms such as blurred vision, scotoma, transient ischemic attacks with visual loss, progressive loss in visual acuity, and sudden blindness, which are frequent in PAPS patients or may occur as presenting manifestation. In such case it is necessary a complete physical exam and laboratory work up.

Anterior segment symptoms are also common. Telangiectasis at conjunctival vessels, keratitis limbal, or filamentary and neovascular glaucoma were sometimes reported, but in many patients the anterior segment was completely normal in spite of serious posterior segment severe disease.

Differential diagnosis should consider diabetic retinopathy, sarcoid, and hemato-logical neoplasia as well as stroke and accelerated artheriosclerosis and, of course, systemic rheumatic diseases such as SLE, Sjögren syndorme, or systemic progres-sive sclerosis and some infections. These cases are considered, of course, secondary APS.

Increased medical awareness has made it possible to recognize more cases. Reports on eye disease linked to aPL have become frequent in the literature. Aspirin and long-term anticoagulation help many patients and it is common to achieve significant visual improvement and stop visual loss progression and vasocclusive disease with minimal adverse effects.

References

1. Shapiro SS, Thiagarajan P. Lupus anticoagulants. Progr Hemost Thromb 1982;6:263–285.
2. Harris EN, Gharavi AE, Hughes GRV. Antiphospholipid antibodies. Clin Rheum Dis 1985;1:591–609.
3. Triplett DA, Brandt JT, Musgrave KA, Orr CA. The relationship between lupus anticoagulants and antibodies to phospholipid. JAMA 1988;259:550–554.
4. Mackworth-Young CG, Loizu S, Walport MJ. Primary antiphospholipid syndrome: features of patients with raised anticardiolipin antibodies and no other disorder. Ann Rheum Dis 1989;48:362–367.
5. Alarcón-Segovia D, Sanchez-Guerrero J. Primary antiphospholipid syndrome. J Rheumatol 1989;16:482–428.
6. Asherson RA, Khamashta MA, Ordi-Ros J, et al. The "primary" antiphospholipid syndrome: major clinical and serological features. Medicine (Baltimore) 1989;68:366–374.
7. Sammaritano LR, Gharavi AE, Lockshin MD. Antiphospholipid antibody syndrome: immunologic and clinical aspects. Semin Arthritis Rheum 1990;20:81–96.
8. Khamashta MA, Cervera R, Asherson RA, et al. Association of antibodies against phospholipids with heart valve disease in systemic lupus erythematosus. Lancet 1990;335:1541–1543.
9. Reyes López PA, Casanova JM, Amigo MC. The anticardiolipin syndrome – a clinical study. In: Ring J, Pryzbilla B, eds. New trends in allergy III. Berlin: Springer-Verlag; 1991:382–394.
10. Amigo M-C, Garcia-Torres R, Robles M, et al. Renal involvement in primary antiphospholipid syndrome. J Rheumatol 1992;19:1181–1185.
11. Hachulla E, Leys D, Deleume JF, Pruvo JP, Devulder B. Manifestations neurologiques associees aux anticorps antiphospholipides. Ou que reste-t-il du neurolupus?. Rev Med Interne 1995;16:121–130.
12. Badui E, Soloni S, Martinez E, et al. The heart in the primary antiphospholipisyndrome. Arch Med Res 1995;26:115–120.
13. Cervera R, Asherson RA, Lie JT. Clinicopathologic correlation of the antiphospholipid syndrome. Semin Arthritis Rheum 1995;24:262–272.
14. Hughes GRV, Harris EN, Gharavi AE. The anticardiolipin syndrome. J Rheumatol 1986;13:486–489.
15. Levin SR, Crofts JW, Lesser GR, Floberg J, Welch KMA. Visual symptoms associated with the presence of a lupus anticoagulant. Ophthalmology 1988;95:686–692.
16. Kleiner RC, Najarian LV, Schatten S, et al. Vaso-occlusive retinopathy associated with antiphospholipid antibodies (lupus anticoagulant retinopathy). Ophthalmology 1989;96:896–904.
17. Gerber SL, Cantor LB. Progressive optic atrophy and the primary antiphospholipid syndrome [letter]. Am J Ophthalmol 1990;1:443–444.
18. Merry P, Acheson JF, Asherson RA, Hughes GR. Management of retinal vein occlusion [letter]. Br Med J 1988;296:294.
19. Asherson RA, Merry P, Acheson JF, et al. Antiphospholipid antibodies: a risk factor for occlusive ocular vascular disease in systemic lupus erythematosus and the "primary" antiphospholipid syndrome. Ann Rheum Dis 1989;48:358 356.
20. Dunn JP, Noorily SW, Petri M, Finkelstein D, Rosenbaum JT, Jabs DA. Antiphospholipid antibodies and retinal vascular disease. Lupus 1996;5:313–322.
21. Wiechens B, Schroder JO, Potzsch B, Rochels R. Am J Ophthalmol 1997;123:848–850.
22. Susuki A, Okamoto N, Watanabe M, Kiritoshi H, Motokura M, Fakuda M. The time course of white retinal arterioles in two cases of antiphospholipid antibody syndrome. Nippon Ganka Gakkai Zasshi 1998;102:455–461.
23. Ihara M, Tanaka H, Nishimura Y. Primary antiphospholipid syndrome with recurrent transient ischemic attacks: report of a case and its successful treatment. Intern Med 1998;37:704–707.
24. Leo-Kottler B, Klein R, Berg PA, Zrenner E. Ocular symptoms in association with antiphospholipid antibodies. Graefes Arch Clin Exp Ophthalmol 1998;236:658–668.
25. Dori D, Gelfand YA, Brenner B, Miller B. Cilioretinal artery occlusion: an ocular complication of primary antiphospholipid syndrome. Retina 1997;17:555–557.
26. Malaviya AN, Marouf R, AI-Jarallah K, et al. Hughes syndome: a common problem in Kuwait Hospitals. Br J Rheumatol 1996;35:1132–1136.
27. Zierhut M, Klein R, Berg P, Turmer KH, Raphael BR. Retinal vasculitis and antiphospholipi antibodies. Ophthalmologe 1994;91:772–776.
28. Dori D, Gerfand YA, Brenner B, Miller B. Cilioretinal artery occlusion: an ocular complication of primary antiphospholipid syndrome. Retina 1997;17:555–567.

29. Wiechens B, Schroder JO, Potzsch B, Rochels R. Primary antipospholipid antibody syndrome and retinal occlusive vasculopathy. Am J Ophtalmol 1997;123:848–850.
30. Suzuki A, Okamoto N, Watanabe M, Kiritoshi H, Motokura M, Fukuda M. The time course oft white retinal arterioles in two cases of antiphopholipid antibody syndrome. Nippon Granka Gakkai Zasshi 1998;102:455–461.
31. Boets EP, Chaar CG, Ronday K, Keunen JE, Breedveld FC. Chorrioretinopathy in primary antiphospholipid syndrome: a case report. Retina 1998;18:382–385.
32. Leo-Kottler B, Klein R, Berg PA, Zrenner E. Ocular symptoms in association with antiphospholipid antibodies. Arch Clin Exp Ophthalmol 1998;236:658–668.
33. Liu E, Nijhawan N, Gladman D, Lam WC, Buys Y. Primary antiphospholipid syndrome and neovascular glaucoma. Can J Ophthalmol 1999;34:349–352.
34. Suzuki A, Okamoto N, Ohnishi M, Watanabe M, Motokura M, Fukuda M. White thread-like retinal arterioles associated with antiphospholipid antibody syndrome. Jpn J Ophthalmol 1999;43:553–558.
35. Hsiao YC, Jou JR, Lin SY, Lin SL. Primary antiphospholipid syndrome manifested as venous stasis retinopathy. Zhonghua Yi Xue Za Zhi (Taipei) 2000;63:498–502.
36. Bolling JP, Brown GC. The antiphospholipid antibody syndrome. Curr Opin Ophthalmol 2000;11:211–213.
37. Ang LP, Yap EY, Fam Hb. Bilateral choroidal infarction in a patient with antiphsopholipid syndrome: a case report. Clin Exp Ophthalmol 2000;28:326–328.
38. Smith JR, Chang H, Chee S. Primary antiphospholipid syndrome masquerading as diabetic retinopathy. Jpn J Ophthalmol 2001;45:105–108.
39. Nogueria Goriba A, Martin Sanchez MD. Syndrome.
40. Srinivasan S, Fern A, Watson WH, McColl MD. Reversal of nonarteritic anterior ischemic optic neuropathy associated with coexisting primary antiphospholipid syndrome and Factor V Leiden mutation. Am J Ophthalmol 2001;131:671–673.
41. Vielpeau I, Le Hello C, Legris A, Salsou E, Lecoq PJ. Retinal vascular occlusion and prumary antiphospholipid syndrome. Report of 2 cases. J Fr Ophtalmol 2001;24:955–960.
42. Champion BL, Choy F, Schriber L, Roche J, Rowe DB. Isolated fascicular oculomotor nerve palsy as the initial presentation of the antiphospholipid syndrome. J Clin Neurosci 2002;9:691–694.
43. Hartnett ME, Laposata M, Van Cott E. Antiphsopholipid antibody syndrome in a six-year-old female patient. Am J Ophthalmol 2003;135:542–544.
44. Monshizadeh R, Werner M, Richard H, Tabandeh H, Bhatti Mt. Vitreous hemorrhage as the presenting sign of antiphospholipid syndrome. Can J Ophthalmol 2003;38:607–609.
45. Cobo-Soriano R, Sanchez-Ramon S, Aparicio MJ, et al.Anthiphospholipid antibodies and retinal thrombosis in patients without risk factors: a prospective case-control study. Am J Ophthalmol 1999;128:725–732.
46. Demirci FY, Kucukkaya R, Akarcay K, et al. Ocular involvement in primary antiphospholipid syndrome. Int Ophthalmol 1998;22:323–329.
47. Miserocchi E, Baltatzis S, Foster CS. Ocular features associated with anticardiolipin antibodies: a descriptive study. Am J Ophtalahmol 2001;131:451–456.
48. Durrani Om, Gordon C, Murray PI. Primary anti-phospholipid antibody syndrome (APS): current concepts. Surv Ophthalmol 2002;47:215–238.
49. Castañon C, Amigo MC, Bañales JL, Nava A, Reyes PA. Ocular vaso-occlusive disease in primary antiphospholipid syndrome. Ophthalmology 1995;102:256–262.
50. Gharavi AE, Harris EN, Asherson RA, Hughes GRV. Anticardiolipin antibodies: isotype distribution and phospholipid specificity. Ann Rheum Dis 1987;46:1–6.
51. Nava A, Bañales JL, Reyes PA. Effect of heat inactivation and sheep erythrocyte adsorption on the titer of anticardiolipin antibodies in primary antiphospholipid syndrome and healthy blood donor's sera. J Clin Lab Anal 1992;6:148–150.
52. Novotny HR, Alvis DL. A method of photographing fluorescence in circulating blood in the human retina. Circulation 1961;24:82–86.

15   Primary Antiphospholipid Syndrome

Tonia L. Vincent and Charles G. Mackworth-Young

Introduction

The emergence of the antiphospholipid syndrome (APS) over the last 30-odd years has been one of the most striking developments in clinical autoimmunity. The identification of a pure or primary variant of the syndrome has been central to this story, not least in enabling us to establish the place of this remarkable condition in the wide spectrum of autoimmune disease.

Circulating antiphospholipid antibodies (aPL), as detected by the false-positive biological test for syphilis, have been known for more than 40 years [1], and their ability to cause prolongation of the partial thromboplastin or kaolin clotting time generated the term *lupus anticoagulant* (LA) [2]. Although the phenomenon was initially described in an systemic lupus erythematosus (SLE) patient associated with a hemorrhagic disorder, by the 1960s it was apparent that the presence of the LA was paradoxically linked to the risk of thrombosis [3]. Following this, associations with thrombocytopenia [4] and recurrent miscarriage [5–7] were established. Not all of these patients had SLE – so the term lupus anticoagulant was thus misleading, not only because of its procoagulant associations in vivo, but also because some patients had no evidence of lupus.

In vitro studies showed that the LA activity was mediated by antibodies [8]. The association of false-positive tests for syphilis led to the suggestion that these antibodies may bind to phospholipids. This was supported by an earlier study, which demonstrated that LA activity could be partially abolished by pre-absorption of test serum with cardiolipin [9].

Direct confirmation came in 1983 with the development of a sensitive immunoassay for anticardiolipin activity in serum [10]. Antibodies detected by this method were subsequently shown to exhibit LA activity [11]. Derivatives of this assay still perform a pivotal role in the diagnosis of the APS.

Defining APS

The direct detection of anticardiolipin antibodies (aCL) enabled Hughes and coworkers to make the first formal description of the APS [12, 13]. They recognized a group of patients with SLE who had raised levels of these antibodies and clinical features including recurrent venous thrombosis, central nervous system disease,

155

and recurrent miscarriage. Serologically, the majority of these patients demonstrated aPL. By 1985 it had become apparent that some of such patients exhibited few or no features of underlying connective tissue disease, and the concept emerged that this syndrome could exist as a separate entity [14–17].

In 1989 three units published clinical series establishing the primary antiphospholipid syndrome (PAPS) [18–20]. They described a group of patients in whom recurrent thrombosis, miscarriage, and thrombocytopenia were associated with aCL; although several patients were positive for anti-nuclear antibodies, none fulfilled classification criteria for the diagnosis of SLE.

APS as a Clinical Spectrum

From these early reports four categories of APS or Hughes syndrome could be defined:

(i) APS associated with underlying connective tissue disease, most usually SLE; (ii) patients with APS with no underlying features of connective tissue disease, the primary APS; (iii) patients with APS and lupus-like disease who have features of connective tissue disease but who do not fulfill classification criteria for the diagnosis of SLE; (iv) APS due to other causes, such as drugs, malignancy, and infection. Many of these patients exhibit increased aCL in the absence of an overt clinical syndrome. When clinical disease is apparent it is usually mild and transient.

These are a heterogeneous group of patients and as such are likely to represent a spectrum of disease rather than discrete disease entities. This is supported by documented development of overt SLE in patients with an original diagnosis of PAPS. In a 5-year follow up by Asherson et al [21], 19 patients with APS (9 with associated SLE; 7 with lupus-like disease; and 3 with PAPS) were studied. During this interval, 3 patients with lupus-like disease progressed to a diagnosis of SLE, and 1 patient with PAPS developed lupus-like disease.

In some instances this transition may take many years. The same unit [22] performed a retrospective study of 80 patients seen over a 10-year period with PAPS. Two cases developed SLE more than 10 years following the initial presentation of PAPS and 1 developed lupus-like disease. Andrews et al [23] described 2 patients with PAPS developing SLE after 8 and 10 years. These findings and similar anecdotal experience mean that clinicians should be mindful of the long transition times from PAPS to SLE-associated APS, even though the studies would suggest that this is a relatively uncommon event.

Differentiation Between SLE-associated APS and PAPS

There are both clinical and serological features that help differentiate between these groups of patients. Vianna et al [24] conducted a multicenter study of primary and secondary APS. Of 114 patients, 56 had SLE-associated APS and 58 had PAPS. They found that both groups of patients had similar clinical presentations with the exception of endocardial valve disease, which occurred in 63% of lupus patients versus 37% of patients with PAPS ($P < 0.005$). Other more predictable differences included autoimmune hemolytic anemia (21% vs. 7%; $P < 0.05$), neutropenia (11% vs. 0%;

$P < 0.01$), ANA positivity (81% vs. 41%), and low C4 levels, all of which were significantly more common in patients with SLE-associated APS. No patient with PAPS had antibodies to extractable nuclear antigens or dsDNA.

The female:male ratio in this study was 7:1 for SLE-associated APS and 4.2:1 for PAPS. Other studies have also documented this relatively low female:male ratio in PAPS compared to SLE, where it is 9:1: Asherson et al [18] reported a ratio of 2:1; and Font et al [25] found a ratio of 5:1. Given that fetal loss may result in more females presenting with APS than males, these findings suggest that female sex is considerably less of a predisposing factor for APS than for SLE.

The question arises as to whether there is a difference in the aCL-associated features between patients with PAPS and those with SLE. It might be supposed that the inflammation of active SLE might be an added risk factor for the development of thrombosis in those patients with raised aCL levels. On the other hand, with individuals who have raise aCL levels and no associated connective tissue disease, there is almost certainly an ascertainment bias in identifying individuals with thrombosis and/or fetal loss. Thus, it has been difficult for formal studies to address the issue.

The largest cohort of individuals with definite APS so far described were reported in a pan-European study of 1000 patients [26]. A little more than 53% of these had PAPS, and in 36.2% the condition was associated with SLE. The latter group had a greater incidence of arthritis, livedo reticularis, leucopenia, and thrombocytopenia than the patients with PAPS. All of these are features seen in pure SLE. No clear difference in APS features was reported between the two groups. The general consensus is that the clinical spectrum of APS is similar in SLE and PAPS (see below). This is reflected in the broad similarity of aCL specificities found in the two conditions.

Antibody Specificity

The past few years have seen major advances in our understanding of the antibodies present in APS, in particular their ligand-binding specificities. Indeed many so-

Table 15.1. Clinical and serological features of primary antiphospholipid syndrome.

| | Mackworth-Young et al [19] | | Asherson et al [18] | | Alarcon-Segovia et al [20] | |
	Number	%	Number	%	Number	%
No. of patients	20		70		9	
M:F ratio	NS		26:44		1:8	
Age range	17–53		21–59		16–43	
aCL IgG	14/20	70	60/70	86	8/9	89
aCL IgM	12/20	60	27/70	39	5/9	56
LA	NS		60/70	86	5/5	100
Thrombosis						
Venous	7/20	35	38/70	54	6/9	67
Arterial	5/20	25	31/70	44	5/9	56
Pregnancy loss	12/15	80	24/70	34	4/4	100
Thrombocytopenia	6/20	30	32/70	46	4/9	44
Migraine	4/20	20	NS		NS	
Livedo reticularis	1/20	5	14/70	20	5/9	56

LA = lupus anticoagulant; NS = not specified.

called anti-phospholipid antibodies may not directly bind phospholipid at all, but associated plasma proteins. As with other autoimmune conditions, work in this field has major implications for our understanding of the pathogenesis(reviewed in [27]). It also has the potential for improving the specificity and sensitivity of laboratory assays for both diagnosis and prognosis.

A large number of ligand-binding specificities have been described in APS [27]. Studies in this area have included patients with SLE-associated APS and with PAPS. No significant differences have so far emerged between these two variants of the condition. The subject is covered in detail elsewhere in this volume. The following summarizes some of the main findings.

Antibodies to Phospholipids

As in SLE-associated APS, the serum of patients with PAPS generally contains antibodies which have specificity for anionic phospholipids (such as cardiolipin and phosphatidyl serine). Some cross-reactivity is sometimes seen with neutral phospholipids (such as phosphatidyl choline), but this is much less common than in patients who have raised aPL levels in the context of infections [28].

Antibodies to β_2-glycoprotein I

Initially, aCL assays were performed in the presence of serum. Removal of serum factors resulted in a drop in detection of aCL, suggesting that serum proteins might be involved in the binding of the antibodies to cardiolipin. Considerable interest was generated when β_2-glycoprotein I (β_2-GPI) was identified as a cofactor for the binding of aCL [29], and was shown to potentiate the anticoagulant activity of aCL [30]. β_2-GPI is a 50 kD heavily glycosylated protein which binds negatively charged molecules such as phospholipids. It is thought to act as a natural inhibitor of thrombosis by inhibiting the conversion of prothrombin to thrombin, the activation of the intrinsic clotting cascade, and protein C activation [31].

Different populations of aCL exist. Although some bind phospholipid in the absence of β_2-GPI, if high sensitivity microtiter plates are employed most aCL can be shown to bind to β_2-GPI [32–35]. This may be through an epitope on native, unbound β_2-GPI ; or through the revealing of a cryptic epitope on the β_2-GPI molecule [36]. Furthermore, there is evidence for the binding of aPL to different domains of β_2-GPI , although binding to domain I may predominate (reviewed in [36]). Those antibodies which bind to cardiolipin in the absence of serum factors can have their binding disrupted by addition of human β_2-GPI , suggesting competition at this phospholipid site [35]. These conflicting results may simply reflect the existence of different subpopulations of aPL within the sera of individuals with APS. What is clear is that, for the majority of so-called aPL that are detected by ELISA in the serum of patients with APS, anionic phospholipid such as cardiolipin is not the antigen to which those antibodies are actually binding.

Antibodies to Prothrombin

While anti-prothrombin antibodies may be responsible for the in vitro phenomenon of the LA, in vivo their presence may be associated with a tendency to increased coagulation. This is an area of controversy, with some groups reporting an association between the presence of anti-prothrombin antibodies and clinical or hematological features of APS [37–39], and other groups finding no association [40–42]. This may be explained by different detection methods and by the presence of antibodies with different epitope specificities [43], resulting in different functional properties [44, 45].

Antibodies to Platelets

There is now considerable evidence for platelet activation in APS. This may occur primarily through the binding of antibodies to β_2-GPI [27]. Specific antiplatelet antibodies have been described in APS. These are frequently seen in SLE, but may also be detected in PAPS. Two studies of platelet antibodies looked exclusively at patients with PAPS. They reported conflicting results as to the relationship with thrombocytopenia.

Godeau et al [46] studied 25 PAPS patients of whom 15 had thrombocytopenia and 10 had normal platelet counts. They found 73% of thrombocytopenic patients had serum platelet antibodies. The most common specificity was for the surface glycoprotein GpIIbIIIa. Only 10% of non-thrombocytopenic patients were platelet antibody positive.

In a study by Panzer et al [47], 22 patients with PAPS were examined for platelet antibodies. Fifteen of 22 had raised levels for such antibodies (mainly GPIIbIIIa) but they found no correlation with the presence of thrombocytopenia, LA activity, or history of thromboembolic disease.

Others

Several other ligand binding specificities have been described in APS [27]. These include antibodies to complement factor H, which has high homology to β_2-GPI [48], and antibodies to clotting factors X and V, which have LA activity. Some are not detectable in standard assays used in APS and include antibodies to a number of regulatory proteins of the coagulation and fibrinolytic pathways, for example, protein C, protein S, thrombomodulin, annexin V, and kininogens [35]. The ways in which these antibodies might contribute to the features of APS are discussed elsewhere [27].

Antibody Sensitivity and Specificity In PAPS

Diagnosis

To date, solid-phase assays for aCL have provided the main laboratory test in the diagnosis of SLE-associated APS and PAPS. More recently, interest has grown in assays for co-factor antibodies, the detection of which appears to improve diagnostic accuracy. Cabiedes et al [49] studied the prevalence of anti–β_2-GPI antibodies in patients with SLE. Thirty-five out of 39 patients with associated APS had antibodies to β_2-GPI, compared to only 2 out of 55 SLE patients with no evidence of APS ($P < 0.0001$). Najmey et al in 1997 [50] conducted a meta-analysis on the use of anti–β_2-

GPI antibodies in the diagnosis of APS. They selected studies where anti–β_2-GPI antibodies had been measured and where clinical details of patients were available. Studies included patients with both SLE and PAPS. A total of 90 individuals were included, of which 65 had two or more clinical manifestations of APS. Anti–β_2-GPI antibodies were present in 89% of APS patients compared to 44% of those who failed to fulfill criteria for the syndrome. No significant difference was found in levels of anti–β_2-GPI antibodies between PAPS and SLE-associated APS.

These observations of the diagnostic specificities of β_2-GPI antibodies in the diagnosis of APS have been mirrored by two studies in PAPS. Cabral et al [51] studied 15 patients with PAPS, 13 aCL-positive syphilis controls, and 76 healthy controls. They found antibodies to β_2-GPI in 12 out of 15 patients with PAPS compared to none in the syphilis or healthy control groups ($P < 0.0001$). Day et al [52] studied the prevalence of these antibodies in patients with PAPS or SLE-associated APS. They demonstrated a high prevalence of IgG anti–β_2-GPI antibodies in PAPS (58%) compared to SLE-associated APS (33%; $P = 0.008$). They suggested that using a combination of anti–β_2-GPI antibodies, aCL, and the LA test would improve diagnostic accuracy.

Clinical Disease Prediction

It has long been known that aCL titer, isotype, and ligand specificity predict clinical sequelae in APS in the context of SLE. For instance, fetal loss is associated with high aCL titers [53] and the presence of IgG, but not IgM or IgA aCL, have good diagnostic accuracy in identifying a preceding history of thrombosis [54]. Viard et al [55] have demonstrated a higher level of thrombosis in those with anti–β_2-GPI antibodies compared to aCL, and Lopez-Sotol ct al [56] showed that IgM aCL is more often associated with hemolytic anemia at presentation, whereas raised IgG antibodies are more likely to be associated with thrombosis, thrombocytopenia, and pregnancy loss.

Most clinicians in the field feel that a similar pattern of association holds true for PAPS. However, there are relatively few data. Levine et al [57] showed that high aCL titers were associated with a shorter time to recurrence of cerebral ischaemia compared to low titers. Prothrombin antibodies have been shown to be predictive of risk of myocardial infarct in middle-aged men without SLE [58].

Classification Criteria for PAPS

Classification criteria for APS were first suggested by Harris et al [15] in 1987. They initially included:

(i)   thrombosis (venous or arterial) or
(ii) miscarriage (at least two)
and
(iii) LA or aCL (> 20 units, IgG or IgM), identified on two occasions more than 8 weeks apart.

Following this, Alarcon-Segovia et al [59] proposed more detailed criteria which took into consideration of both the number of aCL-related manifestations and aCL titers (Table 15.2).

Table 15.2. Preliminary classification criteria for antiphospholipid syndrome in patients with systemic lupus erythematosus .

A. Clinical manifestations associated with aPL.
  Livedo reticularis
  Thrombocytopenia
  Recurrent fetal loss
  Venous thrombosis
  Hemolytic anemia
  Arterial occlusion
  Leg ulcer
  Pulmonary hypertension
  Transverse myelitis

B. Classification groups and APS categories

ACL level	Number of clinical manifestations		
	2	1	0
High (> 5 SD)	definite	probable	doubtful
Low (> 2, < 5 SD)	probable	doubtful	negative
Negative (< 2 SD)	doubtful	negative	Negative

Adapted from Alarcon-Segovia, 1992 [59].

These criteria do not take into account the presence of antibodies of other rele-vant specificities, such as β_2-GPI and prothrombin antibodies. Such criteria may therefore fail to recognize small but significant groups of patients. Indeed, there are clearly documented cases in the literature of patients with the clinical features of APS who have raised levels of β_2-GPI antibodies but no detectable levels of aCL by standard antiphospholipid assays [60, 61]. It is therefore likely that in the future such antibodies will be included in the classification criteria.

It is generally accepted that criteria for the diagnosis of PAPS should include: (i) fulfillment of criteria for APS and (ii) exclusion of the diagnosis of an underlying connective tissue disease, in particular SLE.

In practice this can be difficult. Several of the clinical criteria for the classification of SLE are shared by the APS. For example, thrombocytopenia and pleuritic chest pain are clinical manifestations of both SLE and APS even though the underlying pathology may be different [62]. This led Piette et al [63] to propose specific exclu-sion criteria for primary APS (Table 15.3). The presence of any of the listed clinical features would exclude the diagnosis of PAPS. They stipulate that a follow up of longer than 5 years after the first clinical manifestation is necessary to rule out the subsequent emergence of SLE. This is, of course, an arbitrary period. In practice it seems sensible to make a diagnosis of PAPS in patients with appropriate criteria, while accepting that an associated connective tissue disease, such as SLE, may present in time.

Stringent adherence to these guidelines will necessarily identify a large group of patients who have neither SLE nor PAPS, and whose condition can be viewed as falling into the category of lupus-like APS. In a proportion of such individuals – as in those with true primary APS – a definitive diagnosis of SLE may emerge at a later date.

Clinical Presentation

APS is largely a non-inflammatory autoimmune disorder. In the most part, thrombo-sis is the most important underlying pathological process and accounts for many of

Table 15.3. Exclusion criteria for diagnosis of primary antiphospholipid syndrome.

The presence of any of these criteria excludes the diagnosis of primary antiphospholipid syndrome:
  Malar rash
  Discoid rash
  Oral or pharyngeal ulceration, excluding nasal septum ulceration or perforation
  Arthritis
  Pleuritis, in the absence of pulmonary embolism or left-sided heart failure
  Pericarditis, in the absence of myocardial infarction or uremia
  Persistent proteinuria greater than 0.5 g/day, due to biopsy-proven immune complex-related glomerulonephritis
  Lymphopenia $< 1.0 \times 10^9$/L
  Antibodies to native DNA (detected by radio-immunoassay or Crithidia fluorescence)
  Antibodies to extractable nuclear antigens
  Anti-nuclear antibodies $> 1:320$
  Treatment with drugs known to induce aPL

A follow up longer than 5 years after the first clinical manifestation is necessary to rule out the subsequent emergence of SLE.

Reproduced from Piette, 1993 [63].

the clinical features of all forms of APS. The way in which it presents is similar in PAPS and SLE-associated APS, although in the former the syndrome is often not defined until a clinically apparent thrombosis has occurred. With patients who already have SLE there is usually a heightened awareness of the possibility that features of APS may develop. There have been a large number of studies and case reports documenting clinical features in patients with PAPS. Allowing for differences in the selection and reporting of cases, there is no reason to suppose that the spectrum of clinical features in PAPS is significantly different from that seen in SLE-associated APS. All of the standard features of APS – such as venous or arterial thrombosis, fetal loss, thrombocytopenia, neurological disease, migraine, and livedo reticularis – are well described in PAPS. Some of these areas are worth considering in more detail.

Thrombosis

In most other prothrombotic diseases – for example, protein C and S deficiency, homocysteinuria, and antithrombin III deficiency – thromboses are usually restricted to the venous or to the arterial vasculature. APS is unusual because both systems may be affected. In any given patient, however, one arterial event is likely to predispose to another arterial event; the same is true for venous thrombosis. These observations apply to PAPS as well as to SLE-associated APS. Histologically, these are generally bland thromboses with no evidence of vascular endothelial damage or vasculitis [64], although vasculitis has been reported in some patients, especially with lupus-associated APS [65].

Arterial and venous thromboses have been described in virtually every organ system. Some examples of these occurring in PAPS are summarized in Table 15.4.

Although large and small vessel thrombosis can account for many of the organ restricted clinical presentations, certain organ-specific features are less well characterized. Some of these will be considered further.

Cardiovascular System

One of the most striking lesions seen in APS is the aseptic vegetation on cardiac valves. Such vegetations, which are partly thrombotic, probably account for most

Table 15.4. Thrombotic manifestations reported in primary antiphospholipid syndrome.

Organ	No. of patients	Clinical manifestations	Author
Liver	10	Budd-Chiari syndrome	Asherson, 1991 [66]
			Pomeroy, 1984 [67]
	1	Hepatic artery occlusion	Mor, 1989 [68]
	1	Portal hypertension	Lee, 1997 [69]
	1	Inferior vena cava thrombosis	Tatrai, 1996 [70]
Kidney	1	Hypertension, renal artery thrombosis	Asherson, 1991 [71]
	1	Renal infarction and hypertension	Sonpal, 1992 [72]
Adrenal	1	Hypoadrenalism	Grottolo, 1998 [73]
	1	Bilateral infarction	Marie, 1997 [74]
Heart	1	Large vessel occlusion	Takeuchi, 1998 [75]
Lungs	3	Primary pulmonary hypertension	Nagai, 1997 [76]
			Sandoval, 1996 [77]
CNS	40	CVA	
		Amaurosis fugax	
		Ischemic optic neuropathy	
		Retinal artery occlusion	Levine, 1990 [78]
	1	Arterial and venous thrombosis	Keller, 1996 [79]
	2	Superior sagital sinus thrombosis	Nagai, 1998 [76]
			Khoo, 1995 [80]

cases of Libman Sachs endocarditis seen in SLE. The advent of sensitive echocardiography has increased the frequency of diagnosis of such lesions. They have been well described in PAPS. As in SLE, they are usually asymptomatic. Badui et al [81] found them in 13 out of 20 women with PAPS. Most of these (10 patients) were mitral, and all caused regurgitation. They authors also found electrocardiogram (ECG) abnormalities in 12 patients, and a raised pulmonary artery pressure in 1. Other cardiac abnormalities have been described by Coudray et al [82]. They studied 18 patients with PAPS who were asymptomatic for cardiac disease but who demonstrated abnormal relaxation and impaired filling dynamics of the left ventricle on pulsed Doppler echocardiography. It may well be that such cardiac pathology is due in part to coronary ischemia, but this has not yet been established.

One retrospective study found 21% of patients under 45 years with acute myocardial infarction had raised aCL levels [83]. These findings have been the subject of some controversy, but raise the possibility that a significant proportion of young patients with myocardial infarction may have a form of PAPS.

One area of recent interest in the antiphospholipid field is the association between raised levels of aCL or related antibodies and arterial disease, in particular arterosclerosis. This is considered elsewhere in this book. In patients with inflammatory disorders such as SLE, there are other risk factors for the development of atheroma, including the inflammatory disease itself, and corticosteroid administration. However, there does appear to be a definite association with aCL themselves. For instance, one group found an increase in carotid artery intima media thickness in patients with PAPS compared to controls [84].

Central Nervous System

Neurological involvement is an important cause of morbidity and mortality in PAPS. A wide range of clinical syndromes in the CNS have been described. Some, such as stroke and chorea, are clearly associated with raised aCL, whilst others are less well established, for example, migraine and Guillain-Barré syndrome. In some instances it is likely that in situ thrombosis is responsible for the clinical manifestations, whereas in others embolic phenomena are likely to be important. The 1990 Antiphospholipid Antibodies in Stroke Study Group (APASS) study [85] reported 16 of 72 patients with cerebral ischemia who also had predominantly left-sided cardiac valve lesions.

Several CNS syndromes have been associated with raised levels of aCL even though many of these patients fail to fulfill current classification criteria for PAPS. In patients with cerebral ischemia, an increased prevalence of aPL – 6.8% – has been found in unselected patients with stroke [86], and this figure rises to 46% if patients less than 50 years of age are selected [87]. The 1993 APASS study [88] evaluated 255 consecutive first ischemic stroke patients and 255 matched controls for the presence of aCL as an independent risk factor for stroke. The prevalence of aCL in the stroke group was 9.7% compared with 4.3% in controls. They determined an odds ratio of 2.3 after adjustment for other known risk factors for ischemic events. None of these patients had SLE.

A study by Verrot et al [89] looked at 163 patients with idiopathic epilepsy. They found 19% positive for IgG aCL, but none fulfilled clinical criteria for APS. The absence of any ischemic damage on MRI scan suggested that thromboembolism was an unlikely cause of the epilepsy. This view is not shared by Inzelberg et al [90], who claim that within an SLE population most patients with seizures have evidence of ischaemic injury on magnetic resonance imaging (MRI).

Sneddon first described the clinical association of cerebro-vascular lesions and livedo reticularis in 1965 [91]. Patients with this syndrome exhibit a range of neurological manifestations from headache, dizziness, and focal neurological deficits to progressive cognitive defects and dementia. Kalashnikova et al [92] recognized the association between aPL and the syndrome. Although not all patients express these antibodies, those that do can be considered to have a subset of PAPS.

Chorea is usually a transient clinical manifestation that can occur in the presence of aPL. Both SLE-associated and PAPS-associated disease is recognized [17]. In patients with raised aPL levels, these movement disorders may be induced by oestrogens, for example, the oral contraceptive pill [93] or by pregnancy [94].

Recurrent Abortion

Ten to 15% of all recognized pregnancies result in abortion. By far the majority of these occur in the pre-embryonic (less than 5 weeks post menstrual date) or early embryonic (between 5 and 10 weeks post menstrual date) periods. Thereafter, fetal loss is rare. In a study by Goldstein [95], 232 women with apparently normal early pregnancies were examined. More than 13% had pregnancy loss, of which 87% occurred in the pre-embryonic or embryonic periods.

Several studies have examined the frequency of raised aCL in such individuals who have recurrent miscarriages but who are otherwise healthy (Table 15.5). The reported prevalence of aCL in this population varies from 7% to 42%. By far the majority of these patients with raised aCL levels may be considered to have PAPS rather than SLE-associated APS. The broad range of results is likely to reflect inconsistent aCL and LA tests, variability in the clinical criteria used in assessment of recurrent miscarriages, and differences in patient selection. What is clear, however, is that a significant population of these women do have raised aCL levels.

Table 15.5. The prevalence of anticardiolipin antibody positivity in healthy women with recurrent abortions.

Author	Patients		Type of aPL	No. of abortions	SLE
	Total no.	%			
Lockwood et al, 1986 [96]	55	27	IgG aCL or IUGR or stillbirth	>2	ND
Cowchock et al, 1986 [97]	61	13.1	IgG of IgM aCL	>2	3*
Unanser et al, 1987 [98]	99	42% 10%	IgG or IgM aCL High titer IgG	>3	1
Petri et al, 1987 [99]	44	11	IgG aCL	>3	ND
Granger et al, 1997 [100]	387	16	IgG aCL or LA	>2	4

IUGR = intra-uterine growth retardation; ND = not determined.
*Serology suggestive of SLE.

These studies also failed to delineate accurately the stage of pregnancy loss. Oshiro et al [101] have shown that 50% of pregnancy losses in aCL- or LA-positive recurrent miscarriers (n = 76) were fetal deaths (>10 weeks) compared to only 15% in aCL-negative recurrent miscarriers (n = 290). In other words, aCL is more strongly associated with late abortion (sensitivity of 76%) compared to early losses (sensitivity of 6%). This is not to say that aCL antibodies are not also associated with early losses, but more common causes of early loss, such as genetic, hormonal, and anatomical causes, are numerically more important. Low titer IgG and IgM antibodies do not confer a greater miscarriage risk compared to normal controls in some studies [102], whereas in others a significantly greater proportion of recurrent miscarriage has been found [103].

Comparison of pregnancy loss in PAPS and SLE- associated APS is difficult because of increased losses in lupus per se due to features such as renal impairment. Furthermore, there is likely to be considerable selection bias against patients with connective tissue diseases in recurrent miscarriage clinics in which most of these studies have been performed. It is likely that most aCL-associated recurrent miscarriage falls into the PAPS group. However, it is not an uncommon finding for recurrent miscarriage to predate the diagnosis of SLE, suggesting that at least some of these patients show an evolution from PAPS into SLE-associated APS [104].

Other pregnancy complications, such as intrauterine growth retardation, premature delivery, and pre-eclampsia, are seen in PAPS, as in SLE-associated APS.

Thrombocytopenia

Thrombocytopenia is a common manifestation of both SLE-associated APS and PAPS but is generally mild. In a patient with lupus it is often difficult to determine whether thrombocytopenia is APS related because low platelet counts are a frequent manifestation of SLE itself. Both platelet autoantibodies and platelet activation have been implicated in the pathogenesis of thrombocytopenia in APS, and platelet activation may also play a role in the development of thrombosis. Fanelli et al [105] have found high levels of CD62 and CD63 (markers of platelet activation) on platelets in patients with PAPS. Emmi et al [1066] have confirmed these high levels of CD62 positive platelets in 16 patients with PAPS. They found that the level of CD62 positivity in patients with neurological disease was significantly higher than in PAPS patients without neurological manifestations. They also showed a linear relationship in all patients between the aCL IgG level and the CD62-positive platelet percentage. In PAPS – as in SLE-associated APS – thrombocytopenia is usually mild (platelet counts are rarely lower than 80 x 10^9/L), and not usually of clinical importance.

Catastrophic APS

This syndrome has been described in PAPS as well as SLE-associated APS and is considered further elsewhere in this book.

Progression of PAPS to SLE

It has been the experience of many physicians in the field that a small proportion of patients with PAPS may later develop SLE. Two groups reported an incidence of 4% to 10% [22, 107], while two other groups found no such progression [18, 108]. In a more recent study of 14 children with PAPS, three developed SLE or a lupus-like syndrome during a median follow up of 6 years [109]. These results should be interpreted with care, since the follow-up periods were probably not long enough to assess the frequency of progression, which may take several years. It is certainly important for physicians looking after patients with PAPS to be aware that the disease may "spread" to involve SLE or an SLE-like disorder at any stage.

Treatment in PAPS

The principles of managing patients with PAPS are broadly similar to those for patients with SLE-associated APS. They are covered elsewhere in this book.

Conclusion

PAPS has emerged as an important disease entity. Depending on the organ systems involved, it can produce a highly variable clinical picture, with severity ranging from mild asymptomatic disease (often undiagnosed) to major life-threatening events. It may be regarded as the pure form of a condition which is also frequently seen in the context of other autoimmune diseases. In particular it is intricately linked to APS seen in the context of SLE; and these two variants of the condition appear to behave in a similar fashion. Defining PAPS provides us with the opportunity to study the disease in the absence of other co-morbid conditions such as SLE. Advances in our understanding of the pathogenesis of PAPS should facilitate the development of improved treatment and outlook for patients with all forms of the APS.

References

1. Moore JE, Mohr CF. Biologically false positive serologic tests for syphilis, type incidence and cause. JAMA 1952;150:467–473.
2. Feinstein DI, Rapaport SI. Acquired inhibitors of blood coagulation [review]. Prog Hemost Thromb 1972;1:75–95.
3. Bowie WEJ, et al. Thrombosis in SLE despite circulation anticoagulant. J Clin Invest 1963;62:413–430.
4. Margolius A, Jackson DP, Ratnoff OD. Circulation anticoagulants: a study of 40 cases and a review of the literature. Medicine (Baltimore) 1961;40:145–202.
5. Nilsson IM, et al. Intrauterine death and circulating anticoagulant ("antithromboplastin"). Acta Med Scand 1975;197;153–159.
6. Firkin BG, Howard MA, Radford N. Possible relationship between lupus inhibitor and recurrent abortion in young women [letter]. Lancet 1980;2:366.
7. Carreras LO, et al. Arterial thrombosis, intrauterine death and "lupus" antiocoagulant: detection of immunoglobulin interfering with prostacyclin formation. Lancet 1981;1:244–246.
8. Yin ET, Gaston LW. Purification and kinetic studies on a circulating anticoagulant in a suspected case of lupus erythematosus. Thromb Diath Haemorrhag 1965;14:88–115.
9. Laurell AB, Nilsson IM. Hypergammaglobulinaemia, circulating anticoagulant and biologic false positive Wassermann reaction. J Lab Clin Med 1957;49:694–707.
10. Harris EN, et al. Anticardiolipin antibodies: detection by radioimmunoassay and association with thrombosis in systemic lupus erythematosus. Lancet 1983;2:1211–1214.
11. Violi F, et al. Anticoagulant activity of anticardiolipin antibodies. Thromb Res 1986;44:543–547.
12. Boey ML, et al. Thrombosis in systemic lupus erythematosus: striking association with the presence of circulating lupus anticoagulant. Br Med J 1983;287:1021–1023.
13. Hughes GR. Thrombosis, abortion, cerebral disease, and the lupus anticoagulant. Br Med J 1983;287:1088–1089.
14. Hughes GR. The anticardiolipin syndrome [editorial]. Clin Exp Rheumatol 1985;3:285–286.
15. Harris EN, et al. Clinical and serological features of the 'antiphospholipid syndrome' (APS). B J Rheumatol 1987:19.
16. Mackworth-Young CG, David J, Louizou S, Walport MJ, et al. Primary antiphospholipid syndrome: features of patients with raised anticardiolipin antibodies and no other disorder [abstract]. Ann Rheum Dis 1987:26:94.
17. Asherson RA. A 'primary' antiphospholipid syndrome? J Rheumatol 1988;15:1742–1746.
18. Asherson RA, et al. The "primary" antiphospholipid syndrome: major clinical and serological features. Medicine (Baltimore) 1989;68;366–374.
19. Mackworth-Young CG, Loizou S, Walport MJ. Primary antiphospholipid syndrome: features of patients with raised anticardiolipin antibodies and no other disorder. Ann Rheum Dis 1989;48:362–327.
20. Alarcon-Segovia D, Sanchez-Guerrero J. Primary antiphospholipid syndrome [published erratum appears in J Rheumatol 1989;16:]. J Rheumatol 1989;16:482–428.
21. Asherson RA, et al. Antiphospholipid syndrome: five year follow up. Ann Rheum Dis 1991; 50:805–810.
22. Mujic F, et al. Primary antiphospholipid syndrome evolving into systemic lupus erythematosus. J Rheumatol 1995;22:1589–1592.
23. Andrews PA, Frampton G, Cameron JS. Antiphospholipid syndrome and systemic lupus erythematosus Lancet 1993;342:988–989.
24. Vianna JL, et al. Comparison of the primary and secondary antiphospholipid syndrome: a European Multicenter Study of 114 patients. Am J Med 1994;96:3–9.
25. Font J, et al. The 'primary' antiphospholipid syndrome: antiphospholipid antibody pattern and clinical features of a series of 23 patients. Autoimmunity 1991;9:69–75.
26. Cervera R, et al. Antiphospholipid syndrome: clinical and immunologic manifestations and patterns of disease expression in a cohort of 1,000 patients. Arthritis Rheum 2002;46:1019–1027.
27. Mackworth-Young CG. Antiphospholipid syndrome: multiple mechanisms. Clin Exp Immunol 2004;136:393–401.
28. Loizou CG, et al. Heterogeneity of binding reactivity to different phospholipids of antibodies from patients with systemic lupus erythematosus (SLE) and with syphilis. Clin Exp Immunol 1990;80:171–176.

29. Galli M, et al. Anticardiolipin antibodies (ACA) directed not to cardiolipin but to a plasma protein cofactor [see comments]. Lancet 1990;33:1544–1547.
30. McNeil HP, et al. Anti-phospholipid antibodies are directed against a complex antigen that includes a lipid-binding inhibitor of coagulation: beta 2-glycoprotein I (apolipoprotein H). Proc Natl Acad Sci U S A 1990;87:4120–4124.
31. Harris EN, Pierangeli S. Anticardiolipin antibodies: specificity and function. Lupus 1994;3:217–222.
32. Matsuura E, et al. Anticardiolipin antibodies recognize beta 2-glycoprotein I structure altered by interacting with an oxygen modified solid phase surface. J Exp Med 1994;179:457–462.
33. Roubey RA, et al. "Anticardiolipin" autoantibodies recognize beta 2-glycoprotein I in the absence of phospholipid. Importance of Ag density and bivalent binding. J Immunol 1995;154:954–960.
34. Arvieux J, et al. Measurement of anti-phospholipid antibodies by ELISA using beta 2-glycoprotein I as an antigen. J Immunol Methods 1991;143:223–229.
35. Roubey RA. Immunology of the antiphospholipid antibody syndrome. Arthritis Rheum 1996; 39:1444–1454.
36. Giles IP, et al. How do antiphospholipid antibodies bind beta 2-glycoprotein 1? Arthritis Rheum 2003;48:2111–2121.
37. Sorice M, et al. Anti-prothrombin but not "pure" anti-cardiolipin antibodies are associated with the clinical features of the antiphospholipid antibody syndrome. Thromb Haemost 1998;80:713–715.
38. Nojima J, et al. Anti-prothrombin antibodies combined with lupus anti-coagulant activity is an essential risk factor for venous thromboembolism in patients with systemic lupus erythematosus. Br J Haematol 2001;114:647–654.
39. Nojima J, et al. Acquired activated protein C resistance is associated with the co-existence of anti-prothrombin antibodies and lupus anticoagulant activity in patients with systemic lupus erythematosus. Br J Haematol 2002;118:577–583.
40. Pengo V, et al. Autoantibodies to phospholipid-binding plasma proteins in patients with thrombosis and phospholipid-reactive antibodies. Thromb Haemost 1996;75:721–724.
41. Forastiero RR, et al. Relationship of anti beta2-glycoprotein I and anti prothrombin antibodies to thrombosis and pregnancy loss in patients with antiphospholipid antibodies. Thromb Haemost 1997;78:1008–1014.
42. Amengual O, Atsumi T, Koike T. Specificities, properties, and clinical significance of antiprothrombin antibodies. Arthritis Rheum 2003;48:886–895.
43. Horbach DA, et al. The contribution of anti-prothrombin-antibodies to lupus anticoagulant activity—discrimination between functional and non-functional anti-prothrombin-antibodies. Thromb Haemost 1998;79:790–795.
44. Galli M, et al. Different anticoagulant and immunological properties of anti-prothrombin antibodies in patients with antiphospholipid antibodies. Thromb Haemost 1997;77:486–491.
45. Horbach DA, et al. Lupus anticoagulant is the strongest risk factor for both venous and arterial thrombosis in patients with systemic lupus erythematosus. Comparison between different assays for the detection of antiphospholipid antibodies. Thromb Haemost 1996;76:916–924.
46. Godeau B, et al. Specific antiplatelet glycoprotein autoantibodies are associated with the thrombocytopenia of primary antiphospholipid syndrome. Br J Haematol 1997;98:873–879.
47. Panzer S, et al. Specificities of platelet autoantibodies in patients with lupus anticoagulants in primary antiphospholipid syndrome. Ann Hematol 1997;74:239–242.
49. Cabiedes J, Cabral AR, Alarcon-Segovia D. Clinical manifestations of the antiphospholipid syndrome in patients with systemic lupus erythematosus associate more strongly with anti-beta 2-glycoprotein-I than with antiphospholipid antibodies. J Rheumatol 1995;22:–1899–1906.
48. Kertesz Z, et al. Characterization of binding of human beta 2-glycoprotein I to cardiolipin. Biochem J 1995;310:315–321.
51. Cabral AR, Cabiedes J, Alarcon-Segovia D. Antibodies to phospholipid-free beta 2-glycoprotein-I in patients with primary antiphospholipid syndrome. J Rheumatol 1995;22:1894–1898.
50. Najmey SS, et al. The association of antibodies to beta 2 glycoprotein I with the antiphospholipid syndrome: a meta-analysis. Ann Clin Lab Sci 1997;27:41–46.
52. Day HM, et al. Autoantibodies to beta2-glycoprotein I in systemic lupus erythematosus and primary antiphospholipid antibody syndrome: clinical correlations in comparison with other antiphospholipid antibody tests. J Rheumatol 1998;25:667–674.
53. Loizou S, et al. Association of quantitative anticardiolipin antibody levels with fetal loss and time of loss in systemic lupus erythematosus. Q J Med 1988;68:525–531.
54. Escalante A, et al. Accuracy of anticardiolipin antibodies in identifying a history of thrombosis among patients with systemic lupus erythematosus. Am J Med 1995;98:559–565.

56. Lopez-Soto A, et al. Isotype distribution and clinical significance of antibodies to cardiolipin, phosphatidic acid, phosphatidylinositol and phosphatidylserine in systemic lupus erythematosus: prospective analysis of a series of 92 patients. Clin Exp Rheumatol 1997;15:143-149.

55. Viard JP, Amoura Z, Bach JF. Association of anti-beta 2 glycoprotein I antibodies with lupus-type circulating anticoagulant and thrombosis in systemic lupus erythematosus [see comments]. Am J Med 1992;93:181-186.

57. Levine SR, et al. Recurrent stroke and thrombo-occlusive events in the antiphospholipid syndrome. Ann Neurol 1995;38:119-124.

58. Vaarala O, et al. Antibodies to prothrombin imply a risk of myocardial infarction in middle-aged men. Thromb Haemost 1996;75:456-459.

59. Alarcon-Segovia D, et al. Preliminary classification criteria for the antiphospholipid syndrome within systemic lupus erythematosus. Semin Arthritis Rheum 1992;21:275-286.

60. Cabral AR, et al. The antiphospholipid/cofactor syndromes: a primary variant with antibodies to beta 2-glycoprotein-I but no antibodies detectable in standard antiphospholipid assays. Am J Med 1996;101:472-481.

61. Alarcon-Segovia D, et al. The antiphospholipid / cofactor syndromes. II. A variant in patients with systemic lupus erythematosus with antibodies to b_2-glycoprotein I but no antibodies detectable in standard antiphospholipid assays. J Rheumatol 1997;24:1545-1551.

62. Piette JC, et al. Systemic lupus erythematosus and the antiphospholipid syndrome: reflections about the relevance of ARA criteria [editorial] [see comments]. J Rheumatol 1992;19:1835-1837.

63. Piette JC, et al. Exclusion criteria for primary antiphospholipid syndrome [letter]. J Rheumatol 1993;20:1802-1804.

64. Johannsson EA, Niemi KM, Mustakillio KK. A peripheral vascular syndrome overlapping with SLE: recurrent venous thrombosis and hemorrhagic capillary proliferation with circulating anticoagulants and false-positive reactions for syphilis. Dermatologica 1977;15:257-267.

65. Alegre VA, Gastineau DA, Winkelmann RK. Skin lesions associated with circulating lupus anticoagulant. Br J Dermatol 1989;120:419-429.

66. Asherson RA, Khamashta MA, Hughes GR. The hepatic complications of the antiphospholipid antibodies [editorial]. Clin Exp Rheumatol 1991;9:341-344.

67. Pomeroy C, et al. Budd-Chiari syndrome in a patient with the lupus anticoagulant. Gastroenterology 1984;86:158-161.

68. Mor F, et al. Hepatic infarction in a patient with the lupus anticoagulant. Arthritis Rheum 1989;32:491-495.

69. Lee HJ, Park JW, Chang JC. Mesenteric and portal venous obstruction associated with primary antiphospholipid antibody syndrome. J Gastroenterol Hepatol 1997;12:822-826.

70. Tatrai T, Kiss G, Sevcic K. [Inferior vena cava thrombosis developing in primary antiphospholipid syndrome]. Orv Hetil 1996;137:135-137.

71. Asherson RA, George EN, Hughes GRV. Hypertension, renal artery stenosis and the 'primary' antiphospholipid syndrome. J Rheumatol 1991;18:1413-1415.

72. Sonpal GM, Sharma A, Miller A. Primary antiphospholipid antibody syndrome, renal infarction and hypertension. J Rheumatol 1993;20:1221-1223.

73. Grottolo A, et al. Primary adrenal insufficiency, circulating lupus anticoagulant and anticardiolipin antibodies in a patient with multiple abortions and recurrent thrombotic episodes. Haematologica 1988;73:517-519.

74. Marie I, et al. Acute adrenal failure secondary to bilateral infarction of the adrenal glands as the first manifestation of primary antiphospholipid antibody syndrome [letter]. Ann Rheum Dis 1997;56:567-568.

75. Takeuchi S, Obayashi T, Toyama J. Primary antiphospholipid syndrome with acute myocardial infarction recanalised by PTCA. Heart 1998;79:96-98.

76. Nagai S, et al. Superior sagittal sinus thrombosis associated with primary antiphospholipid syndrome - case report. Neurol Med Chir 1998;38:34-39.

77. Sandoval J, et al. Primary antiphospholipid syndrome presenting as chronic thromboembolic pulmonary hypertension. Treatment with thromboendarterectomy. J Rheumatol 1996;23:772-775.

78. Levine SR, et al. Cerebrovascular and neurologic disease associated with antiphospholipid antibodies: 48 cases. Neurology 1990;40:1181-1189.

79. Keller E, et al. [Coincident arterial and venous cerebral thrombosis in primary antiphospholipid syndrome]. Rofo Fortschr Geb Rontgenstr Neuen Bildgeb Verfahr 1996;165:300-302.

80. Khoo KB, et al. Cerebral venous sinus thrombosis associated with the primary antiphospholipid syndrome. Resolution with local thrombolytic therapy. Med J Aust 1995;162:30-32.

81. Badui E, et al. The heart in the primary antiphospholipid syndrome. Arch Med Res 1995;26:115-120.
82. Coudray N, et al. M mode and Doppler echocardiographic assessment of left ventricular diastolic function in primary antiphospholipid syndrome. Br Heart J 1995;74:531-535.
83. Hamsten A, et al. Antibodies to cardiolipin in young survivors of myocardial infarction: an association with recurrent cardiovascular events. Lancet 1986;1:113-116.
84. Ames PR, et al. Premature atherosclerosis in primary antiphospholipid syndrome: preliminary data. Ann Rheum Dis 2004. In press.
85. APASS, The Antiphospholipid Antibodies in Stroke Study Group. Clinical and laboratory findings in patients with antiphospholipid antibodies and cerebral ischaemia. Stroke 1990;21:1268-1273.
86. Montalban J, et al. Antiphospholipid antibodies in cerebral ischemia. Stroke 1991;22:750-753.
87. Brey RL, et al. Antiphospholipid antibodies and cerebral ischemia in young people. Neurology 1990;40:1190-1196.
88. APASS, The Antiphospholipid Antibodies in Stroke Study Group. Anticardiolipin antibodies are an independent risk factor for first ischemic stroke. Neurology 1993;43:2069-2073.
89. Verrot D, et al. Prevalence and signification of antinuclear and anticardiolipin antibodies in patients with epilepsy. Am J Med 1997;103:33-37.
90. Inzelberg R, Korczyn AD. Lupus anticoagulant and late onset seizures [see comments]. Acta Neurol Scand 1989;79:114-118.
91. Sneddon IB. Cerebral vascular lesion in livedo reticularis. Br J Dermatol 1965;77:180-185.
92. Kalashnikova LA, et al. Anticardiolipin antibodies in Sneddon's syndrome. Neurology 1990;40:464-467.
93. Asherson RA, et al. Systemic lupus erythematosus, antiphospholipid antibodies, chorea, and oral contraceptives [letter]. Arthritis Rheum 1986;29:1535-1536.
94. Lubbe WF, Walker EB. Chorea gravidarum associated with circulating lupus anticoagulant: successful outcome of pregnancy with prednisone and aspirin therapy. Case report. Br J Obstet Gynaecol 1983;90:487-490.
95. Goldstein SR. Embryonic death in early pregnancy: a new look at the first trimester. Obstet Gynecol 1994;84:294-297.
96. Lockwood CJ, et al. Anti-phospholipid antibody and pregnancy wastage. Lancet 1986;2:742-743.
97. Cowchock S, Smith JB, Gocial B. Antibodies to phospholipids and nuclear antigens in patients with repeated abortions. Am J Obstet Gynecol 1986;155:1002-1010.
98. Unander AM, et al. Anticardiolipin antibodies and complement in ninety-nine women with habitual abortion. Am J Obstet Gynecol 1987;156l:114-119.
99. Petri M, et al. Antinuclear antibody, lupus anticoagulant, and anticardiolipin antibody in women with idiopathic habitual abortion. A controlled, prospective study of forty-four women. Arthritis Rheum 1987;30:601-606.
100. Granger KA, Farquharson RG. Obstetric outcome in antiphospholipid syndrome. Lupus 1997;6:509-513.
101. Oshiro BT, et al. Antiphospholipid antibodies and fetal death. Obstet Gynecol 1996;87:489-493.
102. Silver RM, et al. Anticardiolipin antibodies: clinical consequences of "low titers". Obstet Gynecol 1996;87:494-500.
103. Aoki K, et al. Specific antiphospholipid antibodies as a predictive variable in patients with recurrent pregnancy loss. Am J Reprod Immunol 1993;29:82-87.
104. Derue G, et al. Foetal loss in systemic lupus: association with anticardiolipin antibodies. J Obstet Gynaecol 1985;5:207-209.
105. Fanelli A, et al. Flow cytometric detection of circulating activated platelets in primary antiphospholipid syndrome. Correlation with thrombocytopenia and anticardiolipin antibodies. Lupus 1997;6:261-267.
106. Emmi L, et al. Possible pathogenetic role of activated platelets in the primary antiphospholipid syndrome involving the central nervous system. Ann N Y Acad Sci 1997;823:188-200.
107. Silver RM, et al. Clinical consequences of antiphospholipid antibodies: an historic cohort study. Obstet Gynecol 1994;83:372-377.
108. Vianna JL, et al. Comparison of the primary and secondary antiphospholipid syndrome: a European Multicenter Study of 114 patients [see comments]. Am J Med 1994;96:3-9.
109. Gattorno M, et al. Outcome of primary antiphospholipid syndrome in childhood. Lupus 2003;12:449-453.

16 Catastrophic Antiphospholipid Syndrome

H. Michael Belmont

Introduction

The syndrome of multiple vascular occlusions associated with high titer anti-phospholipid antibodies (aPL) is known as catastrophic antiphospholipid syndrome (CAPS). Although antiphospholipid syndrome (APS) is typically characterized by thrombotic events that either occur singly or, when recurrent, are seen many months or even years apart, some patients with this syndrome may develop wide-spread, non-inflammatory vascular occlusions.

The first reports of patients with multiple non-inflammatory vascular occlusions appeared in 1974, by Dosekun [1], and in 1987, by Ingram [2]. However, it was not until Greisman reported in 1991 on two patients with *"acute, catastrophic, wide-spread non-inflammatory visceral vascular occlusions associated with high titer antiphospholipid antibodies"* that the full spectrum of clinical features associated with aPL became appreciated [3]. This spectrum was outlined in an editorial by Harris and Bos [4] that accompanied the Greissman report [3]. The authors described two additional patients with "acute disseminated coagulopathy-vasculopathy associated with antiphospholipid syndrome" and identified three cohorts of patients with these antibodies. They recognized that aPL may be "asymptomatic" and observed in patients free of thrombosis or associated with one or two episodes of thrombosis typically involving only one artery or vein at a time with long periods (months to years) free of occlusive events. Alternatively, aPL may confer a risk for an ominous disorder characterized by multiple, typically three or more, wide-spread thrombotic occlusions often with marked ischemic changes in the extremities, livido reticularis, as well as renal, cerebral, myocardial, pulmonary, and other visceral organ thrombotic vasculopathy. Asherson, describing 10 such patients in an article published in 1992, first proposed the term *catastrophic APS* [5].

Over the past 12 years, several reviews of CAPS have been published [6–9]. It is estimated that CAPS comprises 1% of cases of APS syndrome. To date, approximately 250 cases are described in the literature. In 2000, an international registry of patients with CAPS was created by the European Forum on Antiphospholipid Antibodies and can be referenced via the internet at http://www.med.ub.es/MIMMUN/FORUM/CAPS.HTM, consisting of 220 patients as of August 1, 2004 [10]. Additionally, a set of classification criteria for CAPS was presented at the 10th International Congress on Antiphospholipid Antibodies in 2002 at Taormina, Sicily (Table 16.1) [11–13].This chapter will describe the clinical, therapeutic, and pathogenic aspects of this condition.

Table 16.1. Criteria for the classification of catastrophic antiphospholipid antibody syndrome.

Criteria for the classification of catastrophic antiphospholipid antibody syndrome:
1. Evidence of involvement of three or more organs, systems, or tissues.
2. Development of manifestations simultaneously or in less than a week.
3. Confirmation by histopathology of small vessel occlusion in at least one organ or tissue.[†]
4. Laboratory confirmation of the presence of aPL (lupus anticoagulant or aCL).

Definite catastrophic antiphospholipid antibody syndrome
   All four criteria.

Probable catastrophic antiphospholipid antibody syndrome
   All four criteria, except only two organs, systems, or tissues are involved.
   All four criteria, except for the absence of laboratory confirmation at least 6 weeks apart because of the early death of a
      patient never previously tested for aPL before the catastrophic event.
   Criteria 1, 2, and 4 antiphospholipid.
   Criteria 1, 3, and 4, and the development of a third event in more than a week, but less than a month, despite
      anticoagulation.

Usually, clinical evidence of vessel occlusions, confirmed by imaging techniques when appropriate. Renal involvement is
defined by a 50% rise in serum creatinine, severe systemic hypertension (greater than 190/110 mm Hg), or proteinuria
(greater than 500 mg/24 hours).
[†]For histopathologic confirmation, significant evidence of thrombosis must be present, although vasculitis may coexist
occasionally. If the patient has not been previously diagnosed as having APS, the laboratory confirmation requires that the
presence of aPL must be detected on two or more occasions at least 6 weeks apart (not necessarily at the time of the event),
according to the proposed clinical criteria for the classification of definite APS.

Clinical Aspects

Patients with catastrophic APS can be broadly categorized into those with systemic lupus erythematosus (SLE), "lupus-like" illness satisfying two to three of the modified ACR criteria, primary APS, or secondary to an another autoimmune, connective tissue disease such as rheumatoid arthritis, scleroderma, dermatomyositis, polychondritis, primary, systemic necrotizing vasculitis, inflammatory bowel disease, or Behcet's syndrome [14–21].

Demographic Characteristics

Amongst 220 patients with catastrophic APS in the registry, 156 (70%) are females and 64 (30%) males (2.5:1 female:male ratio) with an age range of 9 to 74 years and an average of 36 years. Thirteen (6%) patients developed the clinical picture before the age of 16 and 19 (9%) after the age of 60. Ninety-one (41%) patients who developed acute, multi-organ involvement suffered from primary APS, 79 (36%) from SLE, 12 (5%) from "lupus-like" illness, and 9 (4%) from other connective tissue disease.

Preceding Thrombotic History

A slight majority (112/220, 50%) of the patients had a prior history of thrombophilia and thrombotic event. A total of 42 (19%) of the 220 patients had a history of venothromboembolic phenomena, including deep venous thrombophlebitis

(DVT), pulmonary embolism, superior and inferior vena cava thrombosis, or Budd-Chian syndrome (hepatic vein thrombosis).

In addition to venous events, previous major arterial occlusions occurred in 29 (13%) of the CAPS patients. Femoral, popliteal, and digital artery peripheral arterial occlusions were reported, as well as myocardial infarctions, cerebral events as transient ischemic attacks or completed cerebral vascular accidents, adrenal infarction, renal infarction, and mesenteric and splenic artery thrombosis. Spontaneous fetal losses had occurred in only 18 (8%) of the 156 female patients and thrombocytopenia in 28 (13%). One patient 31 years before developing CAPS had experienced an atypical pre-eclampsia – eclampsia presentation known as the HELLP syndrome (hemolysis, elevated liver enzymes, and low platelets) [19]. Other potential thrombotic manifestations of pre-existing hypercoagulability include non-healing cutaneous ulcers.

Potential Precipitating Factors

In 130 (59%) of the patients, precipitating factors may have contributed to the development of CAPS. These included infections in 33 (15%) patients, postpartum or recent fetal loss in 7 (3%), and minor surgical procedures or surgery in 19 (9%). Additional precipitating clinical features include malignancy, medication, anticoagulation withdrawal, and SLE exacerbation. The biological significance of these risks is uncertain. As this summary data was culled from numerous investigators' published reports, it may contain biases. The likelihood that the authors ascertained potential risks and chose to include the information can not be certain. Only a prospective study which is designed to audit all identified, hypothetical risk factors could reveal which are statistically significant associations reflective of causal biologic etiologies of CAPS.

Clinical Presentation

Presentation of CAPS is often complex as it involves multiple organs concurrently over a short period of time, typically days to weeks. Figure 16.1 shows the clinical manifestations attributed to thrombotic events at the time of CAPS.

In CAPS, the most characteristic involvement is of renal, pulmonary, cerebral, gastrointestinal, and cerebral vessels. In contrast to the non-catastrophic APS, DVT is uncommon. However, atypical occlusive events such as of adrenal, pancreatic, splenic, testicular, and cutaneous vessels typify CAPS.

In the 220 patients, 152 (70%) had renal involvement usually accompanied by hypertension. Pathological material revealed renal microangiopathy with small vessel occlusive disease.

Pulmonary involvement occurred in 142 (65%) of the patients. The spectrum of features included severe dyspnea, frank adult respiratory distress syndrome (ARDS), pulmonary emboli, sometimes multiple, pulmonary infarction, interstitial infiltrates, and intra-alveolar hemorrhage.

The central nervous system was involved in 122 (55%) of patients, often as major cerebral infarctions on computerized tomography (CT) or magnetic resonance

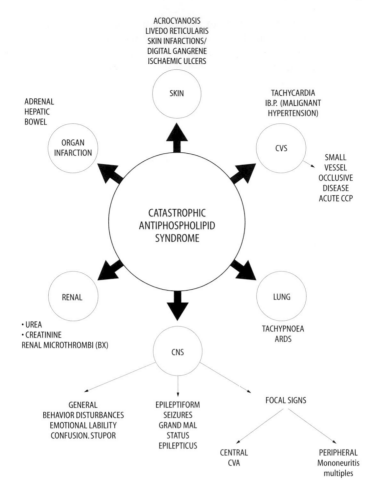

Figure 16.1. Clinical manifestations of catastrophic antiphospholipid syndrome.

imaging (MRI) scans. Additional manifestations include cerebral sinus thrombosis and seizures. Microthrombi and microinfarctions in pathological material obtained from patients suggests that the thrombophilia that characterizes CAPS results in thrombotic events involving the micro-circulation.

Cardiac manifestations were described in 108 (50%) patients, although typical myocardial infarction occurred no more often than diffuse myocardial involvement with congestive heart failure or vale lesions. Again, pathological material revealed multiple myocardial microthrombi.

Ninety-seven (44%) patients had gastrointestinal involvement. Vascular occlusions of mesenteric, portal, and inferior vena cava were common and arterial occlusions were accompanied by gangrene of the bowels and splenic infarctions. Hepatic involvement and pancreatitis were not uncommon. Microthrombi characterized the organs examined at autopsy.

Adrenal thrombosis was present in 23 (11%) patients. Additional unusual features of CAPS include testicular infarction and necrosis of the prostate gland. Another characteristic feature was skin involvement, with 93 (42%) demonstrating livedo reticularis, ulcerations, gangrene, purpura, acrocyanosis, or digital ischemia.

Laboratory Findings

Thrombocytopenia (< 100,000/mm) was reported in 100 (46%) patients, hemolytic anemia in 60 (27%), findings consistent with disseminated intravascular coagulation (DIC) (prolonged coagulation tests with increased fibrinogen degradation factors and hypofibrinogenemia) in 36 (16%), and evidence of microangiopathy with schistocytes (fragmented erythrocytes) reported in peripheral blood smears in 23 (13%) patients. Lupus anticoagulant was detected in 173 (79%) of the patients and anticardiolipin antibodies (aCL) were positive in 190 (86%) patients. The antinuclear antibodies (ANA) was positive in 105 (48%) patients including in high titer.

Outcome

Death occurred in 104 of the 220 (47%) patients and most commonly from cardiac events, predominately from myocardial microthrombi producing cardiac failure, or less often acute myocardial infarction. Respiratory failure especially with ARDS or diffuse alveolar hemorrhage was often a complicating feature in fatal cases. Cerebrovascular involvement was a less common cause of death, although coma, large vessel strokes, multiple small vessel strokes, seizures, and cerebral hemorrhage contributed to significant morbidity. Renal involvement, although a common clinical feature, was not a usual cause of death. Death occurred from gastrointestinal involvement in patients related to esophageal perforation and bowel infarction. Surviving an episode of CAPS is typically associated with a good prognosis, as only 26% develop further APS-related episodes [22], but without features of the catastrophic syndrome. Only a single example of recurrent CAPS has appeared in the literature.

Therapeutic Aspects

In the absence of randomized controlled trials, optimal therapy for patients with catastrophic APS is uncertain. In contrast to the experience with APS where Khamashta [23] reviewed retrospectively, in 147 patients, the efficacy of warfarin, low-dose aspirin, or both in the secondary prevention of thrombosis, no single center, large series of patients with CAPS exists. A more recent prospective randomized trial of 114 APS patients suggested that more moderate-intensity warfarin anticoagulation was no less effective in preventing thrombotic recurrences as compared to high intensity [24]. Treatment is therefore empiric. Because catastrophic APS is a thrombophilic disorder characterized by wide-spread microvasculopathy, the rationale of treatment is to prevent thrombosis by anticoagulation, to prevent the production and circulation of mediators (i.e., aPL, cytokines, complement degradation products, anti-endothelial cell antibodies, etc.) which generate the hypercoagulable state, or to prevent both. In other words, treatment may consist of anticoagulation, immunosuppressives, such as corticosteroids or cytotoxics, or plasmapheresis. The role of antiplatelet agents, prostacyclin, intravenous immunoglobulin, ancrod, defibrotide, and other fibrinolytic treatment is less certain.

Patients treated with the combination of anticoagulation in addition to steroids plus a therapy which can achieve a prompt reduction in aPL titer, either plasmapheresis [25] or intravenous gammaglobulin [26], had the highest survival rate of almost 70% [6–9]. A role for cyclophosphamide is suggested by its use in many of the most severe cases, CAPS accompanying SLE, and knowledge it prevents the rebound production of pathogenic autoantibodies by autoaggresive lymphocytes. Patients have received ancrod, purified fraction of Malayan snake pit viper venom, as well as defibrotide [6–9] and fibrinolytics such as streptokinase [27] with uncertain benefit.

Pathogenic Aspects

Catastrophic APS occurs in a minority of patients with aPL, is characterized by acute, vascular occlusions involving multiple organs, and is an example of a non-inflammatory thrombotic microvasculopathy. The pathogenesis of microvasculopathy in autoimmune disease includes: (1) classic leukocytoclastic vasculitis secondary to subendothelial immune complex deposition in vessel walls; (2) leukothrombosis secondary to intravascular activation of complement, neutrophils, and endothclium in the absence of local immune complex deposition; or (3) thrombosis of vessels secondary to a non-inflammatory vasculopathy [28–30].

Besides APS, other thrombotic microangiopathic syndromes include thrombotic thrombocytopenia purpura (TTP), hemolytic uremic syndrome (HUS), DIC, and HELLP syndrome. The latter is an uncommon complication of pregnancy and, interestingly, Neuwelt described a woman who developed catastrophic APS 31 years after a pregnancy accompanied by HELLP, suggesting a unifying pathophysiologic mechanism [25]. On the other hand, evidence suggests that an inhibitor of von Willebrand factor-cleaving protease (ADAMTS-13) causes the thrombotic microangiopathic hemolytic anemia that characterizes autoimmune associated TTP [31]. The uncatabolized von Willebrand multimers promote disseminated intravascular platelet aggregation.

The diffuse and multiorgan, yet episodic, nature of CAPS occurring in only a minority of patients with likely long-standing circulating aPL is consistent with the hypothesis that an additional biological factor is required for wide-spread microvasculopathy. A candidate target for activation that would then be permissive for the development of APS is endothelial cells [28, 30]. There are groups of immune stimuli that activate endothelial cells and likely contribute to providing preparatory signals for CAPS. These stimuli include cytokines, complement components, and autoantibodies.

Cytokines are likely to be important mediators of endothelial cell activation required for the development of catastrophic APS. Tumor necrosis factor α (TNF-α), interferon α (INF-α), and interleukin-1 (IL-1) each stimulate endothelial cells [32].

It should be noted that while endothelial cells may be acted upon by cytokines produced by other inflammatory cells, they also can be stimulated to produce cytokines such as IL-1, IL-6, IL-8, and TNF-α, which can act as autacoids to upregulate adhesion molecule expression [34].

Several products of the activated complement system (e.g., C3b, iC3b, and C5a) are known to activate the endothelium [33]. Additionally, assembly of the membrane attack complex (MAC), consisting of C5b-9, on endothelial cells results in the up-regulation of adhesion molecules [32]. Specifically, MAC has been shown to participate in the upregulation of endothelial cell tissue factor activity and this expression of tissue factor by the endothelium promotes a procoagulant state that is likely to contribute to the vascular injury typical of catastrophic APS [35]. There is also evidence that C1q is a cofactor required for immune complexes to stimulate endothelial expression of E-selectin, ICAM-1, and VCAM-1 [36]. Finally, the essential role for complement components and neutrophils in APS, especially in the circumstance of placental vasculopathy that underlies fetal loss, is supported by experimental studies where antibodies that block C5a-polymorphonuclear leukocyte C5a receptor interactions prevent complications in pregnant mice which receive human IgG containing aPL antibodies [37–39]. These findings are further confirmed by experience with using C3 convertase inhibitor complement receptor 1–related gene, as well as C3 deficient mice, both of which mitigates fetal loss [38].

Autoantibodies including aPL, anti-endothelial cell, and anti-dsDNA have each been demonstrated to react with endothelial cells in vitro, provide a stimulatory signal, and upregulate adhesion molecules or tissue factor [40, 41]. Antiendothelial cells, for example, have the capacity to increase tissue factor expression. Anti-DNA antibodies stimulate the release of IL-1 and IL-6 from human endothelial cells. In studies, the incubation of endothelial cells with purified IgG containing anti-dsDNA (compared with those incubated with anti-dsDNA–depleted IgG) caused a significant increase of supernatant IL-1 and IL-6 in association with increased mRNA expression of these cytokines. Moreover, using a similar strategy, the upregulation of adhesion molecule expression on endothelial cells by anti-DNA autoantibodies in patients with SLE was demonstrated. Simanitov showed that IgG from patients with aPL is able to enhance endothelial cell adhesion molecule expression and monocyte adherence [42]. This capacity of aPL to activate endothelial cells may be required in catastrophic APS before aPL interacts with platelets or coagulation proteins to mediate diffuse thrombotic microvasculopathy.

The activation of endothelial cells and accompanying upregulation of adhesion molecules and tissue factor is likely pivotal to the development of CAPS. It is the collaboration of cytokines, activated complement components, and autoantibodies that act on endothelial cells to increase its adhesiveness and procoagulant activity that provides the preparatory signals for aPL in CAPS. These same mediators can act on leukocytes and platelets to increase their adhesion to vascular endothelium and to promote microthrombosis and the local release of toxic mediators, including proteases and oxygen-derived free radicals [28, 30, 32]. This interaction between activated endothelial cells, neutrophils, and platelets in the presence of aPL generates the diffuse microvasculopathy that characterizes CAPS. This widespread, thrombotic microvasculopathy is responsible for the clinical features of catastrophic APS by producing tissue injury, which can include pulmonary capillary leak or ARDS, brain capillary leak or "acute cerebral distress syndrome," myocardial dysfunction and potentially systemic inflammatory response syndrome (SIRS) with multi-organ failure [29].

It is now recognized that SIRS may arise both from sepsis and from non-infectious causes, such as immune-mediated organ injury [43]. SIRS is a reaction characterized by widespread inflammation primarily affecting vascular endothelium, however, the same cascade of mediators have been invoked in catastrophic APS [44]. The main endogenous mediators of both include TNF-á and IL-1 with a prominent role for platelet-activating factor, vasodilator prostaglandins, complement activation, and upregulation of adhesion molecules on leukocytes, platelets, and endothelial cells [45]. CAPS and SIRS share similar clinical consequences with multiorgan failure and manifestations, which include impaired renal function, ARDS, cerebral dysfunction, decreased myocardial contractility, and catecholamine unresponsive hypotension.

Summary

CAPS develops in a minority (1%) of patients with aPL and is characterized by acute, vascular occlusion involving three or more organs. The disorder is characterized by a diffuse thrombotic microvasculopathy with a predilection for kidney, lung, brain, heart, skin, and gastrointestinal tract. Treatment is empiric and, although mortality may approach 50%, outcomes appear best for patients that receive combinations of heparin anticoagulation, steroids, plasmapheresis, intravenous gammaglobulin, and, in the setting of SLE disease exacerbation, cyclophosphamide. The etiology of CAPS awaits clarification but likely involves the activation of vascular endothelium to express surface adhesion molecules and possibly tissue factor that interact with circulating cellular inflammatory cells, elements of the phospholipid-dependent coagulation factors, and platelets in the presence of aPL. Improved therapy awaits better understanding of the underlying immunologic, coagulation, and vascular pathology.

References

1. Dosekun AK, et al. Ancrod in systemic lupus erythematosus with thrombosis. Clinical and fibrinolytic effects. Arch Intern Med 1984;144:37–42.
2. Ingram SB, et al. An unusual syndrome of a devastating non-inflammatory vasculopathy associated with anticardiolipin antibodies. Arthritis Rheum 1987;30:1167–1171.
3. Greisman SG, et al. Occlusive vasculopathy in systemic lupus erythematosus-association with anticardiolipin antibody. Arch Intern Med 1991;151:389–391.
4. Harris EN, Bos K. An acute disseminated coagulopathy-vasculopathy associated with the antiphospholipid syndrome. Arch Intern Med 1991;151:231–232.
5. Asherson RA. The catastrophic antiphospholipid syndrome. J Rheumatol 1992;19:508–512.
6. Asherson RA, et al. Catastrophic antiphospholipid syndrome: clinical and laboratory features of 50 patients. Medicine (Baltimore) 1998;77:195–207.
7. Asherson RA, et al. Catastrophic antiphospholipid syndrome: clues to the pathogenesis from a series of 80 patients. Medicine (Baltimore) 2001;80:355–376.
8. Asherson RA, Cervera R. Catastrophic antiphospholipid syndrome. Curr Rheumatol Rep 2003;5:395–400.
9. Asherson RA, Cervera R. Unusual manifestations of the antiphospholipid syndrome. Clin Rev Allergy and Immunol 2003;25:61–78.

10. Asherson RA, et al. Catastrophic antiphospholipid syndrome registry project group. Lupus 2003;12:530–534.
11. Asherson RA, et al. Catastrophic antiphospholipid syndrome: international consensus statement on classification criteria and treatment guidelines. Lupus 2003;12:530–534.
12. Cervera R, Gomez-Puerta JA, Cucho M. Catastrophic antiphospholipid syndrome: analysis of the international consensus statement on preliminary classification criteria for CAPS using the CAPS registry Ann Rheum Dis 62(Suppl)2003; 84.
13. Asherson, RA, et al. Catastrophic antiphospholipid syndrome: proposed guidelines for diagnosis and treatment. J Clin Rheumatol 2003;8;157–165.
14. Le Loet X, et al. Catastrophic antiphospholipid syndrome. Presse Med 1997;26:131–134.
15. Petras T, et al. An adolescent with acute renal failure, thrombocytopenia and femoral vein thrombosis. Nephrol Dial Transplant 1998;13:480–483.
16. Falcini F, et al. Catastrophic antiphospholipid antibody syndrome in pediatric systemic lupus erythematosus. J Rheumatol 1997;24(2):389–392.
17. Provenzale JM, et al. Disseminated thrombosis in primary antiphospholipid syndrome: MR findings. Eur J Radiol 1998;26:244–247.
18. Argento A, DiBenedetto RI. ARDS and adrenal insufficiency associated with the antiphospholipid antibody syndrome. Chest 1998;113:1136–1138.
19. Dasgupta B, et al. Polyarteritis nodosa and the antiphospholipid syndrome. Br Rheumatol 1997;36:1210–1212.
20. Chinnery PF, et al. Fulminant encephalopathy due to the catastrophic primary antiphospholipid syndrome [letter]. Neural Neurosurg Psych 1997;62:300–301.
21. Kane D, et al. Catastrophic antiphospholipid antibody syndrome in primary systemic sclerosis. J Rheumatol 1998;25:810–812.
22. Erkan D, et al. The long term outcome of catastrophic antiphospholipid survivors. Ann Rheum Dis 2003;62:530–533.
23. Khamashta MA, et al. The management of thrombosis in the antiphospholipid-antibody syndrome. N Engl J Med 1995;32:293–297.
24. Crowther M, et al. A comparison of two intensifiers of warfarin for the prevention of recurrent thrombosis in patients with the antiphospholipid antibody syndrome. N Engl J Med 2003;349:1133–1138.
25. Neuwelt CM, et al. Response to repeated plasmapheresis over three years. Arthritis Rheum 1997;40:1534–1539.
26. Yu Z, Lennon VA. Clinical implications of basic research: mechanism of intravenous immune globulin therapy in antibody-mediated autoimmune diseases. N Engl J Med 1999;340:227–228.
27. Kitchens C. Thrombotic storm. Am J Med 1998;164:381.
28. Belmont HM, et al. Pathology and pathogenesis of vascular injury in systemic lupus erythematosus. Interactions of inflammatory cells and activated endothelium. Arthritis Rheum 1996;39:9–22.
29. Golden BD, Belmont HM. The role of microvasculopathy in the catastrophic antiphospholipid syndrome: comment on the article by Neuwelt et al [letter]. Arthritis Rheum 1997;40:1534–1539.
30. Abramson SA, Belmont HM. SLE: mechanism of vascular injury. Hosp Pract 1998;33:107–127.
31. Tsai H-M, Lian EC-Y. Antibodies to von Willebrand factor-cleaving protease in acute thrombotic thrombocytopenic purpura. N Engl J Med 1998;339;1585–1594.
32. Cockwell P, et al. Activation of endothelial cells in thrombosis and vasculitis. Scan J Rheumatol 1997;26:145–150.
33. Arnaout MA, Cohen HR. Complement C3 receptors: structure and function. Mol Immun 1984;21:1191–1199.
34. Berger MD, et al. Calcium requirements for increased complement receptor expression during neutrophil activation J Immunol 1985;135:1342–1348.
35. Kilgore KS, et al. Enhancement by the complement membrane attack complex of tumor necrosis factor-alpha-induced endothelial cell expression of E-selectin and ICAM-I. J Immunol 1995;155:1434.
36. Lozada C, et al. Identification of Clq as the heat-labile serum cofactor required for immune complexes to stimulate endothelial expression of the adhesion molecules E-selectin and intercellular and vascular cell adhesion molecules. Proc Natl Acad Sci USA 1995;92:8378–8382.
37. Salmon JE, Girardi G. The role of complement in the antiphospholipid syndrome. Curr Dir Autoimmun 2004;7:133–148.
38. Salmon JE, et al. Activation of complement mediates antiphospholipid antibody-induced pregnancy loss. Lupus 2003;12:535–538.
39. Girardi G, et al Complement C5a receptors and neutrophils mediate fetal injury in the antiphospholipid syndrome. J Clin Invest 2003;112:1644–1654.

40. Neng Lai LK, et al. Anti-DNA autoantibodies stimulate the release of interleukln-1 and interleukin-6 from human endothelial cells. Journal of Pathology 1996;78:451–458.
41. Lai KN, et al. Upregulation of adhesion molecule expression on endothelial cells by anti-DNA autoantibodies in systemic lupus erythematosus. Clin lmmunol Immunopathol 1996;81:229–238.
42. Simantov R, et al. Activation of cultured vascular endothelial cells by antiphospholipid antibodies. J Clin Invest 1995;96:2211–2219.
43. Bone RC. Why new definitions of sepsis and organ failure are needed? Am J Med 1993;95:348.
44. Nogare D. Septic shock. Am J Med Sci 1991;302:50–65.
45. Waage A, et al. Current understanding of the pathogenesis of gram-negative shock. Infect Dis Clin North Am 1991;5:781–789.

17   Obstetric Antiphospholipid Syndrome

T. Flint Porter, Robert M. Silver, and D. Ware Branch

Introduction

Clinicians first recognized that pregnancy loss was associated with antiphospholipid antibodies (aPL) in the latter third of the last century. The term *antiphospholipid syndrome* (APS) was introduced in 1986 [1] to formalize the association of aPL with pregnancy loss, as well as with thrombotic events. Over a decade of subsequent international laboratory and clinical experience led to the development of an International Consensus Statement on preliminary criteria for definite APS published in 1999 [2]. There is widespread recognition, however, that refining the diagnostic criteria of APS is an ongoing process [3]. In this regard, no area has generated more controversies than obstetric APS, in part because of the substantial differences in patient selection for various studies. The purpose of this chapter is to critically analyze the relationship between aPL and obstetric problems, as well as to outline appropriate management strategies when aPL are found in association with pregnancy loss.

Pathogenesis of Obstetric Problems in APS

The potential complications of pregnancy in women with APS include pregnancy loss (including fetal death and recurrent pre-embryonic and embryonic losses), pre-eclampsia, and placental insufficiency. All have been ascribed to abnormal placental function, probably resulting from maldevelopment of the uteroplacental circulation. Extensive infarction, necrosis, and thrombosis were identified in placentas from failed pregnancies in women with aPL in early reports [4–7]. A large case-control study subsequently confirmed these findings, reporting thrombosis or infarction in 82% of placentas from women with aPL and fetal death [8]. A spiral arterial vasculopathy in decidual vessels also has been linked to aPL-related fetal loss [4, 7]. It must be said, however, that the histological abnormalities seen in APS cases are non-specific. The decidual vasculopathy described in some APS cases, which is characterized by acute atherosis, intimal thickening, fibrinoid necrosis, and an absence of the normal physiologic changes in the spiral arteries, also has been associated with pre-eclampsia and fetal growth restriction [9]. Furthermore, such findings are not always present in gestational tissues of women with APS [10].

How does maldevelopment of the uteroplacental circulation occur in APS? The first investigators in the field assumed that the recognized hypercoagulability of APS was in some way impacting the uteroplacental circulation. Interestingly, initial opinion held that *acute* placental thrombosis in the second or third trimester might be the culprit in APS-related placental insufficiency, or might be the final precipitating event in fetal loss or fetal distress. Numerous possible mechanisms of thrombosis at the level of the maternal decidua and in the intervillous space have been considered. Unfavorable alterations in the prostacyclin–thromboxane pathway [11] and increased tissue factor expression [12, 13] have been implicated. An effect on the protein C pathway is also a possible mechanism, particularly because antigenic and functional levels of protein S decline in normal pregnancy and some pregnant women develop acquired protein C resistance. Recent investigations have shown that aPL disrupt the "antithrombotic shield" on trophoblasts formed by annexin V, a protein with potent anticoagulant activity based on its high affinity binding to anionic phospholipids, which, in turn, displaces coagulation factors from phospholipid surfaces. Importantly, annexin V is very highly expressed by trophoblastic cells, making it a prime candidate for aPL at the level of the placenta. Decreased annexin V has been found on the villi of APS placentas [14], and aPL have been shown to reduce annexin V expression on placental villi and cultured trophoblast [14–16]. Finally, sophisticated techniques have been used to show that monoclonal aPL disrupt the crystal formation of annexin V on phospholipid bilayers [17].

A number of non-thrombotic mechanisms by which aPL might cause placental maldevelopment have also been proposed. Some investigators have found that aPL appear to damage or hamper the normal biology of trophoblasts [18–20]. A particularly attractive candidate mechanism for early pregnancy loss as well as placental insufficiency in later pregnancy is aPL-mediated inhibition of trophoblast invasion [19].

Within the last several years, two lines of experimental evidence suggest a more traditional autoimmune inflammatory role for aPL in the placental damage and maldevelopment. Because aPL also cross-react with oxidized low-density lipoprotein (LDL), a role for oxidant-mediated injury of placental vascular endothelium has been suggested [21]. This is topical because of current interest in oxidative stress as a causative or contributing factor in placental insufficiency, pre-eclampsia, and fetal growth restriction [22]. LDL can be oxidized by trophoblastic cells, as well as other cells present at the maternal–fetal interface [23]. Oxidized LDL itself can inhibit trophoblast invasion in vitro [24]. Inconsistent findings and a lack of direct evidence at the maternal–fetal interface are lingering problems with this concept, at least in terms of adverse fetal outcome. Nonetheless, one can't help but wonder whether aPL might be generated in susceptible individuals by this process of oxidative stress with oxidation of LDL.

Recent work in mice suggests that complement activation is crucial to aPL-related fetal death and fetal growth restriction [25, 26]. This murine model employs passive immunization with polyclonal human aPL IgG or monoclonal aPL and is associated with a substantial rate of fetal death and fetal growth restriction. Local (placental) IgG and C3 deposition are seen with aPL immunization, and there is a robust infiltration with neutrophils. Blocking C3 *convertase* and C5–C5a receptor interactions prevent aPL-mediated pregnancy complications in this model. Also, genetically engineered mice deficient in C3, C4, or C5 and mice depleted of neutrophils are protected. It is worth noting that studies of human placentas from women with APS do not show prominent neutrophil infiltration. Perhaps, however, the damage is already done (at an earlier gestational age) and inflammatory markers and cells are no longer present by the time the placenta is delivered.

Pregnancy Loss Classification, Epidemiology, and Evaluation

Selected Aspects of Conceptus Development

For an understanding of the relationship between aPL and pregnancy loss, it is important to clarify the nomenclature of pregnancy loss. Obstetricians traditionally have grouped all pregnancy losses prior to 20 weeks' gestation (menstrual dates) together as "abortions" and the death of the fetus thereafter as a stillbirth. While this classification has served a somewhat pragmatic role in reproductive record keeping, it ignores precepts of developmental biology and the clinical realities of pregnancy loss.

The development of the conceptus from fertilized egg to live born infant involves numerous complex, inter-related steps. Largely different stages of conceptus development are easily identified and are useful in understanding and studying pregnancy loss. The pre-embryonic period lasts from conception through the 4th week from the first day of the last menstrual period (3 weeks after fertilization). During this period, the early trophoblast differentiates from the tissue destined to become the embryo (the inner cell mass) and accomplishes implantation into the maternal endometrium (days 6–7 after fertilization). The pre-embryo develops into a bilaminar and then trilaminar disk of cells and microscopically observable alterations of the cell disk define the cranial end of the central neural axis of the pre-embryo. Oxygen and nutrient needs are met by diffusion across maternal tissues. The embryonic period is thought to begin around the 5th week of gestation, lasting through the 9th week of gestation. Authorities, according to developmental criteria used, debate the exact beginning and end. During the embryonic period, the trilaminar disk folds to become cylindrical, the head and tail regions become recognizable as cranial and caudal folds, definite segmentation is seen, and all organs form (organogenesis). The fetal period begins at the 10th week of gestation and extends through pregnancy until delivery. This period is characterized by substantial growth and differentiation of previously formed structures with relatively little organogenesis.

There are also distinct phases in the development of the placenta and the maternal–fetal circulation. Careful histological examination [27] and Doppler ultrasound [28] indicate that normal pregnancies are characterized by obstruction of uteroplacental arteries by invading trophoblastic cells which severely limits maternal blood flow into the intervillous tissue during the first 10 to 12 weeks. During this time, the intervillous space is filled with an acellular fluid [27, 29], and the environment is relatively hypoxic [30]. Although there appears to be considerable individual variation, trophoblastic regression and dislocation of arteriolar trophoblastic plugs beginning at 10 weeks' gestation allow initiation of true intervillous blood flow and a concomitant increase in the intervillous oxygen tension. Until this transpires, it is thought that oxygenation of the embryonic tissues occurs largely through diffusion across adjacent tissues, rather than through an organized circulatory delivery.

Classification Aspects of Pregnancy Loss

The classification of pregnancy loss is often made difficult because of the nature of its clinical presentation. The demise of the conceptus usually precedes the symptoms of miscarriage, typically uterine bleeding and cramping, by at least several days, and often by a week or more. For example, the onset of bleeding at 10 to 12 weeks' gestation represents pre-embryonic or embryonic losses in the vast majority of cases. Furthermore, fetal death may not always precede miscarriage, as in cases of cervical incompetence wherein the fetus is usually alive at the time of presentation. Finally, the death of a live-born infant after 20 weeks' gestation usually is recorded as a "neonatal loss" or "neonatal death."

Clinical Aspects of Pregnancy Loss

Human reproduction is inefficient, with an estimated 50% of conceptions failing [31]. The majority of these go unrecognized, occurring prior to or with the expected next menses [32]. The clinical problem of "miscarriage" encompasses recognized pregnancies that progress beyond the expected next menses. Approximately 10% to 12% of pregnancies end in spontaneous abortions prior to 12–14 weeks' gestation (from last menses), most of which are pre-embryonic or embryonic in nature. In a study of 232 women with apparently normal early pregnancies, Goldstein and colleagues [33] showed that 13.4% had pregnancy loss. Nearly 90% occurred in the pre-embryonic or embryonic periods, representing 12% of all pregnancies. Approximately 2% of pregnancies were lost as fetal deaths from 14 to 20 weeks' gestation. The period from 8.5–14 weeks' gestation appeared to be a period of infrequent embryonic or fetal loss with no embryos alive at 8.5 weeks' gestation dying before 14 weeks' gestation, suggesting that pregnancy loss is somewhat biphasic in its distribution. Including both fetal deaths and early neonatal deaths, approximately 5% of all pregnancies end in pregnancy loss from 14 weeks' gestation through term [34–36].

The vast majority of pregnancy losses are sporadic in nature, that is, they occur as an isolated event in a woman with other successful pregnancies. Recurrent pregnancy loss, traditionally defined as the loss of 3 or more consecutive pregnancies, occurs in an estimated 0.5% to 1% of women. Most cases of recurrent pregnancy loss are pre-embryonic or embryonic in nature; recurrent fetal death is much less common. Widely accepted causes of recurrent pre-embryonic or embryonic loss are listed in Table 17.1. Women with 3 successive pre-embryonic or embryonic losses have a recurrence risk of approximately 25% to 30% [37–40]. Some investigators have found that the risk of pre-embryonic or embryonic losses in a next pregnancy increases after 4 or more successive miscarriages.

The risk of recurrent fetal death is less well understood. However, when one fetal death has occurred, the risk increases substantially [41, 42]. In one study of over 350,000 women in Norway, investigators found that 1 previous fetal death between 16–27 weeks increased the risk of recurrence 20-fold, while a fetal death greater than 28 weeks' gestation increased the risk 5-fold. Samueloff [43] reported that the risk fetal death increased 10-fold in patients with a fetal death after 20 weeks' gestation. The commonly accepted causes of fetal death are listed in Table 17.2.

How is all of this important to APS? Harris listed "fetal loss" as the pregnancy loss criterion for APS in his 1987 proposal entitled "The Syndrome of the Black Swan"

Table 17.1. Accepted or suspected causes of pregnancy loss. 📖

Sporadic miscarriage < 10 weeks' gestation
- Chromosomal abnormalities of the conceptus/placenta

Fetal loss
- Parental structural chromosome abnormalities
- Uterine anatomic abnormalities
- Antiphospholipid syndrome
- Thrombophilia, especially factor V Leiden, resistance to activated protein C, prothrombin 20210 mutation, protein S deficiency
- Intrauterine infection, especially viral infections
- Alloimmunization to Rh D antigen and other blood group antigens
- Feto-maternal hemorrhage
- Poorly controlled diabetes mellitus
- Maternal hypertension
- Cervical incompetence

Recurrent pre-embryonic or embryonic pregnancy loss
- Parental structural chromosome abnormalities
- Uterine anatomic abnormalities, including congenital malformations
- Antiphospholipid syndrome
- Numeric chromosome abnormalities of the conceptus
- Molecular genetic abnormalities of the conceptus or placenta
- Hormonal and metabolic disorders
- Luteal phase defects
- Hypersecretion of luteinizing hormone
- Thrombophilia

Table 17.2. Suggested routine evaluation for recurrent pregnancy loss. 📖

History
- Pattern and trimester of pregnancy losses and whether a live embryo or fetus was present
- Exposure to environmental toxins or drugs
- Known gynecologic or obstetric infections
- Features associated with APS
- Genetic relationship between reproductive partners (consanguinity)
- Family history of recurrent miscarriage or syndrome associated with embryonic or fetal loss
- Previous diagnostic tests and treatments

Physical
- General physical examination
- Examination of vagina, cervix, and uterus

Tests
- Hysterosalpingogram or hysteroscopy
- Parental karyotypes
- LA and aCL
- Thrombophilia evaluation (factor V Leiden, prothrombin 20210 mutation)
- Luteal phase endometrial biopsy; repeat in next cycle if abnormal
- Other laboratory tests suggested by history and physical examination

[1], implying that embryonic loss or neonatal death would not qualify. The last 15 years has seen considerable debate regarding the nature of pregnancy loss associated with or attributable to aPL. The 1999 criteria proposed at the International Antiphospholipid Symposium in Sapporo, Japan, probably reflect best the current

consensus [2]. These criteria include any of the following 3 different types of pregnancy loss as a clinical criterion for APS: (1) 1 or more unexplained deaths of a morphologically normal fetus at or beyond the 10th week of gestation with normal fetal morphology documented by ultrasound or direct examination of the fetus; (2) 1 or more premature births of a morphologically normal neonate at or before the 34th week of gestation because of severe pre-eclampsia or placental insufficiency; (3) 3 or more consecutive spontaneous abortions before the 10th week of gestation with maternal anatomic, hormonal abnormalities, and paternal and maternal chromosomal causes excluded.

Evaluation of the Patient with Pregnancy Loss

From the standpoint of determining the cause of pregnancy loss, fetal loss is fundamentally different than pre-embryonic or embryonic loss. In cases of fetal loss, the fetus itself may be examined. In addition, a wide variety of structural malformations and precursors to fetal death (such as hydrops fetalis) may be seen by sonographic examination of the fetus in utero. The finding of a morphologically normal fetus (postmortem changes aside) excludes a chromosomal abnormality in over 95% of cases [38]. In any case, chromosomal abnormalities are relatively infrequent causes of fetal death, especially beyond 15–20 weeks' gestation. The accepted or suspected causes of fetal loss are shown in Table 17.1.

In contrast, the evaluation of a patient suffering recurrent early miscarriage is less direct because morphological clues from the fetus are usually unavailable. Chromosomal abnormalities are common causes of pre-embryonic or embryonic loss, and are modestly common in recurrent pregnancy loss cases [43, 44]. The clinical utility of pathologic evaluation of pre-embryonic and embryonic products of conception is questionable because specimens usually contain only decidual and placental tissue which demonstrate non-specific histological features that provide little insight into the cause of pregnancy loss, cannot be used to distinguish between sporadic and recurrent abortion, and provide no prognostic significance [45]. Early pregnancy sonographic examination of the embryo is unlikely to identify malformations, especially when performed with anything less than state-of-the art equipment and experienced personnel familiar with the morphology of the embryo. A suggested evaluation for recurrent pregnancy loss is shown in Table 17.2.

Pregnancy Loss and Antiphospholipid Antibodies

Type of Pregnancy Loss

aPL are not (frequently) associated with sporadic pregnancy loss at less than 20 weeks' gestation [46]. A number of studies, however, indicate that positive tests for lupus anticoagulant (LA) or IgG or IgM anticardiolipin antibodies (aCL) may be found in up to 20% of women with "recurrent pregnancy loss" or "recurrent abortion" [47–54]. It must be said that recurrent pregnancy loss is defined variably in these studies as either 2 or more consecutive losses or 3 or more consecutive losses. Also, not all required repeatedly positive tests to confirm the diagnosis of APS. In most of these studies, the type of recurrent losses is not stated (i.e., recurrent pre-embryonic or embryonic losses vs. recurrent fetal deaths versus a mixture of the two). Moreover, the rigor with which other common causes of recurrent pregnancy loss have been ruled out is unclear in many studies. Thus, while most authorities agree that aPL are a "cause" of recurrent miscarriage, the frequency with which otherwise healthy women with recurrent miscarriage have repeatedly positive aPL results and all other causes of recurrent miscarriage excluded has not been studied and confirmed by multiple centers.

In one study of a highly selected referral population of 366 women with 2 or more consecutive pregnancy losses, investigators compared the types of prior pregnancy losses in 76 women with and 290 women without LA or with greater than 20 G phospholipid units (GPL) aCL [55] and found that women with moderate-to-high levels of aPL had significantly different pregnancy loss histories compared to women without high levels of aPL. Both groups of women had similar rates of prior pregnancy loss (84%). But, 50% of the prior losses in women with aPL were fetal deaths, compared to less than 15% in women without aPL. More than 80% of women with aPL had at least 1 fetal death, compared with less than 25% of women without aPL ($P < 0.001$). Finally, the specificity of fetal death for the presence of aPL was 76% compared to only 6% for 2 or more pre-embryonic or embryonic losses without fetal death. Unfortunately, studies of fetal death or recurrent fetal death suffer from the same shortcomings as those of recurrent miscarriage with regard to aPL.

If aPL are causative in terms of fetal compromise, why would they result in recurrent early pregnancy loss in some patients and second or third trimester complications in others? To be sure, the relationship between APS cases resulting in adverse outcomes during the pre-embryonic and embryonic period (presenting as recurrent early miscarriage) and those resulting in complications during the fetal period (fetal death or premature delivery due to obstetric complications) is seen as a continuum by some experts. It is possible that the same underlying mechanism (e.g., aPL-mediated hypercoagulability) can operate along the continuum of gestation to cause either predominantly first trimester or predominantly second and third trimester complications. An alternative view holds that women presenting with recurrent pre-embryonic and embryonic losses and aPL represent a largely different patient population. Their pregnancy losses are likely due to different mechanism(s) than later pregnancy complications, perhaps relating to different aPL specificities or aPL operating on a fundamentally different pathophysiological background.

Isotype and Levels of aPL

Many studies of recurrent pregnancy loss and aPL include a substantial proportion of patients positive for low levels of IgG aCL or IgM aCL alone. However, the clinical significance of low positive IgG aCL and isolated IgM aCL is questionable. In one study [56], women with low positive IgG aCL or isolated IgM aCL had no greater risk for aPL-related events than women who tested negative. In addition, their risk for APS-associated complications was markedly lower than the risk in women with LA or less than 20 GPL aCL antibodies. On the other hand, it is intriguing that two studies found a significant proportion of women with recurrent pregnancy loss (primarily pre-embryonic and embryonic losses) had normalized values indicating low levels of IgG aCL antibodies (defined as > 95th or 99th percentiles) [54, 57]. In one of these studies [54], those positive for low levels of IgG aCL antibodies did not have the clinical background typical of a population of women with well-characterized APS (e.g., lupus, thrombosis, etc.).

It may be that low levels of aPL detected by immunoassay are associated with recurrent pre-embryonic and embryonic loss, but that women with LA and moderate-to-high levels of IgG aCL antibodies constitute a different population of patients. Similar contentions may be raised regarding IgM aCL in the absence of LA. To fully understand the significance of low levels of IgG aCL, isolated IgM aCL, or phospholipid-binding autoantibodies other than LA and aCL, study subjects must be meticulously characterized from a clinical standpoint and levels of aPL carefully determined in a way that allows comparison between studies. Of course, repeat testing and the inclusion of appropriate controls are crucial.

Patient Selection in Studies of aPL and Pregnancy Loss

Nowhere is the degree of variability in patient selection more evident or more important than in treatment studies of women with aPL-related pregnancy loss. Two recent reviews have thoroughly discussed this problem [58, 59]. Published treatment studies have identified two major groups of patients found in clinical practice: Group 1 – healthy women whose sole problem is recurrent early pregnancy loss or at least 1 fetal loss; and Group 2 – women with high frequencies of fetal loss (though not necessarily recurrent losses) in addition to systemic lupus erythematosus (SLE), a thrombotic history, or combinations of these.

Thirteen prospective treatment studies of women falling into Group 1 above have been published [60–72]. Direct comparison of most these studies is impossible due to differing definitions for aPL and recurrent pregnancy loss and the gestational age at which the treated pregnancies were enrolled or treatment initiated. Inconsistencies in aPL testing between studies are easily illustrated. Two studies excluded patients with a LA [61, 64], one did not test for LA [60], and three did not test for IgM aCL [60, 65, 72]. Whether patients with low aCL levels fulfilled the serological criterion for APS because LA was present is not specified, and three studies [61, 62, 64] specifically mention exclusion of patients with low aCL levels. The issue of using standardized assays is not well addressed in many studies. Three studies [62, 67, 69] did not report phospholipid dependency of coagulation abnormalities as is required by international guidelines for LA testing. In one study LA was considered present when any of four clotting tests was prolonged, but mixing studies and a neutralization procedure were not performed [65]. In all but two studies [60, 69] published standards were used to define a positive aCL test. The antibody levels allowing inclusion also varied widely. For example, the women included in these studies had at least 5 [66, 67, 70] to 40 [72] GPL units and/or 3 [66, 70] to 21 [61, 64] MPL units.

Some studies started evaluation of pregnancy outcome with a positive pregnancy test [60–62, 64, 65, 69, 72] and categorized first trimester loss, blighted ovum, or absent fetal heart beat as pregnancy loss. Others excluded such patients by virtue of their inclusion after detection of an embryonic heartbeat [66, 68, 70].

Given these differences, it is not surprising that the prevalence of LA varied from 6% [63] to 91% [66] in 10 studies, and the frequency of a positive LA test in absence of aCL varied from 6% [63] to 82% [66]. Positive tests for both LA and aCL were present in from 9% [66] to 67% [72] of patients. Inclusion criteria varied widely between studies. Three studies included patients with at least 2 unexplained losses before 12 weeks gestation or at least 1 pregnancy loss after 12 weeks [62, 63, 69]. Other studies included patients with at least 2 consecutive fetal losses before 32 weeks gestation [65] or at least three consecutive miscarriages [60, 61, 64, 66–68, 70].

It should come as no surprise that studies have reported considerable differences in pregnancy outcomes, given the wide variety of inclusion criteria. Three studies had treatment regimens which included prednisone and aspirin [62, 63, 65]. Live birth rates were 75% for both treatment groups in the one study [62], and 100% in another [63], and 60% of treated pregnancies and in 52% of pregnancies in which placebo was given in a third [65]. A consistent theme among these studies was the association between prednisone use and maternal morbidity and pre-term delivery, often because of pre-term rupture of membranes or pre-eclampsia.

More recent treatment trials of women in Group 1 have studied various regimens of heparin therapy, usually in combination with low-dose aspirin. Three have compared heparin and aspirin to aspirin alone [61, 66, 68] and one study has compared two dosages of heparin combined with low-dose aspirin [64]. Dosing regimens vary widely between studies, making any direct comparisons difficult. Nevertheless, in two studies, more live births (70%–80%) occurred in women treated with heparin and aspirin than among women treated with aspirin alone [61, 66]. Low-dose heparin was as effective as higher dose heparin in a third study [64]. However, a fourth study found that low-molecular-weight heparin was no more effective than aspirin alone [68]. Finally, a fifth study found that low-molecular-weight heparin plus aspirin was as effective as intravenous immune globulin in promoting live births [72]. Rates of maternal thrombosis, pre-eclampsia, and severe placental insufficiency were relatively low in all studies, and did not differ between treatment groups. Our understanding of the treatment of women in Group 1 is further complicated by the fact that a number of studies have found excellent live birth rates and relatively low complication rates in women treated with aspirin alone or supportive care [60, 62, 63, 67, 69].

Group 2 women, those with high frequencies of fetal loss, SLE, a thrombotic history, or combinations of these, have been the focus of three prospective, observational studies [73–75], a retrospective analysis of heparin treatment [76], and one randomized treatment study [77]. As with the studies of patients in Group 1, direct comparison of these studies is virtually impossible due to differences in patient selection, time of initiating treatments, and treatment regimens. Most of these studies demonstrated live births in excess of 60% of treated patients. A majority of women were treated with unfractionated heparin or low-molecular-weight heparin in a variety of dosing regimens. However, in contrast to findings in studies of women in Group 1, studies of women in Group 2 tend to show higher rates of maternal and fetal complications in both treatment and non-treatment groups. Indeed, in one study of well-characterized patients [74], pre-eclampsia occurred in 50% of pregnancies, and pre-term birth prior to 32 weeks' gestation occurred in nearly 40%. It is perhaps reassuring that the only prospective, randomized trial of Group 2 women [77] found a large number of successful pregnancy outcomes with pre-eclampsia and fetal distress in less than 40% of treated women.

Other Complications of Pregnancy in APS

The potential complications of pregnancy in women with APS not only include pregnancy loss, but also pre-eclampsia and placental insufficiency. In addition, pregnant women with APS may suffer thrombosis (including stroke) and complications due to treatment. Those who also have SLE are also at risk for lupus exacerbation during pregnancy.

In case series of women with a history of the most serious complications of APS including fetal loss, SLE, thrombosis, or any combination of these, gestational hypertension–pre-eclampsia is as high as 50%, with a median rate of 32% [74, 75, 78–80]. Placental insufficiency requiring delivery is also relatively frequent in some of these case series [73–75]. Not surprisingly, the rate of pre-term birth in these series ranges from 32% to 65% [74, 75, 78–80].

Women with APS without a history of thrombosis appear to have a substantial risk (i.e., 1% to several percent) of thrombosis during pregnancy [74, 75], and authorities generally recommend thromboprophylaxis and even full anticoagulation [81, 82].

The potential complications of heparin treatment during pregnancy include hemorrhage, osteoporosis with fracture, and heparin-induced thrombocytopenia. The reported rate of osteoporosis and associated fracture is low, though cases have occurred, even with low-molecular-weight heparin [75]. Heparin-induced thrombocytopenia is also infrequent in pregnant women [83].

Management of APS in Pregnancy

Pre-conceptional Counseling

Patients with APS should undergo pre-conceptional assessment, which typically includes a detailed medical and obstetrical history and documentation or confirmation of significant levels of aPL. The patient should be informed of the potential maternal and obstetrical problems, including fetal loss, thrombosis or stroke, pre-eclampsia, fetal growth impairment, and pre-term delivery. In those women who also have SLE, issues related to exacerbation of SLE also should be discussed. All patients with APS should be assessed for evidence of anemia and thrombocytopenia because both may occur in association with APS. Assessment for underlying renal disease (urinalysis, a serum creatinine, 24-hour urine for creatinine clearance, and total protein) may be useful.

Antenatal Surveillance

Women with APS should be evaluated frequently during pregnancy and should be instructed to notify their physician immediately with signs or symptoms of APS-related complications, including thrombosis or thromboembolism. Serial aPL determinations are not useful if the diagnosis of APS has already been confirmed. After 20 weeks' gestation, the primary focus of antenatal visits is the detection of hypertension and/or proteinuria. Starting at 18 to 20 weeks' gestation, serial fetal ultrasound examination of fetal growth should begin and continue every 4–6 weeks in order to identify uteroplacental insufficiency. Fetal surveillance should also include instruction on daily fetal movement counts and initiation of standard tests to assess fetal well-being (i.e., non-stress test, biophysical profile) at 30–32 weeks' gestation. Earlier and more frequent ultrasound examinations and fetal assessment is necessary in patients with a history of adverse obstetric outcomes or contemporary evidence of pre-eclampsia or uteroplacental insufficiency. In the most severe cases, the initiation of fetal surveillance may be justified as early as 24–25 weeks' gestation [84].

Heparin and Other Therapies During Pregnancy

Several treatment regimens have been used in women with APS to improve pregnancy outcome and reduce the risk of thromboembolism. The American College of Chest Physicians (ACCP) has recommended that all women with APS be treated in pregnancy with a combination of low-dose aspirin and subcutaneous, unfractionated heparin or low-molecular-weight heparin (LMWH). Generally speaking, pregnant women with APS and a prior thromboembolic event should receive adjusted-dose anticoagulation while those with APS diagnosed on the basis of obstetric criteria alone, without a prior thrombosis, may be treated with thromboprophylaxis [82]. Other recent experts reviews of treatment regimens have similar recommendations [58, 59]. Table 17.3 provides a summary of treatment regimens.

Women with particularly egregious thrombotic histories, such as recurrent thrombotic events or cerebral thrombotic events, would appear to be at very high risk for thrombosis during pregnancy. In selected such cases, some experts recommend the judicious use of warfarin anticoagulation, rather than heparin.

Clinicians should also realize that otherwise healthy women with recurrent pregnancy loss and low titers of aPL do not require treatment. One controlled trial included a majority of such women and found no difference in live birth rates using either low-dose aspirin or placebo [67].

Anticoagulant coverage of the postpartum period in women with APS and prior thrombosis is critical. Most clinicians and patients prefer switching to warfarin

Table 17.3. Subcutaneous heparin regimens used in the treatment of antiphospholipid syndrome during pregnancy.

Prophylactic Regimens

Recurrent pre-embryonic and embryonic loss; no history of thrombotic events
Standard heparin:	(1) 5000–7500 U every 12 hours in the first trimester, 5000–10,000 U every 12 hours in the second and third trimesters
Low-molecular-weight heparin:	(1) Enoxaparin 40 mg once daily or dalteparin 5000 U once daily, OR
	(2) Enoxaparin 30 mg every 12 hours or dalteparin 5000 U every 12 hours

Prior fetal death or early delivery because of severe preeclampsia or severe placental insufficiency; no history of thrombotic events
Standard heparin:	(1) 7500–10,000 U every 12 hours in the first trimester, 10,000 U every 12 hours in the second and third trimesters
Low-molecular-weight heparin:	(1) Enoxaparin 40 mg once daily or dalteparin 5000 U once daily, OR
	(2) Enoxaparin 30 mg every 12 hours or dalteparin 5000 U every 12 hours

Anticoagulation Regimens–recommended in women with a history of thrombotic events
Standard heparin:	(1) 7500 U every 8–12 hours adjusted to maintain the mid-interval heparin levels in the therapeutic range
Low-molecular-weight heparin:	(1) Weight-adjusted (e.g., enoxaparin 1 mg/kg every 12 hours or dalteparin 200 U/kg every 12 hours) OR

thromboprophylaxis as soon as the patient is clinically stable from delivery. In most cases, an international normal ratio (INR) of 2.5 is desirable. There is no international consensus regarding the postpartum management of women without prior thrombosis in whom the diagnosis of APS is based on a history of fetal death, severe pre-eclampsia, or neonatal death, though all agree there is an increased risk of thrombosis. Postpartum thromboprophylaxis using heparin for 3 to 5 days, especially in the event of cesarean delivery, is recommended in the United Kingdom. In the United States, anticoagulant therapy for 6 weeks after delivery is recommended. For with women with APS diagnosed solely on the basis of recurrent pre-embryonic or embryonic loss, the need for postpartum thromboprophylaxis is uncertain.

References

1. Harris EN. Syndrome of the black swan. Br J Rheumatol 1987;26:324–326.
2. Wilson WA, Gharavi AE, Koike T, et al. International consensus statement on preliminary classi.cation criteria for definite antiphospholipid syndrome: report of an international workshop. Arthritis Rheum 1999;42:1309–1311.
3. Levine JS, Rauch J, Branch DW. Anti-phospholipid syndrome. N Engl J Med 2002;346:752–763.
4. De Wolf F, Carreras LO, Moerman P, Vermylen J, Van Assche A, Renaer M. Decidual vasculopathy and extensive placental infarction in a patient with repeated thromboembolic accidents, recurrent fetal loss, and a lupus anticoagulant. Am J Obstet Gynecol 1982;142:829–834.
5. Branch DW, Scott JR, Kochenour NK, Hershgold E. Obstetric complications associated with the lupus anticoagulant. N Engl J Med 1985;313:1322–1326.
6. Lubbe WF, Butler WS, Palmer SJ, et al. Lupus anticoagulant in pregnancy. Br J Obstet 1984;91:357–363.
7. Nayar R, Lage JM. Placental changes in a first trimester missed abortion in maternal systemic lupus erythematosus with antiphospholipid syndrome: a case report and review of the literature. Hum Pathol 1996;27:201–206.
8. Out HJ, Bruinse HW, Christiaens GCML, et al. Prevalence of aPL in patients with fetal loss. Ann Rheum Dis 1991;50:553–557.
9. Khong TY, DeWolf F, Robertson WB, et al. Inadequate maternal vascular response to placentation in pregnancies complicated by pre-eclampsia and by small for gestational age infants. Br J Obstet Gynecol 1986;93:1049–1059.
10. Salafia CS, Parke AL. Placental pathology in systemic lupus erythematosus and phospholipid antibody syndrome. Rheum Dis Clin North Am 1997;23:85–97.
11. Peaceman AM, Rehnberg KA. The effect of immunoglobulin G fractions from patients with lupus anticoagulant on placental prostacyclin and thromboxane production. Am J Obstet Gynecol 1993;169:1403–1406.
12. Branch DW, Rodgers GM. Induction of endothelial cell tissue factor activity by sera from patients with antiphospholipid syndrome: a possible mechanism of thrombosis. Am J Obstet Gynecol 1993;168:206–210.
13. Dobado-Berrios PM, Lopez-Pedrera C, Velasco F, Aguirre MA, Torres A, Cuadrado MJ. Increased levels of tissue factor mRNA in mononuclear blood cells of patients with primary antiphospholipid syndrome. Thromb Haemost 1999;82:1578–1582.
14. Rand JH, Wu XX, Guller S, Gil J, Guha A, Scher J, Lockwood CJ. Reduction of annexin-V (placental anticoagulant protein-I) on placental villi of women with antiphospholipid antibodies and recurrent spontaneous abortion. Am J Obstet Gynecol 1994;171:1566–1572.
15. Rand JH, Wu XX, Guller S, Scher J, Andree HA, Lockwood CJ. Antiphospholipid immunoglobulin G antibodies reduce annexin-V levels on syncytiotrophoblast apical membranes and in culture media of placental villi. Am J Obstet Gynecol 1997;177:918–923.
16. Vogt E, Ng AK, Rote NS. Antiphosphatidylserine antibody removes annexin-V and facilitates the binding of prothrombin at the surface of a choriocarcinoma model of trophoblast differentiation. Am J Obstet Gynecol 1997;177:964–972.
17. Rand JH, Wu XX, Quinn AS, et al. Human monoclonal antiphospholipid antibodies disrupt the annexin A5 anticoagulant crystal shield on phospholipid bilayers: evidence from atomic force microscopy and functional assay. Am J Pathol 2003;163:1193–1200.

18. Katsuragawa H, Kanzaki H, Inoue T, Hirano T, Mori T, Rote NS. Monoclonal antibody against phos-phatidylserine inhibits in vitro human trophoblastic hormone production and invasion. Biol Reprod 1997;56:50–58.
19. di Simone N, Meroni PL, Del Papa N, et al. Antiphospholipid antibodies affect trophoblast gonadotropin secretion and invasiveness by binding directly and through adhered beta2-glycopro-tein I. Arthritis Rheum 2000;43:140–150.
20. Chamley LW, Duncalf AM, Mitchell MD, Johnson PM. Action of anticardiolipin and antibodies to beta2-glycoprotein-I on trophoblast proliferation as a mechanism for fetal death. Lancet 1998;352:1037–1038.
21. Horkko S, Miller E, Dudl E, et al. Antiphospholipid antibodies are directed against epitopes of oxi-dized phospholipids. Recognition of cardiolipin by monoclonal antibodies to epitopes of oxidized low density lipoprotein. J Clin Invest 1996;98:815–825.
22. Roberts JM, Hubel CA. Oxidative stress in preeclampsia. Am J Obstet Gynecol 2004;190:1177–1178.
23. Bonet B, Hauge-Gillenwater H, Zhu XD, Knopp RH. LDL oxidation and human placental trophoblast and macrophage activity. Proc Soc Exp Biol Med 1998;217:203–211.
24. Pavan L, Tsatsaris V, Hermouet A, Theroud P, Evain-Brion D, Fournier T. Oxidized low-density lipoproteins inhibit trophoblastic cell invasion. J Clin Endocrinol Metab 2004;89:1969–1972.
25. Holers VM, Giradi G, Mo L, et al. Complement C3 activation is required for antiphospholipid anti-body-induced fetal loss. J Exp Med 2002;195:211–220.
26. Giradi G, Berman J, Redecha P, et al. Complement C5a receptors and neutrophils mediate fetal injury in the antiphospholipid syndrome. J Clin Invest 2003;112:1644–1654.
27. Hustin J, Schaaps JP. Echographic and anatomic studies of the maternotrophoblastic border during the first trimester of pregnancy. Am J Obstet Gynecol 1987;157:162–168.
28. Jauniaux E, Hempstock J, Greenwold N, Burton GJ. Trophoblastic oxidative stress in relation to tem-poral and regional differences in maternal placental blood flow in normal and abnormal pregnan-cies. Am J Pathol 2003;162:115–125.
29. Burton GJ, Watson Al, Hempstock J, Skepper JN, Jauniaux E. Uterine glands provide histiotrophic nutrition for the uman fetus during the first trimester of pregnancy. J Clin Endocrinol Metab 2002;87:2954–2959.
30. Jauniaux E, Watson AL, Hempstock J, Bao Y-P, Skepper JN, Burton GJ. Onset of maternal arterial bloodflow and placental oxidative stress: a possible factor in human early pregnancy failure. Am J Pathol 2000;157:2111–2122.
31. Boklage CE. Survival probability of human conceptions from fertilization to term. Int J Fertil 1990;35:75–93.
32. Wilcox AJ, Weinberg CR, O'Connor JF, et al. Incidence of early loss of pregnancy. N Engl J Med 1988;319:189–194.
33. Goldstein SR. Embryonic death in early pregnancy: a new look at the first trimester. Obstet Gynecol 1994;84:294–297.
34. Miller JF, Williamson E, Glue J, Gordon YB, Grudzinskas JG, Sykes A. Fetal loss after implantation: a prospective study. Lancet 1980;ii:554–556.
35. Edmonds DK, Lindsay KS, Miller JF, Williams E, Wood PJ. Early embryonic mortality in women. Fertil Steril 1982;38:447–453.
36. Whitaker PG, Taylor A, Lind T. Unsuspected pregnancy loss in healthy women. Lancet 1983;i:1126–1127.
37. Regan L. A prospective study of spontaneous abortion. In: Beard RW, Sharp F, eds. Early pregnancy loss. London: Springer-Verlag; 1988:23–37.
38. Warburton D, Fraser FC. Spontaneous abortion risks in man: data from reproductive histories col-lected in a medical genetics unit. Am J Hum Genet 1964;16:1–25.
39. Fitzsimmons J, Jackson D, Wapner R, Jackson L. Subsequent reproductive outcome in couples with repeated pregnancy loss. Am J Med Genet 1983;16:583–587.
40. Stirrat GM. Recurrent miscarriage I: Identification and epidemiology. Lancet 1990;336:673–675.
41. Oyen N, Skjaerven R, Irgens LM. Population-based recurrence risk of sudden infant death syndrome compared with other infant and fetal deaths. Am J Epidemiol 1996;144:300.
42. Samueloff A, Xenakis E, Berkus MD, Huff RW, Langer O. Recurrent stillbirth: significance and char-acteristics. J Reprod Med 1993;38:883–886.
43. Stern JJ, Dorfmann AD, Gutierrez-Najar AJ, Cerrillo M, Coulam CB. Frequency of abnormal kary-otypes among abortuses from women with and without a history of recurrent spontaneous abor-tion. Fertil Steril 1996;65:250–253.
44. Sullivan A, et al. Recurrent fetal aneuploidy and recurrent miscarriage. Obstet Gynecol 2004;104:784–788.
45. Fox H. Histological classification of tissue from spontaneous abortions: a valueless exercise? Histopathology 1993;.22:599–600.

46. Infante-Rivard C, David M, Gauthier R, Rivard GE. Lupus anticoagulants, anticardiolipin antibodies, and fetal loss. A case–control study. N Engl J Med 1991;325:1063–1066.
47. Petri M, Golbus M, Anderson R, Whiting-O'Keefe Q, Corash L, Hellmann D. Antinuclear antibody, lupus anticoagulant, and anticardiolipin antibody in women with idiopathic habitual abortion. A controlled, prospective study of forty-four women. Arthritis Rheum 1987;30:601–606.
48. Out HJ, Bruinse HW, Christiaens GCML, et al. Prevalence of aPL in patients with fetal loss. Ann Rheum Dis 1991;50:553–557.
49. Parazzini F, Acaia B, Faden D, Lovotti M, Marelli G, Cortelazzo S. APL and recurrent abortion. Obstet Gynecol 1991;77:854–858.
50. Parke AL, Wilson D, Maier D. The prevalence of aPL in women with recurrent spontaneous abortion, women with successful pregnancies, and women who have never been pregnant. Arthritis Rheum 1991;34:1231–1235.
51. Plouffe L Jr, White EW, Tho SP, et al. Etiologic factors of recurrent abortion and subsequent reproductive performance of couples: have we made any progress in the past 10 years? Am J Obstet Gynecol 1992;167:313–320.
52. MacLean MA, Cumming GP, McCall F, Walker ID, Walker JJ. The prevalence of lupus anticoagulant and anticardiolipin antibodies in women with a history of first trimester miscarriages. Br J Obstet Gynaecol 1994;101:103–106.
53. Yetman DL, Kutteh WH. Antiphospholipid antibody panels and recurrent pregnancy loss: prevalence of anticardiolipin antibodies compared with other aPL. Fertil Steril 1996;66:540–546.
54. Branch DW, Silver RM, Pierangelli SS, van Leeuwen I, Harris EN. APL other than lupus anticoagulant and anticardiolipin antibodies in women with recurrent pregnancy loss, fertile controls, and antiphospholipid syndrome. Obstet Gynecol 1997;89:549–555.
55. Oshiro BT, Silver RM, Scott JR, Yu H, Branch DW. Antiphospholipid antibodies and fetal death. Obstet Gynecol 1996;87:489–493.
56. Silver RM, Porter TF, van Leeuwen I, Jeng G, Scott JR, Branch DW. Anticardiolipin antibodies: clinical consequences of "low titers." Obstet Gynecol 1996;87:494–500.
57. Aoki K, Hayashi Y, Hirao Y, Yagami Y. aPL as a predictive variable in patients with recurrent pregnancy loss. Am J Reprod Immunol 1993a;29:82–87.
58. Branch DW, Khamashta MA. Antiphospholipid syndrome: obstetric diagnosis, management, and controversies. Obstet Gynecol. 2003;101:1333–1344.
59. Derksen RH, Khamashta MA, Branch DW. Management of the obstetric antiphospholipid syndrome. Arthritis Rheum 2004;50:1028–1039.
60. Tulppala M, Marttunen M, Soderstrom-Anttila V, et al. Low-dose aspirin in prevention of miscarriage in women with unexplained or autoimmune related recurrent miscarriage: effect on prostacyclin and thromboxane A2 production. Hum Reprod 1997;12:1567–1572.
61. Kutteh WH. Antiphospholipid antibody-associated recurrent pregnancy loss: treatment with heparin and low-dose aspirin is superior to low-dose aspirin alone. Am J Obstet Gynecol 1996;174:1584–1589.
62. Cowchock FS, Reece EA, Balaban D, Branch DW, Plouffe L. Repeated fetal losses associated with antiphospholipid antibodies: a collaborative randomized trial comparing prednisone with low-dose heparin treatment. Am J Obstet Gynecol 1992;166:1318–1323.
63. Silver RK, MacGregor SN, Sholl JS, Hobart JM, Neerhof MG, Ragin A. Comparative trial of prednisone plus aspirin versus aspirin alone in the treatment of anticardiolipin antibody-positive obstetric patients. Am J Obstet Gynecol 1993;169:1411–1417.
64. Kutteh WH, Ermel LD. A clinical trial for the treatment of antiphospholipid antibody-associated recurrent pregnancy loss with lower dose heparin and aspirin. Am J Reprod Immunol 1996;35:402–407.
65. Laskin CA, Bombardier C, Hannah ME, et al. Prednisone and aspirin in women with autoantibodies and unexplained recurrent fetal loss. N Engl J Med 1997;337:148–153.
66. Rai R, Cohen H, Dave M, Regan L. Randomised controlled trial of aspirin and aspirin plus heparin in pregnant women with recurrent miscarriage associated with phospholipid antibodies (or antiphospholipid antibodies). BMJ 1997;314:253–257.
67. Pattison NS, Chamley LW, Birdsall M, Zanderigo AM, Liddell HS, McDougall J. Does aspirin have a role in improving pregnancy outcome for women with the antiphospholipid syndrome? A randomized controlled trial. Am J Obstet Gynecol 2000;183:1008–1012.
68. Farquharson RG, Quenby S, Greaves M. Antiphospholipid syndrome in pregnancy: a randomized, controlled trial of treatment. Obstet Gynecol 2002;100:408–413.
69. Balasch J, Carmona F, Lopez-Soto A, et al. Low-dose aspirin for prevention of pregnancy losses in women with primary antiphospholipid syndrome. Hum Reprod 1993;8:2234–2239.

70. Backos M, Rai R, Baxter N, Chilcott IT, Cohen H, Regan L. Pregnancy complications in women with recurrent miscarriage associated with antiphospholipid antibodies treated with low dose aspirin and heparin. Br J Obstet Gynaecol 1999;106:102–107.
71. Rai RS, Clifford K, Cohen H, Regan L. High prospective fetal loss rate in untreated pregnancies of women with recurrent miscarriage and antiphospholipid antibodies. Hum Reprod 1995;10:3301–3304.
72. Triolo G, Ferrane A, Ciccia F, et al. Randomized study of subcutaneous low molecular weight heparin plus aspirin versus intravenous immunoglobulin in the treatment of recurrent fetal loss associated with antiphospholipid antibodies. Arthritis Rheum 2003;48:728–731.
73. Lockshin MD, Druzin ML, Qamar T. Prednisone does not prevent recurrent fetal death in women with antiphospholipid antibody. Am J Obstet Gynecol 1989;160:439–443.
74. Branch DW, Silver RM, Blackwell JL, Reading JC, Scott JR. Outcome of treated pregnancies in women with antiphospholipid syndrome: an update of the Utah experience. Obstet Gynecol 1992;80:614–620.
75. Lima F, Khamashta MA, Buchanan NM, Kerslake S, Hunt BJ, Hughes GR. A study of sixty pregnancies in patients with the antiphospholipid syndrome. Clin Exp Rheumatol 1996;14:131–136.
76. Rosove MH, Tabsh K, Wasserstrum N, Howard P, Hahn BH, Kalunian KC. Heparin therapy for pregnant women with lupus anticoagulant or anticardiolipin antibodies. Obstet Gynecol 1990;75:630–634.
77. Branch DW, Peaceman AM, Druzin M, et al. A multicenter, placebo-controlled pilot study of intravenous immune globulin treatment of antiphospholipid syndrome during pregnancy. The Pregnancy Loss Study Group. Am J Obstet Gynecol 2000;182:122–127.
78. Pauzner R, Dulitzki M, Langevitz P, Livneh A, Kenett R, Many A. Low molecular weight heparin and warfarin the treatment of patients with antiphospholipid syndrome during pregnancy. Thromb Haemost 2001;86:1379–1384.
79. Caruso A, de Carolis S, Ferrazzani S, Valesini G, Caforio L, Mancuso S. Pregnancy outcome in relation to uterine artery flow velocity waveforms and clinical characteristics in women with antiphospholipid syndrome. Obstet Gynecol 1993;82:970–977.
80. Huong DLT, Wechsler B, Bletry O, Vauthier-Brouzes D, Lefebvre G, Piette J-C. A study of 75 pregnancies in patients with antiphospholipid syndrome. J Rheumatol 2001;28:2025–2030.
81. American College of Obstetricians and Gynecologists. Thromboembolism in pregnancy. ACOG Prac Bull 2000;19.
82. Ginsberg JS, Greer I, Hirsh J. Use of antithrombotic agents during pregnancy. Chest 2001;119(suppl 1):122S–131S.
83. Fausett MB, Vogtlander M, Lee RM, et al. Heparin-induced thrombocytopenia is rare in pregnancy. Am J Obstet Gynecol 2001;185:148–152.
84. Druzin ML, Lockshin M, Edersheim TG, et al. Second-trimester fetal monitoring and preterm delivery in pregnancies with systemic lupus erythematosus and/or circulating anticoagulant. Am J Obstet Gynecol 1987;157:1503–1510.

18 Infertility and Antiphospholipid Antibodies

Lisa R. Sammaritano

Whether antiphospholipid antibodies (aPL) play a pathogenic role in infertility is highly controversial. aPL have been suggested to represent one potential etiology of infertility, specifically in patients with unexplained implantation failure following in vitro fertilization (IVF). The rationale is appealing, as it represents a logical extension of the demonstrated pathogenicity of aPL in contributing to recurrent spontaneous abortion, where mechanisms other than placental thrombosis and infarction seem to be at play. aPL in this setting are postulated to bind to phospholipids on trophoblast tissue, impairing trophoblast development and preventing normal placentation. Unexplained infertility in patients found to have aPL may represent the earliest form of aPL-mediated obstetric pathology: a disturbance of implantation, leading to failure to achieve biochemical or clinical pregnancy. What evidence supports this? More importantly, is there convincing evidence that makes this clinically relevant, that is, data to support use of current aPL pregnancy therapy to treat patients with failed IVF cycles?

The field of reproductive medicine, like the study of antiphospholipid syndrome (APS), has experienced explosive growth over the last 20 years. Infertility is a common problem, affecting 15% to 20% of couples. By definition, infertility represents the inability of a couple practicing frequent intercourse and not using contraception to conceive a child within 1 year. Causes of infertility are fairly evenly distributed between males and females, and usually fall into one of three major groups: male factor, ovulatory dysfunction, and tubal–peritoneal disease. For this reason, initial work-up includes evaluation of both the male and the female partner. For women, this means hormone tests and direct visualization of the reproductive tract. Routine tests include day-three follicle stimulating hormone (FSH), prolactin, thyroid function tests, cervical cultures, and evaluation of ovulatory function (basal body temperature, urinary lutenizing hormone, transvaginal ultrasound, and/or endometrial biopsy). Tubal patency and uterine morphology are evaluated with a hysterosalpingogram; hysteroscopy and laparoscopy may be required. Low serum progesterone 1 week post-ovulation suggests a luteal phase defect. A postcoital test is sometimes performed to assess cervical mucous and presence of antisperm antibodies [1]. Tests for male factors include semen analysis, specific tests for spermatozoal function such as the hamster egg penetration assay, and hormone levels [2].

A probable etiology for infertility is often uncovered. In general, ovulatory dysfunction accounts for 15% cases, pelvic factors (including endometriosis and adhesions) for 35%, male factors (oligospermia, decreased sperm motility, or abnormal sperm function) for 35%, and abnormal sperm–cervical mucus penetration or antisperm antibodies for 5%. Despite extensive testing, etiology remains unexplained in about 10% to 15% of cases. Importantly, two or more factors are identified in 20% to 40% of couples. Although IVF is an assisted reproductive technique originally developed for patients with Fallopian tube pathology, it is now routinely used for infertility patients with a wide range of etiologies, including those with unexplained infertility [3]. The mechanics of IVF can bypass many potential steps that may be defective.

Briefly, the usual IVF protocol includes ovarian stimulation, retrieval of multiple oocytes, in vitro fertilization, and embryo placement in the uterus. Gonadotropin-releasing hormone (GnRH) analogs are often used to desensitize pituitary gonatotropes to endogenous GnRH and downregulate gonadotropin secretion. Controlled ovarian hyperstimulation is accomplished by administering human menopausal gonadotropin, and ovulation is triggered with human chorionic gonadotropin (hCG) when multiple follicles are mature. Oocytes are usually retrieved through transvaginal ultrasound-guided follicular puncture.

After separation of motile spermatozoa and in vitro capacitation, spermatozoa are added to oocytes and cultured to achieve fertilization. Gamete micromanipulation is used for male factor infertility, usually intracytoplasmic sperm injection (ICSI). Fertilized oocytes are re-examined after incubation to confirm embryonic cleavage has occurred and to assess embryo quality. If indicated, embryo biopsy with prenatal genetic diagnosis may be done to rule out aneuploidy or other genetic defects. Embryo placement (usually 2 to 3 per procedure) is through transcervical transfer to the uterus, and the luteal phase is then maintained with low dose hCG or exogenous progesterone. Within 10–12 days of embryo transfer, implantation can be detected by an increase in serum hCG levels. Diagnosis of clinical pregnancy depends on visualization by ultrasound of a gestational sac containing a fetus with fetal heart activity within the uterine cavity 4–6 weeks after transfer.

Many factors affect IVF outcome. Age is one of the most critical: female fertility begins to decline naturally in the mid-30s and becomes marked after age 40. As patients age, oocyte quality decreases, negatively impacting likelihood of IVF success. In addition, the reported outcomes – including those in many of the aPL studies described below – are often expressed in a number of different ways. *Biochemical pregnancy* is implantation identified by a transient production of hCG but with early loss before sonographic documentation of a fetus. *Clinical pregnancy* is when fetal heart activity is seen. *Ongoing pregnancy* represents currently viable gestations, and *live birth rate* or *deliveries* describes successfully completed pregnancies. Outcome may be expressed as pregnancy rate per cycle or per transfer procedure, or as pregnancy rate per embryo transferred. Control patients are of particular importance in studies of outcome because even in optimal cycles implantation rates per embryo differ between IVF and spontaneous pregnancy. Likelihood of embryo implantation in an IVF cycle is 10%, versus about 25% for a natural cycle. In addition, there are increased rates of ectopic pregnancy and first trimester spontaneous abortion in IVF pregnancies [3].

Recent research has focused on the role of a variety of immunologic factors in reproductive failure, both infertility and recurrent spontaneous abortion (RSA). While alloimmune factors (including T cell embryotoxic cytokines and CD56 natural killer cells) are postulated to play a role primarily in RSA, autoimmune humoral abnormalities (including antiphospholipid, antithyroid, and other autoantibodies), have been suggested to play a role in both RSA and in infertility.

Increased levels of autoantibodies were initially described in patients with infertility due to endometriosis [4], but RSA and infertility patients overall have higher levels of autoantibodies than do fertile woman. Roussev et al [5] determined the frequency of abnormal immunologic tests among 108 women with various types of reproductive failure, including recurrent pregnancy loss, unexplained infertility, endometriosis, premature ovarian failure, and polycystic ovaries. Immunologic tests included aPL, lupus anticoagulant (LA), anti-thyroid antibodies (thyroglobulin and microsomal), embryotoxic factor (ETA), and CD56+ (NK) cells. Sixty-five percent of the patients tested had at least 1 abnormal immune test, compared with 7% of the controls. It is anticipated that RSA patients would have high rates of aPL antibodies, given the association of aPL with both early and late fetal loss. However, aPL was by far the most frequent abnormality among women with unexplained infertility: 42% of patients were positive for aPL, as opposed to lower prevalence of other immune abnormalities (16% patients were positive for CD56+ cells, 16% for ETA, and 9% for anti-thyroid antibodies). A similar study [6] focused on 122 patients with infertility and in vitro fertilization/embryo transfer (IVF/ET) failure: 70% of these patients were positive for 1 or more immune abnormalities, as compared to 10% of normal controls. Geva and colleagues [7] measured anticardiolipin antibodies (aCL), LA, anti-ds DNA antibodies, anti-nuclear antibodies (ANA), rheumatoid factor, and antithyroid antibodies in patients with 3 or more failed IVF cycles, and compared these patients with women who became pregnant in 3 or fewer cycles. Presence of any autoantibody was 22% in the failed IVF groups, as compared with 3% in the group with successful IVF pregnancies. As a result of these and other studies, and despite continued controversy as to their significance, autoantibody testing has become commonplace in patients being evaluated for infertility.

Autoantibodies included in infertility screening often include ANA, aPL, antithyroid antibodies, antisperm antibodies, and antizonal antibodies [8]. ANA, while highly sensitive for the diagnosis of clinical autoimmune disease, are relatively non-specific and are found in a small but definite percentage of the normal population. ANA prevalence in infertility patients referred for IVF, however, ranges from 5% to 43% [8], and some studies suggest a decreased IVF success rate in patients with ANA [9].

Antithyroid antibodies (antithyroglobulin and antithyroid peroxidase), characteristic of autoimmune thyroid disease, are frequently positive in the absence of clinical hypothyroidism. Relationship to RSA is not clear: antithyroid antibodies have been proposed to be associated with increased risk of spontaneous abortion [10], however a later prospective study found no association [11]. Kutteh et al [12] evaluated the prevalence of antithyroid antibodies in 3 distinct groups: patients with recurrent pregnancy loss, patients referred for IVF, and controls. They identified a small but significant increase in women with RSA compared with controls (23% vs. 16%), but there was no difference for the IVF patients versus controls (19% vs. 16%). Further work has shown IVF outcome to be no different in patients with and without antithyroid antibodies (16% vs. 15%) [13].

Antiovarian antibodies may include antibodies against the ooplasm, zona pellucida, and components of the ovary. A high prevalence of antizonal antibodies have been found in patients with failed fertilization in standard IVF, and pregnancy rates improve with use of ICSI [14]. Antisperm antibodies may be found in male or female serum, cervical mucous, or semen, and may interfere with sperm transport,

Table 18.1. Prevalence of antiphospholipid antibodies in patients with infertility.

Study	Study type	Patients	aPLs measured	N	Percent positive
El-Roeiy et al [15]	R	IVF	aCL, aPS, ab to histones ab to nucleotides total Ig, C3, C4	26	39%
Gleicher et al [16]	R	IVF	aCL and panel (6) ab to histones ab to polynucleo (4)total IgG	105	30%
Sher et al [17]	R	IVF	aCL aPL panel (6)	196	53% pelvic 14% male/unexpl
Birdsall et al [18]	P	IVF < or = 28 years old < 3 cycles	aCL, aPS	240	15%
Denis et al [19]	P	IVF	aPL panel (7) 3 isotypes each (21 total)	793	59%
Kowalik et al [20]	R	IVF	aCL, aPS	525	15%
Kutteh et al [21]	P	IVF	aCL aPL panel (4)	191	19%
Eldar-Geva et al [2]	P	IVF	aCL aPL panel (3)	173	30%
Chilcott et al [23]	P	IVF	aCL, LA aPS, a‰2GPI	380	23%

R = retrospective study; P = prospective study; N = number of infertility patients; IVF = in vitro fertilization; aCL = anticardiplipin antibody; aPL = antiphospholipid antibody; aPS = antiphosphatidylserine antibody; aPL panel = aPL antibodies directed against a number of different phospholipids; polynucleo = polynucleotides; aβ₂GPI = anti–β₂-glycoprotein I antibody; LA = lupus anticoagulant; Pelvic = pelvic etiology for infertility; male/unexpl = male factor or unexplained etiology for infertility.

capacitation, acrosomal reaction, fertilization, or implantation. IVF with ICSI also improves outcome in these patients [14].

An increased prevalence of aPL in patients with infertility has been shown in a large number of studies (Table 18.1). Prevalence of aPL in normals, including healthy pregnant women, is about 2% to 5%; in patients with RSA, prevalence is 15% to 20% [24]. Variability in definition and measurement of aPL is likely responsible for the wide variation in reported prevalence in new IVF patients: prevalence ranges from 15% to 59%. The specific aPL measured in these studies range from the generally accepted aCL and LA to large panels of multiple autoantibodies directed against various phospholipids including phosphatidylserine (PS), phosphatydlethanolamine (PE), phosphatidic acid (PA), phosphatidyl glycerol (PG), phosphatidylcholine (PC), and phosphatidylinosital (PI). In general, significance of these broad phospholipids panel results is controversial, and, as expected, they tend to identify a higher prevalence of aPLs [25]. Some authors, however, feel that certain aPLs distinct from aCL and LA are more predictive of IVF failure. Kaider et al [6], for example, identified aPC and aPA as the most common aPLs in patients with IVF failure. In contrast, Eldar Geva and coworkers [22] evaluated 173 patients with assays for all three isotypes of aPLs directed against CL, PS, PA, and PG. They were unable to identify an effect of any aPL on likelihood of IVF success, nor did they find the number of positive antibody tests per patient to be predictive. In a recent prospective controlled trial [23], the investigators evaluated 380 women referred for IVF and screened for aPL including aCL, LA, aPS: 89/380 patients (23%) were positive for aCL or LA, however, none were positive for aPS.

Importance of other aPL is similarly unclear. Several studies have looked at anti–β₂-glycoprotein I antibody (anti–β₂-GPI) in the context of infertility, with conflicting results [26, 27]. Anti–β₂-GPI have been suggested to be more specific for presence of complications in aPL-positive patients. However, several studies in reproductive failure patients found that anti–β₂-GPI do not identify additional aPL-positive RSA patients if initial tests for aCL and LA are negative [28, 29], and have found anti–β_2-GPI to be less sensitive than traditional aPLs in women with recurrent pregnancy loss [30].

Several studies have evaluated significance of anti–β_2-GPI specifically in infertility patients [23, 26, 27, 31]. Stern et al [27] evaluated patients with IVF failure (n = 105) and RSA (n = 97). Although testing was done for IgG and IgM isotypes of anti–β_2-GPI, aCL, aPE, aPS, and aPI in addition to LA and ANA, only positive ANA and IgM anti–β_2-GPI antibodies were significantly increased in patients with IVF failure (and RSA) when compared to fertile controls. Levels in first-time IVF patients were not significantly increased. In contrast, however, Balash and colleagues [26] studied 75 patients with repeated IVF failures and concluded that screening for anti–β_2-GPI in patients with negative aPLs in standard assays was not helpful. Chilcott et al also found anti–β_2-GPI to be less significant than aCL: they identified aCL or LA in 23% of their 380 IVF patients, however, only 3% of those tested for anti–β_2-GPI were positive [23].

If aPL reduces likelihood of successful implantation, the ideal patient population for study would be those patients who have failed multiple IVF cycles (Table 18.2). Studies including only IVF failure patients show roughly the same range of prevalence rates as general infertility patients, from 10% to 32%. However, direct comparison studies do suggest a higher prevalence in patients with implantation failure. As noted above, Stern et al found increased levels of IgM anti–β_2-GPI in patients with failed IVF cycles, while prevalence in new IVF patients was equal to that of controls [27]. Birkenfeld's group reported 32% of their IVF failure patients to be positive for ANA, aCL, or LA, compared with 0% of successful IVF patients and 10% of infertility patients newly referred for IVF [32]. Kaider and coworkers tested for IgG, IgM, and IgA isotypes of 7 different aPLs in women with IVF failure (n = 42) and IVF success (n = 42): 26% of the unsuccessful patients were positive for any aPL, versus only 5% in the success group [33].

While autoantibodies are clearly increased in patients with infertility, whether the antibodies are directly pathogenic and contributing to implantation failure is unclear. They may simply be reflective of a more generalized autoimmune process, for example, or related to the assisted reproduction method itself. Some data suggest that aPL are not induced by the hormonal manipulation necessary for IVF. Most studies evaluate patients before their first IVF cycle and before exposure to ovarian hyperstimulation. In one study, women undergoing treatment with gonadotropins for the first time were tested for aPL throughout the cycle: prior to the initiation of stimulation, during the cycle, and at the end of the cycle [36]. They were compared to women with gonadotropin stimulation at least 60 days earlier, and to normal nonpregnant controls. The IVF cycle did not alter antibody status: 20% of the women tested before ovarian stimulation were positive for aPL; antibody status remained unchanged throughout the treatment cycle. Twenty-four percent of the previously treated women were positive, compared with 4% of the controls.

Experimental data provide a sound theoretical framework supporting a role for aPL in interference with early gestational events. In laboratory animals, the antibodies appear to be pathogenic toward embryonic tissue. Sthoeger et al [37] immunized normal (Balb/c) mice with murine monoclonal aCL to produce an experimental model of APS. Four weeks after active immunization, mice developed severe gestation failure with lowered pregnancy rates and high rates of resorption.

Table 18.2. Prevalence of antiphospholipid antibodies in patients with failed IVF cycles.

Study	Study type	Patients	aPLs	N	IVF failure patients: % aPL-positive	Infertility patients: % aPL-positive	Comments
Birkenfeld et al [32]	R	IVF failure (1 cycle)	aCL, LA, ANA	56	32%	10%	Sig. diff compared to infertility pts
Kaider et al [33]	R	IVF failure (> or = 12 embryos)	aCL, aPL panel (7)	42	26%	N.D.	[Sig diff compared to IVF success pts]
Balash et al [34]	R	IVF failure (> or = 2 cycles)	aCL, LA	40	10%	2%	Sig. diff compared to Infertility pts
Coulam et al [35]	R	IVF failure (> or = 12 embryos)	aCL, aPL panel (7)	312	22%	N.D.	[Sig. diff compared to fertile controls]
Stern et al [27]	P	IVF failure (> or = 10 embryos)	aCL, LA, aPS, aPE, aPI, ANA, aβ2GPI	105	30%	21%	N.S. [Sig. diff compared to fertile controls]
Chilcott et al [23]	P	IVF failure (> or = 1 cycle)	aCL, LA, aPS, aβ2GPI	88	21%	24%	N.S.

R = retrospective study; P = prospective study; N = number of failed IVF patients; IVF = in vitro fertilization; aCL= anticardiplipin antibody; ANA = anticuclear antibody; aPL = antiphospholipid antibody; aPS = antiphosphatidylserine antibody; aPE = ant phosphatidylethanolamine; aPI = antiphosphtydlinosital; aPL panel = aPL antibodies directed against a number of different phospholipids; polynucleo = polynucleotides; aβ2GPI = anti-β_2-glycoprotein I antibody; Infertility pts = infertility patients who have not failed IVF; sig diff = statistically significant difference; N.S.= no significant difference.

Embryos obtained at day 3.5 showed developmental delay and abnormal morphology. In addition, the monoclonal aCL demonstrated specific binding in vitro to trophoectoderm cells of normal embryos. A separate laboratory [38] also showed binding of aPL to normal mouse embryos in vitro by immunofluorescence; subsequent culture of the embryos resulted in significant growth impairment. DiSimone and coworkers similarly demonstrated in vitro binding of aPS to human trophoblast in a dose-dependent manner, adversely affecting trophoblast invasiveness and cytotrophoblast differentiation into syncytium [39]. The same group has further demonstrated changes in transcription and translation of cell adhesion molecules, with resulting altered expression leading to failure of blastocyst implantation [40]. In one IVF center, an association between abnormal human embryo morphology and presence of serum aCL has also been described [41].

There may be additional mechanisms for early pregnancy losses in aPL patients. Shurtz-Swirski et al, for example, have demonstrated an inhibitory effect of human aCL on pulsatile secretion of hCG in human placental cells in vitro [42]. Analysis of the cytokine profile of an experimental murine APS model has shown low production of IL-2, IL-3, and GM-CSF; IL-3 in particular is felt to be particularly important in maintenance of normal pregnancy [43]. Rote and others have also studied effects of monoclonal aPL on trophoblast function in vitro [44]. APS was shown to limit depth of decidual invasion and decrease surface expression of annexin V, leading to increased binding of prothrombin. Finally, Tartakovsky et al [45] used embryo transfer experiments to analyze the relative contribution of maternal versus embryonic dysfunction. Embryos from aCL-immunized and control mice were removed and implanted into surrogate mice, either aCL-immunized or control. The aCL-immunized uterine environment was non-supportive for the development and implantation of normal embryos, and the embryos derived from the aCL-immunized mothers remained deficient even after transfer to a normal uterus. Clearly, aPL can affect implantation and development through both mechanisms.

Given the experimental data, does clinical data also support an effect of aPL on outcome of IVF cycles? This question has been best addressed by two recent studies, a thorough meta-analysis by Hornstein et al [46] and a well-designed observational study by Chilcott et al [23]. Even in early studies, however, statistics have not strongly supported a significant difference in outcome of observed IVF cycles in patients with and without aPL (Table 18.3). While El-Roey et al found a suggestive difference of 5% versus 26% pregnancy rate in IVF patients with and without aPL, the small numbers of patients failed to establish statistical significance [15]. Gleicher's group did not find aPL status to distinguish between IVF success and failure, although increased immunoglobulin levels were associated with a lower IVF pregnancy rate [16]. Chilcott et al evaluated patients referred for IVF for presence of aCL, LA, aPS, and anti-β_2-GPI. Positive tests were repeated for confirmation to avoid transient infection-induced antibody. With 89/380 patients positive for 1 or more aPLs, they found similar pregnancy rates of 9% and 12% for aPL-positive and aPL-negative patients, respectively. While 23% of this population had failed a prior IVF cycle, there was no difference in antibody status between first time and repeat patients [23].

Hornstein et al performed a careful meta-analysis on the available controlled studies published through early 1999 [46]. Although aPL panels varied, all studies met fairly rigorous criteria: IVF outcomes included live birth or clinical pregnancy rates, sera for aPL were collected before the relevant IVF cycle, study design was

Table 18.3. Success rates of in vitro fertilization in patients with and without antiphospholipid antibodies.

Study	Study type	Patients	N [aPL (+) Patients]	Preg rate aPL (+)	Preg rate aPL (−)	Comments
El Roeiy et al [15]	R	IVF	26	5%	26%	N.S.
Gleicher et al [16]	R	IVF	105	33%	26%	N.S. [increased Ig → lower preg rate]
Sher et al [17]	R	IVF	196	16%	28%	N.S.
Birdsall et al [18]	P	IVF	240	39%	28%	N.S. [assoc. with IUGR]
Denis et al [19]	P	IVF	793	66%	68%	N.S. [equal for each aPL type]
Kowalik et al [20]	R	IVF	525	57%	50%	N.S. [no assoc. with isotype]
Kutteh et al [21]	P	IVF	191	35%	40%	N.S.
Chilcott et al [23]	P	IVF	89	9%	12%	N.S.
Hornstein et al [46]	M-A	IVF	703	57%	46%	N.S.

N = number of aPL(+) patients included; R= retrospective study; P = prospective study; M-A = meta-analysis;
Preg rate = pregnancy rate/cycle; IVF = in vitro fertilization; Ig = immunoglobulin; IUGR = intrauterine growth restriction;
N.S.= no significant difference.

either prospective or retrospective cohort, the cohort included women with normal and abnormal aPL values, and data permitted classification of IVF outcome according to normal or abnormal aPL status. A total of 7 studies with 2053 patients were included; 703 (34%) patients had an abnormal aPL test. There was no significant difference in IVF outcome between the aPL-positive and aPL-negative groups: rates of pregnancy were 57% and 46%, respectively. While none of the seven studies individually demonstrated a statistically significant effect, studies evaluating more aPL antibody types were more likely to find a non-significant reduction in the likelihood of IVF success.

Despite a lack of robust supporting data, there are a number of trials of prophylactic treatment for aPL antibodies in patients with IVF failure (Table 18.4). The rationale for use of aspirin and heparin derives from extrapolation from pregnancy failure studies. There is also experimental data to suggest a benefit of heparin, separate from its antithrombotic effects. Ermel and colleagues studied sera from 20 women with aPL and RSA and showed that heparin reduced aPL binding to cardiolipin and phosphatidylserine in a dose-dependent fashion in ELISA studies [50]. In addition, heparin affinity chromatography absorbed over 80% of the IgG aCL in serum. The authors also observed decreases in serum levels of IgG aCL in patients treated with heparin as the dosage of heparin was increased, suggesting that heparin may act by directly binding aPL in vivo. Franklin and Kutteh recently showed that unfractionated and low-molecular-weight heparin equally inhibit ELISA binding of both aCL and aPS antibodies derived from women with RSA [51].

The 1994 study published by Sher et al [17] is the most positive controlled treatment trial so far reported. aPL-positive patients received either aspirin with low-dose heparin, or no treatment. Pregnancy rates with therapy were 49% in the treated aPL-positive group versus 16% in the untreated aPL-positive group. The aPL-negative control patients, however, did not do significantly better than the untreated aPL-positive patients (27%), raising questions about equivalence of the patient populations. While a total of 194 aPL-positive patients were included, treatment was not randomized. Later work by this group suggested an additional benefit

Table 18.4. Effect of therapy on in vitro fertilization outcome in patients with antiphospholipid antibodies.

Study	Patients	N [aPL (+) or (−) patients]	Treatment	Preg rate: aPL (+) treatment group	Preg rate: aPL (+), no Rx (controls)	Preg rate: aPL (−), no Rx (controls)	Comments
Sher et al [17]	IVF	194(+) 171 (−)	Asa / heparin	49%	16%	27%	Sig. diff with Rx [not randomized]
Birkenfeld et al [32]	IVF failure	15(+)	Asa / pred	47%	N.D.	N.D.	No controls
Kutteh et al [21]	IVF	36(+) 151(−)	Asa / heparin	53%	47%	50%	N.S.
Hasegawa et al [47]	IVF	18(+)* 350(−)	Asa / prednl	40%	25%	22%	N.S.
Geva et al [48]	IVF failure	52(+)**	Asa / pred	33%	N.D.	N.D.	No controls
Stern et al [49]	IVF failure	143 (+)	Asa / heparin	15%	18%	N.D.	N.S. Randomized double-blind placebo-controlled

N = number of patients; IVF = in vitro fertilization; Preg rate = pregnancy rate/cycle; Asa = aspirin; pred = prednisone; prednl = prednisolone; Rx = treatment; N.S. = no significant difference between treatment and no treatment groups.
*Included patients with other autoantibodies
**Included patients with aCL, LA, ANA ,anti-ds DNA, and RF.

of IVIG with aspirin and heparin in patients who had failed initial therapy [52]. Most other studies that have included controls, however, have not found a significant benefit to treatment (Table 18.4).

The best designed study to date appears to be the prospective placebo-controlled double-blind study of aspirin and heparin by Stern et al, which included a large number of patients (143 aPL-positive or ANA-positive patients) with a total of 300 IVF cycles [49]. Patients were ages 22–46, with a mean age of 35, and all had failed multiple cycles of IVF. Autoantibody testing included ANA and aPL (aCL, APS, LA, and anti–β_2-GPI). Positive tests for autoantibodies were repeated for confirmation and to rule out transient infection-induced antibodies. Rates of clinical pregnancy did not differ between the two groups: 15% versus 18% success in the treated and untreated groups respectively. While 22% of the patients were ANA positive only, their success rate did not differ from that of the other patients.

With the preponderance of data pointing toward no demonstrated adverse effect of aPL on IVF outcome and, with the recent study above [49], no benefit of aspirin and heparin therapy for IVF cycles in aPL-positive patients, treatment at this time should be limited to controlled studies with rigorous inclusion criteria. Ideally, patients should have aCL, LA, or anti–β_2-GPI in a moderate to high titer (without inclusion of ANA-positive patients or less standard aPLs), with patient age limited to less than 40 years, when IVF success rates drop sharply on the basis of age alone. Although the risk of short-term treatment with aspirin and heparin is commonly minimized, there are unusual cases where the risk is severe. For example, the Centers for Disease Control (CDC) reported a 38-year-old IVF patient with antithyroid antibodies who died from cerebral hemorrhage after treatment with aspirin, heparin, and IVIG due to an unsuspected congenital arteriovenous malformation [53].

Regardless of whether aPL affects IVF outcome, given the increasing availability of IVF and assisted reproduction techniques, patients with a history of aPL and infertility of any etiology have and will continue to undergo this procedure. Although data are limited, patients with aPL do not appear to incur serious risks if they undergo IVF. The major concern for aPL-positive patients (unless they also have SLE) is an increased risk of thrombosis in the setting of elevated levels of estrogen. However, as these levels do not reach those sustained in late pregnancy, risk is not likely increased over that associated with pregnancy itself, the intended outcome of IVF. No thromboses were reported in a series of 10 patients with PAPS who underwent from 1 to 17 cycles of ovarian induction each (total of 47 cycles). Nine of the 10 patients were treated empirically with aspirin during their cycles, however, and 6 with heparin for history of previous thrombosis [54]. In a recent review, Balasch and Cervera report ovulation induction treatment of 17 patients without anticoagulation with no observed thromboses [25]. Huong and coworkers followed 8 primary APS (PAPS) patients and 13 lupus patients – some with aPL – through 114 cycles of ovulation induction therapy, with only 2 episodes of thrombophlebitis [55]. The practice of anticoagulation with low-dose aspirin during the early phase of the cycle to reduce thrombosis risk is unproven but increasingly used. Patients with a history of thrombosis and on warfarin should substitute subcutaneous heparin, holding it temporarily (i.e., for 24 hours) before oocyte retrieval, and restarting soon after.

An additional concern for aPL-positive patients undergoing IVF is the risk of ovarian hyperstimulation syndrome (OHSS), which can predispose to thrombosis.

Severe hyperstimulation is characterized by ascites, nausea and vomiting, hydrothorax, weight gain, and increased hematocrit. Increased prostaglandin production appears to cause peripheral vasodilation with "leaky" blood vessels, leading to intravascular dehydration, third spacing of fluid and development of a hypercoagulable state in conjunction with elevated estrogen levels [3]. With current techniques for monitoring cycles, risk can be lowered but not eliminated [56]. In cases where risk is felt to be excessive, the cycle can be cancelled and fertilized embryos frozen for later transfer.

It is unclear whether pre-existing thrombophilia predisposes to severe OHSS. One study did find an increased prevalence of thrombophilia markers in this population: 17/20 (85%) patients hospitalized for severe OHSS had at least one identifiable marker (5 patients had aPL) compared with 11/41 (27%) control patients [57]. In contrast, a later study [58] did not identify any thrombophilic markers in 20 OHSS patients. Complications of thrombosis due to OHSS have been reported in aPL-positive women. Middle cerebral artery infarct was reported in one 33-year-old aPL-positive woman during OHSS [59]. Similarly, a 28-year-old woman presented with intracardiac thrombosis after multiple ovulation induction cycles and OHSS with aPL discovered at the time of thrombosis [60].

Although early clinical studies and experimental work support a role for aPL pathogenicity in IVF implantation failure, recent studies do not show either a difference in IVF cycle outcome based on aPL status, or a benefit to treatment of aPL-positive patients with heparin and aspirin during IVF. Further controlled studies with more rigorous exclusion criteria and larger numbers of patients may provide more information in the future, but at this time, data do not support use of prophylactic therapy in aPL patients undergoing IVF to improve likelihood of implantation. Anticoagulant therapy may be appropriate to prevent risk of thrombotic complications, however, and is clearly necessary for aPL patients with a history of previous thrombosis.

References

1. Bradshaw KD, Chantilis SJ, Carr BR. Diagnostic evaluation and treatment for the infertile couple. In: Carr BR, Blackwell RE, eds. Textbook of reproductive medicine, 2nd edn. Stamford CT: Appleton and Lange;1998:533–547.
2. McConnell JD. Diagnosis and treatment of male infertility. In: Carr BR, Blackwell RE, eds. Textbook of reproductive medicine, 2nd edn. Stamford CT: Appleton and Lange; 1998:549–564.
3. Steinkampf MP, Davis OK, Rosenwaks Z. Assisted reproductive technology. In: Carr BR, Blackwell RE, eds. Textbook of reproductive medicine, 2nd edn. Stamford CT: Appleton and Lange; 1998;665–678.
4. Gleicher N, El-Roeiy A, Confino E, Friberg J. Reproduction failure because of autoantibodies: unexplained infertility and pregnancy wastage. Am J Obstet Gynecol 1989;160:1376–1380.
5. Roussev RG, Kaider BD, Price DE, Coulam CB. Laboratory evaluation of women experiencing reproductive failure. Am J Reprod Immunol 1996;35:415–420.
6. Kaider AS, Kaider BD, Janowicz PB, Roussev RG. Immunodiagnostic evaluation in women with reproductive failure. Am J Reprod Immunol 1999;42:335–346.
7. Geva E, Amit A, Lerner-Geva L, et al. Autoimmune disorders: another possible cause for in-vitro fertilization and embryo transfer failure. Human Reprod 1995;10:2560–2563.
8. Kutteh WH. Autoimmune factors in assisted reproduction. Minerva Ginecol 2002;54:217–224.
9. Kikuchi K, Shibahara H, Hirano Y, et al. Antinuclear antibody reduces the pregnancy rate in the first IVF-ET treatment cycle but not the cumulative pregnancy rate without specific medication. Am J Reprod Immunol 2003;50:363–367.

10. Mavragani CP, Ionnidis JP, Tzioufas AG, et al. Recurrent pregnancy loss and autoantibody profile in autoimmune diseases. Rheumatology (Oxford) 1999;38:1228–1233.
11. Rushworth PH, Backos M, Rai, R et al. Prospective pregnancy outcome in untreated recurrent miscarries with thyroid autoantibodies. Hum Reprod 2000;15:1637–1639.
12. Kutteh WH, Yetman DL, Carr AC, Beck LA, Scott RT Jr. Increased prevalence of antithyroid antibodies identified in women with recurrent pregnancy loss but not in women undergoing assisted reproduction. Fertil Steril 1999;71:843–848.
13. Kutteh WH, Schoolcraft WB, Scott RT Jr. Antithyroid antibodies do not affect pregnancy outcome in women undergoing assisted reproduction. Hum Reprod 1999;14:2886–2890.
14. Mardesic T, Ulcova-Gallova Z, Huttelova R, et al. The influence of different types of antibodies on in vitro fertilization results. Am J Reprod Immunol 2000;43:1–5.
15. El-Roeiy A, Gleicher N, Friberg J, Confino E, Dudkiewicz A. Correlation between peripheral blood and follicular fluid autoantibodies and impact on in vitro fertilization. Obstet Gynecol 1987;70:163–170.
16. Gleicher N, Liu HC, Dudkiesicz A, et al. Autoantibody profiles and immunoglobulin levels as predictors of in vitro fertilization success. Am J Obstet Gynecol 1994;170:1145–1149.
17. Sher G, Feinman M, Zouves C, et al. High fecundity rates following in vitro fertilization and embryo transfer in antiphospholipid antibody seropositive women treated with aspirin and heparin. Human Reprod 1994;9:2278–2283.
18. Birdsall MA, Lockwood GM, Ledger WL, Johnson PM, Chamley LW. Antiphospholipid antbodies in women having in vitro fertilization. Human Reprod 1996;11:1185–1189.
19. Denis AL, Guido M, Adler RD, et al. Antiphospholipid antibodies and pregnancy rates and outcome in in vitro fertilization patients. Fertil Steril 1997;67:1084–1090.
20. Kowalik A, Vichnin M, Liu HC, Branch W, Berkley AS. Midfollicular anticardiolipin and antiphosphatidylserine titers do not correlate with in vitro fertilization outcome. Fertil Steril 1997;68:298–304.
21. Kutteh WH, Yetman DL, Chantilis SJ, Crain J. Effect of antiphospholipid antibodies in women undergoing in vitro fertilization: role of heparin and aspirin. Human Reprod 1997;12:1171–1175.
22. Eldar-Geva T, Wood C, Lolatgis N, et al. Cumulative pregnancy and live birth rates in women with antiphospholipid antibodies undergoing assisted reproduction. Human Reprod 1999;14:1461–1466.
23. Chilcott IT, Margara R, Cohen H, et al. Pregnancy outcome is not affected by antiphospholipid antibody status in women referred for in vitro fertilization. Fertil Steril 2000;74:848–849.
24. Branch DW, Khamashta MA. Antiphospholipid syndrome: obstetric diagnosis, management, and controversies. Obstet Gynecol 2003;101:1333–1344.
25. Balash J, Cervera R. Reflections on the management of reproductive failure in the antiphospholipid syndrome – the clinician's perspective. Lupus 2002;11:467–477.
26. Balasch J, Reverter JC, Creus M, et al. Human reproductive failure is not a clinical feature associated with β_2-glycoprotein I antibodies in anticardiolipin and lupus anticoagulant seronegative patients (the antiphospholipid/cofactor syndrome). Human Reprod 1999;14:1956–1959.
27. Stern C, Chamley L, Hale L, Kloss M, Speirs A, Baker HW. Antibodies to beta2 glycoprotein I are associated with in vitro implantation failure as well as recurrent miscarriage: results of a prevalence study. Fertil Steril 1998;70:938–944.
28. Lee RM, Emlen W, Scott RT Jr, Branch DW, Silver RM. Anti-β_2-glycoprotein I antibodies in women with recurrent spontaneous abortion, unexplained fetal death, and antiphospholipid syndrome. Am J Obstet Gynecol 1999;181:642–648.
29. Lynch A, Byers T, Emlen W, et al. Association of antibodies to β_2-glycoprotein I with pregnancy loss and pregnancy-induced hypertension: a prospective study in low-risk pregnancy. Obstet Gynecol 1999;93:193–198.
30. Franklin RD, Hollier N, Kutteh WH. β_2 glycoprotein-I as a marker of antiphospholipid syndrome in women with recurrent pregnancy loss. Fertil Steril 2000;73:531–535.
31. Chong P, Matzner W, Ching W. Correlation between beta 2-glycoprotein antibodies and antiphospholipid antibodies in patients with reproductive failure. Am J Reprod Immunol 1998;40:414–417.
32. Birkenfeld A, Mukaida T, Minichiello L, et al. Incidence of autoimmune antibodies in failed embryo transfer cycles. Am J Reprod Immunol 1994;31:65–68.
33. Kaider BD, Price DE, Roussev RG, Coulam CB. Antiphospholipid antibody prevalence in patients with IVF failure. Am J Reprod Immunol 1996;35:388–393.
34. Balasch J, Creus M, Fabregues F, et al. Antiphospholipid antibodies and human reproductive failure. Human Reprod 1996;11:2310–2315.
35. Coulam CB, Kaider BD, Kaider AS, Janowicz P, Roussev RG. Antiphospholipid antibodies associated with implantation failure after IVF/ET. J Assist Reprod Genetics 1997;14:603–608.
36. Franklin RD, Bronson RA, Kutteh WH. Gonadotropins do not induce antiphopholipid antibodies. Am J Reprod Immunol. 1998;40:359–363.

37. Sthoeger ZM, Moses E, Tartovsky B. Anti-cardiolipin antidbodies induce pregnancy failure by impairing embryoinic implantation. Proc Nat Acad Sci U S A 1993;90:6464–6467.
38. Kaider BD, Coulam CB, Roussev RG. Murine embryos as a direct target for some human auto-antibodies in vitro. Human Reprod 1999;14:2556–2561.
39. Di Simone N, Caliandro D, Castellani R, et al. Low-molecular weight heparin restores in-vitro tro-phoblast invasiveness and differentiation in presence of immunoglobulin G fractions obtained from patients with antiphospholipid syndrome. Hum Reprod 1999;14:489–495.
40. Di Simone N, Castellani R, Caliandro D, Caruso A. Antiphospholipid antibodies regulate the expres-sion of trophoblast cell adhesion molecules. Fertil Steril 2002;77:805–811.
41. Azem F, Geva E, Amit A, et al. High levels of anticardiolipin antibodies in patients with abnormal embryo morphology who attended an in vitro fertilization program. Am J Reprod Immunol 1998;39:161–163.
42. Shurtz-Swirski R, Inbar O, Blank M, et al. In vitro effect of anticardiolipin antibodies upon total and pulsatile placental hCG secretion during early pregnancy. Am J Reprod Immunol 1993;29:206–210.
43. Fishman P, Bakemer R, Blank M, et al. The putative role of cytokines in the induction of primary antiphospholipid syndrome. Clin Exp Immunol 1992;90:266–270.
44. Rote NS, Vogt E, DeVere G, Obringer AR, Ng AK. The role of placental trophoblast in the pathophys-iology of the antiphospholipid antibody syndrome. Am J Repro Immunol 1998;39:125–136.
45. Tartakovsky B, Bermas BL, Sthoeger Z, Shearer GM, Mozes E. Defective maternal-fetal interaction in a murine autoimmune model. Human Reprod 1996;11:2408–2411.
46. Hornstein MD, Davis OK, Massey JB, Paulson RJ, Collins MD. Antiphospholipid antibodies and in vitro fertilization success: a meta-analysis. Fertil Steril 2000;73:330–333.
47. Hasegawa I, Yamanoto Y, Suzuki M, et al. Prednioslone plus low-dose aspirin improves the implan-tation rate in women with autoimmune conditions who are undergoing in vitro fertilization. Fertil Steril 1998;70:1044–1048.
48. Geva E, Amit A, Lerner-Geva L, et al. Prednisone and aspirin improve pregnancy rate in patients with reproductive failure and autoimmune antibodies: a prospective study. Am J Reprod Immunol 2000;4:36–40.
49. Stern C, Chamley L, Norris H, Hale L, Baker HWG. A randomized, double-blind, placebo-controlled trial of heparin and aspirin for women with in vitro fertilization implantation failure and antiphos-pholipid or antinuclear antibodies. Fertil Steril 2003;80:376–383.
50. Ermel LD, Marshburn PB, Kutteh WH. Interaction of heparin with antiphospholipid antibodies (APA) from the sera of women with recurrent pregnancy loss (RPL). Am J Reprod Immunol 1995;33:14–20.
51. Franklin RD, Kutteh WH. Effects of unfractionated and low molecular weight heparin on antiphopholipid antibody binding in vitro. Obstet Gynecol 2003;101:455–462.
52. Sher G, Matzner W, Feinman M, et al. The selective use of heparin/aspirin therapy, alone or in com-bination with intravenous immunoglobulin G, in the management of antiphospholipid antibody-positive women undergoing in vitro fertilization. Am J Reprod Immunol 1998;40:74–82.
53. Anonymous. Pregnancy-related death associated with heparin and aspirin treatment for infertility, 1996. JAMA 1998;279:1860–1861.
54. Guballa N, Sammaritano L, Schwartzman S, Buyon J, Lockshin MD. Ovulation induction and in vitro fertilization in systemic lupus erythematosus and antiphospholipid syndrome. Arthritis Rheum 2000;43:550–556.
55. Huong du LT, Wechsler B, Vauthier-Brouzes D, et al. Importance of planning ovulation induction therapy in systemic lupus erythematosus and antiphospholipid syndrome: a single center retrospec-tive study of 21 cases and 114 cycles. Semin Arthritis Rheum 2002;32:174–188.
56. Aboulghar MA, Mansour RT. Ovarian hyperstimulation syndrome: classification and critical analysis of preventive measures. Hum Reprod Update 2003;9:275–289.
57. Dulitzky M, Cohen SB, Inbal A, et al. Increased prevalence of thrombophilia among women with severe ovarian hyperstimulation syndrome. Fertil Steril 2002;77: 463–467.
58. Fabregues F, Tassies D, Reverter RC, et al. Prevalence of thrombophilia in women with severe ovarian hyperstimulation syndrome and cost-effectiveness of screening. Fertil Steril 2004; 81:989–995.
59. Koo EJ, Rha JH, Lee BI, Kim MO, Ha CK. A case of cerebral infarct in combined antiphospholipid antibody and ovarian hyperstimulation syndrome. J Korean Med Sci 2002;17:574–576.
60. Andrejevic S, Bonaci-Nikolic B, Bukilicia M, et al. Intracardiac thrombosis and fever possibly trig-gered by ovulation induction in a patient with antiphospholipid antibodies. Scand J Rheumatol 2002;31:249–251.

19 Transplantation of Solid Organs, Tissues, and Prosthetic Devices in Patients with Antiphospholipid Antibodies

Dawn R. Wagenknecht and John A. McIntyre

Historical Prospective

References to transplantation are found in Greek mythology and in legends and folk tales of the Middle Ages. The first clinical report of a successful transplant was by Bunger in 1823, after he reconstructed a woman's nose by using tissue from her thigh [1]. In the ensuing decades, the success of skin and kidney transplantation was a very controversial topic wherein some investigators reported certain successes whereas others observed only failures [1]. It was not until the age of modern transplantation immunology ascribed to the work of Nobelist Sir Peter Medawar in the 1940s that transplantation became feasible [1]. The foundation for clinical transplantation was established soon after when Murray and colleagues successfully transplanted a kidney from one twin into his identical brother [2]. With these foundations, the ability to successfully transplant tissues and organs became a major medical achievement of the second half of the 20th century.

Advancements in surgical techniques, development of improved immune modulating pharmaceuticals, and a clearer understanding of the immune system vis-à-vis histocompatibility, rejection reactions, and tolerance induction have contributed to ever increasing success rates for solid organ and tissue transplantation. Despite these gains, a small but significant number of allografts fail immediately or within the first weeks after transplant. A frequent observation in these early allograft failures is localized vascular thrombosis within the grafted tissues.

First described in 1969 by Colman and coworkers, immediate thrombosis of renal allografts was suspected to be a result of acute rejection or of an immunologically induced coagulopathy [3]. The thrombosis was limited to the allograft as there was no evidence to suggest systemic coagulation or fibrinolysis. This localization suggests that allografted tissue provides not only a trigger but also a confined location for thrombosis. A literature search using *transplantation* and *thrombosis* as key words revealed reports of thrombosis associated with almost every transplanted organ or tissue with the exception of the cornea. This may not be surprising inasmuch as the cornea is avascular. Indeed, even the transplantation of autologous tissues has been associated with thrombosis [4].

Thromboembolic complications after transplantation have been associated with inherited thrombophilic disorders including deficiencies of antithrombin, protein C and protein S, factor V Leiden, the prothrombin G20210A and MTHFR C585C gene mutations, and dysfibrinogenemias [5, 6]. Acquired disorders associated with transplant related thrombosis include antiphospholipid antibodies (aPL), malignancy, myleoproliferative disorders, heparin-induced thrombocytopenia, and hyperhomocysteinemia. This chapter will confine discussion to a review of aPL in the transplantation literature as it relates to aPL.

aPL Testing

Before proceeding with this review, several points about aPL testing need be brought to the reader's attention. First, publications associating aPL with allograft thrombosis begin in 1988, 20 years after numerous reports showing allograft loss due to thrombosis. Second, assays for aPL are still evolving; functional tests for detection of lupus anticoagulant (LA) were available prior to the solid phase aPL ELISA systems. Standardization efforts continue for both aPL detection assays. Unfortunately, in many of the papers reviewed for this chapter, the LA and ELISA methodologies are omitted or are only partially described, making it difficult to accurately combine patient populations to make broader conclusions. The methodology and reagents used for aPL ELISA testing can have a profound effect on the test result [7]. ELISA procedures that do not consider the presence or absence of known phospholipid (PL)-binding plasma proteins can furnish false negative aPL findings [8]. Assays which use diluent buffers that contain only β_2-glycoprotein I (β_2-GPI) will not detect aPL, which arc dependent upon other PL binding proteins such as prothrombin or protein C. Third, the aPL ELISA is not standardized, thus the criteria for defining aPL positivity can vary between laboratories. For example, some laboratories limit aPL analyses to IgG and IgM anticardiolipin (aCL) as available in commercial kits. Other laboratories also include analysis of IgA aCL. In contrast, our laboratory ELISA is designed to detect all three antibody isotypes for aCL as well as antibodies with additional PL specificities, including antiphosphatidylserine (aPS), antiphosphatidylethanolamine (aPE) and antiphosphatidylcholine (aPC). Finally, as aPL can be associated with subclinical as well as clinical infections; it has been recommended that a patient with a positive aPL finding be retested 6 to 8 weeks later. It is important to discriminate between chronic and temporary presence of aPL, the former thought to be pathogenic, whereas the latter may not be. Few retrospective transplant studies tested serial blood samples from the same patient, however, when serial samples were tested aPL were found in multiple samples.

Analyses of our own data from 5632 consecutive serum samples from patients with aPL associated clinical events revealed that that testing for only IgG and IgM aCL underestimates the number of patients who have aPL [9]. IgA aPL can, and often does, occur independent of IgG and IgM. Further, we observed a significant incremental increase in aPL-positive sera when aPS and aPE are assessed in addition to aCL. Table 19.1 shows the incremental increase of aPL positivity when aPC testing was included in the analysis of 1758 clinical specimens referred for aPL testing. Thus, the aPL findings reported in the majority of the papers cited in this

Table 19.1. Incremental effects of comprehensive ELISA antiphospholipid antibodies clinical testing (n = 1758*).

ELISA aPL test	No. positive	% total
IgG aCL	93	5.3
IgG/IgM aCL	134	7.6
IgG/IgM/IgA aCL	149	8.5
IgG/IgM/IgA aCL, aPS	212	12.0
IgG/IgM/IgA aCL, aPS, aPE	447	25.4
IgG/IgM/IgA aCL, aPS, aPE, aPC	520	29.6

aPL = antiphospholipid antibody; aCL = anticardiolipin; aPS = antiphosphatidylserine; aPE = antiphosphatidylethanolamine; aPC = antiphosphatidylcholine.
*Patient samples referred to our laboratory specifically for aPL testing.

review may actually under estimate the true incidence of aPL-positive patients in the transplant population.

In addition to the laboratory testing, the abbreviations used to describe aPL have not been standardized. aCL antibodies have been abbreviated as ACA, APA, ACL, ACL-Ab, ACLA, aPL, or aCL by different investigators. Similarly, the lupus anticoagulant has been referred to as LA, LAC, or LI (lupus inhibitor). For consistency, we use the abbreviation aPL to represent antiphospholipid antibodies of all specificities; this includes but is not limited to the LA and the ELISA defined aCL, aPS, aPE, and aPC.

Renal Transplantation

A 1988 case report by Liano et al was among the first to describe the presence of an aPL, an LA, in a male patient with end-stage renal disease (ESRD) and a "lupus-like" syndrome [10]. Before renal transplantation and subsequent to steroid therapy, the LA disappeared. Nineteen months post deceased-donor renal transplant, coincident with steroid tapering, the LA returned. The patient suffered a deep vein thrombosis (DVT) of the right leg and echography showed a significant increase in allograft size. Two weeks later the patient died from septic shock. Autopsy revealed an occlusive renal-vein thrombosis and de novo membraneous glomerulonephritis in the transplanted kidney. The return of the LA coexistent with the DVT and renal vein thrombosis could be coincidental, however, LA with a "lupus-like" syndrome is a well-recognized risk factor for thrombosis.

Marcen and colleagues presented 13 LA-positive patients who underwent 16 renal transplants in a 1990 retrospective study [11]. Six of the 16 renal allografts were lost to renal vascular thrombosis. An additional 2 patients who experienced 2 consecutive graft losses were found to be LA positive after each lost a second transplanted kidney. In a total of 6 graft ruptures in 335 transplants, 4 occurred in LA-positive patients. Graft rupture is usually associated with acute rejection, however, there was no evidence of immunological rejection in these 4 cases. The majority of losses occurred within the first 2 weeks post-transplant. The authors emphasized that the presence of an LA could be considered a risk factor for thrombosis in transplant patients. Moreover, immunosuppressive therapy with low dose steroids and cyclosporine A and/or azanthioprine was not effective in suppressing the LA in these patients.

Early reports of the impact of aPL on renal transplant outcome often were in disagreement.

Sitter et al studied 19 successfully transplanted recipients and found the prevalence of IgG and IgM aCL and LA (5%, 5%, and 0%, respectively) did not differ between the transplanted patients and healthy controls [12]. The conclusion stated by these investigators was: "the pathogenetic role of ACA [aCL] for vascular events in end-stage renal patients is far from being established" (p. 81). A similar conclusion was reached by Oymak et al, who investigated IgG aCL in 48 renal transplant patients with a mean transplant time of 36 months [13]. The 9 positive recipients had relatively low levels of aCL. None of the 9 had a history of collagen tissue disease or other autoantibodies. This group reported that the presence of low levels of IgG aCL in renal transplant recipients was not associated with thrombotic events and thus was not a risk factor for thrombosis. A more recent paper arrived at the same conclusion for 4 aCL-positive renal transplant recipients in a study population of 68 with no thrombotic events in an average of 75 months of transplant duration [14]. The authors admitted to not having a statistically valid observation due to the small number of patients. An important note about these reports is that the patients were selected for study because the transplant was successful. In contrast, most of the LA associated renal losses reported by Marcen et al occurred in the first 2 weeks after transplant, before transplant success is defined [11]. This raises the issue that perhaps aPL are most detrimental in the immediate post-transplant period.

A different aPL associated matter was reported by Grandtnerova et al in a longitudinal study wherein patients successfully transplanted for at least 8 months were followed with LA and IgG and IgM aCL studies for a mean of 14 months [15]. The period for serial aCL measurements was 6 to 36 months. A significant association between aCL positivity and slow deterioration of renal allograft function was found in 11 patients as compared to 9 aCL-negative patients. In addition, an association between post-transplant thrombocytopenia and aCL was reported.

The prevalence of hemostatic risk factors for venous and arterial thrombosis and the effects on long-term renal allograft survival and cardiovascular disease was investigated by Marcucci et al [16]. Sixty-three renal transplant recipients (graft duration = 44.6 ± 45.4 months) were compared to 66 age- and sex-matched control subjects. Immunosuppressive therapy for all patients included cyclosporine and steroids; some patients were also prescribed azathioprine. An LA was detected in 15.8% of these successfully transplanted patients compared to 3% of controls ($P < 0.001$); the prevalence of LA was higher in female than in male patients. Four patients and 1 control subject were positive for aCL. The authors suggested that the high prevalence of LA may be a consequence of cyclosporine treatment and proposed a need for further studies. Without pre-transplant aPL testing for comparison, these investigators speculated that the aPL response was secondary to the vascular damage in the transplanted kidney and thus may represent an increased risk factor for long-term allograft survival and cardiovascular disease.

A study of 324 consecutive renal transplant recipients by Ducloux and colleagues also reported an association between cardiovascular disease and aPL (LA and/or aCL) [17]. Patients with a diagnosis of systemic lupus erythematosus (SLE) or primary phospholipid antibody syndrome (PAPS) were excluded from the study. Positive aPL findings were confirmed on a second blood sample collected 4 weeks after initial testing. Patients were followed a mean of 62 months after transplant. Duration of transplant was shorter in aPL-positive compared to aPL-negative patients (61 ± 42 months vs. 79 ± 48 months, $P = 0.02$). Atherosclerotic events occurred more frequently in patients with aPL ($P = 0.0003$) and aCL levels were higher in the patients who experienced these events ($P = 0.003$). Pre-transplant sera were available for 142 of the patients. Eighty-four of these patients had aPL before transplantation; 44% were also aPL positive post-transplant, however, the aPL in 56% disappeared after transplant.

A different approach to investigate hypercoagulability was undertaken by Nampoory and colleagues. For patients who had been on dialysis for at least 6 months, laboratory coagulation findings were followed from pre-transplant through post-transplant [18]. Patients with lupus or other autoimmune diseases, patients administered drugs known to produce aPL, and patients who experienced a thrombotic episode the month prior to enrollment were excluded from study. Thus, the study was designed to screen out patients with aPL associated maladies. Of 82 patients screened, LA was detected in 4, high levels of IgG aCL in 3, IgM aCL in 4, aPS IgG in 8, and IgM aPS in 3. Additional findings were deficiencies in protein C (n = 19), protein S (n = 25), and ATIII (n = 15) with activated protein C resistance found in 16 patients. When dialysis patients with vascular access thrombosis were compared to patients without, there were highly significant differences in relation to the presence of LA and the coagulation protein deficiencies. The difference between these groups with respect to aCL and aPS, however, was not significant. Eighteen patients with hypercoagulability findings during dialysis received a renal transplant; 2 experienced post-transplant thrombotic events and 16 were available for post-transplant evaluation 9.3 ± 4.2 months after surgery. The abnormalities associated with a potential hypercoagulable state for the most part were corrected after transplantation. The number of aCL- and aPS-positive patients in the transplant group was too small for analysis, however, the prevalence of LA was significant as was the correction in APTT values observed post-transplant ($P = 0.002$). These investigators recommended pre-transplantation hypercoagulability screening for hemodialysis patients who are transplant candidates followed by anticoagulation treatment for identified patients to prevent thrombotic events in the post-transplant period.

Fischereder et al investigated the relationship between renal transplant loss and thrombophilia [19]. Post-transplant laboratory testing for protein C or S activity, LA, and factor V Leiden was performed for 132 consecutive renal transplants wherein 1-year graft survival could be assessed. Eighteen patients with thrombophilia were identified (factor V Leiden, 10; LA, 6; protein S deficiency, 2). Twenty-eight transplants were performed for these thrombophilia patients; 11 were lost within the first year compared to 21 of 155 transplants without thrombophilia ($P = 0.0003$). Six of 8 transplants performed in LA-positive recipients failed. The authors therefore concluded that the presence of an LA or other laboratory markers of thrombophilia predict a poor prognosis for renal transplant. A drawback of this retrospective study is the inability to know if the LA were present at the time of transplant.

The aPL specificity as determined by ELISA for the majority of the renal transplant literature cited above is limited to aCL. We initiated a retrospective two center study to assess pre-transplant aPL status of renal patients who lost their grafts within 16 days after transplant [20]. Of 1331 patients transplanted between 1990 and 1997 at Methodist Hospital of Indiana and LifeLink Foundation, Tampa, Florida, we identified 73 (5.5%) with primary non-function. Frozen and stored final cross-match serum samples were available for 56 patients. For a control group, we tested the final cross-match sera from the next consecutive renal transplant patient. Both groups were compared to 252 healthy blood donors. In contrast to previously discussed studies, we tested for IgG, IgA, and IgM aCL, aPS, and aPE. aPL were detected in pre-transplant sera from 32 patients (57%) with early non-function versus 19 control patients (35%) with function ($P = 0.0234$). No single aPL specificity had greater predictive value for allograft failure, and the predominant aPL isotypes were: IgG > IgA > IgM. Because patients awaiting renal transplant are regularly screened for HLA antibody development, historic serum samples were available from 11 patients with primary graft failure. Selected serum samples were spaced 3 months apart and 2 to 5 historic samples were screened for each of the 11 patients. Historic sera from 10 primary non-function patients were without exception positive for the same aPL observed in the final cross-match serum. For 1 patient, 3 of 4 historic sera were aPL positive. These data indicate that pre-transplant screening will identify patients at risk for early renal allograft failure.

In our study, there were no significant differences between the function versus non-function recipients for age, sex, cause of renal failure, panel reactive antibodies, HLA match, cyclosporine levels, or use of OKT3 [20]. Of significant note was that every patient with aPL at the time of transplant who did not receive hemodialysis for ESRD lost their grafts ($P = 0.002$). This group included patients who were transplanted before dialysis was necessary as well as patients treated with continuous ambulatory peritoneal dialysis (CAPD). Inasmuch as it is not uncommon for hemodialysis patients to receive a dialysis treatment just prior to transplant surgery, these data suggest that residual heparin acquired during dialysis may have a protective effect in the immediate transplant period.

Although there no were data for aPL or other laboratory indicators of thrombophilia, an earlier retrospective study of Irish renal transplant recipients reported an increased rate of renal allograft thrombosis in CAPD patients within 16 days of surgery [21]. None of the 99 kidneys transplanted to hemodialysis patients failed due to primary renovascular thrombosis, whereas 9.3% of 97 allografts given to the CAPD patients were lost due to thrombosis ($P < 0.01$). The authors cited data from the European Dialysis and Transplant Association registry for 1990–1991 that showed that loss from primary renovascular thrombosis in patients treated in the United Kingdom was reported as 7.1% in CAPD patients compared to 1.8% in hemodialysis patients. Without identifying specific reasons for increased thrombotic complications in their CAPD transplant group, the authors suggested that anticoagulant treatment might be appropriate in the peri-opertive period.

Subsequent to our observation of aPL related graft loss, routine aPL screening preceding transplantation was instated for all renal transplant candidates at Methodist Hospital of Indiana. Once identified, aPL-positive patients received low-molecular-weight heparin in surgery that was continued post-transplant until the aPL was no longer detectable. Most patients were aPL negative within 3 months after transplant. Heparin treatment for the first 15 aPL-positive recipients, including 2 CAPD patients, resulted in successful outcomes [22].

Direct evidence to implicate aPL in thrombotic graft loss was demonstrated by recovery of aPE from a transplanted nephrectomy specimen [23]. This was the second kidney in 3 years rejected by the patient within hours of surgery. Frozen serum samples were available for retrospective aPL testing for both transplants. Final cross-match serum from the first transplant contained IgA aPE. The allograft diuresed briefly but the patient was returned to dialysis on the third post-transplant day. At the time of second transplant, the patient's serum contained IgG aPE, aCL, aPS, and IgA aPE. The second kidney diuresed in the immediate post-operative period, but a renogram taken 12 hours after transplant showed no blood flow. Upon removal, the only aPL recovered from this patient's second failed kidney was IgG aPE. Immunohistochemical studies of the second allograft showed extensive vascular and perivascular fibrin deposition involving most of the peritubular capillary plexus [24]. ELISA results from serial serum samples showed a drop in aPE immediately post-transplant with a concomitant rise in aPE levels after removal of the thrombosed kidney allograft. These findings suggest that circulating aPE may have targeted the alloactivated vascular endothelium of the allograft, thereby creating a thrombogenic condition.

Humar and colleagues at the University of Minnesota identified 16 patients who lost their first renal allograft in less than 1 month due to thrombosis [25]. Five of the 16 recipients underwent a hematological workup and 3 were found to have aPL. At the time of re-transplant, low-dose heparin was started post-operatively and continued for 3 to 5 days post-transplant. Coumadin or aspirin subsequently replaced heparin and was continued for no less than 3 months post-transplant. These aPL-positive recipients had neither bleeding problems nor thrombosis of their allografts. The 5 aPL-positive patients notwithstanding from the 16 receiving a second transplant, 63% had graft function at 5 years follow up. Both graft and patient survival of the 16 re-transplant patients were equivalent to primary allograft rates at the University of Minnesota.

Antiphospholipid Antibody Syndrome (APS)

Two PAPS patients with ESRD following advanced thrombotic angiopathy were reported by Mondragon-Ramirez et al [26]. Both patients had IgG aCL and 1 was also LA positive. After receiving live unrelated renal transplants, both patients experienced recurrence of the disease in the transplanted kidneys. Despite intensive anticoagulant therapy in the immediate post-transplant period, 1 kidney stopped functioning the second day and the other lost normal function 4 days post-transplant. The authors concluded that more experience is needed with renal transplantation in the setting of PAPS and questioned whether transplantation is an appropriate treatment for these patients.

In a similar case, Chew and coworkers described microangiopathy induced ESRD in a 34-year-old male PAPS patient with high titer IgG aCL [27]. The patient received a haplotype matched kidney from his brother. In preparation for transplant, he was given mycophenolate mofetil and prednisolone daily beginning 2 days prior to transplant. The patient was anticoagulated with warfarin until 2 days prior to surgery. Intra-operatively there was a delay in graft perfusion after vascular anastomosis as evidenced by a mottled appearance of the graft. A wedge biopsy collected at this time showed that 25% of the glomeruli contained thrombi. The patient was given heparin peri-operatively, followed by aspirin, and a 10-day course of anti-lymphocyte serum. On day 3, with a biopsy showing thrombi in the glomeruli, a rise in lactate dehydrogenase, and a fall in platelet count, plasmapheresis was started and continued to day 10. The aCL titers decreased significantly subsequent to plasmapheresis without a rebound upon stopping plasma exchange. A biopsy taken on day 10 post-transplant showed thrombi scattered among the arterioles.

Plasmapheresis was again undertaken for 9 days. On day 23, after a sudden rise in creatinine, a third biopsy indicated cortical infarction without evidence of vascular rejection and on day 138 the patient had an estimated 45% use of his transplanted kidney. The authors concluded that transplantation for patients with high levels of aPL should perhaps be limited to deceased-donor organs.

In a case report, Knight and associates recounted the course of a 46-year-old woman whom, after repeat arteriovenous (A-V) graft thromboses necessitating multiple A-V access procedures, received a 1 haplotype matched kidney from her son [28]. This patient was positive for IgG aCL and was initially LA positive, but upon repeat testing was LA negative. To avoid thrombosis, full heparinization was initiated intra-operatively, but was discontinued on the first post-transplant day due to a markedly elevated phospholipid-dependent clotting assay (PTT). The renal allograft thrombosed several hours after heparin therapy was halted. Examination revealed both the single renal artery and vein were thrombosed. A second, deceased-donor transplant was undertaken 6 months later. Heparin was administered and maintained postoperatively despite excessive bleeding which required two re-explorations of the wound for evacuation of hematomas. The patient was switched to coumadin 2 weeks after transplantation and slowly regained normal kidney function over the course of the first year. Based on this experience, these investigators screen for aPL in any transplant candidate with a history of SLE or recurrent thrombotic complications.

Renal transplant patients diagnosed with APS prior to transplantation were the subject of a study by Vaidya et al [29]. A total of 6 out of 78 patients receiving kidney transplants fulfilled the authors' clinical definition of APS: microrenal angiopathy, more than 2 episodes of A-V shunt thrombosis, cerebrovascular thrombosis, thrombocytopenia, and/or recurrent pregnancy loss with aCL. Three were IgM positive, 1 had IgG, and 2 had both IgG and IgM aCL; none were IgA aCL positive. All 6 APS patients lost their allografts due to thrombosis within the first 7 days. A subsequent paper by this group represented a multi-center study that looked at anticoagulation therapy for APS patients who had high titers of aCL [30]. Their APS criteria were modified from the previous paper from more than 2 A-V shunt thrombosis to more than 6 episodes per year. Eleven APS patients with high titer aCL were transplanted during the study period. Four received anticoagulation therapy and 7 did not. All 7 untreated patients lost their allografts due to thrombosis within the first week; 2 had lost previous grafts within 1 week due to thrombosis. Three of 4 on a coumadin anticoagulation protocol were doing well 1 year post-transplant, but the fourth thrombosed his transplanted kidney within the first week. In the same study there were 37 transplanted aCL-positive patients with no history of thrombotic disorders who were not defined as APS patients and thus served as the control group. No patient in the control group lost his or her allograft as a result of thrombosis, but 10 lost their grafts to acute rejection. This 27% graft loss rate in the control group is extraordinarily high in comparison to contemporary outcome statistics and to the overall 14% loss rate within this cohort. This outcome begs the question of whether aCL without a clinical diagnosis of APS is as benign as the authors contend.

In 2004, Vaidya et al expanded the criteria for APS from previous publications to include a history of lupus without thrombotic events [31]. In this publication only IgG and IgM aCL were discussed. The objective of this study was to investigate the effect of anticoagulant therapy for 9 APS patients who underwent renal transplantation. Two patients were treated with a heparin bolus followed by heparin drip. One lost her graft 2 days post-transplant due to thrombosis, however, the other patient maintains good renal function 5 years post-transplant. The remaining 7 APS patients were treated with coumadin to maintain an international normalized ration (INR) of approximately 1.8. Two of the coumadin treated patients lost their grafts at 2 and 3 days post-transplant due to thrombosis. Three patients returned to dialysis 6 to 22 months post-transplant after coumadin was discontinued due to bleeding complications. Interestingly, these patients had creatinine values of 1.1, 1.5, and 1.8 at the time coumadin was discontinued, suggesting that perhaps the anticoagulant contributed to maintenance of renal function. The remaining 2 coumadin treated patients continue anticoagulant therapy and have good renal function 2 and 3 years post-transplant. The authors concluded that APS patients with ESRD benefit from coumadin therapy without comment on the heparin treated patients. Albeit the numbers are small; 50% of heparin treated patients experienced transplant success compared to 28% of coumadin treated patients. These outcomes suggest that heparin may be a more efficacious treatment for aCL-positive transplant candidates.

Investigators at Brown University presented a study advocating thrombophilia screening for renal transplant candidates with either a personal or strong family history of thrombotic events [32]. Eight of 235 patients who received renal transplants between January 1998 and October 2001 were considered pre-operatively to be high risk for allograft thrombosis due to their clinical histories: aCL IgG or IgM (n = 2), LA (n = 4), APS (n = 1), or having both parents with resistance to activated protein C (n = 1). These 8 patients were anticoagulated with heparin from the time of surgery until they were switched to warfarin on postoperative days 2 to 4. According to the authors, warfarin therapy was continued for 6 months based on data suggesting that renal allograft thrombosis typically occurred within 6 months of transplant. In addition, there were 2 patients with no pre-transplant history who developed DVT post-transplant and were subsequently found to be LA positive. Two of these 10 high-risk patients developed acute rejection 8 and 12 months post-transplant and 1 lost her kidney due to recurrent acute rejection. The most devastating outcomes, allograft loss and renal artery thrombosis, occurred in the 2 patients with no pre-transplant clinical histories of thrombophilia. Although the authors advocate screening all transplant candidates with a history of thrombophilia, these 2 patients illustrate the "smoking guns" that have yet to be detected. Perhaps a more proactive approach to include screening of all transplant candidates would be more beneficial in preventing full or partial allograft loss.

Another study which advocated hypercoagulability screening was unique in that 346 patients transplanted between June 1992 and March 5, 1996 (cohort 1), served as the control group for 502 patients who were transplanted after March 6, 1996, subsequent to screening (cohort 2) [33]. Patients with risk factors defined as 2 or more arteriovenous access thromboses, prior allograft thrombosis, collagen vascular disease, multiple miscarriages, prior DVT, diabetes, autoimmune disease, or Fabry's disease were tested for antithrombin III, proteins S and C deficiencies, activated protein C resistance, and aPL. Initially, aPL testing included IgG and IgM aCL and LA, however, LA screening was discontinued when these investigators found aCL antibodies to be more clinically and economically relevant. Five of the 10 recipients in cohort 2 found to have clinical and laboratory evidence of hypercoagulability were aPL positive. All 10 patients received intravenous heparin within 1 hour of transplant surgery which was continued until discharge, thereafter, the patients received oral warfarin. Fourteen allografts (4.0%) from cohort 1 were lost to thrombosis compared to only 8 (1.6%) allografts in cohort 2. Three of the patients from cohort 1 were re-transplanted with anticoagulant therapy and all achieved long-term graft function. Four of the 5 aPL-positive patients in cohort 2 have maintained excellent graft function. The 1 patient in cohort 2 who experienced allograft thrombosis within 24 hours of transplant had very high IgG aCL (>150 units) and was receiving subcutaneous enoxaparin as opposed to intravenous heparin. Due to this poor outcome, Friedman et al remain cautious about the use of enoxaparin in patients with hypercoagulable states. The resultant recommendation from this study is to screen all transplant candidates for hypercoagulability risk factors and for those with clinical risks, screening should include aCL and activated protein C resistance because the latter represented the majority of the detected hypercoagulable states.

Two studies of post-transplantation aPL findings in renal allograft recipients were published by Ducloux et al [34]. The first report showed that 41 of 120 unselected consecutive renal transplants were aPL positive. Thirty-one were aCL positive, 8 had LA, and 2 patients had both. The mean transplant duration at the time of aPL testing was 67 ± 47 months for the aPL-positive patients and 92.7 ± 57 months for the negative patients. Testing pre-transplant blood from the aPL-positive patients showed that 74% of these patients were aPL positive at the time of transplant. The second paper reported a retrospective analysis of 178 non-SLE renal transplant recipients [35]. The blood sample used for aPL testing was collected after transplantation (median, 70 months). Fifty (28%) patients had aPL post-transplant; 38 were aCL positive (36 IgG, 2 IgM), 9 were LA positive, and 3 had both. In both of these studies the aPL were significantly correlated with duration of hemodialysis, antinuclear antibodies (ANA), and a history of either arterial or venous thrombosis. Transplant duration was significantly shorter for the aPL-positive group. A post-transplant history of venous and arterial thrombosis was significantly more frequent for patients with post-transplant aPL. Pre-transplant blood was available for 55 patients and 64% were aPL positive prior to transplant. Transplant duration and serum creatinine concentrations were not different between patients who remained aPL positive compared to those in whom aPL disappeared post-transplant. Multivariate regression analysis confirmed that both pre- and post-transplant aPL were independent risk factors for thrombosis. The authors raised the question of whether aPL screening before renal transplant would be beneficial and concluded that aPL screening is easy and the risk of thrombosis might be abrogated by the use of prophylactic measures post-transplant.

Renal Transplantation in Patients with SLE

Renal transplantation outcome in patients with lupus nephritis was evaluated in a retrospective study by Radhakrishnan and colleagues [36]. The post-transplant courses of 8 SLE patients who were aCL positive at the time of renal transplantation (4 IgG, 2 IgM, and 2 IgG + IgM aCL; 2 with LA) were compared to 5 transplanted aCL/LA-negative SLE patients. Three patients in each group received living-related donor kidneys; deceased-donor organs were used in the remaining patients. Half of the aCL-positive patients had aPL-related events post-transplant, 3 thrombotic and 1 thrombocytopenic. None of the 5 aCL/LA-negative patients experienced post-transplant thrombosis or thrombocytopenia. The aCL-positive patients had longer post-transplantation hospital stays than did the aCL-negative patients. Some patients received anticoagulation, however, this was not studied in detail. At the conclusion of the study there was no difference between the two groups for number of rejection episodes or renal function at last follow up and all patients had functioning allografts at the time of the report. The authors concluded that aCL-positive SLE patients can be transplanted successfully.

A larger retrospective study of renal transplantation in SLE patients by Stone et al reported a cohort of 85 consecutive, well-documented SLE renal transplant patients tested for aPL by at least 1 test [RPR (biological false positive test for syphilis), dilute Russell Viper Venom Time (dRVVT), aCL IgG/IgM ELISA] [37]. Twenty-five (29.4%) were aPL positive and 15 of these positive patients (60%) had post-transplant events associated with APS. Of these 15 patients, 3 died and 5 lost their transplanted kidney to aPL-associated events within 3 months of transplantation. This represents a 32% failure rate for aPL-positive SLE patients and an overall failure rate of 9.4% (8/85) for patients in this series. These data, in contrast to the previous smaller study [36], indicate that aPL have a significant negative impact on the outcome of renal transplantation in SLE.

A case report by Mathis and Shah described an exaggerated response to heparin in a female SLE patient with high levels of IgG aCL and LA [38]. Unfractionated heparin was started 30 minutes after living-related donor renal transplant surgery with a goal of maintaining the PTT between 50 and 70 seconds. The first PTT was 87.6 seconds, thus heparin was reduced 20%. Five and a half hours later the PTT was 92.6 seconds, necessitating further reduction in heparin, however, the hemoglobin had dropped to 4.8 g/dL. Consequently, heparin was discontinued and transfusions commenced. A retroperitoneal hemorrhage was found by ultrasound. Heparin was reintroduced 48 hours later and doses that previously resulted in bleeding achieved a lesser response. When anti-Xa activity was found to be substantially higher than predicted by the PTT, heparin was discontinued in favor of enoxaparin and warfarin. The patient was discharged with a serum creatinine of 0.9 mg/dL and hemoglobin of 7.8 g/dL. This patient underwent plasmapheresis preoperatively and 5 times post-transplant to remove a B-cell autoantibody. The authors note that patients with a positive cross-match and aPL cannot simply undergo plasmapheresis at transplant for the management of both conditions. This paper suggests that anticoagulation therapy would be required peri-operatively for the aPL, however, the pharmocokinetic variability of anticoagulants may be exaggerated in SLE patients with LA.

Viral Infections and aPL

Baid and co-authors investigated IgG and IgM aCL reactivity in 18 transplant recipients seropositve for hepatitis C virus (HCV) [39]. Pre-transplant sera were aCL positive for 6 of the 18. Of the aCL-positive patients, 5 (4 IgG aCL, 1 IgM aCL) developed biopsy proven, de novo renal thrombotic microangiopathy after transplant (range, 5–120 days). The patient group with renal pathology had significantly higher IgG aCL values than the group without thrombotic microangiopathy ($P = 0.02$); IgM values were not different between the groups. Four of the 5 patients with renal angiopathy died within 5 years compared to no deaths in the other 13 recipients.

An association between aPL and HCV infection was also reported by Ducloux and colleagues [17]. In post-transplant testing of 324 consecutive renal transplant patients, 46% of HCV-positive patients exhibited aPL activity compared to 24% of HCV-negative patients. Due to the low prevalence of HCV in this transplant population, this difference did not reach significance ($P = 0.08$). In contrast, cytomeglovirus serology was positive in the same proportion of patients with and without aPL.

Simultaneous Kidney and Pancreas Transplantation

There is limited data available regarding aPL in simultaneous kidney–pancreas (K-P) transplants. Two cases of K-P transplantation in patients with APS were reported by Wullstein and colleagues [40]. The first was a 47-year-old female who was known to be aCL and LA positive prior to transplant. Upon APS diagnosis the patient was placed on warfarin therapy but was switched to heparin because of bleeding episodes. At the time of transplant surgery heparin was given intravenously; before discharge the patient was switched to warfarin. Eleven weeks later the patient presented with an acute abdomen, which required laparotomy. Warfarin therapy was replaced by heparin during hospitalization. The allografts were not affected by the additional surgery and at 9 months follow up both organs have good function.

The second patient, a 42-year-old male, who had no history of thrombolic events underwent K-P transplant with routine therapy of intravenous heparin for the first week followed by subcutaneous low-molecular-weight heparin until discharge [40]. Thirty-one days post-transplant the patient had a DVT in the left leg. Hypercoagualibility screening revealed an LA but no aCL. The patient received warfarin therapy and 5 months after transplant, the K-P transplant was considered successful.

A second paper by Wullstein et al reviewed outcome data for 47 K-P transplant recipients who underwent routine screening for pro-thrombotic disorders [41]. All recipients were type I diabetics. Immunosuppressive therapy consisted of a single dose of anti-thymocyte globulin, tacrolimus, mycophenolate mofetil, and steriods. Routine anticoagulation therapy consisted of subcutaneous low-molecular-weight heparin for all patients except 1 with known APS who received systemic heparin therapy followed by warfarin. Data were retrospectively analyzed in view of complications (relaparotomy, graft thrombosis, pancreatitis, rejection) and graft function at 3 months post-transplantation. Twenty-five of the patients had abnormal findings in the prothrombotic screenings, however, only 2 patients had aPL and a positive history of APS. For analysis the APS patients were grouped with patients having deficiencies of protein C and S and antithrombin III. The authors concluded that unlike the pro-thrombotic disorders related to genetic mutations, the disorders influenced by external factors had no influence on post-transplant morbidity in this study. Interestingly, at 3 months after K-P transplant the group of patients with any abnormal pro-thrombotic finding had increased glycosolated hemoglobin (HbA1c) compared to patients without pro-thrombotic disorders ($P = 0.023$). The authors propose that partial venous thromboses or microthrombi in the pancreatic grafts may lead to increased HbA1c for patients with pro-thrombotic disorders [41].

Summary of Renal Transplantation in the Presence of aPL

Adverse effects associated with renal transplantation of the aPL-positive patient are summarized in Table 19.2. Negative outcomes have been reported for patients with

Table 19.2. Antiphospholipid antibody positive, renal transplant patient vulnerability.

- High risk for allograft thrombosis during first 2 weeks post-transplant
- aPL-positive CAPD patients at grave risk for renal allograft thrombosis
- aPE eluted from a transplant nephrectomy
- Fibrin deposition in a failed allograft demonstrated by immunohistochemistry
- Slow deterioration of function leading to shorter viable transplant duration compared to aPL negative recipients
- Anticoagulation therapy beneficial, heparin preferred

aPL = antiphospholipid antibody; CAPD = continuous ambulatory peritoneal dialysis; aPE = antiphosphatidylethanolamine.

a pre-transplant diagnosis of APS, leading investigators to recommend anticoagulation therapy post-transplant to neutralize the effects of the aPL [26–30]. A more proactive approach of aPL screening for all renal candidates would identify patients whose first aPL clinical event is renal allograft thrombosis [16, 20, 22]. Patients identified as aPL positive during the pre-transplant laboratory workup can be heparinized during the immediate post-operative period and expect a successful transplant [22, 25].

Orthotopic Liver Transplantation

In hepatic failure, as in renal failure, aPL status of the transplant candidate both before and after transplantation can effect outcome. And as in the renal transplantation literature, the importance of aPL findings is controversial. Talenti and colleagues reported a beneficial consequence of liver replacement in a 46-year-old female patient [42]. The patient had a 30-year history of cryptogenic cirrhosis, and several weeks before undergoing liver transplantation, suffered a cerebral infarction. Laboratory testing at the time of infarction found an LA, moderate IgG aCL, and high titer IgM aCL; IgA aCL was negative. The patient was diagnosed with PAPS, but anticoagulation treatment was avoided because she was awaiting liver transplantation. Two days after transplantation, the patient's aPTT was within normal limits and within the first week her aCL titers fell to normal. At 4 months post-transplant with no reappearance of her pre-transplant aPL, the patient had good liver function.

Living-donor liver transplantation in a 10-year-old male patient with APS induced Budd-Chiari syndrome also proved beneficial in reducing aPL titers [43]. Before transplantation the patient had IgG, IgA, and IgM aCL and was positive for antibodies to a PL binding protein, β_2-glycoprotein I. Anticoagulation therapy began with a heparin drip immediately after surgery; the patient was later switched to baby aspirin and warfarin to maintain an INR of 3. A pathologist's examination of the patient's native liver showed necrosis with organized thrombi that were ascribed to the aPL. Four weeks after transplant a decrease in all aPL titers was seen and 4 months after transplant the patient was doing well without any episode of thrombosis.

In contrast to the previous case reports, Villamil et al reported a case of catastrophic APS following liver transplantation for primary sclerosing cholangitis [44]. Six months prior to transplant a 57-year-old female patient twice suffered from a transient ischemic attack (TIA) and was found to be LA positive but IgG and IgM aCL negative. The patient was treated with aspirin until transplant when low-molecular-weight heparin was added intra-operatively and both were maintained post-operatively. She was doing well until 5 days post-transplant when cellular rejection was diagnosed. On day 7 she developed right hemiparesia and a magnetic resonance imaging (MRI) scan detected an ischemic lesion in the pons. On day 9 the patient had marked bowel dilation with a large subhepatic hematoma; a diagnostic laparotomy showed extensive ischemia of both large and small intestines with no evident source of bleeding. Two days later the patient experienced copious bleeding through her abdominal drains and developed a spontaneous hemothorax with a 7 point fall in hematocrit. Full anticoagulation was stopped and the patient was maintained on aspirin. The patient was intubated for 5 days subsequent to detection of diffuse alveolar infiltrates. When removed from the ventilator she was difficult to arouse despite discontinuation of sedatives more than 48 hours before. A brain MRI showed extensive ischemia of the left hemisphere. On day 64 post-transplantation, the patient, with optimal graft function, was transferred to a neurologic center for rehabilitation.

A prospective study of 12 adult patients with advanced liver disease was designed by Van Thiel and colleagues to determine whether aPL adversely affected vascular thrombosis and whether aPL persist after transplantation [45]. All 12 patients had high levels of IgG and IgM aCL before transplant but 1 month post-transplant none was positive. Two of the patients had a pre-transplant history of peripheral venous thrombosis. In spite of high levels of aCL prior to transplantation, none of the patients was anticoagulated and none experienced thrombotic events during the 2 year post-transplant study duration.

In a large series of pediatric liver recipients, Lallier and his group reported on 73 patients who received 81 hepatic transplants [46]. Vascular complications which included hepatic artery thrombosis (HAT), portal vein thrombosis, or aortic conduit perforation occurred in 13 of the children. For 1 patient, portal vein thrombosis was ascribed to aCL causing a hypercoagulable state.

Pre-transplant sera from 35 liver recipients were assessed by Pascual et al for the presence of IgG and IgM aCL [47]. Seven of the patients presented with HAT post-transplant and 28 did not. Overall, 22 of 35 (63%) had aCL in pre-transplant sera. All 7 HAT patients were aCL positive whereas 15 out of 28 non-HAT recipients had aCL ($P = 0.03$). The patients with HAT tended to have higher IgG and IgM aCL titers than patients free from HAT. Repeat liver transplants were required for 5 of the 7 HAT patients. The authors commented that a negative aCL test has a much higher predictive value than a positive finding.

Four patients with repeated liver allograft loss caused by recurrent HAT were reported by Vivarelli et al [48]. These were the only patients among 24 re-transplantations due to HAT that experienced recurrence. The first patient experienced HAT in his first allograft 7 years after transplantation. Recurrence of HAT 3 days after re-transplantation prompted aPL testing. Due to a high titer IgM anti–ß$_2$-GPI antibody the patient received anti-aggregant prophylaxis with the third liver transplant and was alive and well at the time of the report. HAT developed in the second patient 9 months after transplant. An LA was detected at the time of the first HAT and persisted until 4 months after the third transplant when the patient, who was doing well, tested LA negative. The third patient developed HAT 7 days post-transplant and proceeded to experience HAT in the next 3 transplanted livers. The patient died of sepsis in the post-operative period after his fifth liver transplant. The final patient in the series first experienced HAT 22 months after liver transplanta-

Table 19.3. Effects of antiphospholipid antibodies on the outcome of orthotopic liver transplantation.

- Positive aPL findings corrected after transplantation for some recipients
- Catastrophic APS subsequent to transplantation
- Post-transplantation HAT risks
- Repeat liver transplants due to HAT

aPL = antiphospholipid antibody; APS = antiphospholipid antibody syndrome; HAT = hepatic artery thrombosis.

tion. At that time, high levels of aCL were detected. Subsequently the patient required 2 more transplants with anti-aggregant and anti-thrombotic prophylaxis before he became aCL negative. Including the patients described in detail, the investigators reported 57% of 11 patients re-transplanted due to late HAT were positive for LA and/or aCL. The authors concluded that aPL should be investigated in liver transplant recipients so that adequate anticoagulant, anti-aggregant prophylaxis, or both can be included in post-transplant pharmacotherapy.

After hepatic vessel thrombosis and graft loss occurred in 2 aCL- and LA-positive patients who presented with APS after transplantation, Collier et al retrospectively tested for the presence of IgG aCL [49]. Stored sera collected 2 to 4 weeks post-transplant from 132 patients were analyzed for IgG aCL and compared to the incidence of allograft vascular thrombosis. Twenty-one of the 132 patients experienced hepatic vessel thrombosis. IgG aCL were detected in 9 patients, 2 developed hepatic vessel thrombosis, and 7 did not. This was not a significant finding and authors concluded that the presence of aCL in the absence of an APS diagnosis is an uncommon cause of hepatic vessel thrombosis. However, for patients with a history of pre-transplant thrombotic episodes the authors would consider prescribing post-transplant anticoagulation as a preventative measure. Of note is that HAT occurred in the index patients 7 months and 6 years after transplantation. Similarly, the 4 patients presented by Vivarelli and coworkers presented with HAT 7 days, 9 months, 22 months, and 7 years after liver transplantation [48]. Unfortunately, it is not clear from this report how long the 7 aCL-positive patients without thrombosis were followed. HAT associated with aPL can present many months or years after transplant, thus, one cannot discount the possibility of future graft thrombosis in the aPL-positive patients with patent grafts at the conclusion of this study.

In the setting of liver transplantation, vastly different effects of aPL have been reported. As summarized in Table 19.3, aCL and LA have disappeared subsequent to liver transplantation [42, 43]. In stark contrast are the aPL-positive patients who experienced HAT or catastrophic APS following liver transplantation [44, 47, 49]. The aPL-positive liver transplant patient may benefit from post-transplant anticoagulation therapy, however, aPL associated HAT can occur years after transplant [48, 49].

Heart Transplantation

Heart transplantation literature that addresses the consequences of aPL is limited. A case report by Pengo and associates details a 38-year-old man in need of a heart transplant who was both aCL and LA positive [50]. In preparation for transplantation, the patient underwent 3 consecutive days of plasmapheresis to minimize the possibility of his aPL damaging the vessels of the transplanted heart.

Immunosuppressive therapy with cyclosporine and azathioprine commenced with the plasmapheresis. After the third plasmapheresis, the aCL and LA were reduced. Two days after the last plasmapheresis and while receiving immunosuppressive treatment, the aCL again became positive. Over the next 5 days both the aCL and LA levels rose to basal levels. Unfortunately, due to deterioration of kidney function, immunosuppressive therapy was discontinued and the patient was discharged. The patient died 2 days later and prior to transplantation.

A report from our laboratory contained a retrospective aPL analysis of 105 cardiac transplant recipients tested for IgG, IgA, and IgM aCL, aPS, and aPE [51]. Post-transplantation sera collected a mean of 36 months after the transplant showed 87 (83%) were aPL positive for at least 1 antigen–isotype combination, but many had aPL of more than 1 isotype. In view of the high percentage of aPL-positive patients, we retrospectively tested pre-transplant samples from 79 of the 105 patients. Fifty-two of 79 (66%) pre-transplant sera tested aPL positive with IgA being the most prevalent antibody isotype. Correlation of transplant function or biopsy data with aPL status was not undertaken in this study.

A different aPL related issue was raised for a heart transplant recipient who had a low positive IgM aPL; the specificity of the aPL was not indicated [52]. Flow cyto-metric (FACS) cross-matches are often used to detect recipient anti-donor antibod-ies prior to solid organ transplant. FACS cross-matches with an IgM conjugate using this patient's sera against donor and autologous T lymphocytes resulted in a mean fluorescence channel shift that fluctuated between 30–50 channels. In our opinion, this is a low or borderline level positive. The authors concluded that the IgM reactivity detected by FACS was caused by the aPL. In theory, an aPL can bind to lymphocytes. The binding detected by FACS may be a consequence of viability of the lymphocytes inasmuch as non-viable cells or cells undergoing apoptosis express more anionic PL on the surface, thus, if apoptotic cells were used in the FACS cross-match, a low level binding might not be surprising. Because this aPL-positive serum was not subjected to absorption with phospholipid vesicles to show loss of FACS activity, the question remains if the aPL and the FACS antibodies are one in the same.

On the other hand, we reported the case of a heart transplant candidate who had IgG antibody detected by FACS to 100% of a panel of lymphocyte donors [53]. In preparation for transplant, the patient was given intravenous immunoglobulin (IvIg) until his anti-HLA antibodies were no longer detected by FACS. The patient was transplanted successfully 2 weeks after achieving FACS negative cell panel reac-tivity. Although not included in the published report, this patient also had high titer IgG aCL and aPS which were unaffected by IvIg treatment and which remained pos-itive into the post-transplant period. These data indicate that the IgG detected by FACS was not an aPL.

Left Ventricular Assist Systems (LVAS)

The use of ventricular assist devices either as a bridge to heart transplant or as a permanent replacement in heart failure patients has been plagued by a high inci-dence of thromboembolic complications [54]. We became interested in LVAS patients because of their propensity to develop allo-antibodies, usually anti-HLA, following multiple blood and platelet transfusions [53]. Because these patients are serially tested for sensitization to HLA antigens, frozen sera were available for longitudinal aPL testing. Serial serum samples from 10 LVAS recipients were tested for aCL, aPS, and aPE with IgG, IgM, and IgA conjugates. The majority (60%) of these 10 patients were aPL negative prior to LVAS placement, however, 90% sero-converted to aPL positive after LVAS placement [55]. This finding prompted us to ask whether the aPL were a result of platelet activation due to placement of the LVAS and subsequent change in hemodynamics, or was the LVAS, as a foreign body, directly stimulating aPL production such that the aPL then reacted with platelets? [56]. Either circumstance could be related to the association of aPL and thrombosis after LVAS placement in these patients. The data demonstrated that LVAS recipients exposed to Thrombogen®, a topical bovine component of fibrin glue, developed antibodies to this agent. Further studies showed that Thrombogen® contained PL-binding plasma proteins that supported aPL ELISA reactivity for both anionic (aCL, aPS) and zwitterionic (aPE) PL [57, 58].

The specificity and the platelet reactivity of LVAS patient aPL were similar if not identical to the aPL found in other aPL-positive patients who experienced thrombosis [56]. As a result of the studies with Thrombogen®, the cardiothoracic surgeons at Methodist Hospital of Indiana discontinued or markedly decreased the use of bovine thrombin during LVAS placement. Subsequently, no aPL sero-conversion was found in 5 non-exposed patients. Further, no post-placement thromboembolic events occurred in the 5 non-exposed patients compared to half of 6 exposed patients who experienced either a cerebrovascular accident (n = 2) or a TIA (n = 1).

Valve Replacement

The impact of aPL on cardiac valve replacement has been documented recently in a number of papers that address the outcome of both aortic and mitral valves. Case reports and a single retrospective review describe post-surgical events experienced by patients who received either tissue (homografts) or mechanical valve replacements.

Aortic Valves

Thrombosis of an aortic valve homograft in a patient with LA was reported by Unger and colleagues [59]. The 33-year-old woman had an uneventful post-operative course until she experienced a large thrombus on the aortic aspect of the graft 8 months after surgery. Acenocoumarol treatment was initiated and disappearance of the thrombus followed. Fifty months later the patient experienced a second thrombus of the aortic valve homograft. Unfractionated heparin was administered followed by acenocoumarol resulting in complete disappearance of the thrombus after 3 months. One year later the patient was doing well.

In contrast to the above report, Matsuyama et al reported a 42-year-old woman with a 10-year history of high titer aCL and APS who had an uneventful post-operative course subsequent to prosthetic aortic valve placement [60]. Oral warfarin and low doses of prednisolone were started on the first post-operative day. Without special consideration to reducing the elevated aPL levels, the patient experienced no hemostatic or thrombolic problems in the year following surgery.

Mitral Valves

One hour after placement of a mechanical mitral valve, a 31-year-old woman with a history of APS with LA and aCL became hypotensive with a profoundly ischemic ECG [61]. Suspecting catastrophic APS, the patient was administered intravenous heparin and placed on bypass to support her circulatory collapse. Following 4 plasma exchanges in 36 hours, the patient's IgG aCL levels fell to normal and her myocardial function improved. By the time of discharge 7 weeks post-operatively, the patient's IgG aCL had risen again to greater than 100 G phospholipid (GPL) units. No additonal follow up was provided for this patient.

The case of a 46-year-old female SLE patient with an LA was reported by Brownstein and co-workers [62]. The patient who developed symptoms of cardiac tamponade 8 days after placement of a mechanical mitral valve required surgical evacuation of a mediastinal hematoma. The patient recovered from this procedure but due to persistent rhythm disturbances required implantation of a pacemaker. The patient was discharged on post-operative day 16 taking anticoagulant therapy of aspirin and coumadin.

Kato et al reported a case of a 48-year-old woman previously diagnosed with SLE, APS, and chronic renal failure who was admitted for replacement of a bioprosthetic valve placed 9 years before [63]. Two days after replacement surgery, when heparinization was stopped the patient suddenly had an epileptic fit and ischemic necrosis of the fingers and toes. The patient was treated with aspirin and warfarin. The necrosis gradually disappeared and the patient was discharged 3 months after surgery. The authors concluded that strict management of anticoagulant therapy is required for patients with APS undergoing valve replacement.

A single case of a patient with SLE and APS undergoing mitral valve replacement with a biological prosthesis was reported by da Silva and colleagues [64]. This patient died 9 months later subsequent to massive intra-cardiac thrombosis and prosthesis dysfunction. Two additional cases of mitral valve replacements using tissue valves were among 10 patients with aPS who received mitral valve replacements presented by Berkun et al [65]. One of the patients who received a homograft underwent reoperation 15 months later because of partial detachment of the aortic homograft. The other patient who received a tissue valve was not specifically delineated; there were 4 deaths among the 10 patients and only 4 patients had uneventful outcomes during 8 years of follow up. These investigators concluded that to reduce operative risks APS patients should be considered for earlier operative intervention and that mechanical valves are probably the better choice for these patients.

Summary of Cardiac Replacement and aPL

aPL findings in the settings of heart transplantation, valve replacements, and in mechanical assist devices are summarized in Table 19.4. A high incidence of aPL have been reported in pre- and post-transplant blood of heart transplant patients. While there was no correlation with transplant function or biopsy findings in the aPL-positive patients, there may be an association with aPL development and the use of fibrin glues and bovine thrombin used during cardiac surgery [51, 57, 58]. Further, thrombotic events after both tissue and prosthetic valve replacement surgery have been reported for aPL-positive patients [61, 64, 65]. IvIg treatment for

Table 19.4. Antiphospholipid antibody risks associated with heart transplantation and cardiac prosthetic devices.

- High incidence of aPL pre- and post-transplant
- aPL not abrogated by IvIg treatment
- aPL in LVAS recipients related to use of bovine fibrin glues and thrombin sprays
- High incidence of cerebrovascular events in LVAS recipients
- Thrombotic events subsequent to tissue and prosthetic valve replacement

aPL = antiphospholipid antibody; IvIg = intravenous immunoglobulin; LVAS = left ventricular assist system.

a cardiac transplant patient did not decrease aPL titers, thus careful management of anticoagulant therapy is advised for aPL-positive patients [53, 63].

Lung and Heart-Lung Transplantation

The choice between transplanting the lung alone or the heart and lung enblock for patients with pulmonary dysfunction often depends upon donor availability and other surgical and medical considerations [66]. Three SLE patients with pulmonary hypertension who underwent heart–lung transplant were reported by Asherson et al [67]. Two aPL-negative recipients were considered transplant successes for up to 1 year after transplantation. The only recipient with aPL, LA, and extremely high aCL died during the transplant surgery.

A review of 11 years of lung transplantation experience at Papworth Hospital in Cambridge, United Kingdom, included 2 SLE patients with aCL among 19 who underwent lung transplantation [68]. Overall, 9 patients died, including the aCL-positive SLE patients, both of whom died as a consequence of mesenteric thrombosis resulting in bowel infarction and multi-organ failure. The first patient died 60 days after heart–lung transplant and the second died 18 days after single lung re-transplantation 20 months after the initial heart–lung transplant was complicated by progressive obliterative bronchiolitis. The authors concluded that patients with SLE, particularly those with aCL, should probably not be considered candidates for lung transplantation.

In series of 72 patients with chronic thromboembolic pulmonary hypertension reported by Simonneau and co-investigators, 38 patients were tested for LA. Nine (24%) were found to be LA positive [66]. Eight patients in this series were selected for lung or heart–lung transplantation. One patient died the day after transplant and another died 2 years after transplantation from obliterative bronchiolitis. The remaining 6 patients were alive 5 months to 5 years after transplantation. Unfortunately, it is not possible to discern in this paper which patients may have had LA activity.

In a retrospective review of medical records for 72 single-lung transplants, Nathan and colleagues found 7 symptomatic events of pulmonary embolism in 6 patients [69]. All pulmonary embolism events occurred in men who were diagnosed with idiopathic pulmonary fibrosis. Twenty-three patients had the diagnosis of idiopathic pulmonary fibrosis, thus 27% of these patients had a pulmonary embolism compared to none of the patients with other diagnoses ($P < 0.001$). The length of hospital stay at transplant was longer, but not remarkably so, for the patients who went on to have a pulmonary embolism compared to those who did not. At the time of the events all patients were oxygen independent, ambulatory outpatients. There were no laboratory data provided for these patients.

Table 19.5. Antiphospholipid antibody related morbidity and mortality in lung transplantation patients.

- Increased incidence of aPL in idiopathic pulmonary fibrosis patients
- aPL associated with pulmonary embolism and catastrophic APS

aPL = antiphospholipid antibody; APS = antiphospholipid antibody symdrome.

A study published soon after by Magro and coworkers tested patients with idiopathic pulmonary fibrosis for aPE, aCL, aPS, and anti-β_2-glycoprotein I [70]. This paper reported that 100% of the 18 patients tested positive for 1 or more aPL. When this study was pointed out to Nathan and Barnett in a letter to the editor, they agreed that the findings of Magro should be verified in prospective studies [71]. All new idiopathic pulmonary fibrosis patients seen by Nathan and colleagues are now prospectively tested for aPL [71]. If the high prevalence of aPL is confirmed, this would define a group of patients who would benefit from anticoagulation therapy in the pre- and post-transplant settings [72].

In lung transplantation as in renal transplantation, aPL have been associated with significant morbidity and mortality [67–69]. A brief summary of aPL associated events subsequent to lung transplantation is presented in Table 19.5.

Vascular Bypass Grafts

The previously discussed transplant tissues were allogeneic in origin. Vascular bypass grafting affords a look at the effects of aPL on autologous and prosthetic grafts. Table 19.6 summarizes aPL risks for patients undergoing vascular bypass procedures.

Cardiac Bypass

Dauerman and colleagues presented a case study of a 56-year-old woman with IgG aCL and a factor XII deficiency who underwent a technically unremarkable triple cardiac bypass [73]. Within 1 hour of arriving in the intensive care unit the patient suffered multiple cardiac arrests. Coronary angiography showed thrombotic occlusion of the distal anastamoses of the 3 grafted vessels. Intracoronary thrombolysis was accomplished with rapid injection of urokinase into each of the grafts. With a total dose of 550,000 units of urokinase, the vessels were opened and the patient did not experience bleeding. Repeat angiography 3 days later showed all grafts were patent. The patient, maintained on heparin and later warfarin, had no further cardiac events during 3.5 years of follow up.

Table 19.6. Vascular bypass graft risks for antiphopholipid antibody positive patients.

- Thrombotic occlusion and thrombocytopenia subsequent to cardiac bypass surgery
- Shorter duration of patency after peripheral bypass
- Increased thrombotic events in dialysis patients with A-V grafts compared to patients with A-V fistulas
- APL-positive patients recieving prosthetic grafts may be at higher risk of thrombotic events than those with autologous grafts

aPL = antiphospholipid antibody; A-V = arterio-venous.

The outcome of repeat coronary bypass 14 years after initial bypass was presented by Nakayama et al [74]. The 69-year-old male had been treated with procainamide and warfarin for frequent episodes of premature ventricular beats since the original bypass. Warfarin was discontinued 4 days before the repeat bypass, which was unremarkable until the second post-operative day when the platelet count dropped significantly. The patient developed shock after therapeutic platelet transfusion. A platelet transfusion on post-operative day 8 was followed by a return of shock. Concurrently, thromboses were noted in the grafts to the coronary arteries, right brachiocephlic vein, superior vena cava, and peripheral veins. Heparin was administered to treat the systemic thrombosis and consumptive thrombocytopenia. After thrombectomy, the patient was found LA positive and aCL negative. The LA was negative 2 months after the episodes of graft occlusion, however, the patient died of heart failure 2 months later. These investigators concluded that aPL status should be determined for patients who develop unreasonable thrombocytopenia after bypass, especially for patients with a history of procainamide use.

Peripheral Bypass

In a cross-sectional study of 234 general vascular surgery patients, Taylor et al tested for IgG, IgM, IgA, aCL, and LA prior to surgery [4]. Arterial reconstructions for these patients included bypasses, aneurysm repair, and revascularizations. Sixty patients (25.6%) were aPL positive (53 aCL, 5 LA, and 2 both); none had other hypercoagulable disorders. Ten aCL patients (19%) had IgA only. A significant number of aPL-positive patients had undergone previous peripheral arterial surgery ($P < 0.04$); further, a higher proportion of these patients had undergone previous lower extremity revascularization ($P = 0.047$). aPL-positive patients were 5.6 times more likely to have had an occlusive failure of a previous procedure ($P = 0.003$) and a shorter duration of patency before occlusion ($P = 0.03$) than aPL-negative patients. This study highlights the importance of including IgA in the ELISA as the number of aCL-positive patients was substantially increased.

A second prospective study by this group reached different conclusions [75]. The prospective study followed 262 patients who received elective infrainguinal bypass procedures. As in the original study, patients were tested for IgG, IgM, and IgA aCL, and LA using blood collected prior to surgery. Laboratory results were not known at the time of surgery and thus did not influence surgical treatment. Eighty-three patients (32%) had hypercoagulable states related to aPL (70 aCL, 11 LA, and 2 aCL with LA). Primary patency rates were not significantly different between the aPL-positive (43%) and -negative patients (59%, $P = 0.087$). The aPL-positive and -negative groups were well matched with the exception that aPL-positive patients received post-operative warfarin twice as often as aPL-negative patients. Many more patients were maintained on warfarin in the prospective study than in the retrospective study ($P = 0.002$) [75]. In addition, routine use of aspirin before and after surgery may have contributed to the decrease in thrombotic events for aPL-positive patients in the second prospective study. Comparing the outcome data, the authors noted that aPL may have an adverse effect on prosthetic grafts as opposed to autologous grafts inasmuch as many of the failed grafts in the original retrospective study were prosthetic, whereas none of the grafts in the prospective study were prosthetic [75]. Unfortunately, the patients who received autografts were not analyzed independently for aCL and LA [4, 75]. It would be of interest to analyze separately autologous versus prosthetic grafts as well as include the additional findings for the aPS, aPE, and aPC ELISA.

In contrast to the above study that failed to confirm an earlier report of a relationship between aPL and bypass graft outcome, a more recent paper by Nielsen and coworkers found that IgM and IgG aCL appeared to associate with an increased risk of autologous infrainguinal bypass failure [76]. Although the number of aCL-positive patients in this study of 80 vein graft patients was limited to 7 (IgG 2, IgM 5), patency at 6 months was 14% versus 57% in aCL-negative patients ($P = 0.03$). Four of the 7 patients thrombosed their graft within 3 months and another 2 developed stenosis. The presence of aCL and diabetes independently contributed towards the overall risk of graft failure in this study ($P = 0.008$ and 0.006, respectively). We have reported a high incidence of aPL in diabetic patients (81%), and for those diabetic patients with proliferative retinopathy, IgA aPE was detected with 68% prevalence [77].

Thrombophilia screening for 124 lower-limb revascularization patients presented by Ray et al included testing for low levels of protein C, protein S, or antithrombin III and for LA [78]. Seventy-five patients had occluded (31 recent, 44 old occlusions) and 49 had patent revascularization procedures. Coagulation abnormalities were found in 40% with the most common abnormality, LA, occurring in 34 (27%) patients. Seven of 10 patients retested for LA after a median interval of 3 months remained positive. Caludicants who did not undergo revascularization had a similar frequency and distribution of coagulation abnormalities as patients with patent vascularization procedures. Within the group of patients with patent bypasses, there were no significant differences in the prevalence of abnormalities between those with autogeneous vein bypasses and those with prosthetic grafts (18% vs. 27%). The LA was nearly 4 times more prevalent in patients with old rather than recent occlusions. Further, each of 9 patients with LA in combination with low protein C or protein S levels had a prosthetic graft, causing these investigators to speculate that LA may appear as a consequence of exposure to the prosthetic material.

Hemodialysis Access Grafts

Support for the idea that aPL appearance may be precipitated by the use of prosthetic material has been demonstrated in hemodialysis patients. In a retrospective study of 91 patients who had received a minimum of 6 months of uninterrupted dialysis, Prakash and colleagues found IgG aCL positivity in 22% of patients with arteriovenous grafts compared to 6% positivity in patients with arteriovenous fistulas [79]. One-hundred-forty-two thrombotic events of the arteriovenous graft occurred in 74 patients compared to no thrombotic events in 17 patients with arteriovenous fistulas over the 30-month study period.

In a study limited to dialysis patients who received synthetic, PTFE (Gore-Tex®) grafts, LeSar et al reported 91 surgical procedures for initial placement of vascular access or repair of complications in 34 patients [80]. Twelve patients had hypercoagulable abnormalities defined by LA, aCL, aPS, activated protein C resistance, or deficiencies in protein C, protein S, or antithrombin III. Elevated aPL were found in 83% of these patients and 58% had multiple abnormalities. Hypercoagulability was the only determinable cause in 28 (42%) cases of thrombotic complications. Two patients in this group had frequent PTFE graft thromboses but had normal hypercoagulable workups according to the methods used. This raises an issue about expanding the testing to include additional antibody isotypes and phospholipid antigens, that is, aPE and aPC and IgA.

Bone Marrow Transplantation (BMT)

Reports of LA and solid-organ graft failures were followed by reports of coagulation-associated failures in patients who received allogeneic as well as autologous BMT. In a study by Conlan and coworkers, 46 patients with refractory malignant lymphoma admitted for autologous stem cell transplantation were evaluated for hemostatic abnormalities [81]. Low-to-moderate titer aCL were present in 29% of 35 patients tested (5 IgG, 3 IgM, 2 IgG + IgM). LA (dRVVT) was documented in 7 of 43 patients tested (16%), 3 also were aCL positive. Although the authors implicated these abnormal findings as possible causes or contributors to thrombotic complications frequently seen during autologous BMT, the aPL status was not related to BMT outcome.

Development of an LA following BMT occurred in 38 of 1292 patients from a single program [82]. This study was a retrospective review of autologous and allogenic BMT patients cross-referenced with the coagulation laboratory testing results to identify patients with LA as defined by a prolonged PTT. More frequently detected in children than adults, the LA were usually detected in the first or second month following transplant. Significant associations were noted between the LA and busulfan plus cytoxan treatment as a preparatory regimen, receiving cyclosporine or T-cell depleted marrow and with viral infections. Four of the 38 patients experienced thrombotic complications. Gastrointestinal bleeding occurred in 13 of the patients, and it was the bleeding episodes that prompted requests for coagulation testing and subsequent identification of the LA. As the investigators pointed out, the true incidence of LA in their BMT population was not known because routine coagulation studies were not performed for all patients.

In 1998, a BMT case report was published detailing aCL associated thrombotic complications. This was a case of a 4-month-old patient with Omenn syndrome (SCID variant) who underwent a BMT from a HLA identical sibling [83]. Day 59 post-BMT the child suffered a major cerebral vascular accident (CVA) and developed severe pulmonary hypertension. A persistently elevated aCL was detected. The presence of central line-derived microemboli was suspected. Anticoagulation was initiated, but discontinued 6 months later when aCL was no longer positive. Retrospective analysis of pre-BMT serum from the recipient found low titers of aCL; the donor tested negative. The authors emphasized the importance of screening for aCL whenever thrombotic events are suspected.

Disappearance of aPL after BMT

Four case reports have been published reporting disappearance of aPL subsequent to allogenic and even after autologous BMT. The case published by Olalla et al reported the disappearance of an LA subsequent to BMT with an HLA-identical sibling donor [84]. In this case, a 23-year-old female diagnosed with chronic myeloid leukemia (CML) had a persistent LA at least 15 months prior to transplant, which fully resolved by day 27 post-transplant. She remains hematologically normal 4 years and 8 months after BMT.

Musso and colleagues reported disappearance of aCL and LA subsequent to autologous BMT in a 19-year-old female SLE patient with secondary APS [85]. The patient's clinical history included both arterial and venous thrombosis, thrombocytopenia, and autoimmune hemolytic anemia (AIHA, Evans' syndrome). Eventually, after several relapses of AIHA, she was conditioned to receive autologous CD34 positive progenitor cells from peripheral blood. After mobilization of peripheral blood precursor cells, the aCL became borderline positive and the LA disappeared. Eight months post-transplant she was well and in a normal hematological state without further treatment, suggesting that either the conditioning regime or autologous BMT affected LA and aCL activity in this patient.

Hashimoto and colleagues recorded the course of a 27-year-old female SLE patient who had endured 7 years of monthly plasmapheresis to prevent symptoms of APS [86]. In spite of the intense treatment she suffered myocardial necrosis attributed to damage caused by APS. The patient was found to have aCL at the time of APS diagnosis 9 years before. Based on the progressive nature of the cardiac disease the patient underwent autologous BMT in an attempt to abrogate the effects of APS. aCL levels had decreased from 84.2 to 25.5 U/mL (normal < 10 U/mL) at the 6-month follow up. Twenty-one months after BMT the patient has no recurrent APS symptoms and has experienced improvement in cardiac status.

A female with a clinical history of recurrent episodes of pulmonary hemorrhage, thrombocytopenia, central and peripheral nervous system involvement, and severely disabling diffuse calcinosis, mostly in the hip joints and pelvic muscles, was diagnosed at age 15 with APS when IgG and IgM aCL were detected [87]. In light of rising aCL titers, pulmonary hypertension, ischemic necrosis of the digits, and the child becoming bedridden due severe mobility limitations secondary to the calcinosis, Elhasid and colleagues offered her autologous BMT as a mode of treatment. Gradually the patient's mobility improved as the calcinosis nodules liquefied after transplant. While the aCL levels remained slightly elevated, 2 years after autologous BMT the patient was free from clinical and laboratory evidence of disease activity. The pathogenesis for the disappearance of the massive calcinosis is not clear, however, the authors speculate it is possibly associated with vigorous anti-inflammatory and immunosuppressive therapy provided with BMT.

The clinical outcomes of BMT are reminiscent of the experimental outcome documented for autoimmune-prone mice given bone marrow from autoimmune-resistant mice discussed below [88]. These data support the idea that LA and aCL arise from an aberrant clone of immunocompetent marrow cells and that ablation of this clone by irradiation or chemotherapy can destroy the aberrant cells for successful autologous or allogeneic transplantation.

A recent and unique paper by Mengarelli et al describes prospective aCL and LA studies of 32 patients undergoing allogeneic BMT [88a]. The aim of this prospective study was to investigate levels of aPL in subjects with hematological malignancies undergoing allogenic BMT. LA and aCL were measured prior to the conditioning regimen and at specific intervals post BMT for 6 months. No significant changes in aPL status or levels were observed during the first 3 months post-transplant, however, between 3 and 6 months a significant difference in the incidence of IgG aCL was seen. All recipients of unrelated marrow became IgG aCL positive versus 35% of recipients who received related marrow. LA and IgM aCL mean values did not change. None of the patients experienced a thrombotic diathesis. No correlation between aCL and the conditioning regimen or the type of graft versus host disease

(GVHD) was apparent. Upon examination, aCL seroconversion was associated with CMV infection such that the authors concluded that aCL positivity was significantly associated with, if not a result of, CMV infection. Interestingly, the ELISA used for these studies tested for β_2-glycoprotein I independent aCL, the type of aCL which has been proposed to be associated with infections and not associated with thrombotic events. Support for a relationship between CMV infection and aCL production is found in a recent publication from Gharavi and colleagues [89].

Morio et al described hepatic veno-occulsive disease (VOD) leading to death in a male patient who received HLA-identical bone marrow from his brother [90]. The LA in this patient was detected only after transplant, which implies that the LA was caused either by conditioning therapy or marrow transfusion. Interestingly, neither this patient nor any of those patients presented by Conlan had prolongation of the aPTT [81, 90].

Hepatic VOD resulting in liver dysfunction is a common complication of BMT. Hepatic dysfunction in conjunction with central nervous system (CNS) and pulmonary dysfunction comprises a systemic disorder known as multiple organ dysfunction syndrome (MODS). Vessel destruction by fibrous obliteration in both VOD and MODS is the proposed consequence of pre-transplant chemo-radiation and activation of the hemostatic system. Because aPL are associated with venous and arterial thrombosis which may lead to vessel occlusion, Fastenau and colleagues designed a study to determine if aPL-positive BMT candidates were prone to develop VOD and/or MODS more frequently than aPL negative patients [91]. Pre-transplant blood samples collected prior to chemo-radiation were assayed to determine the incidence of aPL in 112 BMT patients, 57 who developed and 55 who did not develop VOD or MODS post-transplant. In contrast to previously discussed aPL studies which were limited to ELISA detection of aCL, Fastenau tested for aPS and aPE and included testing for IgA aPL as well as differentiating between those aPL that were dependent upon or independent of PL-binding plasma proteins. This study showed that there was no significant difference ($P = 0.480$) in the incidence of aPL between those BMT patients who went on to develop VOD/MODS (57/112) versus those that did not (55/112).

GVHD

An association between aPL and another post-transplant complication, GVHD, was reported by Sohngen and colleagues in a 54-year-old man who received HLA-identical marrow from his sister for treatment of chronic myleomonocytic leukemia [92]. His post-BMT clinical course was complicated by VOD, acute GVHD, and hematemesis secondary to an ulcer in the gastric mucosa. Seven months later after cyclosporine GVHD prophylaxis was tapered, the patient experienced severe chronic GVHD and a significant drop in platelet count. At this time IgG aCL and LA were detected in his blood. Therapy with high dose IvIg and prednisone was not effective. After reinstitution of cyclosporine, the platelet count returned to normal; clinical signs of chronic GVHD and all autoantibodies vanished. The authors concluded that LA as well as other autoantibodies might contribute to chronic GVHD.

A larger, dual center study of chronic GVHD was reported by Quaranta and associates [93]. Eighty-nine BMT recipients who presented with chronic GVHD 106 to 1507 days post-infusion were tested for a number of allo- and autoantibodies as part of an investigation for an association between chronic GVHD and primary biliary cirrhosis. The sera from the patients with GVHD were found to have a variety of autoantibodies including IgG, IgA, and IgM aCL, which were positive in 9 patients (10.1%). The authors did not address the significance of aPL in the setting of chronic GVHD.

An LA in the absence of aCL was detected in a 28-year-old man who received a matched-related allogenic BMT for treatment of aplastic anemia [94]. The patient's immediate post-transplant course was uneventful; engraftment was documented on day 16 and he was discharged from the hospital on day 24. The patient returned on day 34 with symptoms of gastric GVHD. The patient had a normal aPTT prior to transplant but at presentation with acute GVHD, an LA was detected. There was no clinical evidence of thrombosis or systemic bleeding. Methylprednisolone therapy was started and his gastrointestinal symptoms improved. The LA remained abnormal after 6 days of steriod therapy. His acute GVHD flare subsided with initiation of a 4-week course of infliximab. Follow-up 4 months later found the aPTT normal. These authors offer three possible mechanisms for de novo development of the LA in this patient. First, damage of the cell membranes by direct allograft effect (gastrointestinal GVHD). Second, damage of cell membranes secondary to the cytotoxic effects of chemotherapy, namely cyclophosphamide. And the third possibility was the combined effects of the first two proposed mechanisms.

An unsolved mystery in autoimmune conditions as well as in transplantation is the stimulus or trigger for development of aPL. Many investigators concur that genetic components are involved, but there is also the proposal that aPL production is the consequence of a second "hit" or signal. In certain experimental situations, the second (or environmental) signal appears to be recognition of and response to cells that undergo apoptosis. In studies reported by Mevorach apoptosis of murine thymocytes was induced by irradiation, the apoptotic cells then were intravenously injected into syngeneic, age-match recipients [95, 96]. The recipient mice, initially aPL naïve, were bled at intervals post-transplant and were shown to produce aPL and autoantibodies to ssDNA that were self-limiting after 10 weeks. Repeat injection of apoptotic cells induced a second round of aPL production.

These data are intriguing inasmuch as the appearance of aPL may represent a physiological overload mechanism that has the purpose of opsonizing excess cells undergoing programmed cell death and to remove them from the circulation without bringing about inflammatory responses and necrosis [97]. Inasmuch as the primary diseases leading to transplantation may have exposed these patients to excessive numbers of apoptotic cells, the immunological defect in aPL-positive patients may be related to the loss of regulation of this overload network. Production of aPL may be a normal response to infection and/or normal apoptotic processes, but failure to downregulate the aPL production could promote a chronic thrombogenic state. In short, persistent presence of aPL may reflect a situation wherein a regulatory mechanism for keeping aPL under control has been compromised; consequently the patient continues to produce aPL and is at risk for aPL-associated thrombosis.

Lessons from Mice

The clinical accounts suggestive of aPL being a risk factor in BMT prompted several basic experiments using mice that develop systemic autoimmunity involving autoantibodies such as aCL and other lupus-associated features. Transplantation of T-cell depleted marrow from autoimmune-prone W/BF$_1$ mice into irradiated autoimmune-resistant B6C3F$_1$ mice resulted in induction of aCL and lupus-like disease [88]. In reciprocal experiments T-cell depleted marrow from B6C3F$_1$ mice was transplanted to W/BF$_1$ mice, whereupon the lupus-like symptoms and aCL production were prevented in the W/BF$_1$ mice. These results imply that production of aCL is at least partly due to genetic abnormalities within radiosensitive bone marrow stem cells. Moreover, the transplanted B6C3F$_1$ mice that went on to develop cardiovascular disease (CVD) had higher titers of aCL than the transplanted B6C3F$_1$ mice who did not develop CVD ($P < 0.01$). The question that remains unanswered is: Did the CVD stimulate the production of aCL or did the presence of aCL result in CVD?

A second study examined the incidence of gastrointestinal (GI) vasculitis in the same strains of autoimmune-prone and -resistant mice [98]. Similar to the previous experiments, these investigators found that T-cell depleted marrow from W/BF$_1$ mice caused fatal GI vasculitis in recipient B6C3F$_1$ mice. In contrast, transfer of B6C3F$_1$ T-cell depleted marrow to irradiated W/BF$_1$ mice was protective. Mice engrafted with W/BF$_1$ marrow that developed vasculitis had significantly higher titers of aCL than engrafted mice without GI vasculitis ($P < 0.005$).

Additional experiments using marrow transfered from BALB/c mice to lethally irradiated W/BF$_1$ mice by Adachi and coworkers reported that post-transplant, thrombocytopenia, leukocytosis, renal dysfunction, and hypertension were ameliorated in the transplanted W/BF$_1$ mice [99]. Non-treated mice died of myocardial infarction or renal failure by age 7 months, whereas 60% of transplanted mice survived more than 1 year. The treated mice showed no signs of myocardial infarction, which was attributed to lower levels of aCL subsequent to transplantation.

In contrast to the above studies which resolved the natural production of autoimmune disease, Blank et al demonstrated transfer of APS through BMT [100]. Whole cell marrow from mice with an experimentally induced APS transferred to naïve BALB/c mice resulted in development of experimental APS in the recipients. Intrestingly, T-cell depleted marrow failed to transfer the disease as aPL production was not induced, nor was a high rate of fetal resorptions observed in recipients of T-cell depleted marrow.

Explanations for the incongruent results between this study with those mentioned previously are not straightforward. Genetic variations among the different strains of mice used in these various studies may contribute to the variant results.

BMT Summary

Although aPL have been associated with post-BMT thrombotic events, aPL also have been detected subsequent to post-transplant bleeding episodes [82, 83]. A large study of pre-transplant blood samples collected before chemo-radiation therapy failed to find a correlation between aPL and post-transplant VOD or MODS [91]. In fact, allogenic as well as autologous BMT has resulted in abrogation of aPL and APS [84–87]. Summarized in Table 19.7, the risks of BMT for the aPL-positive patient are not as pathognomonic as reported for solid organ transplant recipients.

Table 19.7. Antiphospholipid antibody associated findings in bone marrow transplant.

- LA may develop in the first months after BMT
- aPL may disappear after BMT
- CMV infection associated with aCL seroconversion post-BMT
- No aPL association with development of VOD or MODS
- aPL associated with GVHD
- Autoimmunity can be transferred by BMT in mice
- The sequela of autoimmune disease can be corrected with BMT

LA = lupus anticoagulant; aPL = antiphospholipid antibody; BMT = bone marrow transplant; CMV = cytomegalovirus; VOD = veno-occlusive disease; MODS = multiple organ dysfunction syndrome

Summary

From the data provided in the majority of the solid organ and tissue transplant publications, the presence of aPL should be considered a significant risk factor for any potential transplant candidate. The greatest risk is found in the first 6 months after transplantation [101]. For some patients, however, the hypercoagulable state persists throughout life and thrombotic loss of the transplanted organ can occur years after transplantation surgery [48, 49]. Peritoneal dialysis patients awaiting renal transplantation appear to be at utmost risk. Treatment for aPL associated risks remains focused on anticoagulation therapy. The use of immunosuppressive agents has not proven to have a dramatic effect on aPL titers and has little effect on clinical events [102]. Given the serious psychological and economic impact of irreversible thrombosis in a transplanted organ, the modest expense of pre-transplant aPL screening should be readily justified.

In the United States in 2003, the average cost of a kidney transplant lost to aPL associated thrombosis was estimated to be $117,317 (range, $62,000–$204,000) [103]. The expense of losing a transplanted heart or liver to aPL associated thrombosis not only includes healthcare dollars, but often includes loss of a patient's life. The encouraging news is that once aPL are identified pre-transplant, prophylactic anticoagulation appears capable of averting aPL associated allograft events.

The effects that aPL have relative to BMT are altogether different than those ascribed to solid organs and tissues. By definition, the transplantation of allogeneic bone marrow serves to reconstitute the recipient with a completely new and in cases of allogenic BMT, a genetically different repertoire of antibody producing cells. Previously aPL-positive bone marrow recipients have become aPL negative subsequent to transplantation, assuming that the marrow donor was aPL negative. These observations are the basis for contemporary experimental approaches to curing certain autoimmune diseases with BMT. Similarly, as has been shown in experimental mouse models, an aPL-negative patient, provided cells from an aPL-positive donor, could become aPL positive and suffer increased risk for thrombosis.

Clearly, much remains to be discovered in laboratory exploration of the pathobiology of aPL as well as in instituting methods to neutralize their procoagulant effects at the bedside.

References

1. Converse JM, Cassan P. The histological background of transplantation. In: Rapaport FT, Dausset J, eds. Human Transplantation. 1968:3–10.
2. Murray JE, Merrill JP. Renal homotransplantation in identical twins. Surgical Forum 1955;6:432.
3. Colman RW, Braun WE, Busch G, et al. Coagulation studies in the hyperacute and other forms of renal allograft rejection. N Eng J Med 1969;281:685–691.
4. Taylor LM, Chitwood RW, Dalman RL, et al. Antiphospolipid antibodies in vascular surgery patients. A cross-sectional study. Ann Surg 1994;220:544–551.
5. Irish A. Hypercoagulability in renal transplant recipients. Identifying patients at risk of renal allograft thrombosis and evaluating strategies for prevention. Am J Cardiovasc Drugs 2004;4:139–149.
6. Kujovich JL. Thrombophilia and thrombotic problems in renal transplant patients. Transplantation 2004;77:959–964.
7. Wagenknecht DR, Sugi T, McIntyre JA. The evolution, evaluation and interpretation of antiphospholipid antibody assays. Clin Immunol Newsletter 1995;15:28–38.
8. McIntyre JA, Wagenknecht DR, Sugi T. Phospholipid binding plasma proteins required for antiphospholipid antibody detection – An overview. Am J Reprod Immunol 1997;37:101–110.
9. McIntyre JA, Wagenknecht DR. Antiphospholipid antibodies. Risk assessments for solid organ, bone marrow and tissue transplantation. Rheum Dis Clin North Am 2001;27:611–631.
10. Liano F, Mampaso F, Martin FG, et al. Allograft membranous glomerulonephritis and renal-vein thrombosis in a patient with a lupus anticoagulant factor. Nephrol Dial Transplant 1988;3:684–689.
11. Marcen R, Pascual J, Quereda C, et al. Lupus anticoagulant and thrombosis of kidney allograft vessels. Transplant Proc 1990;22:1396–1398.
12. Sitter T, Spannagl M, Schiffl H. Anticardiolipin antibodies and lupus anticoagulant in patients treated with different methods of renal replacement therapy in comparison to patients with systemic lupus erythematosus. Ann Hematol 1992;65:79–82.
13. Oymak O, Erdem Y, Yalcin AU, et al. Increased prevalence of anticardiolipin antibodies in renal transplant recipients. Nephron 1995;71:469–470.
14. Fabrizi F, Sangiorgio R, Pontoriero G, et al. Antiphospholipid (aPL) antibodies in end-stage renal disease. J Nephrol 1999;12:89–94.
15. Grandtnerova B, Gregova H, Mocikova H, et al. Anticardiolipin antibodies after kidney transplantation in patients with connective tissue disease. Transplant Proc 1999;31:228–229.
16. Marcucci R, Zanazzi M, Bertoni E, et al. Risk factors for cardiovascular disease in renal transplant recipients: new insights. Transpl Int 2000;13(suppl 1):S419–S424.
17. Ducloux D, Bourrinet E, Motte G, et al. Antiphospholipid antibodies as a risk factor for atherosclerotic events in renal transplant recipients. Kidney Int 2003;64:1065–1070.
18. Nampoory MR, Das KC, Johny KV, et al. Hypercoagualibility, a serious problem in patients with ESRD on maintenance dialysis, and its correction after kidney transplantation. Am J Kidney Dis 2003;42:797–805.
19. Fischereder M, Gohring P, Schneeberger H, et al. Early loss of renal transplants in patients with thrombophilia. Transplantation 1996;65:936–939.
20. Wagenknecht DR, Becker DG, LeFor WM, et al. Antiphospholipid antibodies are a risk factor for early renal allograft failure. Transplantation 1999;68:241–246.
21. Murphy BG, Hill CM, Middleton D, et al. Increased renal allograft thrombosis in CAPD patients. Nephrol Dial Transplant 1994;9:1166–1169.
22. Wagenknecht DR, Fastenau DR, Torry RJ, et al. Risk of early renal allograft failure is increased for patients with antiphospholipid antibodies. Transplant Int 2000;134:S78–S81.
23. Wagenknecht DR, Carter CB, McIntyre JA. Antiphospholipid antibodies are implicated in early renal allograft failure. Clin Hemost Rev 1998;12:19.
24. Wagenknecht DR, Fastenau DR, Torry RJ, et al. Antiphospholipid antibodies are a risk factor for early renal allograft failure: isolation of antiphospholipid antibodies from a thrombosed renal allograft. Transplant Proc 1999;31:285–288.
25. Humar A, Key N, Ramcharan T, et al. Kidney retransplants after initial graft loss to vascular thrombosis. Clin Transplantation 2001;15:6–10.
26. Mondragon-Ramirez G, Bochicchio T, Garcia-Torres R, et al. Recurrent renal thrombotic angiopathy after kidney transplantation in two patients with primary antiphospholipid syndrome (PAPS). Clin Transplant 1994;8:93–96.

27. Chew CG, Bannister KM, Mathew TH, et al. Thrombotic microangiopathy related to anticardiolipin antibody in a renal allograft. Nephrol Dial Transplant 1999;14:436–438.

28. Knight RJ, Schanzer H, Rand JH, et al. Renal allograft thrombosis associated with the antiphospholipid antibody syndrome. Transplantation 1995;60:614–615.

29. Vaidya S, Wang CC, Gugliuzza C, et al. Relative risk of post-transplant renal thrombosis in patients with antiphospholipid antibodies. Clin Transplant 1998;12:439–444.

30. Vaidya S, Sellers R, Kimball P, et al. Frequency, potential risk and therapeutic intervention in end-stage renal disease patients with antiphospholipid antibody syndrome. Transplantation 2000;69:1348–1352.

31. Vaidya S, Gugliuzza K, Daller JA. Efficacy of anticoagulation threapy in end-stage renal disease patients with antiphospholipid antibody syndrome. Transplantation 2004;77:1046–1049.

32. Morrissey PE, Ramirez PJ, Gohh RY, et al. Management of thrombophilia in renal transplant patients. Am J Transplant 2002;2:872–876.

33. Friedman GS, Meier-Kriesche HU, Kaplan B, et al. Hypercoagulable states in renal transplant candidates: impact of anticoagulation upon incidence of renal allograft thrombosis. Transplantation 2001;72:1073–1078.

34. Ducloux D, Pellet E, Chalopin J-M. Prevalence and clinical significance of antiphospholipid antibodies in renal transplant recipients. Transplant Proc 1997;29:2400–2401.

35. Ducloux D, Pellet E, Fournier V, et al. Prevalence and clinical significance of antiphospholipid antibodies in renal transplant recipients. Transplantation 1999;67:90–93.

36. Radhakrishnan J, Williams GS, Appel GB, et al. Renal transplantation in anticardiolipin antibody-positive lupus erythematosus patients. Am J Kid Dis 1994;23:286–289.

37. Stone JH, Amend W, Criswell LA. Antiphospholipid antibody syndrome in renal transplantation: occurrence of clinical events in 96 consecutive patients with systemic lupus erythematosus. Am J Kid Dis 1999;34:1040–1047.

38. Mathis AS, Shah NK. Exaggerated response to heparin in a post-operative renal transplant recipient with lupus anticoagulant undergoing plasmapheresis. Transplantation 2004;77:957–958.

39. Baid S, Pascual M, Williams WWJ, et al. Renal thrombotic microangiopathy associated with anticardiolipin antibodies in hepatitis C-positive renal allograft recipients. J Am Soc Nephrol 1999;10:146–153.

40. Wullstein C, Woeste G, Zapletal C, et al. Prothrombotic disorders in uremic type-1 diabetics undergoing simultaneous pancreas and kidney transplantation. Transplantation 2003;76:1691–1695.

41. Wullstein C, Woeste G, Zapletal C, et al. Simultaneous pancreas-kidney transplantaion in patients with antiphospholipid syndrome. Transplantation 2003;75:562–563.

42. Talenti DA, Falk GW, Carey WD, et al. Anticardiolipin antibody-associated cerebral infarction in cirrhosis: clearance of anticardiolipin antibody after liver transplantation. Am J Gastroenterol 1994;89:785–788.

43. Yasutomi M, Egawa H, Kobayashi Y, et al. Living donor liver transplantation for Budd-Chiari syndrome with inferior vena cava obstruction and associated antiphospholipid antibody syndrome. J Pediatr Surg 2001;36:659–662.

44. Villamil A, Sorkin E, Basta MC, et al. Catastrophic antiphospholipid syndrome complicating orthotopic liver transplantation. Lupus 2003;12:104–143.

45. Van Thiel DH, George M, Brems J, et al. Antiphospholipid antibodies before and after liver transplantation. Am J Gastroenterol 2003;98:460–465.

46. Lallier M, St-Vil D, Dubois J, et al. Vascular complications after pediatric liver transplantation. J Ped Surg 1995;30:1122–1126.

47. Pascual M, Thadhani R, Laposata M, et al. Anticardiolipin antibodies and hepatic artery thrombosis after liver transplantation. Transplantation 1997;64:1361–1364.

48. Vivarelli M, La Barba G, Legnani C, et al. Repeated graft loss caused by recurrent hepatic artery thrombosis after liver transplantation. Liver Transpl 2003;9:629–631.

49. Collier JD, Sale J, Friend PJ, et al. Graft loss and the antiphospholipid syndrome following liver transplantation. J Hepatol 1998;29:999–1003.

50. Pengo V, Biasiolo A, Marson P, et al. Immunosuppressive treatment in a heart transplantation candidate with antiphospholipid syndrome. Clin Rheumatol 1996;15:504–507.

51. McIntyre JA, Wagenknecht DR, Faulk WP. Antiphospholipid antibodies in heart transplant recipients. Clin Cardiol 1995;18:575–580.

52. Lye WC, Henell KR, Norman DJ. Antiphospholipid antibodies causing positive flow crossmatches and interfering with T-cell immunophenotyping. Transplant Proc 1992;24:1683–1684.

53. McIntyre JA, Higgins N, Britton R, et al. Utilization of intravenous immunoglobulin to ameliorate alloantibodies in a highly sensitized patient with a cardiac assist device awaiting heart transplantation. Transplantation 1996;62:691–623.
54. Griffith BP, Kormos RL, Nastala CJ, et al. Results of extended bridge to transplantation: window into the future of permanent ventricular assist devices. Ann Thorac Surg 1996;61:396–398.
55. Fastenau DR, Wagenknecht DR, McIntyre JA. Increased incidence of antiphospholipid antibodies in left ventricular assist system recipients. Ann Thorac Surg 1999;68:137–142.
56. Matsubayashi H, Fastenau D, McIntyre JA. Changes in platelet activation associated with left ventricular assist system placement. J Heart Lung Transplant 2000;19:462–468.
57. Fastenau DR, Hormuth DA, McIntyre JA. Antiphospholipid antibodies in left-ventricular assist system recipients after exposure to topical bovine thrombin. Transplant Proc 1998;31:141–142.
58. Fastenau DR, McIntyre JA. Immunochemical analysis of polyspecific antibodies in patients exposed to bovine fibrin sealant. Ann Thorarc Surg 2000;69:1867–1872.
59. Unger P, Plein D, Pradier O, et al. Thrombosis of aortic valve homograft associated with lupus anticoagulant antibodies. Ann Thorac Surg 2004;77:312–314.
60. Matsuyama K, Ueda Y, Ogino H, et al. Aortic valve replacement for aortic regurgitation in a patient with primary antiphoshpolipid syndrome. Jpn Circ J 1999;63:725–726.
61. Dornan RIP. Acute postoperative biventricular failure associated with antiphospholipid antibody syndrome. Br J Anaesth 2004;92:748–754.
62. Brownstein L, Bartholomew TP, Silver DG, et al. A case report of mitral valve replacement in a patient with lupus antibody syndrome. Perfusion 2003;18:373–376.
63. Kato Y, Isobe F, Sasaki Y, et al. Secondary mitral valve replacement in antiphospholipid syndrome and chronic renal failure. Jpn J Thorac Cardvasc Surg 2001;49:728–731.
64. Da Silva AN, Ferreira LD, Monaco CG, et al. Intracardiac thrombosis and mitral prosthesis dysfunction in systemic lupus erythematosus. A case report. Rev Port Cardiol 2003;22:213–219.
65. Berkun Y, Elami A, Meir K, et al. Increased morbidity and mortality in patients with antiphospholipid syndrome undergoing valve replacement surgery. J Thorac Cardiovasc Surg 2004;127:414–420.
66. Simonneau G, Azarian R, Brenot F, et al. Surgical management of unresolved pulmonary embolism. A personal series of 72 patients. Chest 1995;107:52S–55S.
67. Asherson RA, Higenbottam TW, Xuan Dinh AT, et al. Pulmonary hypertension in a lupus clinic: experience with twenty-four patients. J Rheumatol 1990;17:1292–1298.
68. Yeatman M, McNeil K, Smith JA, et al. Lung transplantation in patients with systemic diseases: an eleven-year experience at Papworth Hospital. J Heart Lung Transplant 1995;15:144–149.
69. Nathan SD, Barnett SD, Urban BA, et al. Pulmonary embolism in idiopathic pulmonary fibrosis transplant recipients. Chest 2003;123:1758–1763.
70. Magro CM, Allen J, Pope-Harman A, et al. The role of microvascular injury in the evolution of idiopathic pulmonary fibrosis. Am J Clin Pathol 2003;119:556–567.
71. Nathan SD, Barnett SD. Reply to letter to the editor: Idiopathic pulmonary fibrosis in transplantation. Chest 2003;124:2404.
72. Jankowich MD. Idiopathic pulmonary fibrosis in transplantation. Chest 2003;124:2404.
73. Dauerman HL, Cutlip DE, Selke FW. Intracoronary thrombolysis in the treatment of graft closure immediately after CABG. Ann Thorac Surg 1996;62:280–283.
74. Nakayama M, Kumon K, Yagagi N, et al. Antiphospholipid antibody syndrome in a case with redo coronary artery bypass grafting under cardiopulmonary bypass. Jpn J Surg 1998;28:423–426.
75. Lee RW, Taylor LM, Landry GJ, et al. Prospective comparison of infrainguinal bypass grafting in patients with and without antiphospholipid antibodies. J Vascular Surg 1996;24:524–531.
76. Nielsen TG, Nordestgaard BG, von Jessen F, et al. Antibodies to cardiolipin may increase the risk of failure of peripheral vein bypasses. Eur J Endovasc Surg 1997;14:177–184.
77. Gargiulo P, Goldberg J, Romani B, et al. Qualitative and quantitative studies of autoantibodies to phospholipids in diabetes mellitus. Clin Exp Immunol 1999;118:30–34.
78. Ray SA, Rowley MR, Loh A, et al. Hypercoagulable states in patients with leg ischaemia. Br J Surg 1994;81:811–814.
79. Prakash R, Miller CC, Suki WN. Anticardiolipin antibody in patients on maintenance hemodialysis and its association with recurrent arteriovenous graft thrombosis. Am J Kidney Dis 1995;26:347–352.
80. LeSar CJ, Merrick HW, Smith MR. Thrombotic complications resulting from hypercoagulable states in chronic hemodialysis vascular access. J Am Coll Surg 1999;189:73–81.

81. Conlan MG, Haire WD, Kessinger A, et al. Prothrombotic hemostatic abnormalities in patients with refractory malignant lymphoma presenting for autologous stem cell transplantation. Bone Marrow Transplant 1991;7:475–479.

82. Greeno EW, Haake R, McGlave P, et al. Lupus inhibitors following bone marrow transplant. Bone Marrow Transplant 1995;15:287–291.

83. Qasim W, Gerritsen B, Veys P. Anticardiolipin antibodies and thromboembolism after BMT. Bone Marrow Transplant 1998;21:845–847.

84. Ollalla JI, Ortin M, Hermida G, et al. Disappearance of lupus anticoagulant after allogeneic bone marrow transplantation. Bone Marrow Transplant 1999;23:83–85.

85. Musso M, Porretto F, Crescimanno A, et al. Autologous peripheral blood stem and progenitor (CD34+) cell transplantation for systemic lupus erythematosus complicated by Evans Syndrome. Lupus 1998;7:492–494.

86. Hashimoto N, Iwasaki T, Sekiguchi I, et al. Autologous hematopoietic stem cell transplantation for refractory antiphospholipid syndrome causing myocardial necrosis. Bone Marrow Transplant 2004;33:863–866.

87. Elhasid R, Rowe JM, Berkowitz D, et al. Disappearance of diffuse calcinosis following autologous stem cell transplantation in a child with autoimmune disease. Bone Marrow Transplant 2004;33:1257–1259.

88. Mizutani H, Engelman RW, Kinjoh K, et al. Prevention and induction of occlusive coronary vascular disease in autoimmune $(W/B)F_1$ mice by haploidentical bone marrow transplantation: Possible role for anticardiolipin autoantibodies. Blood 1993;82:3091–3092.

88a. Mengarelli A, Minotti C, Palumbo G, et al. High levels of antiphospholipid antibodies are associated with cytomegalovirus infection in unrelated bone marrow and cord blood allogeneic stem cell transplantation. Br J Haematol 2000;108:126–131.

89. Gharavi AE, Pierangeli S, Harris EN. New developments in viral peptides and APL induction. J Autoimmun 2000;15:227–230.

90. Morio S, Oh H, Hirasawa A, et al. Hepatic veno-occlusive disease in a patient with lupus anticoagulant after allogeneic bone marrow transplantation. Bone Marrow Transplant 1991;8:147–149.

91. Fastenau D, Haire W, Schneider J, et al. The pre-conditioning incidence of antiphospholipid antibodies is not significantly increased in patients with bone marrow transplant-related organ dysfunction. Bone Marrow Transplant 1998;22:681–684.

92. Sohngen D, Heyll A, Meckenstock G, et al. Antiphospholipid syndrome complicating chronic graft-verses-host disease after allogenic bone marrow transplantation. Am J Hematol 1994;47:143–144.

93. Quaranta S, Shulman H, Ahmed A, et al. Autoantibodies in human chronic graft-versus-host disease after hematopoietic cell transplantation. Clin Immunol 1999;91:106–116.

94. Kharfan-Dabaja MA, Morgensztern D, Santos E, et al. Acute graft-versus-host disease (aGVHD) presenting with an acquired lupus anticoagulant. Bone Marrow Transplant 2003;31:129–131.

95. Mevorach D. The immune response to apoptotic cells. Ann N Y Acad Sci 1999;887:191–198.

96. Mevorach D, Zhou JL, Song X, et al. Systemic exposure to irradiated apoptotic cells induces autoantibody production. J Exp Med 1998;188:387–392.

97. Manfredi AA, Rovere P, Galati G, et al. Apoptotic cell clearance in systemic lupus erythematosus. I. Opsonization by antiphospholipid antibodies. Arthritis Rheum 1998;41:205–241.

98. Mizutani H, Engelman RW, Kinjoh K, et al. Gastrointestinal vasculitis in autoimmune-prone (NZW X BXSB)F_1 mice: association with anticardiolipin autoantibodies. Proc Soc Exp Biol Med 1995;209:279–285.

99. Adachi Y, Inaba M, Amoh Y, et al. Effect of bone marrow transplantation on antiphospholipid antibody syndrome in murine lupus mice. Immunobiology 1995;192:218–230.

100. Blank M, Krause I, Lanir N, et al. Transfer of experimental antiphospholipid syndrome by bone marrow cell transplantation. Arthritis Rheum 1995;38:115–162.

101. Kazory A, Ducloux D. Acquired hypercoagulable state in renal transplant recipients. Thromb Haemost 2004;91:646–654.

102. Joseph RE, Radhakrishnan J, Appel GB. Antiphospholipid antibody syndrome and renal disease. Curr Opin Nephrol Hypertens 2001;10:175–181.

103. McIntyre JA, Wagenknecht DR. Antiphospholipid antibodies and renal transplantation: a risk assessment. Lupus 2003;12:555–559.

20   Antiphospholipid Syndrome in Children

Lori B. Tucker and Rolando Cimaz

Introduction

The scientific and clinical understanding of the phenomenon of antiphospholipid antibodies (aPL) has grown enormously since the first descriptions of an inhibitor of in vitro clotting tests in the serum of some patients with systemic lupus erythematosus (SLE) by Conley and Hartman [1], and the subsequent connection of these inhibitors to the occurrence of thromboses [2]. The lupus anticoagulant (LA) described in these early studies was found to be an antibody directed against phospholipids [3]. Extensive studies of adult populations have further identified the primary clinical associations of aPL: recurrent venous and arterial thromboses, thrombocytopenia, and recurrent fetal losses. Other less common or minor clinical findings described in adults with aPL include valvular heart disease, early myocardial infarction, pulmonary hypertension, renovascular microthrombotic disease, hemolytic anemia, transverse myelitis, chorea, and livedo reticularis [4].

In comparison to the enormous amount of information concerning aPL in adults, there has been relatively less research in the area of aPL in pediatrics [5–10]. aPL and their associated clinical features are now recognized to occur in children, although not commonly. Pathogenic mechanisms involved in pediatric antiphospholipid syndrome (APS) appear to be the same as in adults. However, because pediatric patients generally do not have many of the prothrombotic risk factors that can be present in adults, there are clearly differences in the spectrum of clinical findings. The presence of aPL and associated clinical events have been well-described in some children with SLE but occurs in those without SLE as well. In children, one of the most common reported clinical problems associated with aPL is that of cerebral ischemic stroke, in general a relatively rare occurrence in childhood. The less common thrombotic events in children found to have aPL have mainly been the subject of individual case reports.

This chapter will review the current state of knowledge of aPL in pediatrics. The focus of the chapter will be clinical; to date, there is no information to suggest that aPL in children are immunochemically different from those found in adults.

aPL in Healthy Children

aPL can be found in children without any discernible disease. Such naturally occurring aPL are usually present in low titer and could be the result of previous infections and/or vaccinations, common events in the pediatric populations [11–13]. A number of studies have addressed the of aPL in healthy children. Findings have been variable, with results ranging from 2% to 82% of healthy children having measurable aPL [12, 14–19]. This wide range may be related to methodological issues such as inappropriate study groups, different definitions of cut-off values, and lack of uniformity in assay methods. Kontiainen et al looked for anticardiolipin antibodies (aCL) in 173 children who had minor surgical or psychosomatic problems and found a surprisingly high frequency of positive aCL (82%). However, a much lower percentage of these children (5%) had aCL of a moderate-high titer [45 G phospholipid units (GPL) or higher] [17]. The significance of such a high percentage of well children testing positive for low titer aCL is unknown. A similar study looking at children with functional disorders was performed by Rapizzi et al, who found positive aCL in 26% of the children in the study group [12]. In contrast, the other smaller previously mentioned studies have reported quite low frequencies of aCL (under 5%) in healthy children. Avèin et al have examined aPL in a group of 61 apparently healthy children at regular preventive visits and found aCL positivity in 11% and anti–β_2-glycoprotein I (β_2-GPI) in 7%, respectively [13]. In addition, mean values of IgG and IgM aCL were comparable between different age groups, while the mean value of IgA aCL was significantly higher in adult blood donors than in preschool children and adolescents. Moreover, it was found that the mean value of IgG anti–β_2-GPI was highest in preschool children and in this group it was significantly higher than in adolescents and blood donors. This novel finding was attributed by the authors to a possible faulty immune response to nutritional exposure to β_2-GPI in infancy. In particular, because β_2-GPI molecule has been remarkably conserved during the evolution of animal species [20], it is possible that ingestion of bovine β_2-GPI found in different milk or meat products could act as an oral immunization agent and induce transitory production of anti–β_2-GPI in infants, in whom the intestinal mucosa is more permissive for large molecules [21].

LA have also been described in healthy children [11, 22, 23]. They are usually discovered incidentally in pre-operative evaluations of children scheduled for surgeries such as tonsillectomy, who present with prolonged activated partial thromboplastin time (aPTT). In many cases no definite diagnosis is established, and the aPTT spontaneously corrects to the normal range. In one series, positive LA were identified in 7% of 61 apparently healthy children (Avèin et al, unpublished data), and, similarly to previous studies [11, 22, 23], no correlations between LA and aCL/anti–β_2-GPI were observed.

The clinical significance of positive aPL or LA discovered incidentally in children is unknown. In the study by Male et al [11], 95 children identified in a single pediatric tertiary care center and who were found to have a positive LA were followed over a 27-year time period. Eighty-four percent of these children had a LA diagnosed incidentally, in most cases during pre-operative screening tests, when routinely coagulation profiles are performed. One of these patients was found to have SLE. However, in follow up, none of these asymptomatic children developed bleeding, thrombosis, or autoimmune disease. This study suggests that most children with a LA discovered incidentally during laboratory screening will not have any clinical manifestations of APS, both at the time of diagnosis and in further follow up.

Studies of children with aPL that have included healthy controls are summarized in Table 20.1.

Table 20.1. Incidence of antiphospholipid antibodies in healthy children. 📖

Reference	No. patients	% + aPL (IgG; IgM if available)
Caporali [14]	42	IgG 0%; IgM 5%
Singer [35]	20	IgG 10%
Kratz [18]	20	IgG 0 ; IgM 5%
Kontiainen [17]	173	IgG 82%
Rapizzi [12]	100	IgG 26%; IgM & A 1%
Avcin [13]	61	IgG 11%

Clinical Associations of aPL in Childhood

Although the first description of aPL was in patients with SLE, it is well known that aPL can be found in individuals with a number of other conditions. Infections, certain medications, and other autoimmune conditions can be associated with the development of aPL, although not all may be associated with clinical events.

aPL have been described in adult patients with a broad range of *infections*, including acute common viral infections (24, 25). Infection-related aPL differ immunochemically from those seen in patients with autoimmune disease and have not been associated with the typical clinical features of aPL, such as thrombosis. Kratz et al [18] studied a group of 88 children with primarily upper airway infections and found that 30% were positive for aPL . The majority of the aPL identified were of IgM isotype, as would be expected in an acute infection. In the same study, 20% to 25% of a group of children with a variety of disorders including malignancies and inherited metabolic conditions (but excluding autoimmune diseases) were also positive for aPL. None of the children with positive aPL and infection, metabolic disease, or other conditions in this study developed thrombosis, consistent with findings in adult populations. Therefore, it is important for clinicians to remember that aPL can be found incidentally in children after any common viral infection [26, 27]. Because most children suffer from frequent viral infections, all positive aPL titers should be verified on at least 2 occasions, preferably at a time when the child has not had a recent infection. In one study of children with *HIV infection*, 82% of the patients were found to have IgG aCL [28]; these results are similar to those described in adults with HIV as well. *Varicella virus* infection has also been associated with unusual complications linked to aPL, that is, post-varicella purpura fulminans and thromboses [29]. However, healthy children with acute varicella infection have an increased prevalence of LA, unassociated with thrombosis or other clinical problems [30].

There is some evidence that aPL can be associated with *immunizations*. Recently, Blank et al induced the production of anti–β_2-GPI antibodies in mice immunized with *Haemophilus influenzae* or tetanus toxoid [31]. These antibodies were affinity-purified from the immunized mice and passively infused intravenously into naïve mice, where they induced typical APS manifestations. The aPL response to common childhood immunizations has not been studied so far in humans, but this is certainly a point to take into account when interpreting test results in recently immunized subjects.

There has been controversy concerning a possible association of aPL and clinical findings in *acute rheumatic fever* (ARF). Figueroa et al reported that 80% of their patients with active ARF had aCL compared with 40% of those with inactive ARF [32]. The control subjects in this study, however, were adults. No correlation could be established between the presence of chorea and aCL positivity. The authors reported a correlation of carditis and IgM aCL; however, this conclusion was based on the results from only 6 children with carditis (100% positives for IgM aCL) compared with 8 children without carditis (37% of whom were positive for IgM aCL). A second study of children with ARF [33] could not substantiate elevated aCL levels in children with ARF compared with healthy children as controls, and there was no correlation of aCL with disease activity.

aPL have been associated with a variety of *neurological manifestations*. Central nervous system involvement is frequently described in children with both the primary and secondary APS. The presence of aPL has been examined in several small groups of children with tic disorders who do not have recognized autoimmune disease. Although one study [34] showed the presence of LA and aCL in 4/9 children with *Tourette's syndrome*, a larger study done by Singer et al [35] did not show a significant increase in prevalence of aPL in 21 children tested, compared with healthy age-matched control subjects. Several investigators have reported that the prevalence of aPL-associated *cerebral ischemia* is particularly high in pediatric populations, ranging from 16% to 76% [36–39]. In view of these data, the screening of all children with ischemic stroke for aPL seems to be justified.

The association between *migraine* and aPL in children is not clear [40]. A recent study has shown that the prevalence of aPL does not appear to be increased in an unselected group of children with migraine. In this study, the prevalence of aPL, anti-β_2-GPI and LA did not differ significantly between patients with migraine, tension-type headaches, and healthy children [41]. These data suggest that aPL are not a significant factor related to migraine in children.

There is recent interesting data suggesting a potential role for aPL in the development of childhood *seizure* disorder in some patients. aPL have been reported in a case report [42] as well as in a series of children with partial seizures [43]. We have studied prospectively the presence of aPL in 142 pediatric patients with epilepsy and found positive aCL in 11%, anti-β_2-GPI in 18%, and antiprothrombin antibodies in 20% of patients [44]. In total, nearly 30% of the patients with epilepsy in this study tested positive for at least one subtype of aPL. A possible role in the pathogenesis of some forms of epilepsy can be hypothesized. In fact, microthrombotic central nervous system damage, or direct interaction of aPL with neuronal cell membranes could be the basis for development of epileptic seizures. A more recent study has independently confirmed these findings [45].

The presence of IgG aCL has been shown in 24% of a group of 29 children and adolescents with insulin-dependant *diabetes mellitus* [46]. Patients with aCL had a shorter disease duration than those without aCL; however, there were no other autoantibodies or specific clinical associations among these patients.

Interesting is the finding by Ambrožič et al of a high prevalence of IgG anti-β_2-GPI in *atopic dermatitis* of childhood [47], but not in other allergic disorders. These antibodies did not bind to β_2-GPI associated with cardiolipin, and no clinical signs of APS were present in the patients. Again, an interaction between dietary β_2-GPI and the human immune system was hypothesized.

The prevalence of aPL among children with *juvenile idiopathic arthritis* (JIA) has ranged from 8% to 53% in a small number of studies [14–16, 19, 48–50]. However, there has not been any association of thrombosis or other aPL-related clinical events in aPL-positive children with JIA, nor does there appear to be any association with JIA type or other characteristics of the disease. There is only one reported case of a child with JIA who developed a deep vein thrombosis (DVT) and was found to be positive for LA; however, this child was also immobilized due to a lower limb fracture and therefore had an additional risk factor for development of DVT [49]. Therefore, aPL in children with JIA may be an incidental finding. More recently, aPL have been also studied prospectively in childhood arthritis [51]. The values of aCL, anti-β_2-GPI and LA were prospectively followed in 28 patients from the beginning of the disease. Thirteen (46.4%) of them were positive for aCL already at the first referral, but during the follow up the frequency of aCL decreased from 46.4% to 28.6%. For anti–β_2-GPI, the difference in the frequency between the children with JIA and healthy children was not statistically significant. Serial determination of aPL levels in JIA patients revealed frequent fluctuations. None of the patients was persistently positive for LA. Associations between aCL, anti–β_2-GPI, or LA and disease activity could not be established, and no patient with positive aCL, anti–β_2-GPI, or LA showed any clinical feature of APS. The production of aCL in JIA could therefore be associated with an infectious trigger.

Although aPL are generally considered a risk factor for promoting thrombosis, hemorrhagic LAs have been described in adults. This association in the pediatric age has been described by Lee et al [52], and by Becton et al, who reported 6 previously healthy children with sudden onset of bleeding (epistaxis, hemarthrosis) due to transient LA (4 also with aCL) and hypoprothrombinemia [53].

Antiphospholipid-associated Clinical Events

The major clinical events associated with aPL are arterial or venous thrombosis, thrombocytopenia, and recurrent fetal loss. Minor, or less common, clinical events also associated with aPL include livedo reticularis, migraine, chorea, transverse myelitis, cardiac valvular abnormalities, Coombs' positivity, and hemolytic anemia. Most of these clinical findings have been described in children, although some are quite rare. Recurrent fetal losses are obviously not a pediatric problem, although potentially present in teenagers [54]. aPL-associated events have been described in children of all ages, even some as young as a few months of age.

Thrombosis

Thrombosis, either of arterial or venous vessels, is a central pathogenic phenomenon leading to a long list of clinical problems that have been related to the presence of aPL. In contrast to the situation in adulthood, thrombosis in general is a very uncommon clinical problem in pediatrics. This may be related to fewer general risk factors for thrombosis, such as advanced atherosclerosis, cigarette smoking, or contraceptive usage. Therefore, the finding of elevated aPL in children with thrombotic conditions suggests that the presence of aPL is one of the most common precipitating factors for this clinical problem when it occurs in children. Venous and arterial thromboses have been reported in children. Table 20.2 illustrates specific types of thrombotic, and in particular neurologic, problems reported in the literature in children with aPL (excluding those with SLE).

Table 20.2. Antiphospholipid associated clinical events in children (not associated with SLE). 📖

Reference	No. patients	Neurologic events	Thrombotic events	Additional comments
Bernstein [59]	2	–	Iliac vein, DVT, partial Budd-Chiari	–
Falcini [61]	1	Chorea	Myocardial infarction	Thrombocytopenia, livedo reticularis
Vlachoyianno-poulous [82]	1	Chorea	DVT	–
Roddy [55]	1	Infantile stroke	–	–
Ravelli [56]	1	–	SVC thrombosis	–
Hasegawa [71]	1	Spinal cord infarction	–	–
Schoning [36]	8	Ischemic stroke	–	–
Toren [34]	19	Ischemic stroke (1) Tourette's syndrome (3)	DVT (3)	Thrombocytopenia (10) IgA nephritis (1) Vasculitis (1)
Angelini [62]	10	Cerebral ischemia	–	–
Olson [64]	2	Ischemic stroke	–	Family + for primary APS
Manco-Johnson [93]	14	Ischemic stroke	Pulmonary embolism, central venous, arterial	–
Di Nucci [63]	1	Ischemic stroke	–	–
Baca [38]	10	Ischemic stroke	–	–
Von Scheven [58]	5	Ischemic stroke, chorea		Pulmonary embolism Digital ischemia, Addison disease
Brady [60]	1	–	Portal vein thrombosis	–
Nuss [57]	3	–	Pulmonary embolism, DVT	–
Ohtomo [72]	1	–	–	Renal thrombotic microangiopathy
Male [11]	5	TIA (1)	DVT (4)	–
Gattorno [16]	14	Cerebral stroke (5)	DVT (6), peripheral artery occlusion (2), myocardial infarction (1)	–

DVT = deep vein thrombosis; TIA = transient ischemic attack; SVC = superior vena cava

Venous occlusions due to aPL can occur in any blood vessel. Deep vein thrombosis is the most common venous thrombotic condition reported in children associated with aPL. In some cases the DVT was accompanied by pulmonary embolism [57]. Pulmonary hypertension related to microthromboembolic phenomenon is rare but reported in children [58], and therefore APS should be included in the differential of a child presenting with idiopathic pulmonary hypertension. aPL can also be a precipitant of Budd-Chiari syndrome, the thrombotic occlusion of the inferior vena cava and hepatic veins. There are a number of reports of children with Budd-Chiari syndrome who have elevated aPL [59] and it is possible that other children with this syndrome may have associated aPL but have not yet been tested. One case of isolated portal vein thrombosis has been reported secondary to APS [60]. Addison's disease and hypoadrenalism are also known to be caused by infarction of the adrenal glands due to aPL; this has also been reported in children [58]. Myocardial infarction at a young age should prompt the clinician to search for aPL, as there have been rare reports of this association in children [61].

Cerebral ischemic stroke is the most common neurologic event reported in association with aPL, and the most common arterial thrombotic condition. Increasingly, it is becoming clear that a significant proportion of children who suffer from idiopathic stroke, at any age, have elevated aPL levels [37, 62–64]. Angelini and colleagues [62] reported that among an unselected group of 13 children with idiopathic cerebral ischemia, 76% had moderate-to-high titer aPL. Of great interest is the finding that 50% of these children had multiple ischemic events. A study by Schöning et al confirms these findings [36]. These data suggest that aPL in children may rarely be associated with a condition similar to multi-infarct dementia in adults [65, 66].

Two large series of idiopathic cerebral venous and sinovenous thrombosis in children also have identified aPL as an important risk factor [67, 68]. In children with sinovenous thrombosis, the frequency of prothrombotic disorders is 12% to 50%, and the presence of aCL is the most common acquired disorder. In one of these studies [67], 32% of 123 children who underwent testing for prothrombotic disorders had at least one abnormality; the presence of aPL was the most common acquired disorder, with 10 children positive for IgG aCL and the presence of a LA in 4.

In a recent study of 65 unrelated children with ischemic stroke, multiple thrombophilia risk factors were studied and compared with 145 controls [39]. About half of the patients were found to have at least 1 thrombophilia marker, compared with only 25.5% of controls. Protein S, protein C, and antithrombin deficiency, as well as heterozygous FII G20210A and homozygous MTHFR 677T status were not statistically related to stroke. In contrast, the presence of aPL was associated with a greater than 6-fold risk of stroke [odds ratio (OR) = 6.08; 95% confidence interval (CI), 1.5-24.3], and the heterozygosity for factor V Leiden increased the risk of stroke by almost 5-fold (OR = 4.82; 95% CI, 1.4-16.5). Other aPLs may be risk factors for ischemic stroke; for example, stroke in a 20-month-old boy has been described in the presence of anti-β_2-GPI but with absent aCL and LA [69]. Similarly, Ebeling et al reported 6 children presenting with cerebral ischemic strokes prior to the age of 1 year, who were found to have elevated IgG antibodies to β_2-GPI; 4 of the 6 did not have aCL or LA [70].

There are other less common arterial thrombotic conditions reported in children with aPL. Renal artery thrombosis, retinal artery thrombosis, and myocardial infarction have been reported in rare situations in children with high titers of aPL . Transverse myelitis, seen rarely in children with systemic lupus, appears to be a possible thrombotic complication of aPL [71]. Renal thrombotic microangiopathy, a rare finding in adults with APS, has been also described in an adolescent with primary APS who presented with severe hypertension, renal impairment, and a history of Raynaud's phenomenon [72].

Other Clinical Features

Thrombocytopenia is one of the major clinical associations of aPL reported in adults. Patients with SLE and thrombocytopenia have a high incidence of aPL positivity, as do those with Evans' syndrome (hemolytic anemia and thrombocytopenia) [73]. aPL were found as well in 30% of patients with chronic ITP [74]. Thrombocytopenia has been reported in children with primary APS and in two thirds of children with SLE and aPL [75, 76]. Toren et al reported thrombocytopenia in 52% of children with primary APS [77]. Ura et al described a 3-year-old child with immune thrombocytopenic purpura and aPL who later developed clinical findings suggesting APS [78].

Hematologic abnormalities other than thrombocytopenia may also occur in patients who have aPL. Patients with autoimmune hemolytic anemia and Evans' syndrome have been reported to have a high frequency of associated aPL. In one report of 12 SLE patients with aPL and Evans' syndrome, 2 of the patients had childhood-onset SLE [73]. Another recent report [79] described a 14-year-old girl with Evans' syndrome, initially manifested as severe menorrhagia, and high titer aPL, whose severe cytopenias improved with steroids. Interestingly, her thrombocytopenia never resolved completely until low-dose aspirin was administered. Gattorno et al reported 2 adolescent girls presenting with autoimmune hemolytic anemia who later developed thrombosis and were found to be aPL positive [16].

Chorea, a well-known manifestion of adult APS [80], has been reported in aPL-positive children as well [81–84]. In the Euro-Phospholipid project [85], chorea was more prevalent in childhood-onset APS than in adults, with an odds ratio of 17.8.

Among other manifestations, *livedo reticularis* is also mentioned frequently in children with APS as a concomitant clinical finding, and *optic neuropathy* has been described in primary APS [86]. Finally, *catastrophic APS* can occur in children and neonates as well [87–91].

aPL in Childhood-onset SLE

aPL have been reported in a high frequency of adult patients with SLE. Adult patients with SLE and associated aPL have a high risk of thromboembolic events of all types, cardiac valvular disease, thrombocytopenia, and other autoimmune cytopenias. Similarly, studies examining children with SLE have reported finding aPL in 19% to 87% of patients (Table 20.3). In 9 reported series of aPL in children with SLE, the mean prevalence rates for aCL and LA were 45% and 22%, respectively. Gedalia et al screened a general pediatric rheumatology population (n = 106) for presence of aCL, and patients with SLE had the greatest frequency of positivity (37%) when compared to other diagnoses; however, most of these positive tests were low levels of IgG aCL, and no clinical complications were seen [92]. In some cases, a thrombosis associated with aPL has been the presenting sign for the diagnosis of SLE [93]. Conclusions from studies of pediatric patients with SLE are limited by small numbers of patients included and variation in laboratory testing methods for aPL.

Investigators have attempted to show whether the presence of a positive aPL in children with SLE is associated with specific clinical events, with varying results. In

Table 20.3. Antiphospholipid antibodies in pediatric systemic lupus erythematosus (case series).

Reference	No. patients	% aPL +	% aCL +	% LA +
Molta [101]	37	38	19	11
Montes de Oca [100]	120	19	–	19
Shergy [99]	32	50	50	–
Gattorno [16]	19	90	79	42
Ravelli [94]	30	87	87	20
Berube [95]	59	–	19	24
Massengill [97]	36	67	50	6
Seaman [75]	29	65	66	62
Gedalia [92]	36	–	37	–
Campos [107]	57	35	33	7
Levy [96]	149	–	–	16

looking at thrombosis in pediatric patients with SLE, studies show a wide variation in incidence, ranging from 7/29 (24%) [75] to 1/30 (3%) [94]. In most studies, there appears to be a clear association of aPL with thrombotic events. Several studies suggest that the presence of a LA confers a higher risk for thrombosis than aCL antibodies [16, 75, 95]. Berube et al [95] showed a significant relationship of a positive LA test to thrombotic events in children with SLE, with a less significant trend of relationship of a positive aCL to thrombosis. Levy et al reported a significant association between thromboembolic events and the presence of LA in a group of children with SLE [96]. Thromboembolic events occurred in 54% of the children with SLE who had a positive LA, and 31% of these had recurrent events. However, Ravelli et al [94] did not find an association of thrombotic events with aPL positivity in a group of 30 children with SLE, 87% of whom were positive for at least 1 aPL . In a recent study, Massengill et al [97] studied a group of 36 children with lupus nephritis, finding 67% positive for aPL and 22% having had a thrombotic event; however, aPL positivity was not significantly increased among the patients with thrombosis. The types of thrombotic events reported in these studies and in case reports include DVTs, ischemic stroke, retinal artery occlusion, renal artery thrombosis, pulmonary embolism, transverse myelitis, and superior vena cava thrombosis [98–104]. These reports should alert clinicians caring for children with SLE to investigate all patients who present with these clinical findings for the presence of aPL , particularly because therapeutic management will be affected if the child is aPL positive.

The implication of finding a positive aPL in a child with SLE who has not developed any clinical problem which could be related to the aPL is less clear. Many physicians are treating such patients with low-dose aspirin. However, most clinicians are reluctant to give oral anticoagulation unless a documented thrombosis has occurred. This is particularly relevant in the pediatric age, where continuous anticoagulation may be more risky than in adulthood, because of a longer expected lifespan and a higher possibility of traumatic bleeding during sports and play. For this reason, others would not treat (even with low-dose aspirin), other than in the presence of concomitant risk factors (e.g., prolonged immobilization). This controversial issue has yet to be resolved with convincing evidence.

Some studies have examined the association of aPL in pediatric SLE patients and central nervous system (CNS) disease of SLE. Shergy et al [99] reported that the highest titers of aCL seen among a group of 32 children with SLE were found in those with CNS disease, although overall there was no significant difference in the prevalence of aCL in patients with CNS disease and those without. Ravelli et al commented that of 9 patients who developed increasing high titers of IgG aCL during follow up, 6 had neuropsychiatric manifestations [94]. Although these data are suggestive that children with SLE and aPL, particularly those with high titer aPL, may be at higher risk of developing aPL-related CNS disease, larger prospective studies are needed to determine this risk.

In several studies, aPL titers were determined in serial samples over time and attempts were made to correlate disease activity or treatment with aPL titers. In every instance, aPL titers were found to fluctuate widely over time in the same patient [16, 75, 97, 99]. It was unclear from these small studies whether increases of aPL accompanied active disease. Some patients with aPL who were treated aggressively with cyclophosphamide for their disease activity were found to have decreased or negative aPL titers after their treatment course [16, 75].

Recently, there has been the suggestion that lupus headaches may occur more frequently in children with SLE who have aPL. In a cohort of 63 children with SLE, followed for a mean of 3.6 years, headaches were reported in 43% of the patients, and occurred preferentially among patients with elevated levels of aPL ($P < 0.02$) [105].

There is also evidence that the presence of aPL may be an important risk factor predicting poor outcome in children with SLE. In a recent study, Brunner et al have retrospectively assessed disease activity and damage in 66 patients with newly diagnosed childhood-onset SLE [106]. Potential risk factors for damage such as age, race, sex, medications, duration of disease, hypertension, body mass index, aPL, kidney disease, and acute thrombocytopenia were collected. The single best predictor of damage was cumulative disease activity over time, but other possibly important risk factors were corticosteroid treatment, acute thrombocytopenia, and the presence of aPL.

Primary APS in Children

The actual prevalence of APS in pediatrics is not known although many of the children reported in the literature with aPL-related clinical problems would fulfill these criteria for the diagnosis of APS. Primary APS may be less common in childhood than in adults, as most major pediatric rheumatology centers may only follow 1 or 2 such patients. However, although the incidence of thrombosis in children is significantly less than in adults, the proportion of aPL-related thrombosis in children may be higher than previously thought. Manco-Johnson and Nuss identified LA in 25% of 78 consecutive children who were diagnosed with thromboses in their institution [93]. Given the likelihood that aPL can precipitate thrombotic event, special concern is needed particularly when dealing with aPL-positive children who are heterozygous for a congenital prothrombotic disorder (e.g., deficiencies of antithrombin, protein C, protein S, or factor V Leiden mutation) and in the presence of other acquired prothrombotic conditions such as catheters, surgery, infections, or oral contraception. Von Scheven et al also reported on clinical characteristics of 9 patients with APS, 5 of who had primary APS [58]. Clinical features of these 5 patients included digital ischemia, stroke, chorea, adrenal insufficiency, and pulmonary vaso-occlusive disease.

The long-term outcome of primary antiphospholipid syndrome (PAPS) in the pediatric age was recently studied [109]. Features of unselected patients with PAPS who had disease onset before the age of 16 years were retrospectively analyzed in three Italian referral centers. Clinical and laboratory manifestations were assessed to establish whether, at the end of follow up, the final diagnosis was still PAPS or whether they had developed definite SLE or lupus-like syndrome. Fourteen patients, 9 boys and 5 girls, were included in this study, with the presenting clinical manifestation of APS between 3 and 13 years of age (median, 9 years) and followed for 2–16 years (median, 6 years). Six patients presented with DVT, 5 with cerebral stroke, 2 with peripheral artery occlusion, and 1 with myocardial infarction. During follow up, 4 patients had 1 or more recurrences of vascular thrombosis. At last observation, 10 patients could still be classified as having PAPS, 2 had developed SLE, 1 lupus-like syndrome, and 1 Hodgkin's lymphoma. These data suggest that some children who present with the features of PAPS may progress to develop SLE or lupus-like syndrome.

Transplacental Passage of aPL and Neonatal Complications

Evidence exists that in pregnant women with APS, aCL can cross the placenta and be detected in cord blood [110, 111]. However, studies on the outcome of infants born to mothers with APS have shown that except for prematurity and its potential associated complications, these neonates had no other clinical manifestations [110, 112–115]. Three of these studies [110, 113, 114] have examined a total of 129 newborns born to women with aPL detected during or before pregnancy. No significant aPL-related clinical pathology was detected in these studies. In one study [114], mothers were treated with calcium heparin during the pregnancy, and although there was an increased rate of prematurity, no other problems were seen in these infants. In the study by Botet et al [113], 33 pregnancies were studied. All the women were treated with low-dose aspirin, and a higher than expected rate of prematurity was found but no other problems.

These are quite surprising results because it is known that during the first month of life, the risk of thrombotic complications is approximately 40 times greater than at any other age during childhood [116]. Furthermore, premature infants are known to have reduced levels of antithrombin [117], which may additionally increase the risk of thrombosis. Therefore, one would expect high frequency of neonatal thrombosis in infants born to mothers with APS. One possible explanation for this discrepancy may be that the aPL IgG subclasses have a different capacity of crossing the placenta and that the placental transfer of IgG2, which appears to be responsible for most clinical pathogenicity of aPL [118], is actually low. Alternatively, it can be hypothesized that there are some differences in host susceptibility such as intact vessel wall in the neonates, which do not favor thrombus formation.

In contrast to these encouraging data, there is an increasing number of case reports describing neonates or infants who have suffered from aPL-associated thrombosis. Several infants had been reported with aPL-related cerebral ischaemia. Silver et al [119] described 2 infants with middle cerebral artery infarction whose mothers had elevated aCL after delivery. They hypothesized that maternal aCL might have been responsible for intrauterine thromboembolic stroke, but their conclusions were invalidated by the delay between delivery and the laboratory examinations. Sheridan-Pereira et al described an infant with aortic thrombus whose mother had a positive LA [120]. Teyssier et al [121] reported the occurrence of cerebral ischemia and bilateral massive adrenal hemorrhage in a neonate who was aCL positive during the neonatal period and 7 months later. De Klerk et al [122] described a LA-positive neonate who had middle cerebral artery infarct and was born to an apparently healthy mother. Contractor et al [123] described a neonate with thromboses of the renal vein and of the vena cava. The infant and mother were both positive for IgG aCL, with antibodies disappearing in the infant after 4 months of age, supporting the transplacental transfer of aCL antibodies in this case. Recently, neonatal cerebral ischemia with elevated maternal and infant aCL have been reported in additional cases [124, 125]. Several reports have described neonatal APS cases with other complications including aortic thrombosis [126], renal vein thrombosis (123), mesenteric thrombosis [127], Blalock-Taussig shunt thrombosis [128], and a neonatal catastrophic APS with multiple thromboses [89]. Additionally, Hage et al [129] described a case of hydrops fetalis with fetal renal vein thrombosis and suggested that transplacentally transferred maternal aPL may induce typical complications already in the fetus.

It is possible that in aPL-positive infants the clinical complication appears only in the presence of a second hit (e.g., incannulation of umbilical vessels, genetic predisposition for thrombosis, etc.).

Treatment of APS and aPL-related Events in Children

The treatment of children with APS or aPL-related events in children has been similar to that used in adults; however, there are no standard recommendations for therapy based on long-term observation of the outcome of APS in children. Currently, we recommend no therapy in asymptomatic individuals who are identified with aPL or LA and who have no evidence of autoimmune disease, while long-term oral anticoagulation is suggested for individuals who have had a thrombosis associated with positive aPL or LA, whether or not the patient has SLE or any other autoimmune disease.

Most children receive some form of treatment when they present with an aPL-associated event, but type and duration of therapy are variable. For example, of 33 case reports of aPL-associated thromboses, 12 received anticoagulation (heparin, warfarin, or urokinase), 8 aspirin, and 16 immunosuppressives [29]. The differences in treating adult and pediatric patients with anticoagulants consist in a major bleeding risk during the young age, and also in the different plasma concentrations of pro- and anticoagulant proteins in different age groups. Therefore, the pediatric requirements for heparin or warfarin, as well as the side effects of these drugs, differ between children and adults.

It has been recommended by experts that for a child who has aPL but is asymptomatic no therapy should be instituted [6]. The study by Male et al would substantiate this approach, as all asymptomatic patients identified with LA in their study remained well on follow up [11]. Antithrombotic therapy is clearly recommended for children who present with thrombosis and have aPL and/or LA; however, the duration and intensity of this therapy is a question. Several authors have suggested "intermediate intensity anticoagulation therapy" for such patients. The effectiveness of such therapy and the length of treatment required are unknown. Many clinicians are hesitant to recommend long-term aggressive anticoagulation of children given that the potential risks for hemorrhage in active children may exceed the risk of recurring thrombosis. A report by Baca et al [38] describing 10 children with cerebral infarctions in association with aPL provides a picture of the current state of confusion and lack of consistency in treating such patients. In their study, one child had a lupus-like disease and was treated with intravenous methylprednisolone and cyclophosphamide. All aCL-positive patients were treated with low-dose aspirin and no recurrences of cerebral infarctions or other thromboses were seen over a 15-month follow up, despite the fact that no patient underwent oral anticoagulation. However, firm conclusions can be drawn only with a longer follow up. Until large-scale, multi-center studies are undertaken to determine the natural history of children who have had a thrombosis or clinical problem due to aPL, the necessity for treatment is unknown and certainly the type and duration of treatment can not be rationally determined.

References

1. Conley CL, Hartman RC. A hemorrhagic disorder caused by circulating anticoagulant in patients with disseminated lupus erythematosus. J Clin Invest 1952;31:621–622.
2. Bowie EJ, Thompson JH, Pascuzzi CA, et al. Thrombosis in systemic lupus erythematosus despite circulating anticoagulants. J Lab Clin Med 1963;62:416–430.
3. Harris EN, Gharavi AE, Boey ML, et al. Anticardiolipin antibodies: Detection by radioimmunoassay and association with thrombosis in systemic lupus erythematosus. Lancet 1983;ii:1211–1214.
4. Ames PRJ, Khamashta MA, Hughes GRV. Clinical and therapeutic aspects of the antiphospholipid syndrome. Lupus 1995;4:S23–S25.
5. Tucker LB. Antiphospholipid syndrome in childhood: the great unknown. Lupus 1994;3:367–369.
6. Ravelli A, Martini A. Antiphospholipid antibody syndrome in pediatric patients. Rheum Dis Clin North Am 1997;23:657–676.
7. Ravelli A, Martini A, Burgio GR. Antiphospholipid antibodies in paediatrics. Eur J Pediatr 1994;153:472–479.
8. Szer IS. Clinical development in the management of lupus in the neonate, child, and adolescent. Curr Opin Rheumatol 1998;10:431–434.
9. Lee T, von Scheven E, Sandborg C. Systemic lupus erythematosus and antiphospholipid syndrome in childrenand adolesents. Curr Opin Rheumatol 2001;13:415–421.
10. Avčin T, Cimaz R, Meroni PL. Do we need international consensus statement on classification criteria for the antiphospholipid syndrome in paediatric population? Lupus 2001;10:897–898.
11. Male C, Lechner K, Eichinger S, et al. Clinical significance of lupus anticoagulants in children. J Pediatr 1999;134:199–205.
12. Rapizzi E, Ruffatti A, Tonello M, et al. Correction for age of anticardiolipin antibodies cut-off points. J Clin Lab Anal 2000;14:87–90.
13. Avčin T, Ambrožič A, Kuhar M, et al. Anticardiolipin and anti-β_2 glycoprotein I antibodies in sera of 61 apparently healthy children at regular preventive visits. Rheumatology 2001;40:565–573.
14. Caporali R, Ravelli A, De Gennaro F, et al. Prevalence of anticardiolipin antibodies in juvenile arthritis. Ann Rheum Dis 1991;50:599–601.
15. Siamopoulou-Mavridou A, Mavridis AK, Terzoglou C, et al. Autoantibodies in Greek juvenile chronic arthritis patients. Clin Exp Rheumatol 1991;9:647–652.
16. Gattorno M, Buoncompagni A, Molinari AC, et al. Antiphospholipid antibodies in paediatric systemic lupus erythematosus, juvenile chronic arthritis and overlap syndromes: SLE patients with both lupus anticoagulant and high-titre anticardiolipin antibodies are at risk for clinical manifestations related to the antiphospholipid syndrome. Br J Rheumatol 1995;34:873–881.
17. Kontiainen S, Miettinen A, Seppälä I, et al. Antiphospholipid antibodies in children. Acta Paediatr 1996;85:614–615.
18. Kratz C, Mauz-Körholz C, Kruck H, et al. Detection of antiphospholipid antibodies in children and adolescents. Pediatr Hematol Oncol 1998;15:325–332.
19. Serra CRB, Rodrigues SH, Silva NP, et al. Clinical significance of anticardiolipin antibodies in juvenile idiopathic arthritis. Clin Exp Rheumatol 1999;17:375–380.
20. Matsuura E, Igarashi M, Igarashi Y, et al. Molecular definition of human β_2-glycoprotein I (β_2-GPI) by cDNA cloning and interspecies differences of β_2-GPI in alteration of anticardiolipin binding. Int Immunol 1991;3:1217–1221.
21. Avčin T, Kveder T, Rozman B. The antiphospholipid syndrome [letter]. N Engl J Med 2002;347:145–146.
22. Gallistl S, Muntean W, Leschnik B, et al. Longer aPTT values in healthy children than in adults: no single cause. Thromb Res 1997;88:355–359.
23. Siemens HJG, Gutsche S, Brückner S, et al. Antiphospholipid antibodies in children without and in adults with and without thrombophilia. Thromb Res 2000;98:241–247.
24. Vaarala O, Palosuo T, Kleemola M. Anticardiolipin responses in acute infections. Clin Immunol Immunopathol 1986;41:8–15.

25. Asherson RA, Cervera R. Antiphospholipid antibodies and infections. Ann Rheum Dis 2003;62:388–393.
26. Lehmann HW, Plentz A, Von Landenberg P, et al. Intravenous immunoglobulin treatment of four patients with juvenile polyarticular arthritis associated with persistent parvovirus B19 infection and antiphospholipid antibodies. Arthritis Res Ther 2004;6:R1–R6.
27. Ertem D, Acar Y, Pehlivanoglu E. Autoimmune complications associated with hepatitis A virus infection in children. Pediatr Infect Dis J 2001;20:809–811.
28. Carreno L, Monteagudo I, Lopez-Longo FJ. Anticardiolipin antibodies in pediatric patients with human immunodeficiency virus. J Rheumatol 1994;21:1344–1346.
29. Sammaritano LR, Piette JC. Pediatric and familial antiphospholipid syndromes. In: Asherson RA, Cervera R, Piette JC, Shoenfeld Y, eds. The antiphospholipid syndrome II: autoimmune thrombosis. New York: Elsevier; 2002:297–316.
30. Kurugol Z, Vardar F, Ozkinay F, et al. Lupus anticoagulant and protein S deficiency in otherwise healthy children with acute varicella infection. Acta Pediatr 2000;89:1186–1189.
31. Blank M, Krause I, Fridkin M, et al. Bacterial induction of autoantibodies to β_2 glycoprotein I accounts for the infectious etiology of antiphospholipid syndrome. J Clin Invest 2002;109:797–804.
32. Figueroa F, Berrios X, Gutierrez M, et al. Anticardiolipin antibodies in acute rheumatic fever. J Rheumatol 1992;19:1175–1180.
33. Narin N, Kutukculer N, Narin F, et al. Anticardiolipin antibodies in acute rheumatic fever and chronic rheumatic heart disease: is there a significant association? Clin Exp Rheumatol 1996;14:567–569.
34. Toren P, Toren A, Weizman A, et al. Tourette's Disorder: is there an association with the antiphospholipid syndrome? Biol Psychiatry 1994;35:495–498.
35. Singer HS, Krumholz A, Giuliano J, et al. Antiphospholipid antibodies: an epiphenomenon in Tourette syndrome. Mov Disord 1997;12:738–742.
36. Schöning M, Klein R, Krägeloh-Mann I, et al. Antiphospholipid antibodies in cerebrovascular ischemia and stroke in childhood. Neuropediatrics 1994;25:8–14.
37. Takanashi J, Sugita K, Miyazato S, et al. Antiphospholipid antibody syndrome in childhood strokes. Pediatr Neurol 1995;13:323–326.
38. Baca V, Garcia-Ramirez R, Ramirez-Lacayo M, et al. Cerebral infarction and antiphospholipid syndrome in children. J Rheumatol 1996;23:1428–1431.
39. Kenet G, Sadetzki S, Murad H, et al. Factor V Leiden and antiphospholipid antibodies are significant risk factors for ischemic stroke in children. Stroke 2000;31:1283–1288.
40. Angelini L, Zibordi F, Zorzi G, et al. Neurological disorders, other than stroke, associated with antiphospholipid antibodies in childhood. Neuropediatrics 1996;27:149–153.
41. Avčin T, Markelj G, Niksic V, et al. Estimation of antiphospholipid antibodies in a prospective longitudinal study of children with migraine. Cephalalgia 2004;24:831–837.
42. Spreafico R, Binelli S, Bruzzone MG, et al. Primary antiphospholipid syndrome (PAPS) and isolated partial seizures in adolescence. A case report. Ital J Neurol Sci 1994;15:297–301.
43. Angelini L, Granata T, Zibordi F, et al. Partial seizures associated with antiphospholipid antibodies in childhood. Neuropediatrics 1998;29:249–253.
44. Cimaz R, Romeo A, Scarano A, et al. Prevalence of anti-cardiolipin, anti-β2 glycoprotein I, and anti-prothrombin antibodies in young patients with epilepsy. Epilepsia 2002;43:52–59.
45. Eriksson K, Peltola J, Keranen T, et al. High prevalence of antiphospholipid antibodies in children with epilepsy: a controlled study of 50 cases. Epilepsy Res 2001;46:129–137.
46. Lorini R, d'Annunzio G, Montecucco C, et al. Anticardiolipin antibodies in children and adolescents with insulin-dependent diabetes mellitus. Eur J Pediatr 1995;154:105–108.
47. Ambrožič A, Avčin T, Ichikawa K, et al. Anti-β_2 glycoprotein I antibodies in children with atopic dermatitis. Int Immunol 2002;14:1–8.
48. Leak AM, Colaco CB, Isenberg DA. Anticardiolipin and anti-ss DNA antibodies in antinuclear positive juvenile chronic arthritis and other childhood onset rheumatic diseases. Clin Exp Rheumatol 1987;5:18.
49. Caporali R, Ravelli A, Ramenghi B, et al. Antiphospholipid antibody associated with thrombosis in juvenile chronic arthritis. Arch Dis Child 1992;67:1384–1386.
50. Andrews A, Hickling P. Thrombosis associated with antiphospholipid antibody in juvenile chronic arthritis. Lupus 1997;6:556–557.
51. Avčin T, Ambrožič A, Božič B, et al. Estimation of anticardiolipin antibodies, anti-β_2 glycoprotein I antibodies and lupus anticoagulant in a prospective longitudinal study of children with juvenile idiopathic arthritis. Clin Exp Rheumatol 2002;20:101–108.

52. Lee MT, Nardi MA, Hu G, et al. Transient hemorrhagic diathesis associated with an inhibitor of prothrombin with lupus anticoagulant in a $1^1/_2$-year-old girl: report of a case and review of the literature. Am J Hematol 1996;51:307–314.
53. Becton DL, Stine KC. Transient lupus anticoagulants associated with hemorrhage rather than thrombosis: the hemorrhagic lupus anticoagulant syndrome. J Pediatr 1997;130:998–1000.
54. Best IM, Anyadike NC, Bumpers HL. The antiphospholipid syndrome in a teenager with miscarriages, thrombosis, and diabetes mellitus. Am Surgeon 2000;66:748–750.
55. Roddy SM, Giang DW. Antiphospholipid antibodies and stroke in an infant. Pediatrics 1991;87:933–935.
56. Ravelli A, Caporali R, Montecucco C, et al. Superior vena cava thrombosis in a child with antiphospholipid syndrome. J Rheumatol 1992;19:502–503.
57. Nuss R, Hays T, Chudgar U, et al. Antiphospholipid antibodies and coagulation regulatory protein abnormalities in children with pulmonary emboli. J Pediatr Hematol Oncol 1997;19:202–207.
58. von Scheven E, Athreya B, Rose CD, et al. Clinical characteristics of antiphospholipid antibody syndrome in children. J Pediatr 1996;129:339–345.
59. Bernstein ML, Salusinsky-Sternbach M, Bellefleur M, et al. Thrombotic and hemorrhagic complications in children with the lupus anticoagulant. Am J Dis Child 1984;138:1132–1135.
60. Brady L, Magilavy D, Black DD. Portal vein thrombosis associated with antiphospholipid antibodies in a child. J Pediatr Gastroenterol Nutr 1996;23:470–473.
61. Falcini F, Taccetti G, Trapani S, et al. Primary antiphospholipid syndrome: a report of two cases. J Rheumatol 1991;18:1085–1087.
62. Angelini L, Ravelli A, Caporali R, et al. High prevalence of antiphospholipid antibodies in children with idiopathic cerebral ischemia. Pediatrics 1994;94:500–503.
63. Di Nucci GD, Mariani G, Arcieri P, et al. Antiphospholipid syndrome in young patients. Two cases of cerebral ischemic accidents. Eur J Pediatr 1995;154:334.
64. Olson JC, Konkol RJ, Gill JC, et al. Childhood stroke and lupus anticoagulant. Pediatr Neurol 1994;10:54–57.
65. Pope JM, Canny CHL, Bell DA. Cerebral ischemic events associated with endocarditis, retinal vascular disease, and lupus anticoagulant. Am J Med 1991;90:299–309.
66. Coull BM, Bourdette DN, Goddnight SH Jr, et al. Multiple cerebral infarctions associated with antiphospholipid antibodies. Stroke 1987;18:1107–1112.
67. deVeber G, Andrew M, Adams C, et al. Cerebral sinovenous thrombosis in children. N Engl J Med 2001;345:417–423.
68. Heller C, Heinecke A, Junker R, et al. Cerebral venous thrombosis in children: a multifactorial origin. Circulation 2003;108:1362–1367.
69. Katsarou E, Attilakos A, Fessatou S, et al. Anti-β2 glycoprotein I antibodies and ischemic stroke in a 20-month-old boy. Pediatrics 2003;112:188–190.
70. Ebeling F, Petaja J, Alanko S, et al. Infant stroke and β2 glycoprotein 1 antibodies: six cases. Eur J Pediatr 2003;162:678–681.
71. Hasegawa M, Yamashita J, Yamashima T, et al. Spinal cord infarction associated with primary antiphospholipid syndrome in a young child. J Neurosurg 1993;79:446–450.
72. Ohtomo Y, Matsubara T, Nishizawa K, et al. Nephropathy and hypertension as manifestations in a 13-year-old girl with primary antiphospholipid syndrome. Acta Paediatrica 1998;87:903–907.
73. Deleze M, Oria CV, Alarcon-Segovia D. Occurrence of both hemolytic anemia and thrombocytopenic purpura (Evans' Syndrome) in systemic lupus erythematosus. Relationship to antiphospholipid antibodies. J Rheumatol 1988;15:611–615.
74. Harris EN, Gharavi AE, Hegde U, et al. Anticardiolipin antibodies in autoimmune thrombocytopenic purpura. Br J Haematol 1985;59:231–234.
75. Seaman DE, Londino V, Kent Kwoh C, et al. Antiphospholipid antibodies in pediatric systemic lupus erythematosus. Pediatrics 1995;96:1040–1045.
76. Sakai M, Shirahata A, Akatsuka J, et al. Antiphospholipid antibodies in children with idiopathic thrombocytopenic purpura. Rinsho Ketsueki 2002;43:821–827.
77. Toren A, Toren P, Many A, et al. Spectrum of clinical manifestations of antiphospholipid antibodies in childhood and adolescence. Pediatr Hemat Oncol 1993;10:311–315.
78. Ura Y, Hara T , Mori Y, et al. Development of Perthes' disease in a 3-year-old boy with idiopathic thrombocytopenic purpura and antiphospholipid antibodies. Pediatr Hemat Oncol 1992;9:77–80.
79. Avčin T, Jazbec J, Kuhar M, et al. Evans syndrome associated with antiphospholipid antibodies. J Pediatr Hematol Oncol 2003;25:73–74.

80. Cervera R, Asherson RA, Font J, et al. Chorea in the antiphospholipid syndrome. Clinical, radiologic, and immunologic characteristics of 50 patients from our clinics and the recent literature. Medicine (Baltimore) 1997;76:203–212.
81. Besbas N, Damarguc I, Ozen S. Association of antiphospholipid antibodies with systemic lupus erythematosus in a child presenting with chorea: a case report. Eur J Pediatr 1994;153:891–893.
82. Vlachoyiannopoulos PG, Dimou G, Siamopoulou-Mavirdou A. Chorea as a manifestation of the antiphospholipid syndrome in childhood. Clin Exp Rheumatol 1991;9:303–305.
83. Al-Matar M, Jaimes J, Malleson P. Chorea as the presenting clinical feature of primary antiphospholipid syndrome in childhood. Neuropediatrics 2000;31:107–108.
84. Okun MS, Jummani RR, Carney PR. Antiphospholipid- associated recurrent chorea and ballism in a child with cerebral palsy. Pediatr Neurol 2000;23:62–63.
85. Cervera R, Piette JC, Font J, et al. Antiphospholipid syndrome: clinical and immunologic manifestations and patterns of disease expression in a cohort of 1,000 patients. Arthritis Rheum 2002;46:1019–1027.
86. Besbas N, Anlar B, Apak A, et al. Optic neuropathy in primary antiphospholipid syndrome in childhood. J Child Neurol 2001;16:690–693.
87. Falcini F, Taccetti G, Ermini M, et al. Catastrophic antiphospholipid antibody syndrome in pediatric systemic lupus erythematosus. J Rheumatol 1997;24:389–392.
88. Asherson RA, Crevera R, Piette JC, et al. Catastrophic antiphospholipid syndrome: clues to the pathogenesis from a series of 80 patients. Medicine (Baltimore) 2001;80:355–377.
89. Tabbutt S, Griswold WR, Ogino MT, et al. Multiple thromboses in a premature infant associated with maternal phospholipid antibody syndrome. J Perinatol 1994;14:66–70.
90. Orsino A, Schneider R, DeVeber G, et al. Childhood acute myelomonocytic leukemia (AML-M4) presenting as catastrophic antiphospholipid syndrome. J Pediatr Hematol Oncol 2004; 26:327–330.
91. Hudson N, Duffy CM, Rauch J, et al. Catastrophic hemorrhage in a case of pediatric primary antiphospholipid syndrome and factor II deficiency. Lupus 1997;6:68–71.
92. Gedalia A, Molin A, Garcia CO, et al. Anticardiolipin antibodies in childhood rheumatic disorders. Lupus 1998;7:551–553.
93. Manco-Johnson M, Nuss R. Lupus anticoagulant in children with thrombosis. Am J Hematol 1995;48:240–243.
94. Ravelli A, Caporali R, Di Fuccia G, et al. Anticardiolipin antibodies in pediatric systemic lupus erythematosus. Arch Pediatr Adolesc Med 1994;148:398–402.
95. Berube C, Mitchell L, Silverman E, et al. The relationship of antiphospholipid antibodies to thromboembolic events in pediatric patients with systemic lupus erythematosus. Pediatr Res 1998;44:351–356.
96. Levy DM, Massicotte MP, Harvey E, et al. Thromboembolism in paediatric lupus patients. Lupus 2003;12:741–746.
97. Massengill SF, Hedrick C, Ayoub EM, et al. Antiphospholipid antibodies in pediatric lupus nephritis. Am J Kidney Dis 1997;29:355–361.
98. Dungan DD, Jay MS. Stroke in an early adolescent with systemic lupus erythematosus and coexistent antiphospholipid antibodies. Pediatrics 1992;90:96–98.
99. Shergy WJ, Kredich DW, Pisetsky DS. The relationship of anticardiolipin antibodies to disease manifestations in pediatric systemic lupus erythematosus. J Rheumatol 1988;15:1389–1394.
100. Montes de Oca MA, Babron MC, Bletry O, et al. Thrombosis in systemic lupus erythematosus: a French collaborative study. Arch Dis Child 1991;66:713–717.
101. Molta C, Meyer O, Dosquet C, et al. Childhood-onset systemic lupus erythematosus: antiphospholipid antibodies in 37 patients and their first degree relatives. Pediatrics 1993;92:849–853.
102. Kwong T, Leonidas JC, Ilowite NT. Asymptomatic superior vena cava thrombosis and pulmonary embolism in an adolescent with SLE and antiphospholipid antibodies. Clin Exp Rheumatol 1994;12:215–217.
103. Baca V, Sanchez-Vaca G, Martinez-Muniz I, et al. Successful treatment of transverse myelitis in a child with systemic lupus erythematosus. Neuropediatrics 1996;27:42–44.
104. Tomizawa K, Sato-Matsumura KC, Kajii N. The coexistence of cutaneous vasculitis and thrombosis in childhood-onset systemic lupus erythematosus with antiphospholipid antibodies. Br J Dermatol 2003;149:439–441.
105. Brunner HI, Jones OY, Lovell DJ, et al. Lupus headaches in childhood-onset systemic lupus erythematosus: relationship to disease activity as measured by the systemic lupus erythematosus disease activity index (SLEDAI) and disease damage. Lupus 2003;12:600–606.

106. Brunner HI, Silverman ED, To T, et al. Risk factors for damage in childhood-onset systemic lupus erythematosus: cumulative disease activity and medication use predict disease damage. Arthritis Rheum 2002;46:436–444.
107. Campos LM, Kiss MH, D'Amico EA, et al. Antiphospholipid antibodies and antiphospholipid syndrome in 57 children and adolescents with systemic lupus erythematosus. Lupus 2003;12:820–826.
108. Asherson RA, Khamashta MA, Ordi-Ros J, et al. The "primary" antiphospholipid syndrome: major clinical and serological features. Medicine (Baltimore) 1989;68:366–374.
109. Gattorno M, Falcini F, Ravelli A, et al. Outcome of primary antiphospholipid syndrome in childhood. Lupus 2003;12:449–453.
110. Zurgil N, Bakimer R, Tincani A, et al. Detection of anti-phospholipid and anti-DNA antibodies and their idiotypes in newborns of mothers with anti-phospholipid syndrome and SLE. Lupus 1993;2:233–237.
111. Cohen SB, Goldenberg M, Rabinovici J, et al. Anti-cardiolipin antibodies in fetal blood and amniotic fluid derived from patients with the anti-phospholipid syndrome. Hum Reprod 2000;15:1170–1172.
112. Pollard JK, Scott JR, Branch DW. Outcome of children born to women treated during pregnancy for the antiphospholipid syndrome. Obstet Gynecol 1992;80:365–368.
113. Botet F, Romera G, Montagut P, et al. Neonatal outcome in women treated for the antiphospholipid syndrome during pregnancy. J Perinat Med 1997;25:192–196.
114. Ruffatti A, Dalla Barba B, Del Ross T, et al. Outcome of fifty-five newborns of antiphospholipid antibody-positive mothers treated with calcium heparin during pregnancy. Clin Exp Rheumatol 1998;16:605–610.
115. Brewster JA, Shaw NJ, Farquharson RG. Neonatal and pediatric outcome of infants born to mothers with antiphospholipid syndrome. J Perinat Med 1999;27:183–187.
116. Andrew M, David M, Adams M, et al. Venous thromboembolic complications (VTE) in children: first analyses of the Canadian Registry of VTE. Blood 1994;83:1251–1257.
117. Andrew M, Paes B, Milner R, et al. Development of the human coagulation system in the healthy premature infant. Blood 1988;72:1651–1657.
118. Sammaritano LR, Ng S, Sobel R, et al. Anticardiolipin IgG subclasses: association of IgG2 with arterial and/or venous thrombosis. Arthritis Rheum 1997;40:1998–2006.
119. Silver RK, MacGregor SN, Pasternak JF, et al. Fetal stroke associated with elevated maternal anticardiolipin antibodies. Obstet Gynecol 1992;80:497–499.
120. Sheridan-Pereira M, Porreco RP, Hays T, et al. Neonatal aortic thrombosis associated with the lupus anticoagulant. Obstet Gynecol 1988;71:1016–1018.
121. Teyssier G, Gautheron V, Absi L, et al. Anticorps anticardiolipine, ischemie cerebrale et hemorragie surrenalienne chez un nouveau-né. Arch Pediatr 1995;2:1086–1088.
122. de Klerk OL, de Vries TW, Sinnige LGF. An unusual cause of neonatal seizures in a newborn infant. Pediatrics 1997;100:E8.
123. Contractor S, Hiatt M, Kosmin M, et al. Neonatal thrombosis with anticardiolipin antibody in baby and mother. Am J Perinatol 1992;9:409–410.
124. Akanli LF, Trasi SS, Thuraisamy K, et al. Neonatal middle cerebral artery infarction: association with elevated maternal anticardiolipin antibodies. Am J Perinatol 1998;15:399–402.
125. Chow G, Mellor D. Neonatal cerebral ischaemia with elevated maternal and infant anticardiolipin antibodies. Dev Med Child Neurol 2000;42:412–413.
126. Finazzi G, Cortelazzo S, Viero P, et al. Maternal lupus anticoagulant and fatal neonatal thrombosis. Thromb Haemost 1987;57:238.
127. Navarro F, Doña-Naranjo MA, Villanueva I. Neonatal antiphospholipid syndrome. J Rheumatol 1997;24:1240–1241.
128. Deally C, Hancock BJ, Giddins N, et al. Primary antiphospholipid syndrome: a cause of catastrophic shunt thrombosis in the newborn. J Cardiovasc Surg 1999;40:261–264.
129. Hage ML, Liu R, Marcheschi DG, et al. Fetal renal vein thrombosis, hydrops fetalis, and maternal lupus anticoagulant. A case report. Prenat Diagn 1994;14:873–877.

21 Ethnic and Geographic Variation in Antiphospholipid Syndrome

Wendell A. Wilson and Elena Cucurull

Introduction

During the past 20 years, studies of antiphospholipid antibodies (aPL) and antiphospholipid syndrome (APS) have been done in many countries and ethno-geographic groups. To date, the large majority of these studies reported data on systemic lupus erythematosus (SLE) populations, and this review largely focuses on the SLE studies. Comparisons among such studies are of interest because they may help to clarify the causes of APS, analogous to the situation in SLE, in which ethnic and geographic factors are clearly related to prevalence and severity of the disease.

Anticardiolipin Antibodies (aCL) Frequency in SLE

Routine screening for aPL now occurs in SLE clinics because of the strong experimental and clinical evidence of the procoagulant nature of aPL and the demonstrations that anticoagulation provides effective secondary prophylaxis of thrombosis or pregnancy loss in patients with aPL. Studies to date have mainly described the prevalence of aCL among populations of SLE patients and have attempted to estimate the prevalence of secondary APS in SLE, mainly using classification criteria for APS that predated the 1999 international (Sapporo) criteria [1]. Relatively few studies listed in Table 21.1 included lupus anticoagulant (LA) in the assay methods for aPL, probably because tests for LA are more technically demanding and require platelet-poor plasma. The studies listed in Table 21.1 thus mainly provide a point prevalence of aCL in various populations.

It is evident from Table 21.1 that aCL occur in all SLE populations studied, but with highly variable point prevalence. It is likely that assay methods [20] and patient selection contribute to this variability in prevalence as further discussed below, but some variations are of interest. IgG aCL prevalence ranged from 2% in an Afro–Caribbean clinic population to 51% in a report from India. Of even greater interest was the fact that among Afro–Caribbean (Jamaican) SLE patients, the prevalence of IgA aCL was relatively high (21%), but it was not clear whether SLE disease parameters, including disease inactivity, was related to the low frequency of IgG aCL. In the same study [4], using the same assay methods, IgG aCL was seen

Table 21.1. Prevalence and isotype distribution of anticardiolipin and lupus anticoagulant in different populations of SLE patients.

Reference	Ethnicity or country (n)	Any aCL isotype (%)	IgG aCL (%)	IgM aCL (%)	IgA aCL(%)	LA (%)	Correlation with thrombosis and/or fetal loss
Cucurull et al [2]	Colombian[a] (160)	25	18	13	15	NA	Yes
Cucurull et al [2]	Spaniard[a] (160)	34	27	15	16	NA	Yes
Cucurull et al [3]	African-American[a] (100)	33	18	7	24	NA	Yes
Molina et al [4]	Afro-Caribbean[a] (136)	21	2	2	21	NA	No
Aguirre et al [5]	Chilean[a] (129)	30	16	14	8	NA	Yes
Alarcon et al [6]	Hispanic[b] (70)	7*	NA	NA	NA	NA	NA
Alarcon et al [6]	African-American[b] (88)	11*	NA	NA	NA	NA	NA
Alarcon et al [6]	Caucasian[b] (71)	5*	NA	NA	NA	NA	NA
Jones et al [7]	Malaysia[c] (200)	16.5	13	2.5	NA	NA	No
Sebastiani et al [8]	Europe[d] (574)	NA	23	14	14	NA	Yes
Sebastiani et al [9]	Italy (64)	44	44	9	NA	NA	Yes
Gourley et al [10]	Ireland (95)	44	31	28	NA	NA	Yes
Sturfelt et al [11]	Sweden (59)	54	47	13	NA	NA	No
Alarcon-Segovia et al [12]	Mexico (500)	53	39	33	16	NA	Yes
Shrivastava et al [13]	India (76)	51	51	7	5	NA	No
Saluja et al [14]	India[e] (76)	27	27	1	NA	NA	Yes
Saxena et al [15]	India[e] (70)	19	NA	NA	NA	16	Yes
Wong et al [16]	China (91)	46	44	1	4	11	No
Ninomiya et al [17]	Japan (349)	35	28	NA	NA	27	Yes
Tsutsumi et al [18]	Japan (308)	NA	12	4	NA	8	Yes
Chahade et al [19]	Brazilian (54)	20	20	5.5	NA	17	NA

[a]In-house ELISA test done at Louisiana State University Health Sciences Center in New Orleans.

[b]LUMINA Study Group: LUpus in MInority populations: NAture vs Nurture. From University of Alabama at Birmingham, University of Texas-Houston Health Science Center, and University of Texas Medical Branch at Galveston.

[c]Population comprised 164 Chinese, 26 Malay, and 10 Indian. No differences were found in the prevalence of raised aCL between the 3 ethnic groups.

[d]Patients from 7 European countries: 97.7% Caucasians, 3.3% other races.

[e]Both studies from All India Institute of Medical Sciences, New Delhi.

*IgG and IgM aCL and/or LA.

NA = data not available.

fairly commonly among African–American and Colombian SLE patients (18% and 21%, respectively). The relative paucity of IgG and IgM aCL in Afro–Caribbean SLE patients warrants further study. In general, most studies from various countries report a mixture of aCL isotypes in individual patients, with IgG aCL being the most common and most closely associated with thromboses and fetal losses. IgA aCL is rarely present alone, except in Afro–Caribbean SLE patients. In African–American SLE patients, IgA aCL is also frequent, but often co-exists with other isotypes. In early studies in the African–American clinic population in New Orleans, we found that IgG aCL was present in 27% of SLE patients during periods of disease activity, compared with only 5% of SLE patients during periods of less active SLE [34]. Thus, disease activity may be an important variable to address in future inter-ethnic studies. SLE in African–Americans and Afro–Caribbean SLE patients is character- ized by a generally worse outcome and a higher prevalence of autoantibodies than in other ethnic or geographic groups, and it would be of interest if aPL are an excep- tion to this pattern in SLE. In a largely Afro–American obstetric pre-natal clinic population [22], the prevalence of IgG aCL was 1.25% which approximates the fre- quency of IgG aCL found in other unselected pre-natal clinic populations [23].

Significance of IgA aCL

It is also of interest that IgA aCL predominated in another Afro–Caribbean clinic population [24, 25]; these were Jamaican patients with tropical spastic paraparesis (TSP), a chronic neurologic disease that appears to be due to an autoimmune response to infection with human T-cell leukemia virus type 1 (HTLV-1). In some clinical respects, TSP resembles the progressive subset of patients with multiple sclerosis. IgA aCL occurred in 30% of TSP patients, but its relevance to clinical fea- tures of TSP has not been studied.

The mechanisms that may underlie the preponderance of IgA aCL in the above Afro–Caribbean clinic populations, are not known. It is known that HTLV-1 infec- tion is not associated with SLE in Jamaica [26]. A black South African population of SLE patients exhibited relatively high frequencies of specific antinuclear antibodies, similar to previous reports in Jamaican and African–American SLE; however, aCL, and IgA aCL in particular, was not studied in the South African SLE patients [27]. However, IgA aCL appear to be frequent in some infections among black South Africans [28]. It is not clear whether the African origin or ancestry of these populations correlates with the autoantibody profile. Afro–Caribbean and African–American populations share similar, diverse geographic ancestral origins mainly in West Africa; in addition, during the post-slavery period, there have been extensive migrations of Afro–Caribbean peoples to the Americas. However, the gene pool in black South Africans may be significantly different from that in West Africa [29]. It would seem likely that methodological, and possibly, environmental factors underlie the variations that occur in the aCL isotypes among these popula- tions. Whether IgA aCL might contribute to a more comprehensive identification of APS in some SLE populations is controversial [21]. Some studies have found no additional benefit from IgA aCL testing in SLE patients who were screened for IgG and IgM aCL, whereas some studies in other geographic or ethnic groups suggest the opposite.

APS in SLE

Most studies that were powered to address this question in Table 21.1 reported an association of aCL with thromboses and pregnancy loss. The exceptions included a 1991 study from China (Hong Kong) that found a 44% prevalence of IgG aCL and an 11% prevalence of LA [17]. This study did not find an association of aPL with thromboses or pregnancy loss a surprising finding, in view of the very strong association of the presence of LA with these complications.

Whether anti–β_2-glycoprotein I (anti–β_2-GPI) assays provide additional information of clinical or other value is the subject of ongoing study. It is clear that there is a small population of patients who do not have IgG or IgM aCL but who are positive for IgG or IgM anti–β_2-GPI. Whether IgA anti–β_2GPI provides further value is also controversial. Clarifications of these areas will require inter-laboratory efforts to standardize anti–β_2-GPI assays and to compare them with more conventional aPL assays [18, 30].

It is clear from the above that the study of the clinical epidemiology of aPL is still in its infancy. Most studies have reported data on only one ethnic and/or geographic group, and comparisons between these studies are confounded by methodologic variations or patient selection. The publication in 1999 of international consensus criteria for APS [1] should facilitate future studies. Studies of ethnic and/or geographic variation in aPL or APS are of interest for the clinical reasons mentioned above, and also because such variation may provide clues to the genetic or environmental causes of APS, as has been the case in SLE.

Genetic Factors in aPL and APS

The genetic factors that lead to aPL production are still unclear, though some evidence points to the possible importance of major histocompatibility complex (MHC) -DQB or -DR alleles in particular [31]. Vascular thromboses and pregnancy losses have many non-aPL causes, and there is evidence that some risk factors for these clinical complications have additive effects with other risk factors. A few studies have addressed the possibility that aPL may interact with genetic risk factors for thrombosis, for example, factor V Leiden, and the prothrombin gene mutation, that vary markedly in prevalence among ethnic groups.

APS and SLE are heterogeneous diseases, in which the basic causes may well turn out to be as heterogeneous as the clinical presentation of these syndromes. In the case of SLE, there is evidence that a large number of genes contribute to causation, with some genes having relevance in many ethnic groups (e.g., C_4A deficiency alleles) and others having less general significance across ethnic groups [32]. With increasing geographic migration and intermingling across geographic and ethnic groups, such variations in disease parameters will become even more difficult to interpret relative to the genetic or environmental causes of these diseases. In addition, in many communities variation in disease parameters that appear to relate to ethnicity may more closely associate with economic variables or educational opportunities. There is as yet very little understanding of the ways by which such social factors affect the biologic mechanisms that influence disease prevalence and outcome in autoimmune diseases such as SLE.

Summary

Geographic and ethnic studies of aPL and APS suggest that IgG aCL prevalence may be lower among Afro–Caribbean (Jamaican) SLE patients, who interestingly have a high prevalence of IgA aCL. It is not clear whether this is generalizable to other SLE populations that have African ancestry. Further multi-ethnic studies that are internally controlled for laboratory methods and SLE disease activity would be useful in confirming these reports, and exploring their clinical significance.

References

1. Wilson WA, Gharavi AE, Koike T, et al. International consensus statement on preliminary classification criteria for definite antiphospholipid syndrome: report of an international workshop. Arthritis Rheum 1999;42:1309–1311.
2. Cucurull E, Espinoza LR, Mendez E, et al. Anticardiolipin and anti-$\beta_2$glycoprotein I antibodies in patients with systemic lupus erythematosus: comparison between Colombians and Spaniards. Lupus 1999;8:134–141.
3. Cucurull E, Gharavi AE, Diri E, et al. IgA anticardiolipin and anti-$\beta_2$glycoprotein I are the most prevalent isotypes in African American patients with systemic lupus erythematosus. Am J Med Sci 1999;31:55–60.
4. Molina JF, Gutierrez-Urena S, Molina J, et al. Variability of anticardiolipin antibody isotype distribution in 3 geographic populations of patients with systemic lupus erythermatosus. J Rheumatol 1997;24:291–296.
5. Aguirre V, Cuchacovich R, Barria L, et al. Prevalence and isotype distribution of antiphospholipid antibodies in Chilean patients with systemic lupus erythematosus (SLE). Lupus 2001;10:75–80.
6. Alarcon GS, Friedman AW, Straaton KV, et al. Systemic lupus erythematosus in three ethnic groups: III A comparison of characteristics early in the natural history of the LUMINA cohort. Lupus 1999;8:197–209.
7. Jones HW, Ireland R, Senaldi G, et al. Anticardiolipin antibodies in patients from Malaysia with systemic lupus erythematosus. Ann Rheum Dis 1991;50:173–175.
8. Sebastiani GD, Galeazzi M, Tincani A, et al. Anticardiolipin and anti-β_2GPI antibodies in a large series of European patients with systemic lupus erythematosus. Prevalence and clinical associations. European Concerted Action on the Immunogenetics of SLE. Scan J Rheumatol 1999;28:344–351.
9. Sebastiani GD, Passiu G, Galeazzi M, et al. Prevalence and clinical associations of anticardiolipin antibodies in systemic lupus erythematosus: a prospective study. Clin Rheumatol 1991;10:289–293.
10. Gourley IS, McMillan SA, Bell AL. Clinical features associated with a positive anticardiolipin antibody in Irish patients with systemic lupus erythematosus. Clin Rheumatol 1996;15:457–460.
11. Sturfelt G, Nived O, Norgerg R, et al. Anticardiolipin antibodies in patients with systemic lupus erythematosus. Arthritis Rheum 1987;30:382–388.
12. Alarcon-Segovia D, Deleze M, Oria CV, et al. Antiphospholipid antibodies and the antiphospholipid syndrome in systemic lupus erythematosus. A prospective analysis of 500 consecutive patients. Medicine (Baltimore) 1989;68:353–365.
13. Shrivastava A, Dwivedi S, Aggarwal A, et al. Anti-cardiolipin and anti-beta$_2$ glycoprotein I antibodies in Indian patients with systemic lupus erythematosus: association with the presence of seizures. Lupus 2001;10:45–50.
14. Saluja S, Kumar A, Khamashta M, et al. Prevalence & clinical associations of anticardiolipin antibodies in patients with systemic lupus erythematosus in India. Indian J Med Res 1990;92:224–227.
15. Saxena R, Saraya AK, Dhot PS, et al. Lupus anticoagulant and anticardiolipin antibodies in systemic lupus erythematosus. Natl Med J India 1994;7:163–165.
16. Ninomiya C, Taniguchi O, Kato T, et al. Distribution and clinical significance of lupus anticoagulant and anticardiolipin antibody in 349 patients with systemic lupus erythematosus. Intern Med 1992;31:194–199.
17. Wong KL, Liu HW, Ho K, et al. Anticardiolipin antibodies and lupus anticoagulant in Chinese patients with systemic lupus erythematosus. J Rheumatol 1991;18:1187–1192.

18. Tsutsumi A, Matsuura E, Ichikawa K, et al. Antibodies to β_2-glycoprotein I and clinical manifestations in patients with systemic lupus erythematosus. Arthritis Rheum 1996;39:1466–1474.
19. Chahade WH, Staub HL, Khamashta M, et al. Antiphospholipid antibodies in a Brazilian population with systemic lupus erythematosus. Clin Exp Rheumatol 1989;7:446–447.
20. Gharavi AE, Pierangeli SS, Wilson WA. Anticardiolipin antibodies: importance, controversies, discrepancies; the need for guidelines and calibrators. Clin Exp Rheumatol 2001;19:237–239.
21. Wilson WA, Faghiri Z, Taheri F, et al. Significance of IgA antiphospholipid antibodies. Lupus 1998;2(suppl 7):S110–S113.
22. Perez MC, Wilson WA, Brown HL, et al. Anticardiolipin antibodies in unselected pregnant women. Relationship to fetal outcome. J Perinatol 1991;11:33–36.
23. Harris EN, Spinnato JA. Should anticardiolipin tests be performed in otherwise healthy pregnant women? Am J Obstet Gynecol 1991;165:1272–1277.
24. Wilson WA, Morgan Ost C, Barton EN, et al. IgA antiphospholipid antibodies in HTLV-1-associated tropical spastic paraparesis. Lupus 1995;4:138–141.
25. Faghiri Z, Wilson WA, Taheri F, et al. Antibodies to cardiolipin and beta2-glycoprotein-1 in HTLV-1-associated myelopathy/tropical spastic paraparesis. Lupus 1999;8:210–214.
26. Murphy EL Jr, De Ceulaer K, Williams W, et al. Lack of relation between human T-lymphotropic virus type I infection and systemic lupus erythematosus I Jamaica, West Indies. J Acquir Immune Defic Syndr 1988;1:18–22.
27. Rudwaleit M, Tikly M, Gibson K, et al. HLA class II antigens associated with systemic lupus erythematosus in black South Africans. Ann Rheum Dis 1995;54:678–680.
28. Loizou S, Singh S, Wypkema E, et al. Anticardiolipin, anti-beta(2)-glycoprotein I and antiprothrombin antibodies in black South African patients with infectious disease. Ann Rheum Dis 2003;62:1106–1111.
29. Hammond MG, Du Toitt ED, Sanchez-Mazas A, et al. HLA in Sub-Saharan Africa: 12th International Histocompatibility Workshop SSAF report. In: Charron D, ed. HLA 1997. Paris: EDK; 1997:345–353.
30. Wilson WA, Gharavi AE, Piette JC. International classification criteria for antiphospholipid syndrome: synopsis of a post-conference workshop held at the Ninth International (Tours) aPL Symposium. Lupus 2001;10:457–460.
31. Wilson WA, Gharavi AE. Genetic risk factors for aPL syndrome. Lupus 1996;5:398–403.
32. Citera G, Wilson WA. Ethnic and geographic perspectives in SLE. Lupus 1993;2:351–353.
33. Dessein PH, Gledhill RF, Rossouw DS. Systemic lupus erythematosus in black South Africans. S Afr Med J 1988;74:387–389.
34. Wilson WA, Perez MC, Michalski JP, et al. Cardiolipin antibodies and null alleles of C4 in black Americans with systemic lupus erythematosus. J Rheumatol 1988;15:1768–1772.

22 Antiphospholipid Syndrome: Differential Diagnosis

Beverley J. Hunt and Paul R. J. Ames

Introduction

Reaching the correct diagnosis is the aim of every physician. This chapter is designed to ensure that the correct diagnosis is achieved in patients whose differential diagnosis includes antiphospholipid syndrome (APS). In the past, APS was often not considered in the differential diagnosis of a thrombotic state, although this has occurred less frequently as the condition is becoming better known and understood. Lack of understanding of the assays can result in interpretation difficulties, particularly if investigators do not appreciate that both lupus anticoagulant (LA) and anticardiolipin antibodies (aCL) are different facets of the same problem, and that both must be performed to exclude the diagnosis.

If physicians read this particular book, then they will consider APS in the differential diagnosis of thrombotic disease, and should be highly skilled at interpreting the antiphospholipid (aPL) assays. However, there is a possibility of "overdiagnosis," which is as important to avoid as non-recognition, for once a diagnosis of APS has been made, the management of thrombosis in APS is not without recognized morbidity and mortality due to bleeding. Thus, in patients with aPL, it is important to establish from the history, examination, and investigations that the associated clinical features are consistent with APS, that the aPL assays are reproducible, and that there is no other explanation for the thrombotic events.

In view of the diverse presentation of APS, we have planned this chapter taking into account the new international consensus statement on preliminary criteria for the classification of the APS [1].

Clinical Criteria

Vascular Thrombosis

"One or more clinical episodes of arterial, venous or small vessel thrombosis in any tissue or organ. Thrombosis must be confirmed by imaging or Doppler studies or histopathology, with the exception of superficial venous thrombosis. For histopathological confirmation, thrombosis should be present without significant evidence of inflammation in the vessel wall."

The Differential Diagnosis of Venous Thrombosis

Any part of the venous circulation may undergo occlusion in APS. Deep and superficial veins of the lower limbs are most frequently involved, followed by pulmonary embolism and arm vessels. In these instances, and in subjects who are relatively young (< 45 years), the differential diagnosis rests on laboratory tests aiming at the identification of congenital or other acquired thrombophilic states. The current venous thrombophilia screen (1999) is shown in Table 22.1. aPL seems to be a common etiological factor in venous thrombosis in unusual sites such as the abdominal circulation. APS has been described as the second most common cause of Budd-Chiari syndrome [2], after myeloproliferative disorders [3], and thrombosis in other abdominal veins are reported in APS. APS should be included in the differential diagnosis of cerebral vein thrombosis, because the presence of aPL in this population ranges from 8% to 55%, and affected patients tend to have younger age at onset and more extensive involvement than patients with conventional thrombophilic states [4, 5]. Consideration should be given to the prothrombin 20210 mutation, present in 2% of Caucasians, that also appears to predispose to thrombosis in the coronary and cerebral venous vessels. The differential effects of hypercoagulable states in different vascular beds is excellently reviewed by Rosenberg and Aird [6]. In the ophthalmology setting, aPL have been detected from 5% to 47% of subjects presenting with retinal vein occlusion, alongside other thrombophilic factors and vasculitis [7–9]. aPL should be included in the differential diagnosis of thrombotic events causing endocrine abnormalities, such as Addison's disease [10–12] and Sheehan's syndrome (hypopituitarism) [13]. Although the differential diagnosis of venous occlusions often relies on detecting a thrombophilic state, some clinical features may point towards systemic disorders with a higher-than-average risk of venous thrombosis. For example, a history of oral and genital ulceration in a young person with venous thrombosis may suggest Behcet's disease, and the presence of peripheral blood eosinophilia could suggest

Table 22.1. Differential diagnosis of venous thromboembolism in antiphospholipid syndrome.

Activated protein C resistance/factor V Leiden (heterozygote and homozygous)

Heterozygous deficiencies of
Antithrombin
Protein C
Protein S
Prothrombin 20210 heterozygous or homozygous states

Increased levels of factor VIII

Myeloproliferative disorders

Dysfibrinogenemia

Very rare
Paroxysmal nocturnal hemoglobinuria

Possible risk factor
Hyperhomocysteinemia

Table 22.2. Risk factors for arterial thrombosis. 📖

Hypertension
Smoking
Fibrinogen levels
Hyperhomocysteinemia
Hyperlipidemia
Diabetes mellitus
Lipoprotein (a)

the hypereosinophilic syndrome, a condition that, like APS, does not spare any vascular bed.

The Differential Diagnosis of Arterial Thrombosis

When compared to the potentially recognized risk factors for venous thrombotic disease, there are fewer factors to consider in arterial thrombotic disease. All the other known risk factors for arterial thrombotic disease tend to produce thrombosis on the background of arteriosclerosis, that is, these patients tend to have recognizable risk factors for atherosclerosis. Evidence is slowly accumulating to support accelerated atherosclerosis in APS, suggesting that management should include treatment of conventional risk factors as well as anticoagulation. The risk factors for arterial thrombosis are summarized in Table 22.2.

Special Arterial Situations

Special consideration should be given to stroke, where up to 18% of young strokes may have aPL [15]. The neurological manifestations of APS are protean (see Chapter 7). Some patients present with multiple cerebral lesions on magnetic resonance imaging, consistent with multiple cerebral infarcts. These types of lesions are also seen in multiple sclerosis and a cerebral autosomal dominant arteriopathy with subcortical infarcts and leucoencephalopathy (CADASIL) [16, 17]. CADASIL is a hereditary cause of stroke, migraine with aura, mood disturbances, and dementia. Thus, if a patient does present with multiple cerebral lesions, a family history of stroke and dementia should be sought. Post-mortem studies of affected patients show multiple small deep infarcts in the brain and a diffuse leukoencephalopathy. The vasculopathy leads to median thickening by an eosinophilic, granular, and electron-dense material of unknown origin. The genetic defect has been mapped to chromosome 19 and can now be detected in the majority of major neuroscience centers.

It may be very difficult to differentiate APS from multiple sclerosis. Clues include a past history of venous thrombosis and pregnancy loss, suggesting APS, while the presence of cerebellar lesions on MRI are more suggestive of multiple sclerosis [18]. Both states can produce oligoclonal bands in the cerebrospinal fluid (CSF). Another differential diagnosis of multiple cerebral lesions can be cerebral vasculitis, and in such cases the diagnosis may only become apparent on cerebral biopsy.

Catastrophic APS

This syndrome has a number of clinical similarities to heparin-induced thrombocytopenia. In heparin-induced thrombocytopenia patients develop thrombosis at any site, both arterial, venous, and microvascular (especially the skin). This is due to the presence of an antibody that binds to the complex of platelet factor 4/heparin [19]. It usually develops within 10–14 days after starting heparin and the first sign is a falling platelet count. It should be differentiated from a transient thrombocytopaenia that occurs in the first few days of heparin therapy, which is probably due to heparin causing platelet activation and is not associated with any clinically harmful effects.

The differentiation of aPL related thrombocytopenia from heparin induced thrombocytopenia would appear almost straightforward, especially from the history, although the differential diagnosis could be tricky on the laboratory side when both conditions coexist [20, 21].

Pregnancy Morbidity

(A) One or more unexplained deaths of a morphologically normal fetus at or beyond the 10th week of gestation, with normal fetal morphology documented by ultrasound or by direct examination of the fetus, or

(B) One or more premature births of a morphologically normal neonate at or before the 34th week of gestation because of severe pre-eclampsia or eclampsia or severe placental insufficiency, or

(C) Three or more unexplained consecutive spontaneous abortions before the 10th week of gestation, with maternal anatomic or hormonal abnormalities and paternal and maternal chromosomal causes excluded.

In studies of populations of patients who have more than 1 type of pregnancy morbidity, investigators are strongly encouraged to stratify groups of subjects according to A, B, or C above.

In the United Kingdom, pulmonary thrombo-embolism is the leading cause of maternal death. Deep vein thrombosis underlies this disorder and is frequently unrecognized. The risk factors for thrombo-embolism in pregnancy remain the same as those outside of pregnancy: congenital and acquired thrombophilias.

APS has also been identified as a cause of first, second, and third trimester losses as well as intra-uterine growth restriction and pre-eclampsia. One of the major advances in the field of thrombophilia in the last few years has been the recognition that other thrombophilic states also predispose to second and third trimester losses, as well as intra-uterine growth restriction and pre-eclampsia. A case-control study revealed that factor V Leiden, the prothrombin 20210 mutation, and homozygous state for the homocysteine MTHFR mutation C677T were strongly associated with late pregnancy complications of placental abruption, pre-eclampsia and eclampsia, and intra-uterine growth restriction in women [22]. Moreover, a recent study has shown that if women with a previous second or third trimester loss and an inherited thrombophilia show a marked improvement in fetal outcome in the next pregnancy if they receive low-molecular-weight heparin throughout the pregnancy [23].

Interestingly, a cohort study following a group of women with factor V Leiden during pregnancy found its presence was unrelated to adverse pregnancy outcome apart from an 8-fold increased risk of venous thromboembolism [24]. It is now clear that aPL are also associated with first trimester losses. It is not clear at the time of writing whether congenital thrombophilia are associated with first trimester losses. The answers should be available in the next few years.

It is important when considering the late pregnancy morbidity associated with aPL to check that the history concurs with that of placental insufficiency, for in the Lupus Pregnancy clinic at St Thomas' Hospital (London) we have a number of women referred with APS on the basis of pregnancy loss and aPL is an incidental finding. These women have proved to have pregnancy loss due to other causes such as premature labor secondary to an incompetent cervix (in these cases the waters break first, labor supervenes, and the fetus may be born alive of a normal birth weight). Thus, history taking and obtaining the post-mortem findings in previous pregnancy losses are very important. In considering the etiology of first trimester losses it is also important that a gynecologist excludes other relevant causes. It thus seems imperative to run a joint clinic with an obstetrician and/or obstetric physician before aPL can be attributed to be the cause of the pregnancy loss.

Hyperhomocysteinemia

This condition deserves a special mention, for it is the only other condition related to pregnancy loss, arterial thrombosis, and possibly venous thrombosis. High plasma levels of homocysteine are the result of the interplay between congenital and environmental factors. There has been a growing interest on mild or moderate hyperhomocysteinemia as a risk factor for arterial and venous thrombosis.

The most common cause of severe homocysteinemia (fasting plasma levels > 100 µmol/L) is the homozygous deficiency of cystathionine-β-synthase, which has a prevalence of 1 in 335,000. Affected individuals present with premature vascular disease and thrombo-embolism as well as ectopic lens, skeletal abnormalities, and mental retardation [25]. Mild to moderate levels (fasting levels between 15–100 µmol/L) are encountered in phenotypically normal subjects with genetic defects in metabolism, acquired conditions, or more frequently a combination of the two. Often, acquired hyperhomocysteinemia may follow deficiencies of folate, cobalamin, and pyridoxine [26], essential co-factors for homocysteine metabolism and may develop in chronic renal insufficiency. Drugs are another important remedial cause. Drugs such as methotrexate interfere with the metabolism of folate, and nitrous oxide interferes with the metabolism of cobalamin and theophylline and affect vitamin B_6.

A common genetic defect leading to hyperhomocysteinemia is a C-to-T substitution at nucleotide 677 in the gene coding for methylenetetrahydrofolate reductase (MTHFR) [27]. The prevalence of the homozygous C677T mutation is between 5% to 20% in subjects of Caucasian origin. These individuals tend not to have elevated plasma levels of homocysteine unless they have an accompanying low serum concentration of folate [28]. Case-control and cross-sectional studies indicate that mild-to-moderate hyperhomocysteinemia is associated with an increased risk of thrombosis [reviewed in 25]. APS patients with homozygous C667T mutation developed thrombosis at an earlier age than heterozygous or non-mutated APS patients [29]. Mild hyperhomocysteinemia appeared also as an independent predictor of carotid intima-media thickness in primary APS [30]. However prospective studies do not unequivocally show that hyperhomocysteinemia is associated with an increased risk of venous thrombosis. Further studies are also required to fully establish the relationship between homocysteine levels, the C677T MTHFR mutation, and late pregnancy complications. Most importantly however, randomized placebo-controlled double-blind trials of the effects of homocysteine–lowering vitamins are urgently needed. They will help define the relationship between mild-to-moderate hyperhomocysteinemia and thrombosis and potentially have an impact on the prevention of thrombosis.

Other Clinical Features of APS

Thrombocytopenia

Thrombocytopenia is a feature in some patients with APS, present in almost 20% of aPL carriers and probably of autoimmune pathogenesis. Thrombocytopenic bleeding is not frequent in APS, unless there is a coexistent factor deficiency, but prolonged bleeding times do occur [31]. Screening for aPL in subjects with thrombocytopenia of uncertain cause is useful, especially in thrombocytopenia of pregnancy, where the risks of hemorrhage from thrombocytopenia and thrombosis and pregnancy morbidity from aPL could jeopardize fetal and maternal outcome. aPL were detected in 60% of thrombocytopenic HIV subjects addicted to parenteral drugs [32], but there does not appear to be a relationship with thrombosis: in HIV aCL have no anti–β_2-glycoprotein I effect.

Skin Involvement

Livedo reticularis appears in a number of rheumatic conditions and hyperviscosity states. The detection of aPL in a subject with livedo reticularis and a stroke may suggest Sneddon's syndrome, hence the finding of aPL positively in someone with isolated livedo reticularis could warrant closer follow up. Likewise, skin necrosis, skin ulcers, chilblains, and vasculitis have been associated with aPL [33], and may identify those patients at higher risk of vascular damage. Pyoderma gangrenosum is frequently associated with systemic diseases but there are cases where aPL was the only abnormal laboratory finding [34].

The Effect of aPL on Other Thrombophilic Assays

In the presence of aPL, some of the other assays for thrombophilia may cause false positive results. It is well recognized that functional assays for protein C and activated protein C resistance may yield falsely low values in the presence of aPL [35]. Similarly, phospholipid-dependent coagulation assays such as factor XII assays may produce reduced levels. This has been studied by Jones et al [36], who found that factor XII antibodies are present in a significant proportion of LA-positive patients and may lead to an erroneous diagnosis of factor XII deficiency.

Reduced levels of free protein S are present in some patients with aPL, and thus could lead to an erroneous diagnosis of genetic protein S deficiency [37, 38]. The mechanism of this reduction of free protein S is obscure, although this could be caused by antibodies to protein S itself, or autoantibodies to β_2-glycoprotein I with C4b-binding protein [39, 40].

Conclusions

APS/Hughes syndrome is an increasingly diagnosed condition. This chapter emphasizes the need for clinicians to consider the full range of differential diagnoses for
each clinical state, so that the correct diagnosis is reached in an individual patient.

References

1. Wilson WA, Gharavi A, Koike T, et al. International consensus statement on the preliminary
   classification criteria for definite antiphospholipid syndrome. Arthritis Rheum 1999;42:1309–1311.
2. Pelletier S, Landi B, Piette JC, et al. Antiphospholipid syndrome as the second cause of non-tumor-
   ous Budd-Chiari syndrome. J Hepatol 1994;21:76–80.
3. De Stefano V, Teofili L, Leone G, Michiels JJ. Spontaneous erythroid colony formation as the clue to
   an underlying myeloproliferative disorder in patients with Budd-Chiari syndrome or portal vein
   thrombosis. Semin Thromb Hemost 1997;23:411–418.
4. Carhuapoma JR, Mitsias P, Levine SR. Cerebral venous thrombosis and anticardiolipin antibodies.
   Stroke 1997;28:2363–2369.
5. Deschiens MA, Conard J, Horellou MH. Coagulation studies, factor V Leiden, and anticardiolipin
   antibodies in 40 cases of cerebral venous thrombosis. Stroke 1996;27:1724–1730.
6. Rosenberg RD, Aird WC. Vascular-bed-specific hemostasis and hypercoagulable states. N Engl J Med
   1999;340:1555–1564.
7. Coniglio M, Platania A, Di Nucci GD, Arcieri P, Modzrewska R, Mariani G. Antiphospholipid-protein
   antibodies are not an uncommon feature in retinal venous occlusions. Thromb Res 1996;83:183–188.
8. Abu el-Asrar AM, al-Momen AK, al-Amro S, Abdel Gader AG, Tabbara KF. Prothrombotic states
   associated with retinal venous occlusion in young adults. Int Ophthalmol 1996;20:197–204.
9. Glacet-Bernard A, Bayani N, Chretien P, Cochard C, Lelong F, Coscas G. Antiphospholipid antibodies in retinal vascular occlusions. A prospective study of 75 patients. Arch Ophthalmol
   1994;112:790–795.
10. Gonzalez G, Gutierrez M, Ortiz M, Tellez R, Figueroa F, Jacobelli S. Association of primary antiphos-
    pholipid syndrome with primary adrenal insufficiency. J Rheumatol 1996;23:1286–1287.
11. al-Momen AK, Sulimani R, Harakati M, Gader AG, Mekki M. IgA antiphospholipid and adrenal
    insufficiency: is there a link? Thromb Res 1991;64:571–578.
12. Lenaerts J, Vanneste S, Knockaert D, Arnout J, Vermylen J. SLE and acute Addisonian crisis due to
    bilateral adrenal hemorrhage: association with the antiphospholipid syndrome. Clin Exp Rheumatol
    199;9:407–409.
13. Pandolfi C, Gianini A, Fregoni V, Nalli G, Faggi L. Hypopituitarism and antiphospholipid syndrome.
    Minerva Endocrinol 1997;22:103–105.
14. Kuzu MA, Ozaslan C, Koksoy C, Gurler A, Tuzuner A. Vascular involvement in Behcet's disease: 8-
    year audit. World J Surg 1994;18:948–953.
15. Nencini P, Baruffi MC, Abbate R, et al. Lupus anticoagulant and anticardiolipin antibodies in young
    adults with cerebral ischaemia. Stroke 1992;23:189–193.
16. Chabriat H, Vahedi K, Iba-Zizen MT, et al. Clinical Spectrum of CADASIL: a study of 7 familes.
    Lancet 1995;346:934–939.
17. Chabriat H, Levy C, Taillia H, et al. Patterns of MRI lesions in CADASIL. Neurology 1998;51:452–457.
18. Cuadrado MJ, Khamashta MA, Ballesteros A, et al. Can Hughes (antiphospholipid) syndrome be dis-
    tinguished from multiple sclerosis. Analysis of 27 patients and review of the literature. Medicine
    (Baltimore) 2000;79:57–68.
19. Warkentin TE, Chong BH, Greinacher A. Heparin-induced thrombocytopenia: towards consensus.
    Thromb Haemost 1998;79:1–7.
20. Gruel Y, Rupin A, Watier H, Vigier S, Bardos P, Leroy J. Anticardiolipin antibodies in heparin-asso-
    ciated thrombocytopenia. Thromb Res 1992;67:601–606.
21. Lasne D, Saffroy R, Bachelot C, et al. Tests for heparin-induced thrombocytopenia in primary
    antiphospholipid syndrome. Br J Haematol 1997;97:939.
22. Kupferminc MJ, Eldor A, Steinman N, et al. Increased frequency of genetic thrombophilia in women
    with complications of pregnancy. N Engl J Med 1999;340:9–13.

23. Gris JC, Mercier E, Quere I, et al. Low-molecular weight heparin versus low-dose aspirin in women with one fetal loss and a constititional threombophilia disorder. Blood 2004;103:3695–3699.
24. Lindqvist PG, Svenssson PJ, Marsal K, et al. Activated protein C resistance and pregnancy. Thromb Haemost 1999;81:532–537.
25. Cattaneo M. Hyperhomocysteinemia, atherosclerosis and thrombosis. Thromb Haemost 1999;81:165–176.
26. Selhub J, Jacques PF, Wilson PWF, Rush D, Rosenberg JH. Vitamin status and intake as primary determinants of homocysteinemia in an elderly population. JAMA 1993;270:2693–2698.
27. Frosst P, Blom HJ, Milos R, et al. A candidate risk factor for vascular disease: a common mutation in methylenetetrahydrofolate reductase. Nat Genet 1995;10:111–113.
28. Ma J, Stampfer MJ, Hennekens CH, et al. Methylenetetrahydrofolate reductase polymorphism, plasma folate, homocysteine, and risk of myocardial infarction in US physicians. Circulation 1996;94:2410–2416.
29. Ames PRJ, Tommasino C, D'Andrea G, Iannaccone L, Brancaccio V, Margaglione M. Thrombophilic genotypes in subjects with idiopathic antiphospholipid antibodies-prevalence and significance. Thromb Haemost 1998;79:46–49.
30. Ames PRJ, Margarita A, Delgado Alves J, Tommasino C, Iannaccone L, Brancaccio V. Anticardiolipin antibody titre and plasma homocysteine level independently predict intima media thickness of carotid arteries in subjects with idiopathic antiphospholipid antibodies. Lupus 2002;11:208–214.
31. Galli M, Finazzi G, Barbui T. Thrombocytopenia in the antiphospholipid syndrome. Br J Haematol 1996;93:1–5.
32. Muniz-Diaz E, Domingo P, Lopez M, et al. Thrombocytopenia associated with human immunodeficiency virus infection. Immunologic study of 60 patients addicted to parenteral drugs. Med Clin (Barc) 1993;101:761–765.
33. Tajima C, Suzuki Y, Mizushima Y, Ichikawa Y. Clinical significance of immunoglobulin A antiphospholipid antibodies: possible association with skin manifestations and small vessel vasculitis. J Rheumatol 1998;25:1730–1736.
34. Chacek S, MacGregor-Gooch J, Halabe-Cherem J, Nellen-Hummel H, Quinones-Galvan A. Pyoderma gangrenosum and extensive caval thrombosis associated with the antiphospholipid syndrome – a case report. Angiology 1998;49:157–160.
35. Atsumi T, Khamashta MA, Amengual O, et al. Binding of the anticardiolipin antibodies to protein C via beta2 glycoprotein I. Clin Exp Immunol 1998;112:325–333.
36. Jones DW, Gallimore MJ, Winter M. Antibodies to factor XII associated with lupus anticoagulant. Thromb Haemost 1999;81:387–390.
37. Ames PRJ, Iannaccone L, Tommasino C, Brillante M, Brancaccio V. Coagulation activation and fibrinolytic imbalance in subjects with idiopathic antiphospholipid antibodies. A crucial role for acquired free protein S deficicency. Thromb Haemost 1996;76:190–194.
38. Parke AL, Weinstein RE, Bona Rd, Maier DB, Walker FJ. The thrombotic diathesis associated with the presence of phospholipid antibodies may be due to low levels of free protein S. Am J Med 1992;93:49.
39. Walker FJ. Does beta-2-glycoprotein I inhibit interaction between protein S and C4b-binding protein? [abstract] Thromb Haemost 1993;69:930.
40. Atsumi T, Khamashta MA, Ames PRJ, Ichikawa K, Koike T, Hughes GRV. Effect of beta-2 glycoprotein I and monoclonal anticardiolipin antibodies on the protein S/C4B binding protein system. Lupus 1997;6:358–364.

Section 2
Laboratory Investigation

23 Anticardiolipin Testing

Silvia S. Pierangeli

Introduction

It is well known that patients affected with antiphospholipid syndrome (APS) are subject to episodes of thrombosis in arteries and/or veins, pregnancy loss (probably secondary to thrombosis of vessels in the placenta), and thrombocytopenia, associated with antiphospholipid (aPL) antibodies [1, 2]. aPL antibodies are autoantibodies directed against anionic phospholipids or protein–phospholipid complexes [3–5], measured in solid-phase immunoassays as anticardiolipin (aCL), or as an activity which prolongs phospholipid-dependent coagulation assays, the so-called lupus anticoagulants (LA) [6, 7]. Diagnosis of APS is based on finding a "moderate-to-high" positive aCL test and/or a LA test with any one of the characteristic clinical features presented above [2, 8].

The aCL test is important to aid the physician in diagnosis of APS [1, 8]. Although a sensitive test, aCL ELISA tests are positive in a variety of disorders, including connective tissue diseases, infectious disorders such as syphilis [9, 10], Q fever, and acquired immune deficiency syndrome (AIDS) [11–13], and some drug induced disorders [14]. It is generally believed that aCL are clinically significant only when present in APS; thus, there have been continuous attempts to modify the assay to make it *more specific* for APS. In addition, based on an early observation that patients with high positive IgG aCL tests were more likely to have APS [15], that ACL are heterogenous and measured using a wide variety of techniques, efforts have been devoted to quantifying the aCL ELISA test in a standardized manner [16–19]. This chapter will discuss the various techniques used in the diagnosis of APS, a series of aCL workshops that have been used to validate and improve measurement of aCL, as well as issues concerning problems and solutions concerning aCL testing. An overview of new and more specific tests for diagnosis of APS is also discussed.

Historical Background of the Anticardiolipin Test

In 1983, a group of investigators at the Hammersmith Hospital in London, England, noticed that some patients with systemic lupus erythematosus (SLE) had a rather uncommon coagulation abnormality called "lupus anticoagulant" [this was due to the abnormal prolongation of the partial thromboplastin time (PTT)] [20, 21]. The investigators also established that instead of abnormal bleeding, these patients were subject to thrombosis [20]. Soon thereafter, the "lupus anticoagulant (LA) phenomenon" was known to be caused by an autoantibody believed to bind phospholipids, because they inhibited two phospholipid dependent coagulation reactions in the clotting-cascade – the prothrombin–thrombin conversion and the activation of factor X activation [22, 23]. In addition, about 25% to 50% of patients with the LA reaction also had a biological false positive test for syphilis (BFP-STS). Antibodies responsible for the BFP-STS were known to bind CL, a negatively charged phospholipid. The LA test had some drawbacks: it was a functional assay affected by a number of variables, including preparation and storage of samples, type of reagent use, etc. In addition, the test lacked sensitivity and could not be readily standardized. Thus, this group of investigators reasoned that use of a solid phase immunoassay with cardiolipin as antigen might be one way of detecting antibodies with LA activity [6]. They thought that such a test would have the advantages of greater sensitivity, more reproducibility, better quantitation, and the possibility of standardization. The group succeeded in establishing a solid phase radioimmunoassay with cardiolipin as antigen, and the antibodies were termed *anticardiolipin antibodies* (aCL) [6]. Hence, the first aCL test was established in 1983 [6]. The test proved more sensitive than the LA assay and enabled diagnosis of a much larger number of patients with APS. Also, the investigators soon noticed that aCL antibodies crossreacted with negatively charged phospholipids, such as phosphatidylserine (PS) and phosphatidylglycerol (PG) [24]. Thus, the name aCL antibodies was changed to aPL [25]. And the disorder with which these antibodies were associated was called the antiphospholipid syndrome (APS) [25].

Widespread adoption of the solid phase aCL assay led to several potential problems. These antibodies were soon reported in several disorders, such as syphilis [9, 10, 26], AIDS [11, 12], connective tissue diseases, as well as in normal individuals who did not have the features of the disorder. "False" positive tests in the aforementioned conditions could be best explained by the sensitivity of the aCL test. However, methods of performing the test also varied and results were questionable in some instances. Fortunately, it was recognized that the majority of the patients with APS tended to have high aCL antibody levels, usually of the IgG isotype (however, some patients were only IgM positive) [27]. To ensure that the aCL test would retain its value in diagnosis APS, it would be necessary to identify antibodies by isotype and to quantify results using some reliable unit of measurement. There was also a need to establish which testing methods were valid as well as standard procedures for performing the solid phase immunoassay. To achieve these goals, several international standardization workshops were conducted following the first one in 1986 [16–19, 28].

Tests Used in Diagnosis of APS

The aCL Test

The aCL test was first established in 1983, using cardiolipin as an antigen, a mixture of gelatin/PBS to dilute patient serum, and radiollabeled anti-human IgG or IgM to detect bound aCL antibodies. The first aCL assay was a radioimmunoassay [6]. Since the test was first developed, several changes and improvements have been made to reduce the background binding, to quantify the results in units and with respect to incubation times and temperatures [25, 27]. The introduction of adult bovine or fetal calf serum was found to enhance antibody binding to cardiolipin. In 1990, three separate groups of investigators determined that this increase in signal probably occurred because of the presence of antibodies specific for β_2-glycoprotein I (β_2-GPI) [4, 28, 29]. β_2-GPI is a 50 kDa protein present in fetal or bovine serum that binds negatively charged phospholipids. It is now clear that sera from patients with APS bind not only negatively charged phospholipids but also other proteins such as β_2-GPI, prothrombin, or protein C alone or in combination with phospholipids [3–5, 31–34].

The aCL test has been widely utilized by physicians since the mid-1980s for diagnosing patients with APS. Establishment of this diagnosis has enabled effective management of patients with recurrent thrombosis or recurrent pregnancy losses. The aCL test is sensitive and is positive in more than 80% to 90% of patients with the disorder. Association of a positive aCL test with clinical manifestations of APS occurs principally with persistent medium-to-high levels of aCL antibodies and IgG is more prevalent than IgM [27]. However, there are reports that IgM and occasionally IgA aCL antibodies are also associated with clinical manifestations of APS [27, 35].

The inter-laboratory agreement is better when the results of the aCL test are reported by ranges of positivity (i.e., low positive, medium positive, or high positive) [17]. It is because antibody levels are so important to diagnosis that considerable effort has been spent in standardizing test procedures and defining antibody levels [16–19, 28].

Standardization of the Anticardiolipin Test

Several international workshops and forums have been conducted in an attempt to standardize the aCL test [15–19, 28]. In the first aCL workshop, the assay methods that enabled valid measurements of aCL antibody levels were determined [15]. In addition, units of measurement were defined, and 6 standards were introduced to assist laboratories worldwide in establishing the aCL assay. The second workshop demonstrated that semi-quantitative measures of aCL antibody levels enabled the best agreement between laboratories [16]. The third and fourth workshops sought to settle controversial issues regarding aCL specificity, but also sought to examine some of the newly introduced commercial kits [17, 18].

Despite these efforts in standardization, a considerable degree of inter-laboratory variation still exits [36, 37]. Recently, in a large cooperative study that included 30 European laboratory investigators demonstrated that discrepancies and lack of inter-laboratory agreement was mainly due to the way laboratories are performing the test, the way the test is calibrated, and how the results are calculated [28]. The study also showed that when laboratories utilized the "standard" aCL ELISA, as previously described elsewhere [38] – what the authors called the "consensus" kit – and calculated the results in a uniform manner, the agreement between laboratories was much improved [28]. Together these workshops have demonstrated that investigators working collaboratively can contribute to improvement of testing methods, and to greater understanding of scientific issues such as those related to clinical significance and specificity of aCL antibodies.

National and international organizations are also contributing to the standardization of the aCL test: the College of American Pathologists enrolls certified laboratories in quality control surveys for aCL testing and requires participation in the program for accreditation purposes.

Calibrators for aCL Testing

Ever since the aCL test was first developed there was uncertainty about results. The test was found to be positive in unexpectedly high percentages of patients with SLE and other autoimmune disorders, and in patients with a bewildering variety of other diseases who had neither thrombosis nor pregnancy losses [9–14, 39]. Many of these "false positive" results occurred in patients with aCL antibody at low levels [40], whereas patients with features of APS tended to have higher levels. Even in the first series of patients published, results were ranked according to level of positivity showed that those with the highest levels were more subjected to thrombotic or pregnancy related complications [15]. Subsequent studies also showed that the higher the level of aCL positive the more likely the diagnosis of APS [41, 42].

It was evident then that it would not be sufficient to report aCL tests as merely positive or negative, but that measurement of aCL levels would provide more specific diagnosis of APS. To enable valid measurement of aCL levels, a unique approach was taken. A set of IgG aCL calibrators was prepared by mixing a high positive IgG serum sample containing a defined antibody concentration and varying concentrations of normal serum. The value of each of the calibrators could be calculated based on the proportions of the high positive IgG serum and normal serum in the mixture. Thus, these calibrators had values independent of any given assay method. This approach accomplished 3 goals. First, it enabled validation of any aCL antibody assay technique, because readings, whether obtain by ELISA or any other method, had to correlate with the calculated calibrator IgG aCL concentration if the assay technique was valid. Second, aCL levels of unknown samples could be derived from the calibration curve, no matter the technique used to measure the calibrators and samples; finally, secondary calibrators could be prepared because their values could be derived from an IgG calibration curve, utilizing the original calibrators. A similar approach was used to prepare IgM immediately thereafter and, subsequently, IgA calibrators in 1993.

Once the initial IgG and IgM aCL calibrators were prepared, they were subaliquot and distributed to laboratories throughout the world. Each laboratory was asked to measure aCL antibodies by whatever method they normally used. Results were returned to a central laboratory. For each laboratory, the readings of the calibrators obtained were compared with the calculated calibrator values and the correlation between readings and calculated values were determined [16, 17]. Utilizing appropriate statistical methods, a determination could be made as to the validity of the assay. It was this approach that first enabled determination that assays using fetal or bovine serum in the diluent for patient samples gave more valid results.

Preparation of Secondary Calibrators

It was originally intended that, once the initial calibrators were made and validated, other laboratories could make secondary calibrators using the initial ones. Because the first group of calibrators had defined values that covered the full range for the ELISA assay, they could be used to establish calibration curves for IgG or IgM aCL and values of secondary calibrators could be derived Although this approach appeared straightforward it was very difficult for individual laboratories to make secondary calibrators reliably because of the tedium of testing dozens of mixtures of positive and negative sera to select a suitable group of secondary calibrators. It also proved difficult to get large enough quantities of positive sera.

Because of the difficulty in preparing secondary calibrators, many laboratories turned to the Antiphospholipid Standardization Laboratory for distribution of calibrators. That laboratory has distributed standard calibrators since the late 1980s. Because of the large demand, three generations of secondary calibrators have been prepared and distributed. The second generation of calibrators was prepared in 1990 (LAPL GM-001). The third set was prepared in 1997 and was called LAPL-GM-100. A fourth set was prepared in March 2001 and was named LAPL GM-200. Each generation used the first group of calibrators for comparison. Each generation of calibrators was carefully prepared and exhaustively tested in our own and other well-recognized laboratories. As another means of demonstrating the performance of these calibrators, results of 6 samples (from the second standardization workshop, the so-called "KAPS" standards) were compared using each generation of calibrators and the results are displayed in Table 23.1 and Table 23.2. It is evident that there was a good correlation of results.

Monoclonal Anticardiolipin Calibrators

Recently, some laboratories have introduced monoclonal aCL calibrators. When serially diluted, these calibrators correlate well with the originally prepared standard calibratrors [43], providing additional evidence that secondary calibrators can be prepared and validated against the original standard calibrators. These mono-

Table 23.1. IgG KAPS standards values utilizing each generation of anticardiolipin antibody calibrators.

Calibrator	Expected GPL units	Observed GPL units using "a" calibrators (n = 15)	Observed GPL units using "b" calibrators (n = 10)	Observed GPL units using "c" calibrators (n = 22)	Observed GPL units using "d" calibrators (n = 5)
G1	100	88 ± 20.0	103 ± 23.0	102.5 ± 15.0	104.6 ± 20.0
G2	20	17 ± 6.0	20.7 ± 10.0	25.6 ± 8.0	25.0 ± 8.9
G3	10	4.5 ± 3.5	8.4 ± 4.3	9.5 ± 4.0	9.8 ± 3.4

"Expected" values were the calculated values for each calibrator and "observed' values were the values obtained in a run when calibration curve was constructed using: "a": first generation of calibrators; "b": LAPL-G001; "c": LAPL-GM100, or "d": LAPL-GM200. Observed values are expressed as mean ± SD.
n = number of runs.

Table 23.2. IgM KAPS standards values utilizing each generation of anticardiolipin antibody calibrators.

Calibrator	Expected MPL units	Observed MPL units using "a" calibrators (n = 12)	Observed MPL units using "b" calibrators (n = 10)	Observed MPL units using "c" calibrators (n = 13)	Observed MPL units using "d" calibrators (n = 5)
M1	100	99.8 ± 12.4	88.0 ± 19.0	120.0 ± 23.0	105.4 ± 15.0
M2	20	14.8 ± 4.5	23.0 ± 5.6	35.0 ± 9.0	32.0 ± 7.9
M3	10	4.3 ± 2.7	6.4 ± 4.6	15.0 ± 8.0	15.8 ± 3.4

"Expected" values were the calculated values for each calibrator and "observed' values were the values obtained in a run when calibration curve was constructed using: "a": first generation of calibrators; "b": LAPL-G001; "c": LAPL-GM100; or "d": LAPL-GM200. Observed values are expressed as mean ± SD.
n = number of runs.

clonal calibrators bind with different avidities to cardiolipin, phosphatidylserine, phosphatidic acid, phosphatidylinositol, and β_2-GPI, and like most polyclonal aPL antibodies, they do not bind to phosphatidylcholine.

A monoclonal antibody standard offers the theoretical advantage of being a single component that can be utilized in perpetuity. On the other hand, issues of its purity and stability over time and their ability to be stored freeze-dried require resolution. The original standard polyclonal calibrators offer the advantage that they are derived from actual patients, possess the polyspecificity of aPL antibodies, and may still be useful in standardizing ELISA assays for yet-to-be-determined antigens. With respect to the last statement, it should be noted that if standards had been prepared from monoclonal antibodies specific only for cardiolipin and negatively charged phospholipids, believed to be only antigen in the 1980s, they would have missed specificity for β_2-GPI and other possible protein antigens.

Whatever calibrator is used, it should be emphasized that there is no substitute for carefully performed assays utilizing validated methods.

Variations of the aCL Assay

Although quantification of aCL levels has been achieved, there exists substantial inter-assay and, even more so, inter-laboratory variations [36, 37]. In assessing aCL results, it is important to note that the error range of individual test results is relatively large at all levels of positivity. In addition, above 80 to 90 G phospholipid (GPL) or MPL units, or below 20 GPL or MPL units, differences in levels cannot be reliably determined because the correlations between optical density readings and aCL concentrations are relatively flat. These are features of the ELISA that cannot be avoided, no matter the care taken in performing the tests.

Any number of variables can contribute to some error and even failure of the assay. These include type of ELISA plates, differences in substrate and conjugate, and in other components of the assay [44, 45]. Many of these problems can occur with any ELISA and are not confined to the aCL test. To further ensure accurate results, our laboratory uses an in-house control with a defined value and error limits in addition to use of calibrators to construct a calibration curve. If the value of the in-house control falls outside of defined limits (often > 1.5–2.0 standard deviations), the run is repeated.

As indicated earlier and because of the difficulty in obtaining precise and reproducible measurement of aCL levels, we recommend reporting the results semi-quantitatively (high positive, medium positive, low positive, or negative), in addition to values report quantitatively in GPL, MPL, or APL units for IgG, IgM, or IgA, respectively [16, 17]. The definition of negative, low, medium, or high is based on the calibration curve. The low range is taken as between 10 GPL (or MPL) units and 20 GPL (or MPL units) when the calibration curve is relatively "flat" [44, 45]. At this range, there is only a small change in optical density (OD) with aCL levels. In the medium range (20–80 GPL or MPL units), the relationship of OD with changes in aCL levels is linear and steep. The cut-off between negative and low positive is taken as 10 GPL or MPL units in our laboratory and represents the 95th percentile of the normal population. Because there are so many disorders that cause low positive aCL results, our efforts have concentrated not on the cut-off point, but on the level that enables best distinction between APS and non-APS patients. This level is at least above 20 GPL (or MPL units) and even more reliably, above 40 GPL or MPL units [41, 42].

As indicated, several retrospective studies support the view that a diagnosis of APS is more likely with medium-to-high aCL levels. Studies by Levine and Escalante and their respective colleagues demonstrated that medium and high levels of aCL antibodies are more significantly correlated with the clinical manifestations of APS [41, 42]. However, given the likelihood that this is a disease with more than one autoantibody, and that these autoantibodies may vary in specificity, a low positive aCL test need not exclude the presence of other pathogenic antibodies. In addition, there are a few patients with high positive aCL results who do not have any manifestations of APS [40]. In the latter instance these patients may still be at risk for APS in the future, because thrombosis requires not only high antibody levels but may require a second vascular event, which may not have occurred as yet in those particular patients.

Recent reports show an apparent large number of individuals with low-to-moderate titers of aCL antibodies, particularly of the IgM isotype, with no clinical signs of APS. Physicians are puzzled with respect to the significance of those results. In order to clarify that questions, we recently carried out a study in which we examined the prevalence of low positive titers of IgM aCL antibodies in a large number (Group 1) of healthy individuals (n = 982) and in a group of 159 individuals older than 60 years of age (Group 2). The possibility of re-defining currently used cut-off values for IgM aCL tests was also examined. IgM aCL antibodies were tested in 3 ELISA assays: "in-house" aCL [38], BINDAZYMET Anti-IgM Cardiolipin EIA (TBS) kit (The Binding Site, Birmingham, U.K.), and in the APhL® ELISA Kit (Louisville APL Diagnostics, Inc., Doraville, GA). The prevalence of low positive results in Group 1 was 4.7%, 1.5%, and 1.1% in the TBS, aCL, and in the APhL® ELISA Kit and in Group 2 was 3.8%, 0.6%, and 0.6% in the TBS, aCL, and APhL® ELISA Kit, respectively. Cut-offs were re-calculated using 95th percentile (11 MPL for TBS, 5 MPL for aCL, and 9 MPL for the APhL® ELISA Kit). The data confirm that the current cut-offs points of the 3 assays are correct. Up to now, low positive results have implied clinical positivity. We suggest based on this study that the low positive range is re-assigned "indeterminate" and recommend that samples falling in this category should be retested to confirm positivity at a later date.

IgA Anticardiolipin

The value of IgA aCL test in diagnosis of APS is uncertain. Recent studies have made data on prevalence and significance of IgA aCL antibodies available [46]. It appears that in patients with SLE, IgA aCL are similar to IgG aCL regarding their thrombogenicity and requirement of the cofactor β_2-GPI for binding to cardiolipin. In a mouse model designed to study thrombus formation, injected IgA immunoglobulins from patients with APS were shown to cause thrombosis and the mean thrombus size using 2 different IgA immunoglobulin preparations were found to be significantly larger compared to control IgA [35].

In an early study, Gharavi and colleagues found that, although IgA aCL antibodies were present in 51% to 55% patients with APS, most were also IgG or IgM positive, suggesting that measurement of IgA aCL would add little to IgG and IgM determination [27]. In unselected patients with SLE, the prevalence of increased titers of IgA aCL has been reported to vary from 1% to 44%. The lowest reported frequency was that found by Selva O'Callahan et al, who detected IgG aCL in only 2 of their 200 patients with SLE [47]. Higher prevalences were reported in the 2 largest SLE patient cohort studies to date. In a recent European study, where the IgG, IgM, and IgA isotypes were estimated in 577 SLE patients, IgA aCL positive was found in 13.9% of the patients [48]. Alarcon-Segovia et al, in a study that included 500 patients with SLE, found that increased titers of IgA aCL in 16.6% of their patients [49]. In another study Spadaro et al found that IgA aCL was positive in 13 (20%) of their 65 SLE patients [50]. In contrast, Weidman et al, found IgA aCL to be positive in 44% of 92 SLE patients, and also found IgA to be the most frequent aCL isotype [51]. The reported frequency for raised IgA aCL was higher (52.5%) in an earlier study by Faghiri et al, where patients were pre-selected for being IgG or IgM aCL positive and/or having APS associated clinical complications [52]. A prevalence of 83.3% was reported by Lopez et al in a group of patients with SLE and thrombocytopenia [53].

The ethnic group composition of patients can influence the isotype distribution of aCL. Molina et al studied African–American, Afro–Caribbean, and Hispanic patients with SLE and found elevated levels of IgA aCL in 16%, 21%, and 14% of them, respectively [54]. The most important finding was that IgA aCL was the only aCL isotype present in 82% of aCL-positive Afro–Caribbean patients. In contrast, IgA aCL was found to be positive only in 4.4% of Chinese patients with SLE [55]. In our experience, positive IgA aCL antibodies in the absence of IgG and/or IgM aCL are very rare in APS patients with or without SLE.

Numerous studies have investigated possible associations between raised levels of aCL and the clinical manifestations of the APS attributed to these autoantibodies. Several of these studies reported a significant association for IgA aCL with 1 or more of the main clinical manifestations of APS. Cucurul et al, studying both aCL and anti–β_2-GPI antibodies in African–American patients with SLE, found an association between thrombotic events and raised levels of both these autoantibodies [56]. However, the number of their patients with thrombotic events was very small; only 5% of their 100 patients had documented evidence of thrombosis [56]. An association between raised IgA aCL levels and thrombocytopenia in patients with SLE or other collagen vascular diseases has also been reported [57]. Finally, an association between IgA aCL and recurrent fetal loss and with unexplained spontaneous abortions has been shown in women with SLE [58, 59].

In summary, IgA aCL antibodies appear to be similar to IgG aCL in terms of thrombogenicity and cofactor requirement. Controversies reported regarding their prevalence and clinical associations still exist, perhaps due to use of nonstandard zed assays and from difference in the design of the studies.

Testing for Antibodies to Other Phospholipids

Early in the development of aCL immunoassays, it was observed that most APS-associated aCL appeared to be broadly cross-reactive with other anionic phospholipids, for example, phosphatidylserine, phosphatidylinositol, phosphatidic acid, and phosphatidylglycerol [24]. Although most aCL-positive APS patient sera react in assays using other anionic phospholipids, aCL-positive sera from patients with infectious diseases, such as syphilis, do not [26]. These infection-associated antibodies are specific for cardiolipin and do not recognize phosphatidylserine or other anionic phospholipids [26].

In the absence of a positive aCL or LA test, an association between positivity on 1 or more ELISAs utilizing phosphatidylserine, phosphatidylinositol, phosphatidylglycerol, or phosphatidic acid and the clinical manifestations of APS is not well established. The use of those phospholipids antigens to coat the ELISA plates has been reported for the detection of aPL antibodies and a number of laboratories include these tests inn their test panel assays [60–72]. In addition, some reports have indicated that APS patients may have antibodies to Zwitterionic phospholipids such as phosphatidylethanolamine (PE) [64–70]. Toschi and colleagues observed that reactivity to non-cardiolipin anionic phospholipids assays was associated with thrombosis and stroke [62]. The largest studies evaluating panels of non-cardiolipin anionic phospholipids have been conducted with obstetric patients. Yetman and Kutteh found that 10% women with recurrent pregnancy loss were negative in the aCL assay but tested positive in other phospholipid assays, including both anionic phospholipids and phosphatidylethanolamine [63]. Aoki et al compared β_2-GPI–dependent aCL ELISA with a panel of phospholipids assays in a large group of women with reproductive failure [72]. The aCL assay was more frequently positive in patients than controls, whereas no difference between patients and controls was observed with any of the other assays alone [72].

In light of those published observations, it may be argued that ELISAs using phosphatidylserine or one of the other anionic phospholipids would be preferable to aCL ELISA in evaluating patients for APS. However, the generally good correlation among ELISAs using different anionic phospholipids with aCL has lead many investigators to conclude that the aCL assay, along with LA testing, are adequate for evaluation of APS [8]. Routine testing of patient samples against panels of other anionic phospholipids is expensive and usually provides little additional clinical information [73]. Furthermore, the value of these tests is still uncertain because no standardized procedure has been established and specific reference material for each aPL assay is not available. Accordingly, it is difficult at best to make a valid clinical decision based on an isolated positive result in one of these assays. Some problems and adopted means of calculating the data have been addressed by incorporating a positive control in the run and stopping the color reaction when the absorbance of the positive control sample reaches approximately 1.0 OD units. A ratio between the OD of the patient sample and the positive control is calculated and values are then reported as negative, low, medium, or high positive depending on the value of the calculated ratio [60]. As mentioned, several international standardization workshops have served to improve the performance and inter-laboratory reproducibility of aCL ELISAs, but there have not been similar efforts focused on assays using other anionic phospholipids.

The Lupus Anticoagulant

The LA test is less frequently positive in APS and is regarded as a more specific test for detection of aPL [74]. This specificity derives from the fact that the LA reaction is found much less frequently in non-APS disorders. The LA test measures the ability of aPL autoantibodies to prolong phospholipid dependent clotting reactions. Although aPL antibodies detected in aCL and LA tests are specific for phospholipids, phospholipids binding proteins, or a complex of these molecules, the 2 tests (aCL and LA) do not necessarily identify the same antibodies [75]. Furthermore, although the majority of the patients with APS had positive aCL and LA tests, approximately 10% to 16% of them are positive for LA and negative for aCL, and 25% are positive for aCL and negative for LA.

More Specific Tests for APS

Although a sensitive test, one of the major drawbacks of this test is that it may be positive in a number of disorders other than APS. aCL antibodies have been reported in numerous infectious diseases including syphilis, HIV, hepatitis C, Q fever, tuberculosis, parvovirus B19 infections, cytomegalovirus, or drug induced [9–14, 76–79]. However, because patients with APS usually have higher aCL levels [15, 41, 42], greater specificity in diagnosis has been enabled by the use of higher cut-off points. Alternatively, recently new assays that utilize phosphatidylserine [71], mixture of negatively charged phospholipids (APhL® ELISA Kit) [80, 81], or β_2-GPI [82–93] have been proposed for a more specific measurement of antibodies present in APS. Some reports now suggest that *both* the aCL and a more specific test (anti-phosphatidylserine, APhL® ELISA, or anti–β_2-GPI, be run in patients suspected of having APS [94].

For more confident diagnosis of APS, more specific tests are required that are also sensitive. Three antigen preparations are likely candidates. The first and most extensively studied is β_2-GPI [82–93]. The second and third are the APhL® phospholipid mixture utilized as the antigen in APhL® ELISA Kit [80, 81] and phosphatidylserine that is used also in several commercial assays [71].

Current studies show that β_2-GPI, particularly when coated on oxidized or "high-binding" polystyrene ELISA plates, is a relatively specific antigen for autoantibodies present in APS patients [82, 83]. Anti–β_2-GPI antibodies have been reported to be associated primarily with thrombosis in patients with APS [86, 87, 90], but studies have also shown these antibodies in patients with pregnancy loss and other manifestations of APS [84, 87, 89, 91–93].

Various methods have been reported for the detection of anti β_2-GPI antibodies [82–85, 87, 88], but only one study reported the adoption of units of measurement for the detection of these antibodies and establishment of ranges of positivity, cut-off levels, and intra- and inter-assay variations [88]. Studies from several laboratories suggest that the sensitivity of the anti–β_2-GPI test for APS vary from 40% to 90% [82–93].

The second antigen is the APhL® phospholipid mixture prepared as a kit by Louisville APL Diagnostics, Inc. (the APhL® ELISA Kit). The author of this review was directly involved in developing both the antigen and the kit, and any evaluation of data presented in this report must be mindful of this fact. The APhL® phospholipid mixture was determined on the basis of testing of aCL-positive sera from a large number of patients with or without APS. Negatively charged phospholipids were tested singly and as mixtures to determine which would best distinguish APS sera from aCL-positive non-APS samples. A mixture of phospholipids was identified that enabled such distinction, while retaining sensitivity for detection of APS. Four published studies have examined this antigen [80, 81, 85, 96]. The largest enrolled 438 patients with various connective tissue diseases, 33 patients with APS, and 200 healthy controls, who were examined using the aCL bench assay and the APhL® ELISA Kit [81]. The sera were prepared and labeled in one center and tested blind in another laboratory; results were analyzed in the center where the samples were labeled. In that study, all patients with APS were positive for aCL antibodies and 30/33 were positive utilizing the APhL® ELISA Kit (90.9% sensitivity). In patients without APS, 45/438 were aCL positive but only 9 of 438 sera were positive in the APhL® ELISA Kit (99.5% specific). These data suggest that the APhL®ELISA

Table 23.3. Clinical sensitivity of two antiphospholipid assays and one anti–β_2-glycoprotein I assay. 📖

Assay	No. APS samples that tested positive / total no. APS samples tested	Sensitivity
aCL ELISA	54/54	100%
APhL® ELISA	53/54	98%
Anti–β_2-GPI	40/54	74%

Positive sample considered when above the cut-off point for each assay. Sensitivity for a given assay was calculated as follows: (# of samples that tested positive/# of samples tested) × 100.

aCL ELISA = anticardiolipin ELISA; APhL® ELISA Kit (Louisville APL Diagnostics, Inc.); anti–β_2-GPI (QUANTA LITE β_2GPI INOVA Diagnostics, Inc.).

Kit may be a sensitive and relatively specific means of identifying patients with APS [81].

In our experience, we have tested 54 APS samples in the aCL ELISA, the APhL® ELISA Kit, and in the anti–β_2-GPI ELISA. The sensitivity for the anti–β_2-GPI assay was 74% (Table 23.3). The specificity of the anti–β_2-GP1 varies among groups of investigators and publications [82–93], depending on the selection patient sera and the technique utilized. In a series of experiments performed by our group, in 184 samples from non-APS patients who had syphilis or other autoimmune disorders. 18 out of 184 samples were positive, yielding a specificity of 82% (Table 23.4). In general, most investigators agree that the anti–β_2-GPI test is more specific than the aCL ELISA for diagnosis of APS. In the same series of experiments the kit that utilizes the APhL® phospholipid mixture was shown to be 98% sensitive and 99% specific. In a most recent study, 69 samples from patients with syphilis, 30 with leishmaniasis (kala-azar), and 33 with leptospirosis were tested in the aCL ELISA, the anti–β_2-GPI ELISA, and in the APhL®ELISA Kit [95]. The results showed that the APhL® ELISA Kit was 96.3%, compared to the aCL ELISA. Interestingly, 36 samples out of the 132 samples tested in this study were also positive in the anti–β_2-GPI ELISA (specificity 70%). This relatively high incidence of anti–β_2-GPI antibodies in this group of infectious diseases sera is not understood and will need further investigation [95, 97].

Finally, there have been increasing number of reports from some various centers suggesting that patients with APS have antibodies that bind proteins other than β_2-GPI in recently developed ELISA tests. These include prothrombin (98, 99), protein C, protein S [100], and annexins. Reports showing the diagnostic value of these assays are still controversial. Determination of the value of ELISA tests utilizing protein antigens other than β_2-GPI will require validation and standardardization of the techniques and testing large numbers of sera from patients with APS as well as with other disorders to determine their diagnostic and predictive values.

Table 23.4. Clinical specificity of two antiphospholipid assays and one anti–β_2-glycoprotein I assay. 📖

Assay	No. of non-APS samples that tested positive / total no. APS samples tested	Specificity
aCL ELISA	74/84	60%
AphL® ELISA	1/184	99.9%
Anti–β_2-GPI	18/84	82%

Positive sample considered when above the cut-off point for each assay. Specificity for a given assay was calculated as follows: (# of non-APS samples that tested positive/# of samples tested) × 100.

aCL ELISA = anticardiolipin ELISA; APhL® ELISA Kit (Louisville APL Diagnostics, Inc.); anti–β_2-GPI (QUANTA LITE β_2GPI INOVA Diagnostics, Inc.)

What Test(s) Should Be Used for Diagnosis of APS?

Correct identification of patients with APS is important because prophylactic anti-coagulant therapy can prevent thrombosis from recurring, and treatment of affected women during pregnancy can result in live births. Because there are many causes of thrombosis and of pregnancy loss, the confirmation of diagnosis of APS is dependent in finding a positive antiphospholipid antibody or LA test. The LA and aCL tests are generally accepted confirmatory tests for APS. Recently, a forum of antiphospholipid experts gathered at a special session during the 8th International Symposium on aPL agreed that these 2 tests should be used primarily in the diagnosis of APS [8]. In summary, a diagnosis of APS can be made with confidence in patients who present with well-documented clinical features (venous or arterial thrombosis and/or pregnancy loss) characteristic of APS, and a moderate-to-high positive IgG aCL (above 40 GPL units) or LA test. However, there are a number of situations in which the anti–β_2-GPI of the APhL® ELISA Kit might be utilized to confirm diagnosis of the APS. These include:

- Patients with venous or arterial thrombosis or with pregnancy loss who are low positive for IgG aCL, or only IgM or IgA aCL positive.
- Patients presenting with equivocal features of APS [94]. Additional examples include patients with idiopathic thrombocytopenia; thrombophlebitis, athero-sclerosis, first trimester pregnancy losses, or instances in which venous or arterial thrombosis or recurrent pregnancy loss may be attributable to factor other than APS.
- Unusual presentations of APS include chorea, transverse myelopathy, livedo reticularis, leg ulcers, or cardiac valvular lesions presenting in the absence of pregnancy loss or thrombosis.
- Patients with clinical features that are very suggestive of APS but are aCL and LA negative.

Summary

The first aCL test was developed in 1983 and subsequently standardized. Although in the last 6 to 7 years new and more specific tests have become available, the aCL ELISA and the LA tests are still the first choice to be used in diagnosis of APS. While there is now doubt that the aCL test is useful in the diagnosis of APS, limitations of the assay have caused uncertainty and misinterpretation of the value of the test. Utilization of validated ELISA kits with well-tested calibrators and an in-house standard may enable more reproducible measurements. Reporting results semi-quantitatively preserves the clinical use of the test without the misinterpretation of a quantitative result that may lack precision, The development of newer tests, such as the β_2-GPI ELISA and the APhL® ELISA Kit utilizing the phospholipid mixture, gives promise to a more specific and reliable diagnosis of APS while retaining good sensitivity. Other tests such as ELISA for prothrombin antibodies and annexin V antibodies are still under development and will require standardization and extensive evaluation.

References

1. Harris EN. Antiphospholipid syndrome. In: Klippel JH, Dieppe PA, eds. Rheumatology. London: Mosby-Year Bool; 1994:32.1–32.6.
2. Harris EN. Syndrome of the black swan. Br J Rheumatol. 1987;26:324–326.
3. Pierangeli SS, Harris EN, Davis SA, DeLorenzo G. β_2Glycoprotein 1 enhances cardiolipin binding activity but it is not the antigen for antiphospholipid antibodies. Br J Haematol 1992;82:565–570.
4. McNeil HP, Simpson RJ, Chesterman CN, Krilis S. Anti-phospholipid antibodies are directed against a complex antigen that includes a lipid binding inhibitor of coagulation: β_2 glycoprotein 1 (apolipoprotein H). Proc Natl Acad Sci U S A. 1990;87:4120–4124.
5. Roubey RAS, Eisenberg RA, Harper MF, Winfield JB. "Anticardiolipin" antibodies recognize β_2 glycoprotein 1 in the absence of phospholipid. J Immunol 1995;154:954–960.
6. Harris EN, Gharavi AE, Boey ML, et al. Anticardiolipin antibodies: detection by radioimmunoassay and association with thrombosis. Lancet 1983;ii:1211–1214.
7. Triplett DA, Brandt JT. Lupus anticoagulants: misnomer, paradox, riddle, epiphenomenon. Hematol Pathol 1988;2:121–143.
8. Wilson WA, Gharavi AE, Koike T, et al. International consensus statement on primary classification criteria for definite antiphospholipid syndrome. Arthritis Rheum 1999;42:1309–1311.
9. Moritsen S, Hoier-Madson M, Wiik A, et al. The specificity of anti-cardiolipin antibodies from syphilis patients and from patients with systemic lupus erythematosus. Clin Exp Immunol 1989;76:178–183.
10. Harris EN, Gharavi AE, Wasley GD, Hughes GRV. Use of an enzyme-linked immunosorbent assay and of inhibition studies to distinguish between antibodies to cardiolipin from patients with syphilis or autoimmune disorders. J Infect Dis 1988;157:23–31.
11. Intrator L, Oksenhendler E, Desforges L, PB. Anticardiolipin antibodies in HIV infected patients with or without autoimmune thrombocytopenia purpura. Br J Haematol 1988;67:269–270.
12. Canoso RT, Zon LI, Groopman JE. Anticardiolipin antibodies associated with HTLV-III infection. Br J Haematol 1987;65:495–498.
13. Galvez J, Martin I, Medino D, Pujol E. Thrombophlebitis in a patient with acute Q fever and anticardiolipin antibodies. Med Clin (Barc) 1997;108:396–397.
14. Canoso RT, Sise HS. Chlorpromazine-induced lupus anticoagulant and associated immunologic abnormalities. Am J Hematol 1982;13:121.
15. Harris EN, Chan JKH, Asherson RA, et al. Thrombosis, recurrent fetal loss and thrombocytopenia. Predictive value of the anti-cardiolipin test. Arch Intern Med 1986;146:2153–2156.
16. Harris EN, Gharavi AE, Patel S, Hughes GRV. Evaluation of the anti-cardiolipin antibody test: report of an international workshop held April 4 1986. Clin Exp Immunol 1987;68:215–222.
17. Harris EN. The second international anticardiolipin standardization workshop/the Kingston Antiphospholipid Antibody study (KAPS) group. Am J Clin Pathol 1990;94:476–484.
18. Harris EN, Pierangeli SS, Birch D. Anticardiolipin wet workshop report: Vth International Symposium on Antiphospholipid Antibodies. Am J Clin Pathol 1994;101:616–624.
19. Pierangeli SS, Stewart M, Silva LK, Harris EN. Report of an anticardiolipin wet workshop during the VIIth International Symposium on antiphospholipid antibodies. J Rheumatol 1998;25:156–162.
20. Boey MD, Colaco CB, Gharavi AE. Thrombosis in SLE: striking association with the presence of circulating "lupus anticoagulant". BMJ 1983;287:1088–1089.
21. Hughes GRV. Thrombosis, abortion, cerebral disease and the lupus anticoagulant. BMJ 1983;287:1088–1089.
22. Shapiro SS, Thiagarajan P. Lupus anticoagulant. Prog Haemost Thromb 1982;6:263–285.
23. Thiagarajan P, Shapiro SS, DeMarco L. Monoclonal immunoglobulin ëM coagulation inhibitor with phospholipid specificity: mechanism of a lupus anticoagulant. J Clin Invest 1980;66: 397–405.
24. Harris EN, Gharavi AE, Loizou S, et al. Crossreactivity of anti-phospholipid antibodies. J Clin Lab Immunol 1985;16:1–6.
25. Harris EN, Gharavi AE, Hughes GRV. Antiphospholipid antibodies. Clin Rheum Dis 1985;11: 591–609.
26. Pierangeli SS, Goldsmith GH, Krnic S, Harris EN. Differences in functional activaty of anticardiolipin antibodies from patients with syphilis and the antiphospholipid syndrome. Infect Immun 1994;62:4081–4084.
27. Gharavi AE, Harris EN, Asherson RA, Hughes GRV. Anticardiolipin antibody isotype ditribution and phospholipid specificity. Ann Rheum Dis 1987;46:1–6.

28. Tincani A, Allegri F, Sanmarco M, et al. Anticardiolipin antibody assay: a methodological analysis for a better consensus in routine determinations – a cooperative project of the European Antiphospholipid Forum. Thromb Haemost 2001;86:575–583.
29. Galli M, Comfurius P, Maasen C, et al. Anticardiolipin (ACA) antibodies directed not to cardiolipin but to a plasma protein cofactor. Lancet 1990;336:1544–1547.
30. Matsuura E, Igarashi Y, Fujimoto M. Anticardiolipin cofactor(s) and differential diagnosis of autoimmune disease. Lancet 1990;336:177–178.
31. Gharavi AE, Harris EN, Sammaritano LR, et al. Do patients wth antiphospholipid syndrome have antibodies to β_2 glycoprotein 1. J Lab Clin Med 1993;122:426–431.
32. Gharavi AE, Sammaritano LR, Bovastro JL, Wilson WA. Specificities and characteristics of β_2 glycoprotein 1 induced antiphospholipid antibodies. J Lab Clin Med 1995;125:775–778.
33. Matsuura E. Igarashi Y, Yasuda T, et al. Anticardiolipin antibodies recognize β_2 glycoprotein 1 structure altered by interacting with an oxygen modified solid phase surface. J Exp Med 1994;179:457–462.
34. Martinuzzo M, Forastiero RR, Carreras LO. Anti-β_2 glycoprotein 1: detection and association with thrombosis. Br J Haematol 1995;89:397–402.
35. Pierangeli SS, Liu X, Barker JH, Anderson G, Harris EN. Induction of thrombosis in a mouse model by IgG, IgM and IgA immunoglobulins from patients with the Antiphospholipid Syndrome. Thromb Haemost 1995;74:1361–1367.
36. Peaceman AH, Silver RK, MacGregor SN, Scool ML. Interlaboratory variation in antiphospholipid antibody testing. Am J Obstet Gynecol 1992;144:1780–1784.
37. Reber G, Arvieux J, Comby D, et al. Multicenter evaluation of nine commercial kits for the quantitation of anticardiolipin antibodies. Thromb Haemost 1995;73:444–452.
38. Harris EN. Annotation: antiphospholipid antibodies. Br J Haematol 1990:74:1–9.
39. Merkel PA., Chang YC, Pierangeli SS, Convery K, Harris EN, Polisson RP. The prevalence and clinical associations of anticardiolipin antibodies in a large inception cohort of patients with connective tissue diseases. Am J Med 1996;101:576–583.
40. Silver RM, Porter TF, Leeuwen IV, et al. Anticardiolipin antibodies: clinical consequences of "low titers". Obstet Gynecol 1996;87:494–500.
41. Escalante A, Brey RL, Mitchell BD, Dreiner U. Accuracy of anticardiolipin antibodies in identifying a history of thrombosis among patients with systemic lupus erythematosus. Am J Med 1995;98:559–567.
42. Levine SR, Salowich-Palm L, Sawaya KL, et al. IgG anticardiolipin titer >40 GPL and the risk of subsequent thrombo-occlusive events and death. Stroke 1997;28:1660–1665.
43. Ichikawa K, Tsutsumu A, Atsumi T, et al. A chimeric antibody with human gamma 1 constant region as a putative standard for assays that detect IgG β_2 glycoprotein I antibodies. Arthritis Rheum 1999;42:2461–2470.
44. Harris EN, Pierangeli SS. Revisiting the anticardiolipin test and its standardization. Lupus 2002;11:269–275.
45. Pierangeli SS, Gharavi AE, Harris EN. Testing for antiphospholipid antibodies: problems and solutions. Clin Obstet Gynecol 2001;44:48–57.
46. Wilson WA, Faghri Z, Taheri Z, Gharavi AE. Significance of IgA antiphospholipid antibodies. Lupus 1998;7(suppl 2):S110–S113.
47. Selva O'Callaghan A, Ordi-Ros J, Monegal-Ferran F, Martinez N, Cortes-Hernandez F, Vilardell-Torres M. IgA anticardiolipin antibodies – relation with other antiphospholipid antibodies and clinical significance. Thromb Haemost 1998;79:282–285.
48. Galeazzi M, Sebastiani GD, Tincani A, et al. HLA class II alleles associations of anticardiolipin and anti-β_2 glycoprotein I antibodies in a large series of European patients with systemic lupus erythematosus. Lupus 2000;9:47–55.
49. Alarcon-Segovia D, Deleze M, Oria CV, et al. Antiphospholipid antibodies and the antiphospholipid syndrome in systemic lupus erythematosus. Medicine (Baltimore) 1989;68:353–365.
50. Spadaro A, Riccieri V, Terracina S, Rinaldi T, Taccari E, Zoppini A. Class specific rheumatoid factors and antiphospholipid syndrome in systemic lupus erythematosus. Lupus 2000;9:56–60.
51. Weidman CE, Wallace DJ, Peter JB, Knight PJ, Bear MB, Klinenberg JR. Studies of IgG, IgM and IgA antiphospholipid antibody isotypes in systemic lupus erythematosus. J Rheumatol 1988;15:74–79.
52. Faghri Z, Taheri F, Wilson WA, et al. IgA is the most prevalent isotype of anticardiolipin and anti-β_2 glycoprotein I antibodies in Jamaican and African-American SLE patients. Lupus 1998;7(suppl 2):S185.
53. Lopez LR, Santos M, Espinoza LR, LaRosa F. Clinical significance of immunoglobulin A vesus immunoglobulins G and M anticardiolipin antibodies in patients with systemic lupus erythematosus: correlation with thrombosis, thrombocytopenia and recurrent abortion. Coag Transf Med 1992;98:449–454.

54. Molina JF, Gutierrez-Urena S, Molina J, et al. Variability of anticardiolipin antibody isotype distribution in 3 geographic populations of patients with systemic lupus erythematosus. J Rheumatol 1997;24:291–296.
55. Wong KL, Liu HW, Ho K, Chan K, Wong R. Anticardiolipin antibodies and lupus anticoagulant in Chinese patients with systemic lupus erythematosus. J Rheumatol 1991;18:1187–1192.
56. Cucurull E, Gharavi AE, Diri E, Mendez E, Kappoort D, Espinoza LE. IgA anticardiolipin and anti-β_2 glycoprotein I are the most prevalent isotypes in African American patients with systemic lupus erythematosus. Am J Med Sci 1999;318:53–60.
57. Tajim C, Suzuki Y, Mizushima Y, Ichikawa Y. Clinical significance of immunoglobulin A antiphospholipid antibodies: possible association with skin manifestations and small vessel vasculitis. J Rheumatol 1998;25:1730–1737.
58. Kalunian KC, Peters JB, Middlekauff HR, et al. Clinical significance of a single test for anti-cardiolipin antibodies in patients with Systemic Lupus Erythematosus. Am J Med 1988;85:602–608.
59. Bahar AM, Kwak JY, Beer AE, et al. Antibodies to phospholipids and nuclear antigens in nonpregnant women with unexplained spontaneous recurrent abortion. J Reprod Immunol 1993;24:213–222.
60. Branch DW, Silver R, Pierangeli S, Harris EN. Antiphospholipid antibodies other than lupus anticoagulant and anticardiolipin antibodies in women with recurrent pregnancy loss, fertile controls, and antiphospholipid syndrome. Obstet Gynecol 1997;89:549–555.
61. Toschi V, Motta A, Castelli C, Paracchini ML, Zerbi D, Gibelli A. High prevalence of antiphosphatidylinositol antibodies in young patients witjh cerebral ischemia of undetermined cause. Stroke 1998;29:1759–1764.
62. Toschi V, Motta A, Castelli C, et al. Prevalence and clinical significance of antiphospholipids antibodies to non-cardiolipin antigens in systemic lupus erythematosus. Hemostasis 1993;23:275–283.
63. Yetman DL, Kutteh WH. Antiphospholpid antibody panels and recurrent pregnancy loss: prevalence of anticardiolipin antibodies compared with other antiphospholipid antibodies. Fertil Steril 1996;66:540–546.
64. Smirnov MD, Esmon CT. Phosphatidylethanolamine incorporation into vesicles selectively enhances factor V inactivation by activated protein C. J Biol Chem 1994;269:816–819.
65. Berard M, Chantome R, Marcelli A, Boffa MC. Antiphosphatidylethanolamine antibodies as the only antiphospholipid antibodies. I. Association with thrombosis and vascular cutaneous diseases. J Rheumatol 1996;23:1369–1374.
66. Karmonihkine M, Berard M, Piette JC, et al. Antiphosphatidylethanolamine antibodies in systemic lupus erythematosuss with tthrombosis. Clin Exp Rheumatol 1992;10:603–605.
67. Sugi T, McIntyre JA. Autoantibodies to phosphatidylethanolamine (PE) recognize a kininogen-PE complex. Blood 1995;86:3083–3089.
68. Boffa MC, Berard M, Sugi T, McIntyre JA. Antiphosphatidylethanolamine antibodies are the only antiphospholipid antibodies detected by ELISA. II. Kininogen reactivity. J Rheumatol 1996;76:1375–1379.
69. Sugi T, McIntyre JA. Phosphatidylethanolamine induces specific conformational changes in the kininogens recognizable by antiphosphatidylethanolamine antibodies. Thromb Haemost 1996;76:354–360.
70. Balada E, Ordi-Ros J, Paredes F, Villarreal J, Mauri M, Vilardell-Torres M. Antiphosphatidylethanolamine contribute to diagnosis of antiphospholipid syndrome in patients with systemic lupus erythematosus. Scand J Rheumatol 2001;30:235–241.
71. Rote NS, Dostal-Johnson D, Branch DW. Antiphosphollipid antibodies and recurrent pregnancy loss: correlation between the activated partial thromboplastin and antibodies against phosphatidylserine and cardiolipin. Am J Obstet Gynecol 1990;163:575–584.
72. Aoki K, Dudkiewics AB, Matsuura E, Novotny M, Kaberlain G, Gleicher N. Clinical significance of β_2 glycoprotein I dependent anticardiolipin antibodies in the reproductive autoimmune failure syndrome: correlation with conventional antiphospholipid antibody detection systems. Am J Obstet Gynecol 1995;172:926–931.
73. Bertolaccini ML, Roch B, Amengual O, Tsumi T, Khamashta MA, Hughes GR. Multiple antiphospholipid tests do not increase the diagnostic yield in antiphospholipid syndrome. Br J Rheumatol 1998;37:1229–1232.
74. Derksen RH, Hasselaar P, Blokzijl L, Gmelig Meyling FH, de Groot PG. Coagulation screen is more specific than the anticardiolipin antibody ELISA in defining a thrombotic subset of lupus patients. Ann Rheum Dis 1988;47:364–371.
75. Walton SP, Pierangeli SS, Campbell A, Klein E, Burchitt B, Harris EN. Demonstration of antiphospholipid antibodies heterogeneity by phospholipid column chromatography and salt gradient elution. Lupus 1995;4:263–271.

76. Violi F, Ferri D, Basili S. Hepatitis C virus, antiphospholipid antibodies, and thrombosis. Hepatology 1997;25:782.
77. Cheng HM, Khairullah NS. Induction of antiphospholipid autoantibody during cytomegalovirus infection. Clin Infect Dis 1997;25:1493–1494.
78. Adebajo AO, Charles P, Maini RN, Hazleman BL. Autoantibodies in malaria, tuberculosis and hepatitis in a west African population. Clin Exp Immunol 1993;92:73–76.
79. Gratacos E, Torres PJ, Vidal J, et al. Prevalence and clinical significance of anticardiolipin antibodies in pregnancies complicated by parvovirus B19 infection. Prenat Diagn 1995;15:1109–1113.
80. Harris EN, Pierangeli SS. A more specific ELISA assay for the detection of antiphospholipid. Clin Immunol 1995;15:26–28.
81. Merkel PA, Chang YC, Pierangeli SS, Harris EN, Polisson RP. Comparison between the standard anticardiolipin antibody test and a new phospholipid test in patients with a variety of connective tissue diseases. J Rheumatol 1999;26:591–596.
82. Matsuura E, Igarashi Y, Triplett DA, Koike T. Anticardiolipin antibodies recognize β_2 glycoprotein 1 structure altered by interacting with an oxygen modified solid phase surface. J Exp Med 1994;179:457–462.
83. Roubey RAS, Eisenberg RA, Harper MF, Winfield JB. Anticardiolipin autoantibodies recognize β_2 glycoprotein I in the absence of phospholipid: importance of antigen density and bivalent binding. J Immunol 1995;154:954–960.
84. Balestrieri G, Tincani A, Spatola L, et al. Anti-β_2-Glycoprotein I antibodies: a marker of antiphospholipid syndrome? Lupus 1995;4:122–130.
85. Arvieux J, Pouzol P, Roussel B, et al. Measurement of anti-phospholipid antibodies by ELISA using β_2 glycoprotein I as an antigen. Br J Haematol 1992;81:568–573.
86. Viard JP, Armoura Z, Bach JF. Association of anti-β_2 glycoprotein with lupus circulating anticoagulant and thrombosis in SLE. Am J Med 1992;93:181–186.
87. Cabiedes J, Cabral A, Alarcon-Segovia D. Clinical manifestations of the antiphospholipid syndrome in patients with systemic lupus erythematosus associate more strongly with anti-β_2 glycoprotein 1 than with antiphospholipid antibodies. J Rheumatol 1995;22:1899–1906.
88. Lewis S, Keil LB, Binder WL, DeBari V. Standardized measurement of major immunoglobulin class (IgG, IgA and IgM) antibodies to β_2 glycoprotein 1 in patients with antiphospholipid syndrome. J Clin Lab Anal 1998;12:293–297.
89. Katano K, Aoki A, Sasa H, Ogasawara M, Matsuure E, Yagami Y. β_2-glycoprotein I-dependent anticardiolipin antibodies as a predictor of adverse pregnancy outcomes in healthy pregnant women. Hum Reprod 1996;11:509–512.
90. Martinuzzo ME, Forastiero RR, Carreras LO. Anti-β_2 glycoprotein 1 antibodies: detection and association with thrombosis. Br J Haematol 1995;89:397–402.
91. Ogasawara M, Aoki K, Matsuura E, Sasa H, Yagami Y. Anti β_2 glycoprotein I antibodies and lupus anticoagulant in patients with recurrent pregnancy loss: prevalence and clinical significance. Lupus 1996;5:587–592.
92. Tsusumi A, Matsuure E, Ichikawa K, et al. Antibodies to β_2-glycoprotein I and clinical manifestations in patients with systemic lupus erythematosus. Arthritis Rheum 1996;39:1466–1474.
93. Chamley LW. Antiphospholipid antibodies or not? The role of β_2 glycoprotein 1 in autoantibody-mediated pregnancy loss. J Reprod Immunol 1997;36:123–142.
94. Harris EN, Pierangeli EN. "Equivocal" antiphospholipid syndrome. J Autoimmun 2000;15:81–75.
95. Santiago M, Martinelli R, Iko A, et al. Anti-β_2 glycoprotein I and anticardiolipin antibodies in leptospirosis, syphilis and Kala-azar. Clin Exp Rheumatol 2001;19:425–430.
96. Day HM, Thiagarajan P, Ahn C, Reveille ID, Tinker KF, Arnett FC. Autoantibodies to β_2 glycoprotein I in systemic lupus erythematosus and primary antiphospholipid syndrome: clinical correlations in comparison with other antiphospholipid antibody tests. J Rheumatol 1998;4:667–674.
97. Santiago M, Martinelli R, Reis MG, et al. Diagnostic performance of anti-β_2 glycoprotein I and anticardiolipin assays for clinical manifestations of the antiphospholipid syndrome. Clin Exp Rheumatol 2004. In Press.
98. Bevers E, Galli M, Barbui T, Comfurius P, Zwaal RFA. Lupus anticoagulant IgG's (LA) are not directed to phospholipids only, but to a complex of lipid-bound human prothrombin. Thromb Haemost 1991;66:629–632.
99. Rao LVM, Hoang AD, Rapaport SI. Difference s in interactions of lupus anticoagulant IgG with human prothrombin and bovine prothrombin. Thromb Haemost 1995;73:668–674.
100. Oosting JD, Derksen RH, Bobbink IW, Hackeng JM, Bouma BN, deGroot P. Antiphospholipid antibodies directed against a combination of phospholipids with prothrombin, protein C or protein S: an explanation for their pathogenic mechanism? Blood 1993;81:2618–2625.

24 Lupus Anticoagulants: Mechanistic and Diagnostic Considerations

Jef M. M. C. Arnout and Jos Vermylen

Introduction

Antiphospholipid syndrome (APS) is defined as the association of antiphospholipid antibodies (aPL) with arterial or venous thrombosis, recurrent foetal loss, thrombocytopenia, or neurological disorders [1–3]. The gradual development of the notion APS started in the 1950ss with the recognition of two laboratory curiosities in a subset of patients with systemic lupus erythematosus (SLE). In these patients, rheumatologists frequently found a chronic biological false positive test for syphilis, whereas hematologists described a non-specific coagulation inhibitor manifested by prolongation of the whole blood clotting time and the prothrombin time, without reduction of any specific clotting factor then measurable [1–3]. The non-specific coagulation inhibitor which appeared not to be associated with a bleeding tendency was named the "lupus anticoagulant" by Feinstein and Rapaport [4] and was regarded as a laboratory curiosity until Bowie et al [5] drew the attention to the high prevalence of thrombotic complications in SLE patients with this "anticoagulant." The LA was later also found to be associated with obstetric complications and thrombocytopenia [6].

Only in the 1980s did it became clear that antibodies interacting with anionic phospholipids are responsible for the in vitro LA effect and the chronic biological false positive syphilis serology [7]. This led to the development of better-defined LA tests and the so-called anticardiolipin test in which antibodies binding to solid phase cardiolipin (aCL) are measured [8, 9]. With these improved assays, the majority of SLE patients with a LA also had elevated aCL levels and a statistically significant relation between these 2 types of aPL was observed. It is now well established that persistently present aCL and LA in patients with SLE are associated with thrombosis and pregnancy morbidity [10]. This association is now termed APS [11]. Some patients with similar clinical symptoms and laboratory findings but not suffering from SLE or a closely related autoimmune disease are diagnosed as having a "primary APS" [12]. The availability of a sensitive assay for aCL has been crucial for the further characterization of aPL. Affinity purification of aCL led to the discovery that, in contrast to what the term aPL suggests, aCL do not bind to cardiolipin per se but to β_2-glycoprotein I bound to anionic phospholipid surfaces [13–15].

Antigenic Targets of aPL

Soon after the discovery that β_2-glycoprotein I was involved in the binding of aCL to cardiolipin, it was reported that a subpopulation of aCL possesses LA activity and that certain LAs are directed against prothrombin. It was also reported that aCL bind to β_2-glycoprotein I even in the absence of PL [16]. The affinity of the interaction of these antibodies with fluid phase β_2-glycoprotein I is, however, low. It is now generally accepted that autoimmune aPL have in common that they are directed against proteins with affinity for PL or negatively charged surfaces. The main anti-

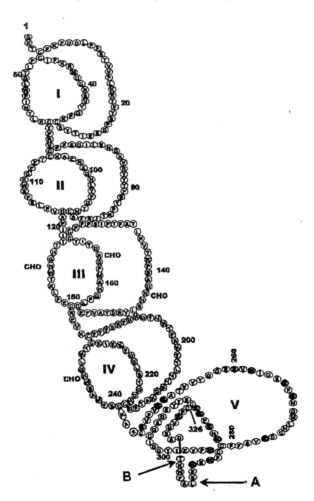

Figure 24.1. Structure of human β_2-glycoprotein I based on amino acid sequence, disulphide mapping, and crystallographic data. The five repeating sushi domains are indicated with roman numbers. CHO denotes N-linked glycosylation sites, 1 denotes amino terminal end, and 326 denotes carboxyterminal end. The hydrophobic flexible loop Ser311–Lys317 is indicated by *arrow A*; the positively charged amino acids interacting with the anionic phospholipid headgroups are marked in grey. *Arrow B* indicates the plasmin sensitive cleavage site at position Lys317–Thr318.

gens are β_2-glycoprotein I and prothrombin, although a number of autoantibodies recognizing other PL binding proteins, like protein C, protein S, annexin V, complement factor H, high- and low-molecular-weight kininogen, prekallikrein, factor XI, tissue factor pathway inhibitor (TFPI), factor VII/VIIa, etc., have been found in sera of patients with APS [17–19].

Relevant Structures of β_2-Glycoprotein I and Prothrombin

β_2-glycoprotein I (apolipoprotein H) is mainly synthesized by hepatocytes and to a lesser extent by endothelial cells and placental cells [20]; its plasma concentration is approximately 3 µmol/L. β_2-glycoprotein I consists of a single polypeptide chain of 326 amino acids and is composed of 5 homologous domains of approximately 60 amino acids, designated short consensus repeats/complement control protein repeats, or "sushi" domains [21, 22]. These are designated as domain I to domain V, from the N terminus to the C terminus (Fig. 24.1). Domains III and IV are heavily glycosylated. Domain V contains a 6-residue insertion and a 19-residue C-terminal tail resulting in a C-terminal loop consisting of 20 amino acids cross-linked by an additional disulfide bond [22]. The crystal structure of β_2-glycoprotein I has been defined [23, 24]. The overall shape is that of an elongated fishhook, domain V being at right angle to the aligned first 4 domains, and making contact with the phospholipid surface. A hydrophobic core consisting of 6 amino acids (Ser311–Lys317) would penetrate deep within the phospholipid bilayer; it is surrounded by 14 positively charged residues, which stabilize the binding to phospholipids via electrostatic interactions with the anionic phospholipid head groups. β_2-glycoprotein I is sensitive to cleavage by plasmin between Lys 317 and Thr318 [25]. The cleaved form binds much less avidly to negatively charged phospholipids. Binding of β_2-glycoprotein I to phospholipid does not involve calcium ions.

Prothrombin is a 579 amino acid long single chain glycoprotein, whose plasma concentration is approximately 1.5 µmol/L. Prothrombin is built up by an amino terminal GLA domain, in which the 10 γ-carboxyglutamic acid residues are concentrated and through which prothrombin binds to negatively charged phospholipid in the presence of Ca^{2+} ions [26]. Two kringle domains, K1 and K2, and a serine protease domain follow the GLA domain [see Fig. 24.2(A)]. The two kringle domains contain a highly conserved pentapeptide CRNPD, shared by all kringle proteases. Prothrombin contains 2 cleavage sites for factor Xa and 2 cleavage sites for thrombin, respectively, located at positions 271 and 320 and positions 155 and 284. Prothrombinase-catalyzed activation of prothrombin occurs by factor Xa mediated consecutive cleavages at positions 320 and 271, resulting in the generation of meizothrombin, prothrombin fragment 1+2, and α thrombin. This is followed by thrombin cleavage at position 155 giving rise to prothrombin fragment 1 and prothrombin fragment 2. Depending on the enzyme and the conditions used, prothrombin can be degraded into various fragments [see Fig. 24.2(B)] that may be used for epitope mapping.

The plasma concentrations of β_2-glycoprotein I and prothrombin are remarkably similar. As will be discussed later, the LA phenomenon depends on surface occupancy. Presumably, micro-molar concentrations of the phospholipid binding proteins are required to allow adequate surface coverage.

Panel A

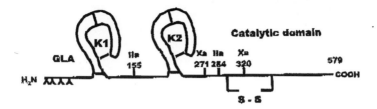

Panel B

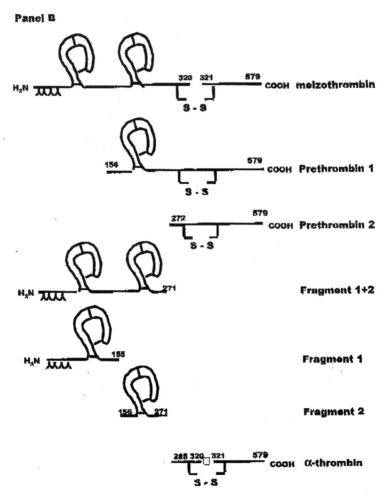

Figure 24.2. Panel (A) shows a simplified structure of prothrombin. The amino terminal GLA domain is followed by two kringle domains and a catalytic domain, stabilized by an internal disulphide bridge. The cleavage sites for thrombin (IIa) and activated factor X (Xa) are indicated. Panel (B) gives the prothrombin fragments that may be formed after digestion by thrombin or activated factor X.

Anticoagulant Mechanism of LA in vitro

The in vitro anticoagulant effect of LA was originally explained by the assumption that these antibodies compete with clotting factors for anionic phospholipids acting as catalytic surface for coagulation reactions. With the discovery of β_2-glycoprotein I and prothrombin as cofactors for aPL, the question rose how antibodies may enhance the binding of these proteins to phospholipids. This question has been addressed first for so-called β_2-glycoprotein I–dependent lupus anticoagulants. A few characteristics of the antibody β_2-glycoprotein I–phospholipid interaction should be noted. β_2-glycoprotein I, although binding with high affinity to pure negatively charged phospholipids such as cardiolipin and phosphatidylserine, has only a weak affinity for physiological procoagulant phospholipids [27], explaining why this protein is at most a poor anticoagulant. To become anticoagulant, the complex of β_2-glycoprotein I and patient anti–β_2-glycoprotein I antibody should have a higher affinity for phospholipid than that of β_2-glycoprotein I alone. However, patient anti–β_2-glycoprotein I antibodies by themselves only have a relatively weak affinity for β_2-glycoprotein I. This makes a scenario unlikely, where antibody binding causes a conformational change in β_2-glycoprotein I that favors phospholipid binding. A second possible scenario is much more plausible (see Fig. 24.3).

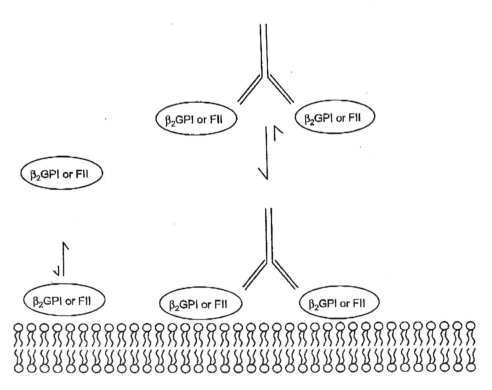

Figure 24.3. LA-positive aPL form stable bivalent immune complexes on PL surfaces. The affinity of the bivalent immune complex for coagulation active PL surfaces is higher than that of the monomeric PL-binding protein such as β_2-glycoprotein I (β_2-GPI) or prothrombin (FII) alone.

Indeed, it has been shown that in the presence of a physiologic procoagulant phospholipid surface, some anti–β_2-glycoprotein I IgGs cross-link 2 phospholipid-bound β_2-glycoprotein I molecules and thereby attach these with high affinity to the surface [28–30]. The surface occupancy by bivalent complexes impedes the clotting reaction and accounts for the LA phenomenon.

Studying a series of murine monoclonal antibodies against human β_2-glycoprotein I, it became apparent that several antibodies, although detected in the aCL assay, did not affect phospholipid dependent clotting tests [30]. Apparently, only LA-positive anti–β_2-glycoprotein I antibodies cross-link 2 β_2-glycoprotein I molecules in such a way that both β_2-glycoprotein I molecules of the bivalent complex can interact efficiently with the phospholipid surface. Because the affinity increases with the number of available binding sites, these particular bivalent complexes have a significantly higher affinity for coagulation active phospholipids than β_2-glycoprotein I alone and remain attached on the surface. This then explains the observation that a significant proportion of patients have antibody binding to immobilized β_2-glycoprotein I (a positive anti-cardiolipin assay), yet lack LA activity in their plasma [31]. Autoimmune anti–β_2-glycoprotein I antibodies are indeed a heterogeneous group of antibodies. Patients further often have polyclonal antibodies with different specificities. It was therefore not surprising that studies on the domain-specific location of the epitopes recognized by these antibodies showed binding to various domains of β_2-glycoprotein I , mainly V, IV, and I [32–34]. However, certain groups claimed that a dominant epitope was located on domain IV [33] while others provided evidence for a dominant epitope on domain I [34,35]. It recently became clear that this discrepancy is due to the orientation of β_2-glycoprotein I on the different micro-titer plates used for binding studies and that the majority of anti–β_2-glycoprotein I antibodies bind to domain I [36]. Clear discrimination at the epitope level between LA-positive and -negative anti–β_2-glycoprotein I antibodies has not yet been reported.

In the same manner, only a proportion of prothrombin dependent aPL show LA activity [37]. Some autoimmune antibodies to prothrombin can markedly enhance binding of prothrombin to negatively charged phospholipid [38, 39], again likely via the formation of bivalent prothrombin antibody complexes [40].

The epitopes recognized by autoimmune antiprothrombin antibodies have not yet been fully characterized. Binding to prethrombin 1, fragment 1+2, and fragment 1 has been reported [38, 41, 42]. Antibodies recognizing prethrombin 1 are likely to be directed against a conformational epitope on kringle 2 because binding usually disappears under reducing conditions and because binding to thrombin appears to be very exceptional. Puurunen et al [42] have described a more precise epitope for anti-prothrombin antibodies located on kringle 2, between amino acid 210 and 229. This amino acid sequence contains a conserved pentapeptide CRNPD shared by all kringle proteins, such as plasminogen and factor XII. Puurunen showed that a high proportion of autoimmune anti-prothrombin antibodies cross-react with plasminogen. Whether this conserved sequence is indeed a dominant epitope on prothrombin is questionable because antiprothrombin antibodies do not cross-react with factor XII, another kringle protein sharing the same conserved pentapeptide [43]. Patient antibodies to prothrombin seem to be polyclonal or oligoclonal in nature as antibodies recognizing various prothrombin fragments may occur simultaneously [38].

aPL and Risk for Thrombosis

Although aPL are mainly measured to fulfill the classification criteria for an APS, they are more and more used to estimate the risk for (recurrent) thrombosis or pregnancy morbidity in a given patient. There is growing consensus that LA are stronger risk factors for thrombosis than aCL. It was firstly shown that the presence of a LA correlates better with a history of thrombotic complications than the presence of aCL. The results from a systematic review of the literature formally established that, in patients with previous thrombosis and/or SLE, the presence of a LA is a stronger risk factor for future thrombotic complications than the presence of aCL [44].

Pathogenic Mechanisms of aPL: Surface Mediated Thrombogenic Characteristics

In view of the strong association between the presence of (certain) aPL and thrombosis, it is tempting to believe that aPL are involved in the thrombogenesis. Several prothrombotic mechanisms have been proposed which have in common that they interfere with surface mediated phenomena.

The formation of bivalent immune complex described above is also a surface-dependent phenomenon because the binding between anti-β_2-glycoprotein I antibodies and its antigenic target in solution is hampered by the intrinsically low affinity nature of this interaction. The observation that LAs are more closely associated with thrombotic events than aCL also provides an argument in favor of the hypothesis that the prothrombotic activity of aPL may be a surface mediated phenomenon.

Anionic enriched PL surfaces, needed for the formation of stable bivalent immune complexes, are hardly available within a healthy vessel because negatively charged PLs are normally sequestered within the inner leaflet of the PL bilayer of the cell membrane. Such surfaces, however, become available during normal haemostatic processes [45–47].

aPL do probably not cause thrombosis by themselves but rather influence the thrombotic process once negatively charged PL becomes exposed. aPL would therefore function as a "second hit." There is indirect clinical support for the concept of a double hit phenomenon. First, not all patients with aPL develop thrombosis but those who do develop thrombosis have a high rate of recurrence. Secondly, arterial events are almost always followed by arterial events and venous thrombosis is most likely followed by another venous thrombosis [48].

There are several "anticoagulant" surface mediated processes with which aPL are thought to interfere. One major anticoagulant pathway involves protein C and protein S [49]. Protein C, activated by thrombin on endothelial thrombomodulin, and protein S bind to negatively charged PL through their GLA domains; activated protein C in association with protein S cleaves factor Va and factor VIIIa on the PL surface and thereby inactivates the intrinsic tenase and prothrombinase reactions. Occupancy of the surface by immune complexes could impede these interactions and thereby promote further thrombin generation and thrombus growth. Indeed,

LAs can induce "activated protein C resistance" [50]. A second anticoagulant mechanism involves tissue factor pathway inhibitor. This protein binds to negatively charged PL and to factor Xa on PL. This protein complex then links to the tissue factor–factor VIIa complex, and shuts off further tissue factor mediated clotting. Again, occupancy of the PL surface by immune complexes may impede this interaction, leading to prolonged thrombin generation [51].

While these interferences of the immune complexes with anticoagulant pathways have been elegantly demonstrated in vitro, it is difficult to unequivocally extrapolate these observations in vivo because the immune complexes could impede assembly of the procoagulant complexes to the same extent and the overall result would then be neutral. However, under certain pathological conditions, this may not be the case. Oxidation is believed to play an important role in inflammatory diseases such as atherosclerosis. In addition it was reported that oxidation of phosphatidylethanolamine containing liposomes potentiates the anticogulant effect of the protein C pathway without affecting the procoagulant pathway. Total IgG from patients with aPL and thrombosis appears to selectively inhibit the anticoagulant effect of phospholipid oxidation [52].

The prothrombotic action of aPL may not be limited to inhibition of surface mediated anticoagulant pathways. Chesterman's group provided evidence that enhanced antibody-mediated deposition of prothrombin on PL may lead to increased thrombin generation in conditions of flow [53].

We suggest that the deposition of immune complexes on slightly activated cells may induce further cell activation, leading to generation of micro-vesicles that paradoxically provide a much larger PL surface resulting in enhanced thrombin generation [54, 55] (see Fig. 24.4).

This pathogenetic model was confirmed in an in vivo model of thrombosis in the hamster in whom slight radical induced endothelial injury of a carotid artery had been provoked after intravenous injection of monoclonal antibodies to human β_2-glycoprotein I [56]. One of the tested antibodies had LA activity in hamster plasma, a second bound immobilized hamster β_2-glycoprotein I but was without LA activity, a third had no affinity for hamster β_2-glycoprotein I. The antibody with LA activity markedly enhanced arterial thrombosis, the second antibody without LA activity hardly enhanced thrombosis, the third antibody being inactive. $F(ab)_2$ fragments of the LA antibody also enhanced thrombosis, whereas Fab fragments were inactive. These findings confirm that bivalency is required for thrombosis enhancement but also that the Fc component of the antibody is not compulsory for this enhancement. Immunohistological examination revealed that the antibody was mainly localized focally within the platelet thrombus, suggesting thrombus growth spreading from the foci of immune complex deposition on activated platelets. These experiments are in agreement with a double hit scenario: following mild endothelial damage, a small platelet thrombus develops (first hit); the slightly activated platelets expose negatively charged PL; this leads to patchy deposition of bivalent β_2-glycoprotein I–antibody complexes; these complexes cause further platelet activation and thrombus growth (second hit).

The fact that Fc receptor activation is not compulsory for the prothrombotic action is intriguing and may suggest that another type of receptor-triggered process is involved. Direct evidence for this was obtained from in vitro experiments under flow conditions showing that recombinant β_2-glycoprotein I–dimer, like β_2-glycoprotein I–antibody dimers, enhances platelet activation and deposition on collagen

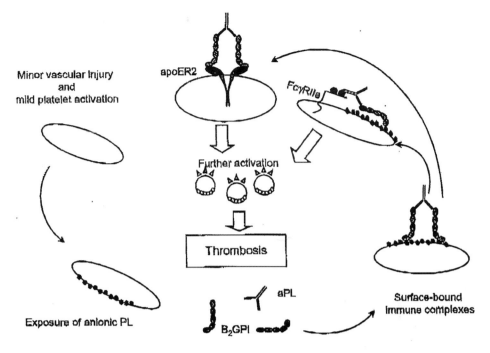

Figure 24.4. Putative pathogenic mechanism in APS: as a consequence of an initial damage, anionic PLs are exposed on cells of the blood, on endothelium, or on trophoblasts. In the presence of aPL and their antigenic targets such as β_2-glycoprotein I bivalent immune complexes with increased affinity for these PL surfaces are formed. The deposition of immune complexes causes further cellular activation probably via cross-linking apolipoprotein E receptor 2 (apoER2) and a signal transducing mechanism involving p38MAP kinase and this in addition to the potential role of the platelet FcγRIIa receptor; for platelets this would lead to release of granule contents and formation of micro-vesicles, which would paradoxically provide a much larger negatively charged PL surface, and therefore enhance rather than inhibit thrombin generation.

surfaces [57]. This platelet deposition appeared to be dependent on cross-linking and activation of the apolipoprotein E receptor 2.

Laboratory Diagnosis of LA

SSC Criteria for LA Testing

According to the recommendations of the SSC, the laboratory diagnosis of a LA should be based on the following criteria: prolongation of a phospholipid dependent clotting test, in particular when the phospholipid content of the test system is low; lack of correction of the prolonged clotting time by addition of a small amount of normal plasma (thereby excluding clotting factor deficiency); correction by the presence of a higher concentration of phospholipid or by use of a reagent that is poorly responsive to the LA effect [58]. Detection of LA is delicate and sometimes impossible when the patient is already treated with heparin or oral anticoagulants.

Because autoimmune aPL are chronic, the presence of a LA should be confirmed on a second sample taken several weeks later. It should be emphasized that a 6-week interval may not be sufficient to distinguish persistent LA from those seen in relation with infectious disease because the latter may persist for several months [59].

It is very hard to give precise recommendations on which assays to use for the detection of LA. Selection of assay systems with optimal sensitivity and specificity is almost impossible due to the lack of a gold standard (a well-defined LA-positive patient population). Given the fact that various assays may detect different types of LA [60, 61] and that not all LA are associated with thrombosis, the best way to select optimal screen assays should be based on clinical trials. According to a recent systematic review of the literature however, the risk of thrombosis at present appears to be independent of the laboratory tests used to identify LA [44].

Discrimination Between LA and Factor VIII Inhibitors

Differentiation between LA and specific factor inhibitors, although extremely important in view of their different clinical consequences, often remains difficult. In a survey of the European Concerted Action on Thrombophilia (ECAT), a sample with a slow acting auto-immune factor VIII inhibitor at 10 Bethesda Units was included [61]. As much as 20% of the participating laboratories interpreted their results as compatible with the presence of a LA. In several cases, this interpretation was based on the combination of a prolonged partial thromboplastin time (aPTT) which did not entirely correct upon mixing with normal plasma and a prolonged confirm aPTT with reduced phospholipids. As clinical laboratories receive less and less information on the clinical condition of the patients from whom samples for LA diagnosis are obtained, the use of factor assays should be encouraged whenever a LA is diagnosed in an aPTT based system. Laboratories should be aware that potent LA and specific factor VIII inhibitors may behave very similarly in vitro (an example is given in Table 24.1). In the presence of a potent LA, the apparent activity of various clotting factors in a one-stage assay may be reduced. However, a high titer factor VIII inhibitor may also cause a false reduction of factors IX, XI, and XII and therefore mimic a LA. Determining factor levels in diluted plasma may be of help to differentiate between a LA and a factor VIII inhibitor. In the first case, the apparent clotting

Table 24.1. An example of the effect of a strong lupus anticoagulant and a high titer FVIII inhibitor on factor assays.

		Plasma predilution in buffer		
		1/10	1/20	1/40
Lupus anticoagulant	FVIII (%)	1.6	8.5	39.9
	FIX (%)	8.3	28.9	57.2
	FXI (%)	5.9	19.7	51.8
	FXII (%)	21.3	44.1	66.4
Factor VIII inhibitor	FVIII (%)	0.5	0.5	0.5
	FIX (%)	12.6	18.2	27.3
	FXI (%)	15.4	21.6	31.3
	FXII (%)	22.5	29.7	35.7

Note that not all LA or factor VIII inhibitors behave similarly.

factor activity increases as higher plasma dilutions are being tested. In the latter case, the factor VIII level remains low in diluted plasma.

Importance of LA Potency or Titer

For aCL, the thrombotic risk seems to increase with the antibody titer. Only few attempts have been made to study the relation between the LA potency or titer and the clinical manifestations of the APS.

A first feasibility study to quantify LA was performed by the Groupe d'Etudes sur l'Hémostase et la Thrombose (GEHT) [60]. The LA potency was determined in samples from 40 patients with APS and 29 LA-positive asymptomatic individuals using LA screening assays calibrated with a normal plasma pool spiked with equimolar combinations of a LA positive anti-β_2-glycoprotein I monoclonal antibody (moab) and an LA-positive anti-prothrombin moab at concentrations ranging from 0 to 60 μg/mL. Eight reagent–instrument combinations were used in this study. Patients with APS had coagulation profiles distinct from those with asymptomatic LA, the former having significantly higher LA titers measured using a calibrated dilute Russell Viper Venom Time (dRVVT). The largest difference was found for the 2 dRVVT assays, which were more responsive to β_2-glycoprotein I–dependent LA. This study not only showed that quantification of LA activity in clinical samples using calibrator plasmas spiked with moabs against protein targets of aPL is feasible, but also suggested that there might be a relation between the titer (or potency) and the risk for thrombosis.

That such relation indeed exists was subsequently confirmed in a prospective study of 678 patients with SLE [62]. In this study, the immediate risk of deep venous thrombosis increased 34% with each 5 seconds prolongation of the dRVVT.

Importance of the Antigenic Target of LA

There is growing evidence that β_2-glycoprotein I–dependent aPL may be more strongly associated with thrombosis than prothrombin-dependent aPL. The results of a 4-year prospective study based on the Italian registry show that the risk for thrombosis is highest in APS patients who in addition to a LA also have medium or high titer aCL [63]. Because autoimmune aCL are β_2-glycoprotein I–dependent aPL, this observation may suggest that the LA associated with thrombosis may be predominantly directed against β_2-glycoprotein I. Galli and coworkers noted that β_2-glycoprotein I–dependent LA more strongly prolong the dRVVT than prothrombin-dependent LA, whereas the effects of these two types of LA on the kaolin clotting time (KCT) are opposite [64]. She also found the dRVVT to be a better predictor of thrombosis than the KCT in a historical cohort of 100 consecutive LA-positive patients [65]. However, it should be noted that there also is evidence for a prothrombotic role of anti-prothrombin antibodies [66, 67].

Two recent reports describe a method to discriminate β_2-glycoprotein I–dependent LA from prothrombin dependent ones. The first method, by Simmelink et al [68], is based on the high affinity interaction between β_2-glycoprotein I and pure cardiolipin. β_2-glycoprotein I and LA dependent on this protein are adsorbed on cardiolipin vesicles which are added to patient plasma. Shortening of a LA sensitive aPTT in the presence of cardiolipin vesicles is an indication for the presence of a

β_2-glycoprotein I–dependent LA. The second method, by Pengo et al [69], is even more elegant and is based on an increased affinity of β_2-glycoprotein I for coagulation active phospholipids when the calcium concentration or the ionic strength in the reaction mixture is lowered [70]. A further prolongation of a LA sensitive screening assay such as the dRVVT or the dilute prothrombin time after lowering the calcium concentration from 10 to 5 mM is an indication for the presence of a β_2-glycoprotein I–dependent LA in a patient sample. On the contrary, the clotting time is slightly shortened with lower calcium concentrations in case of prothrombin containing immune complexes, because calcium is involved in the binding of prothrombin to phospholipids. The availability of relatively simple clotting based assays to differentiate β_2-glycoprotein I from prothrombin dependent LA now makes it possible to more properly address the question whether the risk for thrombosis is to some extent linked to the target antigen of the LA.

Quality Control

Despite internationally accepted guidelines [58] and many efforts to better standardize LA assays, several national and international inter-laboratory surveys and workshops have shown that the accuracy of LA testing still is far from optimal. In the first French interlaboratory survey on LA, only 41% of 4500 laboratories made a correct diagnosis of LA [71]. In the U. K. national external quality assessment scheme (NEQAS), a weak LA was not found by more than 50% of the laboratories and a factor IX deficient plasma was diagnosed as LA positive by 26% of the laboratories [72]. A major shortcoming in this regard is the lack of internationally accepted reference and control materials. For internal quality assessment, laboratories and reagent manufacturers still have to rely on LA-positive patient samples.

A set of LA-positive reference plasmas with a range of potencies has been prepared by the LA working party of the British Society for Haematology [73]. These plasmas were obtained by pooling several LA-positive plasmas and diluting them in LA-negative plasma. However, the supply of such materials is very limited and the fact that each new pool will have different characteristics probably makes this approach less suited to prepare real reference materials.

LA positive anti–β_2-glycoprotein I and anti-prothrombin moabs are now available [74, 75]. These antibodies recognize the same target proteins as human LA and share the same mechanism of action. In addition, they may be combined and can be produced in large quantities with a constant behavior over time. Therefore, normal plasma pools spiked with certain amounts of these moabs have the potential to serve as reference and control materials for LA testing. The Scientific and Standardization subcommittee on LA and phospholipid-dependent antibodies of the International Society on Thrombosis and Haemostasis is currently preparing such international reference materials.

Acknowledgments

The work of J. Arnout is supported by a grant from the Flemish Fund for medical scientific research Levenslijn 7.0032.98 and FWO G.0226.01.

References

1. Moore JE, Mohr CF. Biologically false-positive serologic tests for syphilis: type, incidence, and cause. JAMA 1952;150:467–473.
2. Moore JE, Lutz WB. The natural history of systemic lupus erythematosus: an approach to its study through chronic biologic false-positive reactions. J Chronic Dis 1955;1:297–316.
3. Conley CL, Hartmann RC. A hemorrhagic disorder caused by circulating anticoagulant in patients with disseminated lupus erythematosus. J Clin Invest 1952;31:621–622.
4. Feinstein DI, Rapaport SI. Acquired inhibitors of blood coagulation. Prog Haemost Thromb 1972;1:75–95.
5. Bowie EJW, Thompson JH Jr, Pascuzzi CA, Owen CA Jr. Thrombosis in systemic lupus erythematosus despite circulating anticoagulants. J Lab Clin Med 1963;62:416–430.
6. Laurell AB, Nilsson IM. Hypergammaglobulinaemia, circulating anticoagulant, and biologic false positive Wassermann reaction: a study of 2 cases. J Lab Clin Med 1957;49:694–707.
7. Thiagarajan P, Shapiro SS, De Marco L. Monoclonal immunoglobulin M coagulation inhibitor with phospholipid specificity. Mechanism of lupus anticoagulant. J Clin Invest 1980;66:397–405.
8. Harris EN, Gharavi AE, Boey ML, et al. Anticardiolipin antibodies: detection by radioimmunoassay and association with thrombosis in systemic lupus erythematosus. Lancet 1983;ii:1211–1214.
9. Triplett DA, Brandt JT, Kaczor D, Schaeffer J. Laboratory diagnosis of lupus inhibitors: a comparison of the tissue thromboplastin inhibition procedure with a new platelet neutralization procedure. Am J Clin Pathol 1983;79:678–682.
10. Love PE, Santoro SA. Antiphospholipid antibodies: anticardiolipin and the lupus anticoagulant in systemic lupus erythematosus (SLE) and in non-SLE disorders. Ann Intern Med 1990;112:682–698.
11. Hughes GRV, Harris EN, Gharavi AE. The anticardiolipin syndrome. J Rheumatol 1986;13:486–489.
12. Alarcon-Segovia D, Sanchez-Guerrero J. Primary antiphospholipid syndrome. J Rheumatol 1989;16:482–488.
13. McNeil HP, Simpson RJ, Chesterman CN, Krilis SA. Anti-phospholipid antibodies are directed against a complex antigen that includes a lipid-binding inhibitor of coagulation: beta-2-glycoprotein I (apolipoprotein H). Proc Natl Acad Sci U S A 1990;87:4120–4124.
14. Galli M, Comfurius P, Maassen C, et al. Anticardiolipin antibodies (ACA) directed not to cardiolipin but to a plasma protein cofactor. Lancet 1990;335:1544–1547.
15. Matsuura E, Igarashi Y, Fujimoto M, Ichikawa K, Koike T. Anticardiolipin cofactor(s) and differential diagnosis of autoimmune disease. Lancet 1990;336:177–178.
16. Roubey RAS, Eisenberg RA, Harper MF, Winfield JB. "Anticardiolipin" autoantibodies recognize β_2-glycoprotein I in the absence of phospholipid. Importance of Ag density and bivalent binding. J Immunol 1995;154:954–960.
17. Roubey RA. Update on antiphospholipid antibodies. Curr Opin Rheumatol 2000;12:374–378.
18. Arnout J, Wittevrongel C, Vermylen J. Phospholipid-binding proteins and the antiphospholipid syndrome: a role for complement factor H? Thromb Haemost 1997;(suppl):1.
19. Forastiero RR, Martinuzzo ME, Broze GJ. High titers of autoantibodies to tissue factor pathway inhibitor are associated with the antiphospholipid syndrome. J Thromb Haemost 2003;1:718–724.
20. Caronti B, Calderaro C, Alessandri C, et al. Beta2-glycoprotein I (beta2-GPI) mRNA is expressed by several cell types involved in anti-phospholipid syndrome-related tissue damage. Clin Exp Immunol 1999;115:214–219.
21. Lozier J, Takahashi N, Putnam FW. Complete amino acid sequence of human plasma beta 2-glycoprotein I. Proc Natl Acad Sci U S A 1984;81:3640–3644.
22. Steinkasserer A, Barlow PN, Willis AC, et al. Activity, disulphide mapping and structural modelling of the fifth domain of human beta 2-glycoprotein I. FEBS Lett 1992;313:193–197.
23. Bouma B, de Groot PG, van den Elsen JM, et al. Adhesion mechanism of human beta(2)-glycoprotein I to phospholipids based on its crystal structure. EMBO J 1999;18:5166–5174.
24. Schwarzenbacher R, Zeth K, Diederichs K, Gries A, Kostner GM, Laggner P, Prassl R. Crystal structure of human beta2-glycoprotein I: implications for phospholipid binding and the antiphospholipid syndrome. EMBO J 1999;18:6228–6239.
25. Ohkura N, Hagihara Y, Yoshimura T, Goto Y, Kato H. Plasmin can reduce the function of human beta2 glycoprotein I by cleaving domain V into a nicked form. Blood 1998;91:4173–4179.
26. Mann K. Prothrombin and thrombin. In: Colman RW, Hirsch J, Marder VJ, SlzmanEW, eds. Hemostasis and thrombosis: basic principles and clinical practice. Philadelphia: J.B. Lippincott; 1994:184–199.

27. Harper MF, Hayes PM, Lentz B, Roubey RAS. Characterization of β₂-glycoprotein I binding to phospholipid membranes. Thromb Haemost 1998;80:610–614.
28. Willems GM, Janssen MP, Pelsers MMAL, et al. Role of divalency in the high-affinity binding of anticardiolipin antibody-β₂-glycoprotein I complexes to lipid membranes. Biochemistry 1996;35:13833–13842.
29. Takeya H, Mori T, Gabazza EC, et al. Anti-β₂-Glycoprotein I (β₂GPIÒ) monoclonal antibodies with lupus anticoagulant-like activity enhance the β₂GPI binding to phospholipids. J Clin Invest 1997;99:2260–2268.
30. Arnout J, Wittevrongel C, Vanrusselt M, Hoylaerts M, Vermylen J. Beta-2-glycoprotein I dependent lupus anticoagulants form stable bivalent antibody-beta-2-glycoprotein I complexes on phospholipid surfaces. Thromb Haemost 1998;79:79–86.
31. Galli M, Comfurius P, Barbui T, Zwaal RF, Bevers EM. Anticoagulant activity of beta 2-glycoprotein I is potentiated by a distinct subgroup of anticardiolipin antibodies. Thromb Haemost 1992;68:297–300.
32. Hunt J, Krilis S. The fifth domain of beta 2-glycoprotein I contains a phospholipid binding site (Cys281-Cys288) and a region recognized by anticardiolipin antibodies. J Immunol 1994;152:653–659.
33. George J, Gilburd B, Hojnik M, et al. Target recognition of beta2-glycoprotein I (beta2GPI)-dependent anticardiolipin antibodies: evidence for involvement of the fourth domain of beta2GPI in antibody binding. J Immunol 1998;160:3917–3923.
34. Iverson GM, Victoria EJ, Marquis DM. Anti-beta2 glycoprotein I (beta2GPI) autoantibodies recognize an epitope on the first domain of beta2GPI. Proc Natl Acad Sci U S A 1998;95:15542–15546.
35. McNeeley PA, Dlott JS, Furie RA, et al. Beta2-glycoprotein I-dependent anticardiolipin antibodies preferentially bind the amino terminal domain of beta2-glycoprotein I. Thromb Haemost 2001;86:590–595.
36. Iverson GM, Matsuura E, Victoria EJ, Cockerill KA, Linnik MD. The orientation of beta-2-GPI on the plate is important for the binding of anti-beta2gpi autoantibodies by ELISA. J Autoimmun 2002;18:289–297.
37. Horbach DA, van Oort E, Derksen RH, de Groot PG. The contribution of anti-prothrombin-antibodies to lupus anticoagulant activity – discrimination between functional and non-functional antiprothrombin-antibodies. Thromb Haemost 1998;79:790–795.
38. Rao LV, Hoang AD, Rapaport SI. Mechanism and effects of the binding of lupus anticoagulant IgG and prothrombin to surface phospholipid. Blood 1996;88:4173–4182.
39. Simmelink MJ, Horbach DA, Derksen RH, et al. Complexes of anti-prothrombin antibodies and prothrombin cause lupus anticoagulant activity by competing with the binding of clotting factors for catalytic phospholipid surfaces. Br J Haematol 2001;113:621–629.
40. Field SL, Chesterman CN, Dai YP, Hogg PJ. Lupus antibody bivalency is required to enhance prothrombin binding to phospholipid. J Immunol 2001;166:6118–6125.
41. Akimoto T, Akama T, Kono I, Sumida T. Relationship between clinical features and binding domains of anti-prothrombin autoantibodies in patients with systemic lupus erythematosus and antiphospholipid syndrome. Lupus 1999;8:761–766.
42. Puurunen M, Manttari M, Manninen V, Palosuo T, Vaarala O. Antibodies to prothrombin crossreact with plasminogen in patients developing myocardial infarction. Br J Haematol 1998;100:374–379.
43. Jones DW, Nicholls PJ, Donohoe S, Gallimore MJ, Winter M. Antibodies to factor XII are distinct from antibodies to prothrombin in patients with the anti-phospholipid syndrome. Thromb Haemost 2002;87:426–430.
44. Galli M, Luciani D, Bertolini G, Barbui T. Lupus anticoagulants are stronger risk factors of thrombosis than anticardiolipin antibodies in the antiphospholipid syndrome. A systematic review of the literature. Blood 2003;101:1827–1832.
45. Bevers EM, Comfurius P, Dekkers DW, Zwaal RF. Lipid translocation across the plasma membrane of mammalian cells. Biochim Biophys Acta 1999;1439:317–330.
46. Heemskerk JW, Bevers EM, Lindhout T. Platelet activation and blood coagulation. Thromb Haemost 2002;88:186–193.
47. Siljander P, Farndale RW, Feijge MA, et al. Platelet adhesion enhances the glycoprotein VI-dependent procoagulant response: involvement of p38 MAP kinase and calpain. Arterioscler Thromb Vasc Biol 2001;21:618–627.
48. Rosove MH, Brewer PMC. Antiphospholipid thrombosis: clinical course after the first thrombotic event in 70 patients. Ann Intern Med 1992;117:303–308.
49. Esmon CT. Regulation of blood coagulation. Biochim Biophys Acta 2000;1477:349–360.

50. Galli M, Ruggeri L, Barbui T. Differential effects of anti-beta2-glycoprotein I and antiprothrombin antibodies on the anticoagulant activity of activated protein C. Blood 1998;91:1999–2004.
51. Salemink I, Blezer R, Willems GM, Galli M, Bevers E, Lindhout T. Antibodies to beta2-glycoprotein I associated with antiphospholipid syndrome suppress the inhibitory activity of tissue factor pathway inhibitor. Thromb Haemost 2000;84:653–656.
52. Safa O, Hensley K, Smirnov MD, Esmon CT, Esmon NL. Lipid oxidation enhances the function of activated protein C. J Biol Chem 2001;276:1829–1836.
53. Field SL, Hogg PJ, Daly EB, et al. Lupus anticoagulants form immune complexes with prothrombin and phospholipid that can augment thrombin production in flow. Blood 1999;94:3421–3431.
54. Arnout J. The pathogenesis of the antiphospholipid syndrome: a hypothesis based on parallelisms with heparin-induced thrombocytopenia. Thromb Haemost 1996;75:536–541.
55. Vermylen J, Hoylaerts MF, Arnout J. Antibody-mediated thrombosis. Thromb Haemost 1997;78:420–426.
56. Jankowski M, Vreys I, Wittevrongel C, et al. Thrombogenicity of beta-2-glycoprotein I dependent antiphospholipid antibodies in a photochemically induced thrombosis model in the hamster. Blood 2003;101:157–162.
57. Lutters BC, Derksen RH, Tekelenburg WL, Lenting PJ, Arnout J, De Groot PG. Dimers of 2-glycoprotein I increase platelet deposition to collagen via interaction with phospholipids and the apolipoprotein E receptor 2'. J Biol Chem 2003;278:33831–33838.
58. Brandt JT, Triplett DA, Alving B, Scharrer I. Criteria for the diagnosis of lupus anticoagulants: an update. Thromb Haemost 1995;74:1185–1190.
59. Male C, Lechner K, Speiser W, Pabinger I. Transient lupus anticoagulants in children: stepwise disappearance of diagnostic features. Thromb Haemost 2000;83:174–175.
60. Le Querrec A, Arnout J, Arnoux D, et al. Quantification of lupus anticoagulants in clinical samples using anti-beta2GP1 and anti-prothrombin monoclonal antibodies. Thromb Haemost 2001;86:584–589.
61. Arnout J. Antiphospholipid syndrome: diagnostic aspects of lupus anticoagulants. Thromb Haemost 2001;86:83–91.
62. Somers E, Magder LS, Petri M. Antiphospholipid antibodies and incidence of venous thrombosis in a cohort of patients with systemic lupus erythematosus. J Rheumatol 2002;29:2531–2536.
63. Finazzi G, Brancaccio V, Moia M, et al. Natural history and risk factors for thrombosis in 360 patients with antiphospholipid antibodies: a four-year prospective study from the Italian Registry. Am J Med 1996;100:530–536.
64. Galli M, Finazzi G, Bevers EM, Barbui T. Kaolin clotting time and dilute Russell's viper venom time distinguish between prothrombin-dependent and beta-2-glycoprotein I-dependent antiphospholipid antibodies. Blood 1995;86:617–623.
65. Galli M, Finazzi G, Norbis F, Marziali S, Marchioli R, Barbui T. The risk of thrombosis in patients with lupus anticoagulants is predicted by their specific coagulation profile. Thromb Haemost 1999;81:695–700.
66. Nojima J, Kuratsune H, Suehisa E, et al. Anti-prothrombin antibodies combined with lupus anticoagulant activity is an essential risk factor for venous thromboembolism in patients with systemic lupus erythematosus. Br J Haematol 2001;114:647–654.
67. Zanon E, Saggiorato G, Ramon R, Girolami A, Pagnan A, Prandoni P. Anti-prothrombin antibodies as a potential risk factor of recurrent venous thromboembolism. Thromb Haemost 2004;91:255–258.
68. Simmelink MJA, Derksen RHWM, Arnout J, de Groot PG. A simple method to discriminate between $\beta_2$glycoprotein I- and prothrombin-dependent lupus anticoagulants. J Thromb Haemost 2003;1:740–747.
69. Pengo V, Biasiolo A, Pegoraro C, Iliceto S. A two-step coagulation test to identify anti-beta2-glycoprotein I Lupus anticoagulants. J Thromb Haemost 2004;2:702–707.
70. Harper MF, Hayes PM, Lentz B, Roubey RAS. Characterization of β_2-glycoprotein I binding to phospholipid membranes. Thromb Haemost 1998;80:610–614.
71. Roussi J, Roisin JP, Goguel A. Lupus anticoagulants. First French Interlaboratory Etalanorme Survey. Am J Clin Pathol 1996;105:788–793.
72. Jennings I, Kitchen S, Woods TAL, Preston FE, Greaves M. Clinically important inaccuracies in testing for the lupus anticoagulant: an analysis of results from three surveys of the UK national external quality assessment scheme (NEQAS) for blood coagulation. Thromb Haemost 1997;77:934–937.
73. Gray E, Mackie I, Greaves M. Calibration of the 1st British reference plasma panel for lupus anticoagulants. Br J Haematol 1998;105(suppl 1):97.

74. Arnout J, Vanrusset M, Wittevrongel C, Vermylen J. Monoclonal antibodies against β-2-glycoprotein I: use as reference material for lupus anticoagulant tests. Thromb Haemost 1998;79:955–958.
75. Arnout J, Boon D, Vandervoort P, Vanrusselt M, Vermylen J. A monoclonal antibody against prothrombin fragment 2 behaves like a lupus anticoagulant. Lupus 2002;11:550.

25 β_2-glycoprotein I and Anti–β_2-glycoprotein I Antibodies

Shinsuke Yasuda, Tatsuya Atsumi, and Takao Koike

Introduction

In patients with antiphospholipid syndrome (APS), pathogenic antiphospholipid antibodies (aPL) are not directed against phospholipids itself, but against plasma proteins that bind to negatively charged surface, such as β_2-glycoprotein-I (β_2-GPI) [1–3], prothrombin [4–6], annexin V, protein C, protein S, high- and low-molecular-weight kininogens [7], tissue plasminogen activator [8], factor VII [9], factor XII [10], complement component C4, and complement factor H [11]. Among them, autoantibodies against β_2-GPI have been extensively investigated and recognized as the most relevant, because anti–β_2-GPI autoantibodies are not only a marker of APS [12], but also seem to play pathogenic roles in developing thrombosis [12, 13].

Structure and Physiological Function of β_2-GPI

β_2-GPI, also known as apolipoprotein H, is a 50-kDa phospholipid binding protein present in plasma at an approximate concentration of 200 μg/mL. β_2-GPI has 5 homologous short consensus repeats and 4 glycation sites, forming an elongated fishhook-like 3-dimensional structure. Domains of β_2-GPI structurally resemble each other, except that domain V has an extra C-terminal loop and a positively charged lysine cluster. According to the crystal structure of human β_2-GPI, it was proposed that this large positively charged patch interacts with negatively charged phospholipid with a flexible and partially hydrophobic loop inserted into the lipid layer when it binds to the cell surface [14, 15] (Fig. 25.1). β_2-GPI also binds to other negatively charged molecules such as heparin, DNA, oxidized low-density lipoprotein (LDL) [16, 17], and apoptotic bodies [18].

Because negatively charged molecules trigger the intrinsic coagulation pathway, β_2-GPI was proposed to be a natural anticoagulant. β_2-GPI inhibits prothrombinase and tenase activity on platelets or phospholipid vesicles [19], inhibits factor XII activation [20], and modulates ADP-dependent activation of platelets [21]. Recently, β_2-GPI has been shown to bind directly to factor XI and attenuate its activation [22]. On the other hand, β_2-GPI exerts procoagulant activities by reduction of activated protein C [23]. Data from knockout mice suggests that β_2-GPI may

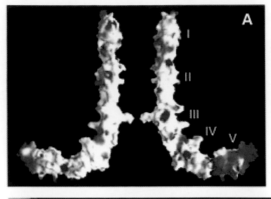

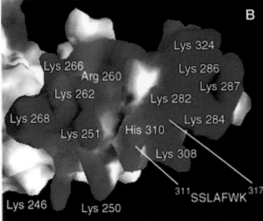

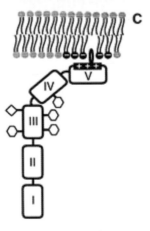

Figure 25.1. Structure of human β_2-GPI and binding model of β_2-GPI and phospholipids. (A) Two views, related by 180° rotation of the electrostatic potential surface of β_2-GPI. (B) Positively charged patch on the aberrant half of domain V. (C) Diagram of the proposed model for binding of β_2-GPI to anionic phospholipids. [Reprinted from Bouma et al. Adhesion mechanism of human beta(2)-glycoprotein I to phospholipids based on its crystal structure. EMBO J 1999;18:5171.]

contribute in thrombin generation in vivo [24]. In spite of these studies concerning roles of β_2-GPI in coagulation/fibrinolysis system, genetic deficiency of β_2-GPI is not a major risk factor of either thrombosis or bleeding in humans [25, 26]. These results were consistent with our cases with β_2-GPI deficiency, which is due to single nucleotide deletion and resulting frame shift in β_2-GPI gene β_2-GPI Sapporo) [27, 28].

Approximately 30% of plasma β_2-GPI resides in the lipoprotein fraction. β_2-GPI binds oxidized LDL, inhibiting the uptake and proteolytic degradation of oxidized LDL by macrophage [16]. β_2-GPI enhances the enzymatic activity of lipoprotein lipase [29] and contributes to triglyceride clearance from plasma [30]. Thus, β_2-GPI may have an anti-atherogenic role in vitro.

Interaction Between β_2-GPI and Anti–β_2-GPI Antibodies

It is generally accepted that anti–β_2GPI antibodies are a group of heterogeneous autoantobodies. The majority of anti–β_2-GPI antibodies present in patients with APS do not bind solid-phase β_2-GPI when coated on plain polystyrene plates. Matsuura et al [31] demonstrated that polyclonal or monoclonal aPL bind directly to β_2-GPI coated on irradiated plates in the absence of cardiolipin. This binding of aPL was inhibited by addition of cardiolipin with β_2-GPI . These authors concluded that aPL recognizes a cryptic epitope in the presence of β_2-GPI , which undergoes conformational change following interaction with irradiated surface or cardiolipin. Conformational change in β_2-GPI upon binding to phospholipids was confirmed by spectroscopy and spectrophotometry [32]. Roubey et al [33] proposed that increased density of β_2-GPI on irradiated polystyrene plates is important for binding of aPL. Because aPL had low affinity to β_2-GPI in a liquid phase and Fab' fragment of patient IgG had low affinity to immobilized β_2-GPI, they concluded that anticardiolipin antibodies (aCL) binding to β_2-GPI on a microtiter plate or anionic phospholipid membrane is dependent upon the bivalency of the autoantibody. Using a dimerized form of mutant β_2-GPI, Sheng et al [34] demonstrated that dimerization of β_2-GPI is important for the binding of autoantibody. Anti–β_2-GPI antibodies that react to β_2-GPI immobilized on plain plates are also detected in APS patients [35]. In the absence of phospholipids, autoantibodies that bind β_2-GPI in solution have also been reported [34, 36, 37]. Anti–β_2-GPI antibodies that are not detectable on cardiolipin-coated plates but detectable on plain plates are reported in children with atopic dermatitis [38].

Thus, there are conflicting data about the reactivity of anti–β_2-GPI antibodies, which may reflect the heterogeneity of autoantibodies and/or the variety of assay conditions used in different laboratories. Although ELISA is commonly used for the detection of anti–β_2-GPI autoantibodies, details of the assays differ significantly. First, β_2-GPI may be coated on plain plates, on irradiated or oxygenated plates, or on anionic phospholipids such as cardiolipin. Second, β_2-GPI used in the assays is derived from human, bovine, or goat. Third, blocking agents or dilution buffers are different. Last, antibodies used for the standard are different, although monoclonal anti–β_2-GPI antibodies have been proposed as international standards [39, 40].

Epitope Mapping on β_2-GPI

Because of potential benefits in the treatment of patients, substantial amount of investigations have been done to specify the domain that bears epitopes for autoimmune anti–β_2-GPI antibodies. Reflecting the heterogeneity of anti–β_2-GPI antibodies, epitopes for the autoantibodies have been reported to reside in all domains of β_2-GPI.

Using a series of domain-deleted recombinant β_2-GPI, Iverson et al [41] showed that the binding of patients' aPL to solid-phase β_2-GPI was inhibited by deletion mutants containing domain I, but not by those lacking domain I. Supporting this report, single amino-acid substitutions in domain I abolished the binding of aPL to β_2-GPI [42]. Using surface plasmon resonance, McNeeley et al [43] compared the binding of native β_2-GPI and deletion mutant that lacks domain I to patient sera, the result indicated that majority of sera from patients recognize domain I of β_2-GPI. Domain IV is also reported to be recognized by autoimmune aPL. Using domain deletion mutants, Igarashi et al [44] and George et al [45] found that a murine monoclonal anti–β_2-GPI antibody binds domains I–IV better than the whole β_2-GPI or domains I–III, concluding that domain IV is a major epitope for aPL. According to our data using phage peptide libraries, antigenic structure for 3 human monoclonal and a murine monoclonal anti–β_2-GPI antibodies were identified in domain IV, although a similar structure was also found in domain I [46]. Binding of anti–β_2-GPI antibodies to solid phase β_2-GPI was significantly reduced by site-directed mutagenesis of W^{235}, a common amino acid component for the epitopes. Using a hexapeptide phage library, Blank et al [47] identified 3 hexapeptides that react specifically with human monoclonal anti–β_2-GPI antibodies. These hexapeptides bore homologous sequence to regions of β_2-GPI in domains I and II, domain III, or domain IV. The importance of domain V as an epitope for aPL as well as as a phospholipid binding site has also been reported [48, 49].

To explain these different results about B cell epitopes, the clinical study by Shoenfeld et al [50] may give us one of the clues. They tested the reactivity of patient sera against six β_2-GPI–related peptides which obtain protein sequences from domain I, domain III, domain IV, inter-linker region of domain IV and V, or domain V. Eighty-seven percent of the patients had antibody reactivity against at least one of these β_2-GPI–related peptides and a high degree of simultaneous reactivity against several β_2-GPI–related peptides was found, suggesting heterogeneous reactivity of aPL against various epitopes of the β_2-GPI molecule.

Clinical Significance of Anti–β_2-GPI Antibodies

Association between the presence of anti–β_2-GPI antibodies and clinical manifestation of APS has been investigated. Reports have shown that IgG and IgM anti–β_2-GPI antibodies with medium or high titers is significantly related to the history of thrombosis [12, 51–60]. Although IgA class anti–β_2-GPI antibodies are not widely investigated, clinical studies found significant association between the presence of this isotype of autoantibodies and thrombosis [61–65]. However, clinical significance of IgA anti–β_2-GPI antibodies has yet to be established because most patients with IgA anti–β_2-GPI antibodies were also positive for IgG and/or IgM isotype [61, 66]. Among IgG subclasses of aCL, IgG_2 aCL is more correlated with thrombosis than the other subclasses [67]. In anti–$β_2$-GPI antibodies found in APS patients, IgG_2 predominance is evident, whereas IgG_1 predominance of aCL related with infectious diseases [68].

In order to evaluate clinical significance of laboratory tests such as lupus anticoagulant, aCL, anti–$β_2$-GPI antibodies and anti-prothrombin antibodies, Galli et al [69] reviewed 32 mainly retrospective literatures from 1988 though 2001, which contains over 5000 patients in total. As previously reported, lupus anticoagulants are stronger risk factor for thrombosis than aCL in patients with APS [70]. Thirty-four of 60 studies showed significant associations (5/17 with arterial thrombosis, 12/21 with venous thrombosis, and 17/22 with any thrombosis), when anti–$β_2$-GPI antibody was measured. Isotype analysis revealed that IgG anti–$β_2$-GPI antibodies were significantly associated with thrombosis in 20 of 33 studies, although only 2 of 10 studies reached significant association when multivariate analysis was introduced. IgM isotype was associated in 7 of 15 studies, IgA in all of 3. When the type (arterial or venous) of thrombosis is concerned, anti–$β_2$-GPI antibodies were not associated with arterial thrombosis, but only marginally with venous thrombosis, whereas aCL were associated with arterial but not venous thrombosis. This discrepancy may be due to the existence of $β_2$-GPI–independent aCL, which are detected mainly in patients with infectious diseases [71–73]. In addition, titers of anti–$β_2$-GPI antibodies differ considerably according to different assay kits, although better concordance is obtained for high titers of autoantibody [74]. We compared clinical significance of $β_2$-GPI–dependent aCL (aCL-$β_2$-GPI) and phosphatidylserine-dependent anti-prothrombin (aPS/PT) antibodies using multivariate analysis [75]. Both antibodies had significant correlation with manifestations of APS, including thrombocytopenia or not, although aPS/PT had stronger correlation than aCL-$β_2$-GPI (Table 25.1). Lopez et al [76] surveyed aPL (aCL, antiphosphatidylserine, anti–$β_2$-GPI, aPT antibodies) of 100 patients with APS and concluded that anti–$β_2$-GPI antibody and antiphosphatidylserine antibody have a stronger predictive value and association for arterial thrombosis. Autoantibodies against $β_2$-GPI/oxidized LDL complex are detected in patients with systemic lupus erythematosus (SLE) and APS. Strong correlation was found between IgG anti–$β_2$-GPI/oxidized LDL antibodies

Table 25.1. Relationship between anti–$β_2$-glycoprotein I antibody/phosphtidylserine dependent antiprothrombin antibody and clinical manifestation of antiphospholipid syndrome.

Category, assay	Odds ratio	95% donfidence interval	P value
Manifestations of APS or thrombocytopenia			
IgG/M aPS/PT	3.36	1.52–7.43	0.0025
IgG/M/A aCL/$β_2$-GPI	3.07	1.38–6.86	0.0059
Manifestations of APS (thrombocytopenia is excluded)			
IgG/M aPS/PT	2.92	1.33-6.40	0.0091
IgG/M/A aCL/$β_2$-GPI	2.06	0.91-4.66	0.0887
Relationship with LA-dRVVT			
IgG/M aPS/PT	9.39	3.74–23.55	< 0.0001
IgG/M/A aCL/$β_2$-GPI	4.01	1.64–9.78	0.0023

Source: Atsumi T, Leko M, Bertolaccini ML, et al. Association of autoantibodies against the phosphatidylserine-prothrombin complex with manifestations of the antiphospholipid syndrome and with the presence of lupus anticoagulant. Arthritis Rheum 2000 Sep;43(9):1982–93; Copyright © 2000; reprinted with permission of Wiley-Liss, Inc.; a subsidiary of John Wiley & Sons, Inc.

and arterial thrombosis in APS [77]. The relative specificity of this novel assay system indicates that β_2-GPI/oxidized LDL/anti–β_2-GPI antibody complex may directly be associated with atherosclerosis.

The importance of anti–β_2-GPI antibodies in pregnancy complications has also been studied. According to some reports, anti–β_2-GPI antibodies are associated with pregnancy complications [78–81]. In one case-control study on women with no antecedent of thromboembolic or autoimmune disease, anti–β_2-GPI antibody as well as LA was identified as an independent risk factor for unexplained early fetal loss [82]. However, others could not find association between this laboratory test and obstetric complications [83, 84]. The significance of IgA anti–β_2-GPI in pregnancy is also uncertain [66, 85, 86]. After reviewing literatures about APS and pregnancy loss, Bruce et al [87] found that it is impossible to draw any conclusion regarding anti–β_2-GPI and clinical features of secondary APS in SLE because of the variation of assay systems.

Possible Role of Anti–β_2-GPI Antibodies

The mechanisms by which anti–β_2-GPI antibodies cause thrombosis remain unknown, although several hypotheses have been proposed. Inhibition of anticoagulant activity in β_2-GPI has been suggested as one of the mechanisms. Anti–β_2-GPI antibodies block the inhibitory effect of β_2-GPI on factor Xa generation on activated platelets [88]. However, anticoagulant activity found in β_2-GPI may not be critical in vivo. Although the affinity of β_2-GPI for anionic phospholipids is lower than other clotting factors, binding of anti–β_2-GPI antibodies increases the affinity of β_2-GPI for negatively charged phospholipids approximately 100 times [89]. Increment of the affinity may modify the physiological function of β_2-GPI, or inhibit the binding of other phospholipid binding proteins. Activated protein C acts as an anticoagulant by degrading factors Va and VIIIa. Anti–β_2-GPI antibodies are reported to inhibit both protein C activation and activated protein C [90] only in the presence of β_2-GPI [91]. Cell-mediated mechanisms have also been reported. Tissue factor expression on endothelial cells is induced by aPL [92–95]. Interaction between dimmers of β_2-GPI and apolipoprotein E receptor 2 on platelets was reported, which result in increased platelet adhesion to collagen probably via induction of thromboxane synthesis [96]. Raschi et al [97] reported an involvement of toll-like receptor family and MyD88 pathway in endothelial activation observed after stimulation by monoclonal anti–β_2-GPI antibodies. Acceleration of atherosclerosis induced by anti–β_2-GPI antibodies has been reported and growing evidence is accumulated in these fields. This point will be discussed in Chapter 40.

Cleavage of β_2-GPI: Implication in aCL Binding and Negative Feedback Pathway in Extrinsic Fibrinolysis

β_2-GPIis proteolytically cleaved between Lys-317 and Thr-318 in domain V (nicked β_2-GPI), being unable to bind to phospholipids [48]. This cleavage is generated by factor Xa or by plasmin, the latter being more effective [98]. Once this cleavage happens to β_2-GPI, it loses the antigenicity for pathogenic aPL [99]. Nicked β_2-GPI

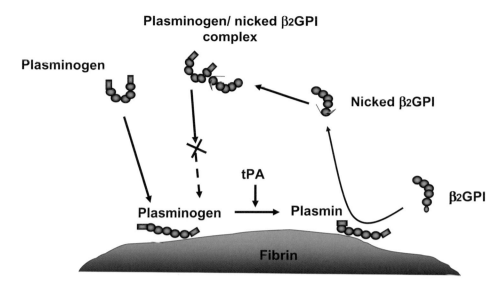

Figure 25.2. Upon formation of intra-vessel blood clot, plasminogen binds fibrin at first via kringle V and is activated by tissue plasminogen activator (tPA) into active plasmin. Then, fibrinolytic system becomes active. Generated plasmin cleaves β_2-GPI into nicked β_2-GPI that binds to plasminogen and inhibits its binding to fibrin, thus playing a role in negative feedback pathway of extrinsic fibrinolysis.

has been identified in plasma of patients under conditions characterized by massive thrombin generation and fibrinolytic turnover, such as disseminated intravascular coagulation (DIC) [100], leukemia, or positive LA. We have shown that ratio of nicked β_2-GPI against total β_2-GPI is elevated in patients with cerebral infarction including asymptomatic lacunar infarct [101]. We demonstrated that nicked β_2-GPI, but not intact β_2-GPI, binds to plasminogen, presumably mediated by the interaction between the lysine cluster on the fifth domain of nicked β_2-GPI and lysine binding site on the fifth kringle domain of plasminogen. Nicked β_2-GPI also suppressed plasmin generation in the presence of tissue plasminogen activator, plasminogen, and soluble fibrin monomer. Nicked β_2-GPI interfered the binding of plasminogen to fibrin, which is the first step in fibrinolysis. Thus, plasmin generated nicked β_2-GPI controls extrinsic fibrinolysis via a negative feedback pathway loop (Fig. 25.2).

Conclusions

Because β_2-GPI was found to be a major antigen for aPL, many studies have been focused on the physiological role of β_2-GPI, on mechanism of thrombosis induced by anti–β_2-GPI antibody, and on clinical significance of this autoantibody. Physiological roles of β_2-GPI have been reported, although "true" property in human has yet to be determined. Several epitopes for anti–β_2-GPI antibodies are known, however, all of the anti–β_2-GPI antibodies may not be pathogenic and anti–β_2-GPI antibodies are heterogeneous. What we learn from these clinical reports would be as follows. First, the standardization of the assay system for aPL is urgent. Second, measurement of aPL using multiple methods is favored in order to establish better assay for diagnosis and/or for prediction of disease activity. Last, more prospective, multi-center studies will be needed after standardization of the assay systems.

Recently, pathogenic roles of anti–β_2-GPI antibodies have been reported in the fields of coagulation and fibrinolysis, atherosclerosis, or signal transduction and cell activation. These findings may contribute to better and specific therapies for patients with APS.

References

1. Matsuura E, Igarashi Y, Fujimoto M, Ichikawa K, Koike T. Anticardiolipin cofactor(s) and differential diagnosis of autoimmune disease. Lancet 1990;336:177–178.
2. Galli M, Comfurius P, Maassen C, et al. Anticardiolipin antibodies (ACA) directed not to cardiolipin but to a plasma protein cofactor. Lancet 1990;335:1544–1547.
3. McNeil HP, Simpson RJ, Chesterman CN, Krilis SA. Anti-phospholipid antibodies are directed against a complex antigen that includes a lipid-binding inhibitor of coagulation: β_2-glycoprotein I (apolipoprotein H). Proc Natl Acad Sci U S A 1990;87:4120–4124.
4. Galli M, Beretta G, Daldossi M, Bevers EM, Barbui T. Different anticoagulant and immunological properties of anti-prothrombin antibodies in patients with antiphospholipid antibodies. Thromb Haemost 1997;77:486–491.
5. Arvieux J, Darnige L, Caron C, Reber G, Bensa JC, Colomb MG. Development of an ELISA for autoantibodies to prothrombin showing their prevalence in patients with lupus anticoagulants. Thromb Haemost 1995;74:1120–1125.
6. Atsumi T, Ieko M, Bertolaccini ML, et al. Association of autoantibodies against the phosphatidylserine-prothrombin complex with manifestations of the antiphospholipid syndrome and with the presence of lupus anticoagulant. Arthritis Rheum 2000;43:1982–1993.
7. Sugi T, McIntyre JA. Autoantibodies to phosphatidylethanolamine (PE) recognize a kininogen-PE complex. Blood 1995;86:3083–3089.
8. Cugno M, Dominguez M, Cabibbe M, et al. Antibodies to tissue-type plasminogen activator in plasma from patients with primary antiphospholipid syndrome. Br J Haematol 2000;108:871–875.
9. Bidot CJ, Jy W, Horstman LL, et al. Factor VII/VIIa: a new antigen in the anti-phospholipid antibody syndrome. Br J Haematol 2003;120:618–626.
10. Jones DW, Mackie IJ, Gallimore MJ, Winter M. Antibodies to factor XII and recurrent fetal loss in patients with the anti-phospholipid syndrome. Br J Haematol 2001;113:550–552.
11. Rampazzo P, Biasiolo A, Garin J, et al. Some patients with antiphospholipid syndrome express hitherto undescribed antibodies to cardiolipin-binding proteins. Thromb Haemost 2001;85:57–62.
12. Tsutsumi A, Matsuura E, Ichikawa K, et al. Antibodies to β_2-glycoprotein I and clinical manifestations in patients with systemic lupus erythematosus. Arthritis Rheum 1996;39:1466–1474.
13. Pierangeli SS, Liu SW, Anderson G, Barker JH, Harris EN. Thrombogenic properties of murine anti-cardiolipin antibodies induced by β_2 glycoprotein 1 and human immunoglobulin G antiphospholipid antibodies. Circulation 1996;94:1746–1751.
14. Bouma B, de Groot PG, van den Elsen JM, et al. Adhesion mechanism of human β_2-glycoprotein I to phospholipids based on its crystal structure. EMBO J 1999;18:5166–5174.
15. Schwarzenbacher R, Zeth K, Diederichs K, et al. Crystal structure of human ?$_2$-glycoprotein I: implications for phospholipid binding and the antiphospholipid syndrome. EMBO J 1999;18:6228–6239.
16. Hasunuma Y, Matsuura E, Makita Z, Katahira T, Nishi S, Koike T. Involvement of β_2-glycoprotein I and anticardiolipin antibodies in oxidatively modified low-density lipoprotein uptake by macrophages. Clin Exp Immunol 1997;107:569–573.
17. Kobayashi K, Kishi M, Atsumi T, et al. Circulating oxidized LDL forms complexes with β_2-glycoprotein I: implication as an atherogenic autoantigen. J Lipid Res 2003;44:716–726.
18. Pittoni V, Ravirajan CT, Donohoe S, Machin SJ, Lydyard PM, Isenberg DA. Human monoclonal anti-phospholipid antibodies selectively bind to membrane phospholipid and β_2-glycoprotein I (β_2-GPI) on apoptotic cells. Clin Exp Immunol 2000;119:533–543.

19. Nimpf J, Bevers EM, Bomans PH, et al. Prothrombinase activity of human platelets is inhibited by β₂-glycoprotein-I. Biochim Biophys Acta 1986;884:142–149.
20. Schousboe I, Rasmussen MS. Synchronized inhibition of the phospholipid mediated autoactivation of factor XII in plasma by β₂-glycoprotein I and anti-β₂-glycoprotein I. Thromb Haemost 1995;73:798–804.
21. Nimpf J, Wurm H, Kostner GM. Interaction of β₂-glycoprotein-I with human blood platelets: influence upon the ADP-induced aggregation. Thromb Haemost 1985;54:397–401.
22. Ieko M, Tarumi T, Takeda M, Naito S, Nakabayashi T, Koike T. Synthetic selective inhibitors of coagulation factor Xa strongly inhibit thrombin generation without affecting initial thrombin forming time necessary for platelet activation in hemostasis. J Thromb Haemost 2004;2:612–618.
23. Mori T, Takeya H, Nishioka J, Gabazza EC, Suzuki K. β₂-glycoprotein I modulates the anticoagulant activity of activated protein C on the phospholipid surface. Thromb Haemost 1996;75:49–55.
24. Sheng Y, Reddel SW, Herzog H, et al. Impaired thrombin generation in β₂-glycoprotein I null mice. J Biol Chem 2001;276:13817–13821.
25. Hoeg JM, Segal P, Gregg RE, et al. Characterization of plasma lipids and lipoproteins in patients with β₂-glycoprotein I (apolipoprotein H) deficiency. Atherosclerosis 1985;55:25–34.
26. Bancsi LF, van der Linden IK, Bertina RM. β₂-glycoprotein I deficiency and the risk of thrombosis. Thromb Haemost 1992;67:649–653.
27. Yasuda S, Tsutsumi A, Chiba H, et al. β₂-glycoprotein I deficiency: prevalence, genetic background and effects on plasma lipoprotein metabolism and hemostasis. Atherosclerosis 2000;152:337–346.
28. Takeuchi R, Atsumi T, Ieko M, et al. Coagulation and fibrinolytic activities in 2 siblings with β₂-glycoprotein I deficiency. Blood 2000;96:1594–1595.
29. Nakaya Y, Schaefer EJ, Brewer HB Jr. Activation of human post heparin lipoprotein lipase by apolipoprotein H (β₂-glycoprotein I). Biochem Biophys Res Commun 1980;95:1168–1172.
30. Wurm H. β₂-Glycoprotein-I (apolipoprotein H) interactions with phospholipid vesicles. Int J Biochem 1984;16:511–515.
31. Matsuura E, Igarashi Y, Yasuda T, Triplett DA, Koike T. Anticardiolipin antibodies recognize β₂-glycoprotein I structure altered by interacting with an oxygen modified solid phase surface. J Exp Med 1994;179:457–462.
32. Subang R, Levine JS, Janoff AS, et al. Phospholipid-bound β₂-glycoprotein I induces the production of anti-phospholipid antibodies. J Autoimmun 2000;15:21–32.
33. Roubey RA, Eisenberg RA, Harper MF, Winfield JB. "Anticardiolipin" autoantibodies recognize β₂-glycoprotein I in the absence of phospholipid. Importance of Ag density and bivalent binding. J Immunol 1995;154:954–960.
34. Sheng Y, Kandiah DA, Krilis SA. Anti-β₂-glycoprotein I autoantibodies from patients with the "antiphospholipid" syndrome bind to β₂-glycoprotein I with low affinity: dimerization of β₂-glycoprotein I induces a significant increase in anti-β₂-glycoprotein I antibody affinity. J Immunol 1998;161:2038–2043.
35. Arvieux J, Regnault V, Hachulla E, Darnige L, Roussel B, Bensa JC. Heterogeneity and immunochemical properties of anti-β₂-glycoprotein I autoantibodies. Thromb Haemost 1998;80:393–398.
36. Roubey RA. Autoantibodies to phospholipid-binding plasma proteins: a new view of lupus anticoagulants and other "antiphospholipid" autoantibodies. Blood 1994;8:2854–2867.
37. Tincani A, Spatola L, Prati E, et al. The anti-β₂-glycoprotein I activity in human anti-phospholipid syndrome sera is due to monoreactive low-affinity autoantibodies directed to epitopes located on native beta2-glycoprotein I and preserved during species' evolution. J Immunol 1996;157:5732–5738.
38. Ambrozic A, Avicin T, Ichikawa K, et al. Anti-β₂-glycoprotein I antibodies in children with atopic dermatitis. Int Immunol 2002;14:823–830.
39. Ichikawa K, Tsutsumi A, Atsumi T, et al. A chimeric antibody with the human gamma1 constant region as a putative standard for assays to detect IgG β₂-glycoprotein I-dependent anticardiolipin and anti-β₂-glycoprotein I antibodies. Arthritis Rheum 1999;42:2461–2470.
40. Ichikawa K, Khamashta MA, Koike T, Matsuura E, Hughes GR. β₂-Glycoprotein I reactivity of monoclonal anticardiolipin antibodies from patients with the antiphospholipid syndrome. Arthritis Rheum 1994;37:1453–1461.
41. Iverson GM, Victoria EJ, Marquis DM. Anti-β₂ glycoprotein I (β₂GPI) autoantibodies recognize an epitope on the first domain of beta2GPI. Proc Natl Acad Sci U S A 1998;95:15542–15546.
42. Reddel SW, Wang YX, Sheng YH, Krilis SA. Epitope studies with anti-β₂-glycoprotein I antibodies from autoantibody and immunized sources. J Autoimmun 2000;15:91–96.
43. McNeeley PA, Dlott JS, Furie RA, et al. β₂-glycoprotein I-dependent anticardiolipin antibodies preferentially bind the amino terminal domain of β₂-glycoprotein I. Thromb Haemost 2001;86:590–595.

44. Igarashi M, Matsuura E, Igarashi Y, et al. Human β_2-glycoprotein I as an anticardiolipin cofactor determined using mutants expressed by a baculovirus system. Blood 1996;87:3262–3270.

45. George J, Gilburd B, Hojnik M, et al. Target recognition of β_2-glycoprotein I (β_2GPI)-dependent anticardiolipin antibodies: evidence for involvement of the fourth domain of beta2GPI in antibody binding. J Immunol 1998;160:3917–3923.

46. Koike T, Ichikawa K, Atsumi T, Kasahara H, Matsuura E. β_2-glycoprotein I-anti-β_2-glycoprotein I interaction. J Autoimmun 2000;15:97–100.

47. Blank M, Shoenfeld Y, Cabilly S, Heldman Y, Fridkin M, Katchalski-Katzir E. Prevention of experimental antiphospholipid syndrome and endothelial cell activation by synthetic peptides. Proc Natl Acad Sci U S A 1999;96:5164–5168.

48. Hunt JE, Simpson RJ, Krilis SA. Identification of a region of β_2-glycoprotein I critical for lipid binding and anti-cardiolipin antibody cofactor activity. Proc Natl Acad Sci U S A 1993;90:2141–2145.

49. Wang MX, Kandiah DA, Ichikawa K, et al. Epitope specificity of monoclonal anti-β_2-glycoprotein I antibodies derived from patients with the antiphospholipid syndrome. J Immunol 1995;155:1629–1636.

50. Shoenfeld Y, Krause I, Kvapil F, et al. Prevalence and clinical correlations of antibodies against six β_2-glycoprotein-I-related peptides in the antiphospholipid syndrome. J Clin Immunol 2003;23:377–383.

51. Guerin J, Feighery C, Sim RB, Jackson J. Antibodies to β_2-glycoprotein I – a specific marker for the antiphospholipid syndrome. Clin Exp Immunol 1997;109:304–309.

52. Martinuzzo ME, Forastiero RR, Carreras LO. Anti β_2 glycoprotein I antibodies: detection and association with thrombosis. Br J Haematol 1995;89:397–402.

53. McNally T, Purdy G, Mackie IJ, Machin SJ, Isenberg DA. The use of an anti-β_2-glycoprotein-I assay for discrimination between anticardiolipin antibodies associated with infection and increased risk of thrombosis. Br J Haematol 1995;91:471–473.

54. Balestrieri G, Tincani A, Spatola L, et al. Anti-β_2-glycoprotein I antibodies: a marker of antiphospholipid syndrome? Lupus 1995;4:122–130.

55. Cabral AR, Cabiedes J, Alarcon-Segovia D. Antibodies to phospholipid-free β_2-glycoprotein-I in patients with primary antiphospholipid syndrome. J Rheumatol 1995;22:1894–1898.

56. Forastiero RR, Martinuzzo ME, Kordich LC, Carreras LO. Reactivity to β_2 glycoprotein I clearly differentiates anticardiolipin antibodies from antiphospholipid syndrome and syphilis. Thromb Haemost 1996;75:717–720.

57. Roubey RA, Maldonado MA, Byrd SN. Comparison of an enzyme-linked immunosorbent assay for antibodies to β_2-glycoprotein I and a conventional anticardiolipin immunoassay. Arthritis Rheum 1996;39:1606–1607.

58. Amengual O, Atsumi T, Khamashta MA, Koike T, Hughes GR. Specificity of ELISA for antibody to β_2-glycoprotein I in patients with antiphospholipid syndrome. Br J Rheumatol 1996;35:1239–1243.

59. Cabiedes J, Cabral AR, Alarcon-Segovia D. Clinical manifestations of the antiphospholipid syndrome in patients with systemic lupus erythematosus associate more strongly with anti-β_2-glycoprotein-I than with antiphospholipid antibodies. J Rheumatol 1995;22:1899–1906.

60. Sanmarco M, Soler C, Christides C, et al. Prevalence and clinical significance of IgG isotype anti-β_2-glycoprotein I antibodies in antiphospholipid syndrome: a comparative study with anticardiolipin antibodies. J Lab Clin Med 1997;129:499–506.

61. Tsutsumi A, Matsuura E, Ichikawa K, Fujisaku A, Mukai M, Koike T. IgA class anti-β_2-glycoprotein I in patients with systemic lupus erythematosus. J Rheumatol 1998;25:74–78.

62. Pasquier E, Amiral J, de Saint ML, Mottier D. A cross sectional study of antiphospholipid-protein antibodies in patients with venous thromboembolism. Thromb Haemost 2001;86:538–542.

63. Fanopoulos D, Teodorescu MR, Varga J, Teodorescu M. High frequency of abnormal levels of IgA anti-β_2-glycoprotein I antibodies in patients with systemic lupus erythematosus: relationship with antiphospholipid syndrome. J Rheumatol 1998;25:675–680.

64. Lee SS, Cho ML, Joo YS, et al. Isotypes of anti-β_2-glycoprotein I antibodies: association with thrombosis in patients with systemic lupus erythematosus. J Rheumatol 2001;28:520–524.

65. Wilson WA, Morgan OC, Barton EN, et al. IgA antiphospholipid antibodies in HTLV-1-associated tropical spastic paraparesis. Lupus 1995;4:138–141.

66. Bertolaccini ML, Atsumi T, Escudero CA, Khamashta MA, Hughes GRV. The value of IgA antiphospholipid testing for diagnosis of antiphospholipid (Hughes) syndrome in systemic lupus erythematosus. J Rheumatol 2001;28:2637–2643.

67. Sammaritano LR, Ng S, Sobel R, et al. Anticardiolipin IgG subclasses: association of IgG2 with arterial and/or venous thrombosis. Arthritis Rheum 1997;40:1998–2006.

68. Amengual O, Atsumi T, Khamashta MA, Bertolaccini ML, Hughes GR. IgG2 restriction of anti-β₂-glycoprotein I as the basis for the association between IgG2 anticardiolipin antibodies and thrombosis in the antiphospholipid syndrome: comment on the article by Sammaritano et al. Arthritis Rheum 1998;41:1513–1515.

69. Galli M, Luciani D, Bertolini G, Barbui T. Anti-β₂-glycoprotein I, antiprothrombin antibodies, and the risk of thrombosis in the antiphospholipid syndrome. Blood 2003;102:2717–2723.

70. Galli M, Luciani D, Bertolini G, Barbui T. Lupus anticoagulants are stronger risk factors for thrombosis than anticardiolipin antibodies in the antiphospholipid syndrome: a systematic review of the literature. Blood 2003;101:1827–1832.

71. Vaarala O, Palosuo T, Kleemola M, Aho K. Anticardiolipin response in acute infections. Clin Immunol Immunopathol 1986;41:8–15.

72. Santiago M, Martinelli R, Ko A, et al. Anti-β₂-glycoprotein I and anticardiolipin antibodies in leptospirosis, syphilis and Kala-azar. Clin Exp Rheumatol 2001;19:425–430.

73. Giordano P, Galli M, Del Vecchio GC, et al. Lupus anticoagulant, anticardiolipin antibodies and hepatitis C virus infection in thalassaemia. Br J Haematol 1998;102:903–906.

74. Audrain MA, Colonna F, Morio F, Hamidou MA, Muller JY. Comparison of different kits in the detection of autoantibodies to cardiolipin and β₂ glycoprotein 1. Rheumatology (Oxford) 2004;43:181–185.

75. Atsumi T, Ieko M, Bertolaccini ML, et al. Association of autoantibodies against the phosphatidylserine-prothrombin complex with manifestations of the antiphospholipid syndrome and with the presence of lupus anticoagulant. Arthritis Rheum 2000;43:1982–1993.

76. Lopez LR, Dier KJ, Lopez D, Merrill JT, Fink CA. Anti-β₂-glycoprotein I and antiphosphatidylserine antibodies are predictors of arterial thrombosis in patients with antiphospholipid syndrome. Am J Clin Pathol 2004;121:142–149.

77. Lopez D, Kobayashi K, Merrill JT, Matsuura E, Lopez LR. IgG autoantibodies against β₂-glycoprotein I complexed with a lipid ligand derived from oxidized low-density lipoprotein are associated with arterial thrombosis in antiphospholipid syndrome. Clin Dev Immunol 2003;10:203–211.

78. Ulcova-Gallova Z, Bouse V, Krizanovska K, Balvin M, Rokyta Z, Netrvalova L. β₂-glycoprotein I is a good indicator of certain adverse pregnancy conditions. Int J Fertil Womens Med 2001;46:304–308.

79. Lee RM, Emlen W, Scott JR, Branch DW, Silver RM. Anti-β₂-glycoprotein I antibodies in women with recurrent spontaneous abortion, unexplained fetal death, and antiphospholipid syndrome. Am J Obstet Gynecol 1999;181:642–648.

80. Falcon CR, Martinuzzo ME, Forastiero RR, Cerrato GS, Carreras LO. Pregnancy loss and autoantibodies against phospholipid-binding proteins. Obstet Gynecol 1997;89:975–980.

81. Faden D, Tincani A, Tanzi P, et al. Anti-β₂ glycoprotein I antibodies in a general obstetric population: preliminary results on the prevalence and correlation with pregnancy outcome. Anti-β₂ glycoprotein I antibodies are associated with some obstetrical complications, mainly preeclampsia-eclampsia. Eur J Obstet Gynecol Reprod Biol 1997;73:37–42.

82. Gris JC, Quere I, Sanmarco M, et al. Antiphospholipid and antiprotein syndromes in non-thrombotic, non-autoimmune women with unexplained recurrent primary early foetal loss. The Nimes Obstetricians and Haematologists Study – NOHA. Thromb Haemost 2000;84:228–236.

83. Lynch A, Byers T, Emlen W, Rynes D, Shetterly SM, Hamman RF. Association of antibodies to β₂-glycoprotein 1 with pregnancy loss and pregnancy-induced hypertension: a prospective study in low-risk pregnancy. Obstet Gynecol 1999;93:193–198.

84. Lee RM, Brown MA, Branch DW, Ward K, Silver RM. Anticardiolipin and anti-β₂-glycoprotein-I antibodies in preeclampsia. Obstet Gynecol 2003;102:294–300.

85. Carmo-Pereira S, Bertolaccini ML, Escudero-Contreras A, Khamashta MA, Hughes GR. Value of IgA anticardiolipin and anti-β₂-glycoprotein I antibody testing in patients with pregnancy morbidity. Ann Rheum Dis 2003;62:540–543.

86. Yamada H, Tsutsumi A, Ichikawa K, Kato EH, Koike T, Fujimoto S. IgA-class anti-β₂-glycoprotein I in women with unexplained recurrent spontaneous abortion. Arthritis Rheum 1999;42:2727–2728.

87. Bruce IN, Clark-Soloninka CA, Spitzer KA, Gladman DD, Urowitz MB, Laskin CA. Prevalence of antibodies to β₂-glycoprotein I in systemic lupus erythematosus and their association with antiphospholipid antibody syndrome criteria: a single center study and literature review. J Rheumatol 2000;27:2833–2837.

88. Shi W, Chong BH, Hogg PJ, Chesterman CN. Anticardiolipin antibodies block the inhibition by β₂-glycoprotein I of the factor Xa generating activity of platelets. Thromb Haemost 1993;70:342–345.

89. Takeya H, Mori T, Gabazza EC, et al. Anti-β₂-glycoprotein I (β₂GPI) monoclonal antibodies with lupus anticoagulant-like activity enhance the β₂GPI binding to phospholipids. J Clin Invest 1997;99:2260–2268.

90. Marciniak E, Romond EH. Impaired catalytic function of activated protein C: a new in vitro mani-
     festation of lupus anticoagulant. Blood 1989;74:2426–2432.
91. Ieko M, Ichikawa K, Triplett DA, et al. β_2-glycoprotein I is necessary to inhibit protein C activity by
     monoclonal anticardiolipin antibodies. Arthritis Rheum 1999;42:167–174.
92. Amengual O, Atsumi T, Khamashta MA, Hughes GR. The role of the tissue factor pathway in the
     hypercoagulable state in patients with the antiphospholipid syndrome. Thromb Haemost
     1998;79:276–281.
93. Branch DW, Rodgers GM. Induction of endothelial cell tissue factor activity by sera from patients
     with antiphospholipid syndrome: a possible mechanism of thrombosis. Am J Obstet Gynecol
     1993;168(1 Pt 1):206–210.
94. Kornberg A, Blank M, Kaufman S, Shoenfeld Y. Induction of tissue factor-like activity in mono-
     cytes by anti-cardiolipin antibodies. J Immunol 1994;153:1328–1332.
95. Conti F, Sorice M, Circella A, et al. β_2-glycoprotein I expression on monocytes is increased in anti-
     phospholipid antibody syndrome and correlates with tissue factor expression. Clin Exp Immunol
     2003;132:509–516.
96. Lutters BC, Derksen RH, Tekelenburg WL, Lenting PJ, Arnout J, de Groot PG. Dimers of β_2-glyco-
     protein I increase platelet deposition to collagen via interaction with phospholipids and the
     apolipoprotein E receptor 2'. J Biol Chem 2003;278:33831–33838.
97. Raschi E, Testoni C, Bosisio D, et al. Role of the MyD88 transduction signaling pathway in endothe-
     lial activation by antiphospholipid antibodies. Blood 2003;101:3495–3500.
98. Ohkura N, Hagihara Y, Yoshimura T, Goto Y, Kato H. Plasmin can reduce the function of human β_2
     glycoprotein I by cleaving domain V into a nicked form. Blood 1998;91:4173–4179.
99. Matsuura E, Igarashi J, Kasahara H, et al. Proteolytic cleavage of β_2-glycoprotein I: reduction of
     antigenicity and the structural relationship. Intern Immunol 2000;12:1183–1192.
100. Horbach DA, van Oort E, Lisman T, Meijers JC, Derksen RH, de Groot PG. β_2-glycoprotein I is pro-
     teolytically cleaved in vivo upon activation of fibrinolysis. Thromb Haemost 1999;81:87–95.
101. Yasuda S, Atsumi T, Ieko M, et al. Nicked β_2-glycoprotein I: a marker of cerebral infarct and a
     novel role in the negative feedback pathway of extrinsic fibrinolysis. Blood 2004;103:3766–3772.

26 Antiprothrombin Antibodies

Maria Laura Bertolaccini

Introduction

In clinical practice, anticardiolipin antibody (aCL) detected by ELISA and lupus anti-coagulant (LA) detected by clotting assays have been standardized for the diagnosis of the antiphospholipid syndrome (APS). However, it is now established that antiphospholipid antibodies (aPL) are a large and heterogeneous family of immunoglobulins, which, despite their name, do not seem to bind phospholipids, but are directed to plasma proteins with affinity for anionic surfaces (i.e., phospholipids).

Amongst these phospholipid binding proteins, the best studied is β_2-glycoprotein I (β_2-GPI), which bears the cryptic epitope(s) for aCL binding. These epitopes are exposed when β_2-GPI binds to negatively charged phospholipids such as cardiolipin, or irradiated plastic plates [1]. Several studies have highlighted the significance of anti–β_2-GPI antibodies (anti–β_2-GPI) as an alternative ELISA with higher specificity than the conventional aCL ELISA [2–4].

Prothrombin, another phospholipid binding protein, was first proposed as a possible co-factor for LA by Loeliger in 1959 [5]. In subsequent years, the interest regarding this protein has increased and several groups have investigated the significance of antiprothrombin antibodies.

Prothrombin

Prothrombin is a single chain glycoprotein, synthetized in the liver, recognized very early as the prime contributor to the blood coagulation process. This protein is found in plasma at a concentration of around 2.5 µmol/L. Its gene spans 21 kilobase pairs [6] on chromosome 11. Mature prothrombin contains 579 amino acid residues with a molecular mass of 72 kD, including 3 carbohydrate chains and 10 γ-carboxyglutamic acid residues [7].

The tenase complex, entailing factor Xa and factor V, calcium and phospholipids as co-factors, physiologically activates prothrombin. Once negatively charged, phospholipids bind prothrombin and tenase converts prothrombin to thrombin, which triggers fibrinogen polymerization into fibrin [8]. In addition, thrombin binds thrombomodulin on the surface of endothelial cells and activates protein C, which then exerts its anticoagulant activity by digesting factor V and depriving in this way the tenase complex from its most important co-factor. Due to this negative feedback pathway prothrombin/thrombin behaves as an "indirect" anticoagulant.

The prothrombin molecule consists of 3 functional domains: Gla, kringle, and catalytic. During its liver byosinthesis, prothrombin undergoes γ carboxylation (10 glutamic acid residues in proximity of its amino terminus). These γ carboxyglutamic residues, known as Gla domains and located on fragment 1 of the prothrombin molecule, are essential for the calcium dependency of phospholipid binding to prothrombin, necessary for the conversion of prothrombin to biologically active α-thrombin. Two kringle domains follow this region and are involved in pro(thrombin) binding to fibrin [6]. Tenase selectively hydrolyses 2 peptide bonds on the catalytic domain of the prothrombin molecule. Cleavage at Arg273–Thr274 results in the liberation of prothrombin fragment 1+2 (residues 1–273) and prothrombin 2 (residues 274–581); further cleavage at Arg322–Ile323 results in the formation of α-thrombin. The latter, one of the most potent enzymes known, not only converts fibrinogen to fibrin but acts upon factors V, VIII, XIII, protein C, platelets, and endothelial cells [9]. The schematic representation of the prothrombin molecule is shown in Figure 26.1.

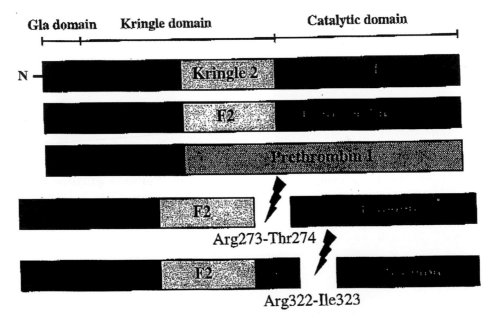

Figure 26.1. Schematic representation of the prothrombin molecule. Cleavage at Arg273–Thr274 results in the liberation of prothrombin fragment 1+2 (residues 1–273) and prethrombin 2 (residues 274–581); further cleavage at Arg322–Ile323 results in the formation of α-thrombin.

Antiprothrombin Antibodies

History

In 1959, Loeligler [5] was the first to describe the "LA co-factor phenomenon" when he described that the addition of normal plasma to that of a patient with LA increased the degree of coagulation inhibition. A low plasma level of prothrombin was also found; suggesting that the co-factor associated with this phenomenon was most likely to be prothrombin. Later, Rapaport et al [10] described the case of a child with LA who underwent recurrent bleeding episodes. Further investigation showed a severe prothrombin deficiency, a prolonged prothrombin time, and a prolonged activated partial thromboplastin time (aPTT). In 1983, Bajaj et al [11] were the first to provide evidence of the presence of non-neutralizing prothrombin-binding antibodies in 2 patients with LA and hypoprothrombinemia. These antibodies bound prothrombin without inhibiting its conversion to thrombin. The authors postulated that hypo-prothrombinemia resulted from the binding of antibodies to prothrombin and rapid clearance of these complexes from the circulation.

In 1984, Edson et al [12] demonstrated prothrombin–antiprothrombin complexes in the plasma of patients with LA but without severe hypo-prothrombinemia in prothrombin crossed immunoelectrophoresis experiments. These findings were later confirmed by Fleck et al [13], who found antiprothrombin antibodies in 72% of the LA-positive patients and showed that these antibodies had LA activity. In 1991, Bevers et al [14] highlighted the importance of antiprothrombin antibodies in causing LA activity. After incubation with cardiolipin containing liposomes, the LA activity remained in 11/16 patients with LA. These 11 samples demonstrated LA activity in a phospholipid-bound prothrombin dependent fashion. Subsequently, Oosting et al [15] showed that 4/22 LA inhibited endothelial cell mediated prothrombinase activity and the IgG fraction containing LA activity bound to phospholipid–prothrombin complex. In 1995, Arvieux et al [16] showed that antiprothrombin antibodies could be detected by a standard ELISA using prothrombin coated onto irradiated plates.

Immunological Characteristics

Antiprothrombin antibodies are commonly detected by ELISA using irradiated plates [16] or in complex with phosphatidylserine [17, 18]. The mode of presentation of prothrombin in solid phase seems to influence its recognition by antiprothrombin antibodies. In fact, antiprothrombin antibodies cannot bind when prothrombin is immobilized onto non-irradiated plates [16, 17], but does so if prothrombin is immobilized on a suitable anionic surface, adsorbed on γ-irradiated plates, or exposed to immobilized anionic phospholipids. An analogy between the behavior of these antibodies and anti–β_2-GPI has been suggested. Antiprothrombin antibodies might be directed against cryptic or neoepitopes (antigens) exposed when prothrombin binds to anionic phospholipids and/or may be low affinity antibodies binding bivalently to immobilized prothrombin. Wu et al [19] observed that human prothrombin undergoes a conformational change upon binding to phosphatidylserine containing surfaces in the presence of calcium. On the other hand, Galli et al [17] demonstrated that antiprothrombin antibodies could be of low affinity and suggested that prothrombin complexed with phosphatidylserine could allow clustering and better orientation of the antigen, offering optimal conditions for antibody recognition.

A high percentage of antiprothrombin antibodies have species specificity for the human protein [14], but a minority react with bovine prothrombin [20]. The epitope(s) recognized by these antibodies are being investigated. Rao et al [21] demonstrated binding of aPT to prethrombin 1 and fragment 1, as well as the whole prothrombin molecule, when using purified IgG preparations from LA-positive patients. One of these antibodies reacted with immobilized thrombin. Malia et al [22] also demonstrated binding of antiprothrombin antibodies to fragment 1+2. Recently, Akimoto et al [23] showed that 61.5% of aPT bound to fragment 1 and 38.4% to prethrombin (fragment 2 + α-thrombin). Overall, these data suggests that the dominant epitopes are likely to be located near the phospholipid binding site of the prothrombin molecule, although they may have a heterogeneous distribution.

It has been reported that most LA depend on the presence of phospholipid bound prothrombin, as well as phospholipid bound β_2-GPI, and the anticoagulant properties of aPT have been studied by several groups. Perpimkul et al [24] showed LA activity due to antiprothrombin antibodies in 9/10 samples from LA-positive patients. Galli et al [17] and Horbach et al [25] reported the existence of 2 types of circulating antiprothrombin antibodies which may be distinguished on the basis of their effect in coagulation assays: (1) functional, which cause LA activity, and (2) non-functional, which do not contribute to the LA activity, probably caused by a different epitope specificity of antiprothrombin antibodies [26]. Recently, a human monoclonal antiprothrombin antibody with LA activity has been raised and a semi-quantitative LA assay has been established in an attempt to help in the standardization of this test [27].

Clinical Significance

Prothrombin appears to be a common antigenic target of aPL [28]. However, its clinical significance is far from clear. Most of the studies available in the literature investigated the clinical significance of aPT detected by ELISA using prothrombin coated on irradiated plates and positive correlations with the clinical manifestations of the APS have been reported [29–31]. Little data are available on antibodies directed to phosphatidylserine–prothrombin complex (aPS-PT).

Antiprothrombin Antibodies and Thrombotic Events

Petri et al [29] reported that aPT have potential predictive value for thrombosis in a cohort of patients with systemic lupus erythematosus (SLE). Subsequent studies failed to show aPT as a risk factor for thromboembolic events, undoubtedly reflecting the heterogeneity and lack of appropriate standardization for the detection of these antibodies. Pengo et al [32] found no correlation between the presence of aPT and thrombosis in 22 APS patients with thrombosis. Galli et al [33] showed aPT in 58% of APS patients; however they found no correlation with thrombotic events. At variance, Puurunen et al [30], Horbach et al [25], and Muñoz-Rodriguez et al [34] reported a positive correlation between aPT and thrombosis in SLE. Puurunen et al [30] found a positive correlation between the presence of aPT and deep vein thrombosis (DVT) in a SLE population. Horbach et al [25] investigated the clinical significance of aPT in 175 patients with SLE and found that both IgG and IgM aPT were more frequent in patients with a history of venous thrombosis. We also reported a correlation between the presence of aPT and the occurrence of vascular events when we studied 207 patients with SLE [31]. These findings were expanded by Muñoz-Rodriguez et al [34], who found an association between the presence of aPT and thrombotic events in a cohort of 177 patients with various autoimmune diseases.

A recent systematic review of the literature [35] showed that no clear associations with thrombosis are found for antiprothrombin antibodies, irrespective of isotype, site, and type of event and the presence of SLE. This may be explained by different detection methods and by the presence of antibodies directed to different epitopes resulting in different functional properties [17, 25, 26].

Vaarala et al [36] showed a predictive value of 2.5-fold increase in the risk of myocardial infarction or cardiac death in middle-aged men with high levels of aPT. A nested case-control study estimated aPT to increase the thrombotic risk in men with DVT or pulmonary embolism [37]. Subsequent studies confirmed the association between aPT and venous thrombosis in patients with and without LA and/or aCL [38, 39]. Recently, Zanon et al [40] reported, after multivariate analysis, that aPT were likely risk factors for recurrent thromboembolism in their population of patients with acute venous thromboembolism.

There are only few papers on the significance of antiprothrombin antibodies when using the phosphatidylserine–prothrombin complex as antigen. In 1997, Galli et al [17] suggested that the prevalence of antiprothrombin antibodies increased from 58% when using prothrombin coated on irradiated plates (aPT) to 90% when prothrombin was coated with phosphatidylserine (aPS-PT). Funke et al [41] reported that aPS-PT conferred an odds ratio (OR) of 2.8 for venous thrombosis and of 4.1 for arterial thrombosis in patients with SLE. Atsumi et al [18] supported these data by showing that the presence of aPS-PT conferred an OR of 3.6 for APS in 265 Japanese patients with systemic autoimmune diseases.

Table 26.1. Antiprothrombin antibodies and thrombosis: data reported in the literature.*bl/TT*bg

Author	Study group	N	Correlation
Petri et al [29]	SLE	100	Yes
Vaarala et al [36]	Myocardial Infarction	106	Yes
Pengo et al [32]	aPL	22	No
Puurunen et al [30]	SLE	139	Yes (DVT)
Horbach et al [25]	SLE	175	Yes (venous)
Galli et al [17]	aPL	59	No
Swadzba et al [42]	SLE + LLD	127	No
Forastiero et al [38]	aPL	233	Yes (venous)
Palosuo et al [37]	DVT + PE	265	Yes
Bertolaccini et al [31]	SLE	207	Yes
Martinuzzo et al [43]	Pulmonary hypertension	54	No
Guerin et al [44]	Autoimmune diseases	265	No
Funke et al [41]	SLE	97	Yes
Sorice et al [45]	SLE	38	Yes (APS)
Lakos et al [46]	Autoimmune diseases	70	Yes
Muñoz-Rodriguez et al [34]	APS	177	Yes
Atsumi et al [18]	Autoimmune diseases	265	Yes
Galli et al [47]	aPL	72	No
Pasquier et al [48]	DVT	241	Yes
Nojima et al [49]	SLE	124	Yes
Previtali et al [50]	Thrombosis	79	No
Simmelink et al [51]	LA positive	46	Yes
Zanon et al [40]	VTE	236	Yes

N = number of patients; SLE = systemic lupus erythematosus; aPL = antiphospholipid antibodies; LLD = lupus-like disease; DVT = deep venous thrombosis; PE = pulmonary embolism; APS = antiphospholipid syndrome; LA = lupus anticoagulant; VTE = venous thromboembolism.

Table 26.1 summarizes data on clinical associations of antiprothrombin antibodies available in the literature.

Antiprothrombin Antibodies and Pregnancy Morbidity

Although several studies supported the association between antiprothrombin antibodies and thrombotic events, the association between these antibodies and pregnancy morbidity is controversial and not fully investigated.

Early reports showed no association between the presence of antiprothrombin antibodies and pregnancy morbidity, defined by 2 or more pregnancy losses before week 13 of pregnancy and/or 1 fetal death [52]. Donohoe et al [53] showed an association between IgM aPT and fetal loss. Akimoto et al [54] reported a specific association between aPT directed to prethrombin 1 and fragment 1 in pregnant women with severe pre-eclampsia and abortion. In a recent retrospective study by von Landenberg et al [55], IgG aPT showed a predictive value of 4.5-fold increased risk for early pregnancy loss in patients with APS, risk that was higher to that of aCL (3.4-fold).

Recently, Tsutsumi et al [56] failed to detect antiprothrombin antibodies by using the phosphatidylserine–prothrombin complex as antigen in 81 women with unexplained recurrent miscarriages, suggesting that testing for these antibodies does not seem to aid in the evaluation of patients with unexplained recurrent miscarriages.

Pathogenic Role of antiprothrombin antibodies

Despite uncertainities regarding the pathogenetic mechanism, there is increasing evidence suggesting that antiprothrombin antibodies play a role in the hypercoagulable state of the APS. The antigen (prothrombin) is not only a molecule involved in coagulation but also it is present in plasma or on cell surfaces that are exposed to plasma, therefore accessible to circulating antibodies. Some effects of antiprothrombin antibodies at the endothelial cell level have been proposed: (1) these antibodies inhibit thrombin mediated endothelial cell prostacyclin release and hamper protein C activation [57]; (2) antiprothrombin antibodies could recognize the prothrombin–phospholipid complex on endothelial cell surface, activating endothelial cell and inducing procoagulant substances [58]; or (3) they could increase the affinity of prothrombin for negatively charged phospholipids [21]. Thus, the prothrombin–antiprothrombin antibodies complex would compete with the binding of other coagulation factors for the available surface, resulting in a prolongation of clotting assays that can be neutralized by the addition of extra phospholipids. This in vitro phenomenon could be extrapolated to an in vivo scenario: membrane binding antibody–prothrombin complexes could decrease the concentration of prothrombin and/or phospholipid sites available for optimal assembly of the prothrombinase complex [59], leading to a hypercoagulable state and consequently to a thrombotic tendency.

The prothrombotic activity of antiprothrombin antibodies has been recently showed in animal models. Haj-Yahja et al [60] showed that immunization with β_2-GPI, prothrombin, or both results in the production of autoantibodies directed towards the immunizing agent. Although the prothrombin immunized group did not develop clinical and/or serological features of APS, thrombus induction was demonstrated when using an ex vivo model in which the aorta of mice immunized with prothrombin developed a visible thrombus after stasis (suture) for 1 minute, providing evidence for the prothrombotic effect of aPT.

The Value of IgA Isotype

There is still controversy as to whether patients with features of the APS, negative to IgG or IgM aPL, have IgA aPL and, if so, their clinical significance [61, 62]. This controversy is based on some experimental work that suggests that IgA aCL are as prothrombotic as the IgG or IgM isotypes [63]. Also, some data on IgA anti–β_2-GPI showed that this isotype is very frequent in SLE patients [64–66] and its presence has been associated with thrombosis [64, 65, 67] and pregnancy loss [68, 69]. We failed to demonstrate the presence of antiprothrombin antibodies (by using either the aPT and/or the aPS-PT system) of the IgA isotype in 134 SLE patients [70], data later confirmed by Atsumi et al [18] in the sera of 265 Japanese SLE patients. However, Matsuda et al [71] studied 60 SLE patients and described 1 patient with no aPL related clinical features but positivity not only for IgA aPS-PT but also for IgG and IgM aPS-PT, aCL, anti–β_2-GPI, and LA. Furthermore, von Landenberg et al [55] showed that IgA aPT was significantly associated with venous thrombosis in patients with APS. However, all patients from this study fulfilled Sapporo criteria for APS [72] (either aCL and/or LA positivity), and the possible additive risk given by the finding of IgA aPT was not analyzed. From these findings, we cannot rule out the existence of IgA aPT and/or aPS-PT in some lupus sera but we could suggest that IgA antiprothrombin antibodies might not be relevant for the recognition of the APS in SLE.

Conclusion

It has been demonstrated that the interaction between aPL and anionic phospholipids is mediated by plasma proteins, one of them identified as prothrombin. Antiprothrombin antibodies are frequently found in patients with aPL but the immunological characteristics and mechanisms of action are not completely understood. As thrombotic mechanisms are multifactorial and complex, further investigations are required to define the role of aPT in the pathogenesis of thrombosis. Knowledge of the behavior of specific aPL would aid in defining specific thrombogenic pathways and improved management of patients with APS. However, in order to accomplish this, standardization of the methods for the detection of these antibodies is mandatory.

References

1. Matsuura E, Igarashi Y, Yasuda T, Triplett DA, Koike T. Anticardiolipin antibodies recognize beta 2-glycoprotein I structure altered by interacting with an oxygen modified solid phase surface. J Exp Med 1994;179:457–462.
2. Roubey RA, Maldonado MA, Byrd SN. Comparison of an enzyme-linked immunosorbent assay for antibodies to beta 2-glycoprotein I and a conventional anticardiolipin immunoassay. Arthritis Rheum 1996;39:1606–1607.
3. McNally T, Mackie IJ, Machin SJ, Isenberg DA. Increased levels of beta 2 glycoprotein-I antigen and beta 2 glycoprotein-I binding antibodies are associated with a history of thromboembolic complications in patients with SLE and primary antiphospholipid syndrome. Br J Rheumatol 1995;34:1031–1036.
4. Amengual O, Atsumi T, Khamashta MA, Koike T, Hughes GRV. Specificity of ELISA for antibody to beta 2-glycoprotein I in patients with antiphospholipid syndrome. Br J Rheumatol 1996;35:1239–1243.

5. Loeliger A. Prothrombin as a co-factor of the circulating anticoagulant in systemic lupus erythematosus? Thromb Diath Haemorrh 1959;3:237–256.
6. Degen SJ, Davie EW. Nucleotide sequence of the gene for human prothrombin. Biochemistry 1987;26:6165–6177.
7. Chow BKC, Ting V, Tufaro F, MacGillivray RTA. Characterization of a novel liver-specific enhancer in the human prothrombin gene. J Biol Chem 1991;266:18927–18933.
8. Mann KG, Nesheim ME, Church WR, Haley P, Krishnaswamy S. Surface-dependent reactions of the vitamin K-dependent enzyme complexes. Blood 1990;76:1–16.
9. Pelzer H, Schwarz A, Stuber W. Determination of human prothrombin activation fragment 1 + 2 in plasma with an antibody against a synthetic peptide. Thromb Haemost 1991;65:153–159.
10. Rapaport SI, Ames SB, Duvall BJ. A plasma coagulation defect in systemic lupus erythematosus arising from hypoprothrombinemia combined with antiprothrombinase activity. Blood 1960;15:212–227.
11. Bajaj SP, Rapaport SI, Fierer DS, Herbst KD, Schwartz DB. A mechanism for the hypoprothrombinemia of the acquired hypoprothrombinemia-lupus anticoagulant syndrome. Blood 1983;61:684–692.
12. Edson JR, Vogt JM, Hasegawa DK. Abnormal prothrombin crossed-immunoelectrophoresis in patients with lupus inhibitors. Blood 1984;64:807–816.
13. Fleck RA, Rapaport SI, Rao LV. Anti-prothrombin antibodies and the lupus anticoagulant. Blood 1988;72:512–519.
14. Bevers EM, Galli M, Barbui T, Comfurius P, Zwaal RF. Lupus anticoagulant IgG's (LA) are not directed to phospholipids only, but to a complex of lipid-bound human prothrombin. Thromb Haemost 1991;66:629–632.
15. Oosting JD, Derksen RH, Bobbink IW, Hackeng TM, Bouma BN, de Groot PG. Antiphospholipid antibodies directed against a combination of phospholipids with prothrombin, protein C, or protein S: an explanation for their pathogenic mechanism? Blood 1993;81:2618–2625.
16. Arvieux J, Darnige L, Caron C, Reber G, Bensa JC, Colomb MG. Development of an ELISA for autoantibodies to prothrombin showing their prevalence in patients with lupus anticoagulants. Thromb Haemost 1995;74:1120–1125.
17. Galli M, Beretta G, Daldossi M, Bevers EM, Barbui T. Different anticoagulant and immunological properties of anti-prothrombin antibodies in patients with antiphospholipid antibodies. Thromb Haemost 1997;77:486–491.
18. Atsumi T, Ieko M, Bertolaccini ML, et al. Association of autoantibodies against the phosphatidylserine-prothrombin complex with manifestations of the antiphospholipid syndrome and with the presence of lupus anticoagulant. Arthritis Rheum 2000;43:1982–1993.
19. Wu JR, Lentz BR. Phospholipid-specific conformational changes in human prothrombin upon binding to procoagulant acidic lipid membranes. Thromb Haemost 1994;71:596–604.
20. Rao LV, Hoang AD, Rapaport SI. Differences in the interactions of lupus anticoagulant IgG with human prothrombin and bovine prothrombin. Thromb Haemost 1995;73:668–674.
21. Rao LVM, Hoang AD, Rapaport SI. Mechanisms and affects of the binding of lupus anticoagulant IgG and prothrombin to surface phospholipids. Blood 1996;88:4173–4182.
22. Malia RG, Brooksfield C, Bulman L, Greaves M. Prothrombin fragment 1-2: the epitope for antiphospholipid antibody expression [abstract]. Thromb Haemost 1997;171:689.
23. Akimoto T, Akama T, Kono I, Sumida T. Relationship between clinical features and binding domains of anti-prothrombin autoantibodies in patients with systemic lupus erythematosus and antiphospholipid syndrome. Lupus 1999;8:761–766.
24. Permpikul P, Rao LV, Rapaport SI. Functional and binding studies of the roles of prothrombin and beta 2-glycoprotein I in the expression of lupus anticoagulant activity. Blood 1994;83:2878–2792.
25. Horbach DA, van Oort E, Donders RC, Derksen RH, de Groot PG. Lupus anticoagulant is the strongest risk factor for both venous and arterial thrombosis in patients with systemic lupus erythematosus. Comparison between different assays for the detection of antiphospholipid antibodies. Thromb Haemost 1996;76:916–924.
26. Horbach DA, van Oort E, Derksen RH, de Groot PG. The contribution of anti-prothrombin-antibodies to lupus anticoagulant activity – discrimination between functional and non-functional antiprothrombin-antibodies. Thromb Haemost 1998;79:790–795.
27. Atsumi T, Ieko M, Ichikawa K, Horita T, Amasaki Y, Koike T. Semi-quantitative anticoagulant test using phosphatidylserine dependent monoclonal antiprothrombin antibody [abstract]. Lupus 2001;10:S9.
28. Galli M, Barbui T. Antiprothrombin antibodies: detection and clinical significance in the antiphospholipid syndrome. Blood 1999;93:2149–2157.
29. Petri M, Miller J, Goldman D, Ebert R. Anti-plasma protein antibodies are predictive of thrombotic events [abstract]. Arthritis Rheum 1994;37:S281.

30. Puurunen M, Vaarala O, Julkunen H, Aho K, Palosuo T. Antibodies to phospholipid-binding plasma proteins and occurrence of thrombosis in patients with systemic lupus erythematosus. Clin Immunol Immunopathol 1996;80:16–22.
31. Bertolaccini ML, Atsumi T, Khamashta MA, Amengual O, Hughes GR. Autoantibodies to human prothrombin and clinical manifestations in 207 patients with systemic lupus erythematosus. J Rheumatol 1998;25:1104–1108.
32. Pengo V, Biasolo A, Brocco T, Tonetto S, Ruffatti A. Autoantibodies to phospholipid-binding plasma proteins in patients with thrombosis and phospholipid reactive antibodies. Thromb Haemost 1996;75:721–724.
33. Galli M. Non beta 2-glycoprotein I cofactors for antiphospholipid antibodies. Lupus 1996;5:388–392.
34. Munoz-Rodriguez FJ, Reverter JC, Font J, et al. Prevalence and clinical significance of antiprothrombin antibodies in patients with systemic lupus erythematosus or with primary antiphospholipid syndrome. Haematologica 2000;85:632–637.
35. Galli M, Luciani D, Bertolini G, Barbui T. Anti-beta 2-glycoprotein I, antiprothrombin antibodies, and the risk of thrombosis in the antiphospholipid syndrome. Blood 2003;102:2717–2723.
36. Vaarala O, Puurunen M, Manttari M, Manninen V, Aho K, Palosuo T. Antibodies to prothrombin imply a risk of myocardial infarction in middle-aged men. Thromb Haemost 1996;75:456–459.
37. Palosuo T, Virtamo J, Haukka J, et al. High antibody levels to prothrombin imply a risk of deep venous thrombosis and pulmonary embolism in middle-aged men – a nested case-control study. Thromb Haemost 1997;78:1178–1182.
38. Forastiero RR, Martinuzzo ME, Cerrato GS, Kordich LC, Carreras LO. Relationship of anti beta2-glycoprotein I and anti prothrombin antibodies to thrombosis and pregnancy loss in patients with antiphospholipid antibodies. Thromb Haemost 1997;78:1008–1014.
39. Forastiero R, Martinuzzo M, Adamczuk Y, Carreras LO. Occurrence of anti-prothrombin and anti-beta2-glycoprotein I antibodies in patients with history of thrombosis. J Lab Clin Med 1999;134:610–615.
40. Zanon E, Saggiorato G, Ramon R, Girolami A, Pagnan A, Prandoni P. Anti-prothrombin antibodies as a potential risk factor of recurrent venous thromboembolism. Thromb Haemost 2004;91:255–258.
41. Funke A, Bertolaccini ML, Atsumi T, Amengual O, Khamashta MA, Hughes GRV. Autoantibodies to prothrombin-phosphatidylserine complex: clinical significance in systemic lupus erythematosus [abstract]. Arthritis Rheum 1998;41:S240.
42. Swadzba J, De Clerck LS, Stevens WJ, et al. Anticardiolipin, anti-beta(2)-glycoprotein I, antiprothrombin antibodies, and lupus anticoagulant in patients with systemic lupus erythematosus with a history of thrombosis. J Rheumatol 1997;24:1710–1715.
43. Martinuzzo ME, Pombo G, Forastiero RR, Cerrato GS, Colorio CC, Carreras LO. Lupus anticoagulant, high levels of anticardiolipin, and anti-beta2-glycoprotein I antibodies are associated with chronic thromboembolic pulmonary hypertension. J Rheumatol 1998;25:1313–1319.
44. Guerin J, Smith O, White B, Sweetman G, Feighery C, Jackson J. Antibodies to prothrombin in antiphospholipid syndrome and inflammatory disorders. Br J Haematol 1998;102:896–902.
45. Sorice M, Pittoni V, Circella A, et al. Anti-prothrombin but not "pure" anti-cardiolipin antibodies are associated with the clinical features of the antiphospholipid antibody syndrome. Thromb Haemost 1998;80:713–715.
46. Lakos G, Kiss E, Regeczy N, et al. Antiprothrombin and antiannexin V antibodies imply risk of thrombosis in patients with systemic autoimmune diseases. J Rheumatol 2000;27:924–929.
47. Galli M, Dlott J, Norbis F, et al. Lupus anticoagulants and thrombosis: clinical association of different coagulation and immunologic tests. Thromb Haemost 2000;84:1012–1026.
48. Pasquier E, Amiral J, de Saint Martin L, Mottier D. A cross sectional study of antiphospholipid-protein antibodies in patients with venous thromboembolism. Thromb Haemost 2001;86:538–542.
49. Nojima J, Kuratsune H, Suehisa E, et al. Anti-prothrombin antibodies combined with lupus anticoagulant activity is an essential risk factor for venous thromboembolism in patients with systemic lupus erythematosus. Br J Haematol 2001;114:647–654.
50. Previtali S, Barbui T, Galli M. Anti-beta2-glycoprotein I and anti-prothrombin antibodies in antiphospholipid-negative patients with thrombosis: a case control study. Thromb Haemost 2002;88:729–732.
51. Simmelink MJ, De Groot PG, Derksen RH. A study on associations between antiprothrombin antibodies, antiplasminogen antibodies and thrombosis. J Thromb Haemost 2003;1:735–739.
52. Falcon CR, Martinuzzo ME, Forastiero RR, Cerrato GS, Carreras LO. Pregnancy loss and autoantibodies against phospholipid-binding proteins. Obstet Gynecol 1997;89:975–980.
53. Donohoe S, Mackie IJ, Isenberg D, Machin SJ. Anti-prothrombin antibodies: assay conditions and clinical associations in the anti-phospholipid syndrome. Br J Haematol 2001;113:544–549.

54. Akimoto T, Akama T, Saitoh M, Kono I, Sumida T. Antiprothrombin autoantibodies in severe preeclampsia and abortion. Am J Med 2001;110:188–191.
55. von Landenberg P, Matthias T, Zaech J, et al. Antiprothrombin antibodies are associated with pregnancy loss in patients with the antiphospholipid syndrome. Am J Reprod Immunol 2003;49:51–56.
56. Tsutsumi A, Atsumi T, Yamada H, et al. Anti-phosphatidylserine/prothrombin antibodies are not frequently found in patients with unexplained recurrent miscarriages. Am J Reprod Immunol 2001;46:242–244.
57. Roubey RA. Autoantibodies to phospholipid-binding plasma proteins: a new view of lupus anticoagulants and other antiphospholipid autoantibodies. Blood 1994;84:2854–2867.
58. Arnout J. The pathogenesis of the antiphospholipid syndrome: a hypothesis based on parallelisms with heparin-induced thrombocytopenia. Thromb Haemost 1996;75:536–541.
59. Roubey RA. Immunology of the antiphospholipid antibody syndrome. Arthritis Rheum 1996;39:1444–1454.
60. Haj-Yahja S, Sherer Y, Blank M, Shoenfeld Y. Anti-prothrombin antibodies cause thrombosis in a novel qualitative ex-vivo animal model. Lupus 2003;12:364–369.
61. Gharavi AE, Harris EN, Asherson RA, Hughes GR. Anticardiolipin antibodies: isotype distribution and phospholipid specificity. Ann Rheum Dis 1987;46:1–6.
62. Lopez LR, Santos ME, Espinoza LR, La Rosa FG. Clinical significance of immunoglobulin A versus immunoglobulins G and M anti-cardiolipin antibodies in patients with systemic lupus erythematosus. Correlation with thrombosis, thrombocytopenia, and recurrent abortion. Am J Clin Pathol 1992;98:449–454.
63. Pierangeli SS, Liu XW, Barker JH, Anderson G, Harris EN. Induction of thrombosis in a mouse model by IgG, IgM and IgA immunoglobulins from patients with the antiphospholipid syndrome. Thromb Haemost 1995;74:1361–1367.
64. Fanopoulos D, Teodorescu MR, Varga J, Teodorescu M. High frequency of abnormal levels of IgA anti-beta2-glycoprotein I antibodies in patients with systemic lupus erythematosus: relationship with antiphospholipid syndrome. J Rheumatol 1998;25:675–680.
65. Tsutsumi A, Matsuura E, Ichikawa K, Fujisaku A, Mukai M, Koike T. IgA class anti-beta2-glycoprotein I in patients with systemic lupus erythematosus. J Rheumatol 1998;25:74–78.
66. Cucurull E, Gharavi AE, Diri E, Mendez E, Kapoor D, Espinoza LR. IgA anticardiolipin and anti-beta2-glycoprotein I are the most prevalent isotypes in African American patients with systemic lupus erythematosus. Am J Med Sci 1999;318:55–60.
67. Abinader A, Hanly AJ, Lozada CJ. Catastrophic antiphospholipid syndrome associated with anti-beta-2-glycoprotein I IgA. Rheumatology 1999;38:84–85.
68. Yamada H, Tsutsumi A, Ichikawa K, Kato EH, Koike T, Fujimoto S. IgA-class anti-beta2-glycoprotein I in women with unexplained recurrent spontaneous abortion. Arthritis Rheum 1999;42:2727–2728.
69. Lee RM, Branch DW, Oshiro BT, Rittenhouse L, Orcutt A, Silver RM. IgA β2 Glycoprotein-I antibodies are elevated in women with unexplained recurrent spontaneous abortion and unexplained fetal death [abstract]. J Autoimmun 2000;15:A63.
70. Bertolaccini ML, Atsumi T, Escudero-Contreras A, Khamashta MA, Hughes GRV. The value of IgA antiphospholipid testing for the diagnosis of antiphospholipid (Hughes) syndrome in systemic lupus erythematosus. J Rheumatol 2001;28:2637–2643.
71. Matsuda J, Sanaka T, Yoshida M, Gotoh M, Gohchi K. Existence of IgA-antiprothrombin antibody in a patient with systemic lupus erythematosus. Eur J Haematol 2002;69:126–127.
72. Wilson WA, Gharavi AE, Koike T, et al. International consensus statement on preliminary classification criteria for definite antiphospholipid syndrome: report of an international workshop. Arthritis Rheum 1999;42:1309–1311.

27 Antiphospholipid Syndrome in the Absence of Standard Antiphospholipid Antibodies: Associations with Other Autoantibodies

Robert A. S. Roubey

Introduction

Although the presence of antiphospholipid antibodies (aPL) is, by definition, a sine qua non of antiphospholipid syndrome (APS), the spectrum of autoantibodies associated with APS is likely to extend beyond standard anticardiolipin and lupus anticoagulant assays. These include autoantibodies to phospholipid-binding proteins, such as β_2-glycoprotein I (β_2-GPI) and prothrombin, as well as antibodies detected in immunoassays using phospholipids other than cardiolipin. These antibodies are present in some patients with clinical manifestations of APS, that is, thrombosis, pregnancy loss, who have negative tests for anticardiolipin antibodies (aCL) and lupus anticoagulant (LA). At the present time such patients would not be classified as having definite APS by international criteria [1], but fall within a broader concept of APS or APS-like conditions. If these other autoantibodies are shown to be associated with the same risks of thrombosis, pregnancy loss, etc., as conventional aPL as research proceeds, then it is likely that consensus serological classification criteria for APS will expand.

This broader serologic view of APS highlights the unusual relationship of conventional aPL tests to the syndrome. APS is currently defined as the association of certain clinical events, for example, thrombosis or recurrent fetal loss, with a persistently positive aCL or LA test. Positivity in an aPL test is, therefore, an essential element of the syndrome, rather than a diagnostic test for the syndrome. There is no independent gold standard for APS by which one can assess the diagnostic sensitivity or specificity of aPL tests. Positive aPL assays are probably best thought of as risk factors for the clinical manifestations of APS. A highly positive aPL assay should not be considered a false positive if the patient does not have a history of thrombosis or another clinical feature of APS. Further, there are no established exclusion criteria for APS. A patient with thrombosis and a positive aPL test would be considered to have APS whether or not other important risk factors for thrombosis were present. In fact, other factors may be critical in determining which individuals with aPL will have a thrombotic event or miscarriage.

Autoantibodies Associated with APS

In considering "aPL-negative" APS, it should be keep in mind that conventional aCL ELISAs and LA assays were developed based on an inaccurate or incomplete understanding of the specificities of the antibodies detected in these tests. Elucidation of these specificities and the discovery of additional autoantibodies associated with thrombosis and/or fetal loss are a work in progress.

Antibodies Detected in Conventional aPL Assays

Before discussing APS-associated antibodies that may not be detected in conventional aPL assays, it is necessary to understand the antibodies that are detected in these tests. The specificities of aPL are reviewed in detail elsewhere in this volume. Briefly, in APS patient sera, the large majority of antibodies detected in aCL ELISAs recognize β_2-GPI, not cardiolipin. β_2-GPI in these assays derives from bovine serum, a common component of the blocking buffer/sample diluent. Antibodies directed against cardiolipin may also be detected in aCL assays, but do not appear to be associated with the clinical manifestations of APS. LA activity in most APS patient plasmas is due to autoantibodies directed against β_2-GPI and/or autoantibodies to prothrombin. Although LA activity is commonly thought of as an intrinsic property of certain antibodies, differences in the various assays used to detect LA may be critically important in determining whether a patient sample will exhibit LA in a particular assay. For example, the LA activity of certain anti–β_2-GPI monoclonal antibodies derived from APS patients was found to be dependent on the concentration of β_2-GPI in the LA assay [2]. Certain antibodies may be detected in one type of LA assay but not another. Galli and colleagues found that the dilute Russell viper venom time was more sensitive to prolongation by anti–β_2-GPI antibodies, whereas the kaolin clotting time was more sensitive to prolongation by anti-prothrombin antibodies [3].

Antibodies Detected in Immunoassays Using Other Anionic Phospholipids

Early in the development of aCL immunoassays, it was observed that most APS-associated "anticardiolipin" antibodies appeared to be broadly cross-reactive with other anionic phospholipids, for example, phosphatidylserine, phosphatidylinositol, phosphatidic acid, and phosphatidylglycerol. With the discovery that bovine β_2-GPI was the key antigen in aCL ELISAs, this apparent cross-reactivity is currently best understood in terms of β_2-GPI binding similarly to the various anionic phospholipids. Bovine serum is commonly used in the assays with other anionic phospholipids and β_2-GPI binds reasonably well to micro-titer plates coated with any negatively charged phospholipid [4]. Accordingly, most anti–β_2-GPI antibodies can be detected in any of the anionic phospholipids ELISAs. The generally good correlation among ELISAs using different anionic phospholipids has led many investigators to conclude that the aCL assay, along with LA testing, are adequate for evaluation of APS. Routine testing of patient samples against panels of other anionic phospholipids is expensive and usually provides little additional clinical information [5–8].

Although most aCL-positive APS patient sera react in assays using other anionic phospholipids, aCL-positive sera from patients with infectious diseases, such as syphilis, do not [9]. These infection-associated antibodies are specific for cardiolipin and do not recognize phosphatidylserine, other anionic phospholipids, or β_2-GPI [10]. In light of this observation, it may be argued that ELISAs using phosphatidylserine or one of the other anionic phospholipids would be preferable to the aCL ELISA in evaluating patient for APS [11]. The justification for the routine use of the aCL ELISA is largely due to the nearly 20 years of clinical experience with this assay. Additionally, several international standardization workshops have served to improve the performance and inter-laboratory reproducibility of aCL ELISAs [12–14]. Similar standardization efforts have not been applied to assays using anionic phospholipids other than cardiolipin.

There are a number of reports in which sera from patients with clinical features of APS are negative in aCL ELISAs, but positive in 1 or more assays utilizing other anionic phospholipids. The molecular basis for this pattern of reactivity and the antigenic specificities of the "non-anticardiolipin" antibodies detected in theses assays are both unclear. When sera are screened for IgG, IgM, and IgA antibodies to a broad panel of different phospholipids, low level reactivity in a single assay may be due to random error, given the large number of individual tests being performed.

Like aCL ELISAs, bovine serum is typically present in assays using other phospholipids. It is not known whether antibodies detected in antiphosphatidylserine, antiphosphatidylinositol, or similar assays are directly binding to phospholipids or to a phospholipid-binding component of bovine or human serum. Detailed studies using highly purified antibodies and antigens, similar to the experiments demonstrating the role of β_2-GPI in the aCL assay, have not been performed. Limited studies using patient sera suggest that at least some antibodies detected in the presence of other phospholipids depend upon the presence of β_2-GPI [15–17]. Why such antibodies would not be detectable in standard aCL assays is not known. The antibodies might be specific for conformational determinants on β_2-GPI that are dependent upon the type of phospholipid. Other factors to be considered include differential clustering patterns of β_2-GPI on different phospholipids, and differences in phospholipid fatty acid composition and/or oxidation status, which could influence how β_2-GPI binds to the phospholipid-coated plate.

In the absence of a positive aCL or LA test, an association between positivity in 1 or more ELISAs utilizing phosphatidylserine, phosphatidylinositol, phosphatidylglycerol, or phosphatidic acid, and the clinical manifestations of APS is not well established [5, 6]. Toschi and colleagues observed that reactivity in non-cardiolipin anionic phospholipid assays was associated with thrombosis and stroke [17, 18]. Interestingly, antibody binding in these assays was β_2-GPI dependent. The largest studies evaluating panels of non-cardiolipin anionic phospholipids have been conducted with obstetrical patients. Yetman and Kutteh found that 10% of women with recurrent pregnancy loss were negative in the aCL assay but tested positive in another phospholipid assay, including both anionic phospholipids and phosphatidylethanolamine (see below) [19]. Aoki et al compared a (β_2-GPI–dependent) aCL ELISA with a panel of phospholipid assays in a large group of women with reproductive failure [20]. The aCL assay was more frequently positive in patients than controls, whereas no difference between patients and controls was observed with any of the other assays alone. Positivity in more than one other assay was more frequent among patients, however, most of these patients were also positive in the aCL assay.

The performance of ELISAs using anionic phospholipids other than cardiolipin is difficult to assess. As noted above, in general, these assays have not been subjected to rigorous inter-laboratory evaluation or national/international standardization efforts. Monospecific reference material for each aPL assay are not widely available. Therefore, it is difficult to make a valid clinical decision based on an isolated positive result in one of these assays.

Antibodies Detected in Immunoassays Using Phosphatidylethanolamine

Phosphatidylethanolamine is a zwitterionic phospholipid normally present in the outer leaflet of cell membranes. It has been shown to play an important role in phospholipid-dependent reactions of the protein C pathway [21]. Anti-phosphatidylethanolamine antibodies may be the only autoantibodies detectable in a small number of patients with clinical features of APS [22–28]. Careful studies of the specificity of anti-phosphatidylethanolamine antibodies demonstrate that they do not bind to phosphatidylethanolamine itself but to a complex of phosphatidylethanolamine and certain proteins present in bovine serum, that is, high- and low-molecular-weight kininogens (HMWK, LMWK) and/or factor XI and prekallikrein, proteins that bind to HMWK [29–32]. β_2-GPI is not involved. These antibodies may exert a thrombogenic effect by enhancing thrombin-induced platelet aggregation [31, 33].

To date, no large studies have demonstrated the clinical utility of the anti-phosphatidylethanolamine ELISA. However, the case reports and antibody studies cited above support further study and efforts toward standardization. On a research basis it is reasonable to consider anti-phosphatidylethanolamine testing in evaluating patients suspected of having APS, but who are negative in the standard aPL assays.

Species-Specific Autoantibodies to Human β_2-GPI

A large body of data indicate that autoantibodies to β_2-GPI are among the most important antibodies associated with APS. Conventional aCL ELISAs and LA assays detect many anti–β_2-GPI antibodies, but have some limitations. An important limitation of standard aCL ELISAs is the species of β_2-GPI. As previously mentioned, the predominant species of β_2-GPI in aCL assay is bovine. Whereas anti–β_2-GPI antibodies from most APS patients recognize β_2-GPI from many species, some recognize only the human protein. Although a small amount of human β_2-GPI is present in aCL assays (from the diluted serum sample being tested), aCL assays may miss these antibodies [34, 35]. Species specificity seems to be occur more frequently among IgM anti–β_2-GPI antibodies than IgG anti–β_2-GPI antibodies. This issue is directly addressed in anti–β_2-GPI ELISAs in which the human protein is the antigen. Several groups have reported on the presence of APS clinical manifestations in patients who are positive in the anti–β_2-GPI assay but negative in aCL and/or LA assays [36–40].

Although the anti–β_2-GPI ELISA is not yet part of the serological criteria for the classification of definite APS or considered as a first-line laboratory test, for clinical purposes most experienced physicians would consider a patient with anti–β_2-GPI antibodies and clinical features of APS to have the syndrome. At present, suspicion of APS in the setting of a negative aCL assay is a reasonable indication for anti–β_2-GPI testing. Interlaboratory evaluation and standardization efforts for the anti–β_2-GPI ELISA are needed and will likely enhance the value of this test in the future.

Autoantibodies to Prothrombin

Autoantibodies directed against prothrombin represent a large proportion of LA antibodies in patients with APS [41–43]. Immunoassays for the detection of anti-prothrombin have recently been developed [43–47]. There are significant methodological differences among the anti-prothrombin ELISAs that have been reported and optimal assay conditions have not been established [48, 49]. Overall, the various anti-prothrombin assays demonstrate that, in certain patients, anti-prothrombin antibodies may be present in the absence of a positive LA assay. This may be due to one or more factors including: (1) use of a LA assay that is relatively insensitive to the effects of anti-prothrombin antibodies; (2) greater analytical sensitivity of immunoassays as compared to coagulation assays (immunoassays may detect lower concentrations of antibody than coagulation reactions); and/or (3) an intrinsic characteristic of certain anti-prothrombin antibodies, for example, fine specificity, that may be responsible for LA activity. The small number of studies to date suggest that LA positivity is more closely associated with thrombosis and fetal loss than a positive anti-prothrombin ELISA [44, 46, 50]. Larger studies and optimization/standardization of anti-prothrombin ELISAs are needed to evaluate the association of anti-prothrombin antibodies with clinical features of APS and determine whether detection of these antibodies in ELISA constitutes a valid basis for aPL-negative APS.

Autoantibodies to Components of the Protein C Pathway

Inhibition of the anticoagulant protein C pathway has long been considered as a possible mechanism predisposing to thrombosis in patients with APS. Recent data suggest that autoantibodies directed against components of this pathway, protein C, protein S, and thrombomodulin, may be associated with clinical features of APS [51–53]. Such antibodies are probably not detectable in standard aCL and LA tests. Additionally, autoantibodies to C4b-binding protein, a complement control protein that regulates free protein S levels and has structural similarity to β_2-GPI, have been reported [54, 55].

Other Autoantibodies

Limited data suggest the possible association of a number of other autoantibodies with thrombosis and fetal loss. These include autoantibodies to tissue factor pathway inhibitor [56], annexin V [57, 58], factor XII [59, 60], vascular heparin sulfate proteoglycan [61], and complement factor H [54]. If the clinical associations are borne out by further study, such antibodies may eventually be included in an expanded serological definition of APS.

Summary

Certain autoantibodies not detected in standard aCL and LA assays may be associated with clinical manifestations of APS. These antibodies are not included in the current serological criteria for the classification of definite APS, although these criteria are likely to be expanded in the future. Autoantibodies to β_2-GPI and prothrombin, detected in protein-based ELISAs, are likely candidates for consideration. At the present time antibodies detected in ELISAs using anionic phospholipids other than cardiolipin are of possible interest, however, evidence for the clinical utility of such assays is weak. Future studies elucidating the specificity of these antibodies and inter-laboratory efforts toward assay standardization are needed. Antibodies detected in anti-phosphatidylethanolamine assays may be associated with clinical features of APS and may directly contribute to a prothrombotic state.

In conclusion, certain patients with clinical features of APS may have 1 or more of the autoantibodies discussed above, in the absence of aCL or LA. While these patients do not meet current classification criteria for definite APS, conceptually they may be included in a broader clinical view of autoantibody-mediated thrombosis and pregnancy loss.

References

1. Wilson WA, Gharavi AE, Koike T, et al. International consensus statement on preliminary classification criteria for definite antiphospholipid syndrome: report of an international workshop [review]. Arthritis Rheum 1999;42:1309–1311.
2. Takeya H, Mori T, Gabazza EC, et al. Anti-β2-glycoprotein I (β2GPI) monoclonal antibodies with lupus anticoagulant-like activity enhance the β2GPI binding to phospholipids. J Clin Invest 1997;99:2260–2268.
3. Galli M, Finazzi G, Bevers EM, Barbui T. Kaolin clotting time and dilute Russell's viper venom time distinguish between prothrombin-dependent and β_2-glycoprotein I-dependent antiphospholipid antibodies. Blood 1995;86:617–623.
4. Jones JV, James H, Mansour M, Eastwood BJ. β_2-Glycoprotein I is a cofactor for antibodies reacting with 5 anionic phospholipids. J Rheumatol 1995;22:2009.
5. Bertolaccini ML, Roch B, Amengual O, Atsumi T, Khamashta MA, Hughes GR. Multiple antiphospholipid tests do not increase the diagnostic yield in antiphospholipid syndrome. Br J Rheumatol 1998;37:1229–1232.
6. Branch DW, Silver R, Pierangeli S, Harris EN. Antiphospholipid antibodies other than lupus anticoagulant and anticardiolipin antibodies in women with recurrent pregnancy loss, fertile controls, and antiphospholipid syndrome. Obstet Gynecol 1997;89:549–555.
7. Amoroso A, Mitterhofer AP, Del Porto F, et al. Antibodies to anionic phospholipids and anti-beta2-GPI: association with thrombosis and thrombocytopenia in systemic lupus erythematosus. Hum Immunol 2003;64:265–273.
8. Fialova L, Mikulikova L, Matous-Malbohan I, Benesova O, Zwinger A. Prevalence of various antiphospholipid antibodies in pregnant women. Physiol Res 2000;49:299–305.

9. Pierangeli SS, Goldsmith GH, Krnic S, Harris EN. Differences in functional activity of anticardiolipin antibodies from patients with syphilis and those with the antiphospholipid syndrome. Infect Immun 1994;62:4081–4084.
10. McNally T, Purdy G, Mackie IJ, Machin SJ, Isenberg DA. The use of an anti-β_2-glycoprotein-I assay for discrimination between anticardiolipin antibodies associated with infection and increased risk of thrombosis. Br J Haematol 1995;91:471–473.
11. Lopez LR, Dier KJ, Lopez D, Merrill JT, Fink CA. Anti-beta 2-glycoprotein I and antiphosphatidylserine antibodies are predictors of arterial thrombosis in patients with antiphospholipid syndrome. Am J Clin Pathol 2004;121:142–149.
12. Harris EN, Gharavi AE, Patel SP, Hughes GRV. Evaluation of the anti-cardiolipin test: report of an international workshop held 4 April 1986. Clin Exp Immunol 1987;68:215–222.
13. Harris EN. Special report. The Second International Anti-cardiolipin Standardization Workshop/the Kingston Anti-Phospholipid Antibody Study (KAPS) group. Am J Clin Pathol 1990;94:476–484.
14. Harris EN, Pierangeli S, Birch D. Anticardiolipin wet workshop report. Fifth international symposium on antiphospholipid antibodies. Am J Clin Pathol 1994;101:616–624.
15. Matsuda J, Saitoh N, Gotoh M, Gohchi K, Tsukamoto M. Prevalence of β_2-glycoprotein I antibody in systemic lupus erythematosus patients with β_2-glycoprotein I dependent antiphospholipid antibodies. Ann Rheum Dis 1995;54:73–75.
16. Matsuda J, Saitoh N, Gohchi K, Gotoh M, Tsukamoto M. Detection of beta-2-glycoprotein-I-dependent antiphospholipid antibodies and anti-beta-2-glycoprotein-I antibody in patients with systemic lupus erythematosus and in patients with syphilis. Int Arch Allergy Immunol 1994;103:239–244.
17. Toschi V, Motta A, Castelli C, Paracchini ML, Zerbi D, Gibelli A. High prevalence of antiphosphatidylinositol antibodies in young patients with cerebral ischemia of undetermined cause. Stroke 1998;29:1759–1764.
18. Toschi V, Motta A, Castelli C, et al. Prevalence and clinical significance of antiphospholipid antibodies to noncardiolipin antigens in systemic lupus erythematosus. Haemostasis 1993;23:275–283.
19. Yetman DL, Kutteh WH. Antiphospholipid antibody panels and recurrent pregnancy loss: prevalence of anticardiolipin antibodies compared with other antiphospholipid antibodies. Fertil Steril 1996;66:540–546.
20. Aoki K, Dudkiewicz AB, Matsuura E, Novotny M, Kaberlain G, Gleicher N. Clinical significance of β_2-glycoprotein I-dependent anticardiolipin antibodies in the reproductive autoimmune failure syndrome: correlation with conventional antiphospholipid antibody detection systems. Am J Obstet Gynecol 1995;172:926–931.
21. Smirnov MD, Esmon CT. Phosphatidylethanolamine incorporation into vesicles selectively enhances factor Va inactivation by activated protein C. J Biol Chem 1994;269:816–819.
22. Karmochkine M, Cacoub P, Piette JC, Godeau P, Boffa MC. Antiphosphatidylethanolamine antibody as the sole antiphospholipid antibody in systemic lupus erythematosus with thrombosis. Clin Exp Rheumatol 1992;10:603–605.
23. Karmochkine M, Berard M, Piette JC, et al. Antiphosphatidylethanolamine antibodies in systemic lupus erythematosus. Lupus 1993;2:157–160.
24. Berard M, Chantome R, Marcelli A, Boffa MC. Antiphosphatidylethanolamine antibodies as the only antiphospholipid antibodies. I. Association with thrombosis and vascular cutaneous diseases. J Rheumatol 1996;23:1369–1374.
25. Wagenknecht DR, Fastenau DR, Torry RJ, et al. Risk of early renal allograft failure is increased for patients with antiphospholipid antibodies. Transpl Int 2000;13(suppl 1):S78–S81.
26. Sanmarco M, Alessi MC, Harle JR, et al. Antibodies to phosphatidylethanolamine as the only antiphospholipid antibodies found in patients with unexplained thromboses. Thromb Haemost 2001;85:800–805.
27. Balada E, Ordi-Ros J, Paredes F, Villarreal J, Mauri M, Vilardell-Tarres M. Antiphosphatidylethanolamine antibodies contribute to the diagnosis of antiphospholipid syndrome in patients with systemic lupus erythematosus. Scand J Rheumatol 2001;30:235–241.
28. Sugi T, Matsubayashi H, Inomo A, Dan L, Makino T. Antiphosphatidylethanolamine antibodies in recurrent early pregnancy loss and mid-to-late pregnancy loss. J Obstet Gynaecol Res 2004;30:326–332.
29. Sugi T, McIntyre JA. Autoantibodies to phosphatidylethanolamine (PE) recognize a kininogen-PE complex. Blood 1995;86:3083–3089.
30. Boffa MC, Berard M, Sugi T, McIntyre JA. Antiphosphatidylethanolamine antibodies as the only antiphospholipid antibodies detected by ELISA. II. Kininogen reactivity. J Rheumatol 1996;23:1375–1379.

31. Sugi T, McIntyre JA. Phosphatidylethanolamine induces specific conformational changes in the kininogens recognizable by antiphosphatidylethanolamine antibodies. Thromb Haemost 1996;76:354–360.
32. Sugi T, McIntyre JA. Certain autoantibodies to phosphatidylethanolamine (aPE) recognize factor XI and prekallikrein independently or in addition to the kininogens. J Autoimmun 2001;17:207–214.
33. Sugi T, McIntyre JA. Autoantibodies to kininogen-phosphatidylethanolamine complexes augment thrombin-induced platelet aggregation. Thromb Res 1996;84:97–109.
34. Arvieux J, Darnige L, Hachulla E, Roussel B, Bensa JC, Colomb MG. Species specificity of anti-β_2-glycoprotein I autoantibodies and its relevance to anticardiolipin antibody quantitation. Thromb Haemost 1996;75:725–730.
35. Arvieux J, Regnault V, Hachulla E, Darnige L, Roussel B, Bensa JC. Heterogeneity and immunochemical properties of anti-β_2-glycoprotein I autoantibodies. Thromb Haemost 1999;80:393–398.
36. Roubey RAS, Maldonado MA, Byrd SN. Comparison of an enzyme-linked immunosorbent assay for antibodies to β_2-glycoprotein I and a conventional anticardiolipin ELISA. Arthritis Rheum 1996;39:1606–1607.
37. Cabiedes J, Cabral AR, Alarcón-Segovia D. Clinical manifestations of the antiphospholipid syndrome in patients with systemic lupus erythematosus associate more strongly with anti-β_2-glycoprotein-I than with antiphospholipid antibodies. J Rheumatol 1995;22:1899–1906.
38. Cabral AR, Cabiedes J, Alarcón-Segovia D. Antibodies to phospholipid-free β_2-glycoprotein-I in patients with the primary antiphospholipid syndrome. J Rheumatol 1995;22:1894–1898.
39. Balestrieri G, Tincani A, Spatola L, et al. Anti-beta$_2$-glycoprotein I antibodies: a marker of antiphospholipid syndrome? Lupus 1995;4:122–130.
40. Martinuzzo ME, Forastiero RR, Carreras LO. Anti-β_2-glycoprotein I antibodies: detection and association with thrombosis. Br J Haematol 1995;89:397–402.
41. Bevers EM, Galli M, Barbui T, Comfurius P, Zwaal RFA. Lupus anticoagulant IgG's (LA) are not directed to phospholipids only, but to a complex of lipid-bound human prothrombin. Thromb Haemost 1991;66:629–632.
42. Permpikul P, Rao LVM, Rapaport SI. Functional and binding studies of the roles of prothrombin and β_2-glycoprotein I in the expression of lupus anticoagulant activity. Blood 1994;83:2878–2892.
43. Arvieux J, Darnige L, Caron C, Reber G, Bensa JC, Colomb MG. Development of an ELISA for autoantibodies to prothrombin showing their prevalence in patients with lupus anticoagulants. Thromb Haemost 1995;74:1120–1125.
44. Forastiero RR, Martinuzzo ME, Cerrato GS, Kordich LC, Carreras LO. Relationship of anti β_2-glycoprotein I and anti prothrombin antibodies to thrombosis and pregnancy loss in patients with antiphospholipid antibodies. Thromb Haemost 1997;78:1008–1014.
45. Galli M, Beretta G, Daldossi M, Bevers EM, Barbui T. Different anticoagulant and immunological properties of anti-prothrombin antibodies in patients with antiphospholipid antibodies. Thromb Haemost 1997;77:486–491.
46. Horbach DA, van Oort E, Derksen RH, De Groot PG. The contribution of anti-prothrombin-antibodies to lupus anticoagulant activity – discrimination between functional and non-functional anti-prothrombin-antibodies. Thromb Haemost 1998;79:790–795.
47. Swadzba J, De Clerck LS, Stevens WJ, et al. Anticardiolipin, anti-β_2-glycoprotein I, antiprothrombin antibodies, and lupus anticoagulant in patients with systemic lupus erythematosus with a history of thrombosis. J Rheumatol 1997;24:1710–1715.
48. Jaekel HP, Trabandt A, Schmid D, et al. Autoantibodies to prothrombin and phosphatidylserine/prothrombin-complexes: do they contribute to the serodiagnosis of primary and secondary anti-phospholipid syndrome? Clin Lab 2004;50:295–304.
49. Amengual O, Atsumi T, Koike T. Antiprothombin antibodies and the diagnosis of antiphospholipid syndrome. Clin Immunol. In press.
50. Horbach DA, Oort EV, Donders RCJM, Derksen RHWM, De Groot PG. Lupus anticoagulant in the strongest risk factor for both venous and arterial thrombosis in patients with systemic lupus erythematosus: comparison between different assays for the detection of antiphospholipid antibodies. Thromb Haemost 1996;76:916–924.
51. Oosting JD, Derksen RHWM, Bobbink IWG, Hackeng TM, Bouma BN, De Groot PG. Antiphospholipid antibodies directed against a combination of phospholipids with prothrombin, protein C, or protein S: an explanation for their pathogenic mechanism? Blood 1993;81:2618–2625.
52. Pengo V, Biasiolo A, Brocco T, Tonetto S, Ruffatti A. Autoantibodies to phospholipid-binding plasma proteins in patients with thrombosis and phospholipid-reactive antibodies. Thromb Haemost 1996;75:721–724.

53. Carson CW, Comp PC, Esmon NL, Rezaie AR, Esmon CT. Thrombomodulin antibodies inhibit protein C activation and are found in patients with lupus anticoagulant and unexplained thrombosis. Arthritis Rheum 1994;37:S296.
54. Guerin J, Sim RB, Feighery C, Jackson J. Antibody recognition of complement regulatory proteins, factor H, CR1 and C4BP in antiphospholipid syndrome patients. Lupus 1998;7(suppl 2):S180.
55. Arvieux J, Pernod G, Regnault V, Darnige L, Garin J. Some anticardiolipin antibodies recognize a combination of phospholipids with thrombin-modified antithrombin, complement C4b-binding protein, and lipopolysaccharide binding protein. Blood 1999;93:4248–4255.
56. Forastiero RR, Martinuzzo ME, Broze GJ. High titers of autoantibodies to tissue factor pathway inhibitor are associated with the antiphospholipid syndrome. J Thromb Haemost 2003;1:718–724.
57. Matsuda J, Saitoh N, Gohchi K, Gotoh M, Tsukamoto M. Anti-annexin V antibody in systemic lupus erythematosus patients with lupus anticoagulant and/or anticardiolipin antibody. Am J Hematol 1994;47:56–58.
58. Arai T, Matsubayashi H, Sugi T, et al. Anti-annexin A5 antibodies in reproductive failures in relation to antiphospholipid antibodies and phosphatidylserine. Am J Reprod Immunol 2003;50:202–208.
59. Aberg H, Nilsson IM. Recurrent thrombosis in a young woman with a circulating anticoagulant directed against factors XI and XII. Acta Med Scand 1972;192:419–425.
60. Jones DW, Gallimore MJ, Harris SL, Winter M. Antibodies to factor XII associated with lupus anticoagulant. Thromb Haemost 1999;81:387–390.
61. Shibata S, Sasaki T, Harpel P, Fillit H. Autoantibodies to vascular heparan sulfate proteoglycan in systemic lupus erythematosus react with endothelial cells and inhibit the formation of thrombin-antithrombin III complexes. Clin Immunol Immunopathol 1994;70:114–123.

Section 3

Basic Aspects

28 Vascular Pathology of Antiphospholipid Antibody Syndrome

Gale A. McCarty

Introduction

Antiphospholipid antibody syndrome (APS) is now recognized as a systemic vasculopathy involving complex interactions between endothelial cells, platelets, and inflammation and coagulation cascades [1–3]. *Vasculopathy* is a term often equated with thrombotic microangiopathy (TMA) but unfortunately continues to be used or confused with vasculitis (where inflammatory cells are present throughout the vessel wall) or perivasculitis (where the infiltrate is adventitial but the vessel wall is intact) [4–14].

The identification of TMA is dependent on many factors: (a) time course from symptomaticity to biopsy, (b) action of naturally occurring anticoagulants, or (c) time course of institution of antithrombotic treatments. TMA may involve changes on the intra-luminal side, through the vessel wall, and into the adventitia. At the light microscopic level, this spectrum involves endothelial cell swelling, thrombosis that is usually bland, but occasionally associated with a reactive cellular infiltrate as part of neoangiogenesis (reactive angioendotheliomatosis). Varying degrees of recanalization, fibrin, and/or platelet deposition in the vessel wall, proliferation of myointimal cells with attendent luminal decrease, medial thickening, and hyalinization usually with preservation of the internal elastic lamina occur, but in some instances discrete vasculitis or perivasculitis is present [1–14].

Limited electron microscopic studies have in some vessels identified indistinct electron dense deposits in sub-endothelial areas that have not yet been fully characterized as representative of antiphospholipid (aPL) antibodies but have been identified as immunoglobulin [2, 4, 6–12]. Some of the confusion in the APS literature is attributable to (a) poor differentiation of perivasculitis versus panvasculitis, (b) misinterpretation of positive fluorescent antibody (FA) studies for immunoglobulins and complement components as definitive of an immune complex vasculitis, when complement and markers of endothelial cell activation have new effector functions [1, 3, 9], (c) occurrence of co-existing vasculitis in secondary APS, most often in systemic lupus erythematosus (SLE), and (d) anatomic differences between arteries and veins versus capillaries, with their lack of limiting vascular smooth muscle cells and attendant inflammatory cell extravasation or spillage beyond capillary network without identifiable capillary necrosis (capillaritis) [4, 6–8, 12].

The major incremental knowledge over the last 4 years comes from the growing awareness of nephropathy in both primary and secondary APS, which in lupus patients do not relate to WHO Classification and its insidious association with hypertension, loss of renal function, cumulative vascular damage, and arterial thrombosis [6–8, 10].

Additionally, advances in the immunobiology of vascular inflammation and relationship of antibody-mediated vasculopathy to atherogenesis and vaso-occlusive disease are important [1, 3, 5]. Vascular pathology and clinicoserologic correlations in 18 patients with primary (1°) and secondary (2°) syndromes are presented in this chapter relative to the current spectra of APS involvement in the literature, which has expanded to include different combinations of vascular damage from reactive endotheliomatosis to calciphylaxis. Because there is no evidence-based approach or systematic reviews for these aspects of APS, small and large case series predominate. A prospectus is offered regarding processes of endothelial cell–platelet interactions in inflammation, injury, and repair that might help to explain the wide spectrum of vasculopathy in APS.

Methods

Biopsy, surgical, or autopsy specimens were obtained from patients seen in academic and consultative practice. The diagnoses of 1° or 2° APS were made by modified Harris and American College of Rheumatology (ACR) criteria, longitudinal aPL enzyme immunoassays (EIAs) done on at least 2 occasions 4–6 weeks apart for IgG/M anticardiolipin (aCL), IgG/M antiphosphatidylserine (aPS) performed in a laboratory certified by the aPL Standardization Laboratory of E. Nigel Harris, MD, simultaneous lupus anticoagulant (LA) profile by activated partial thromboplastin time (aPTT) or a dilute Russell viper venom time (dRVVT) performed according to the Standardization Committee's recommendations, and in 1 patient an anti-prothrombin antibody test [15, 16]. In other patients, a standardized IgG/M/A EIA for aCL, aPS, and antiphosphatidylethanolamine (aPE) were performed in addition to IgG/M aCL [17]. Epidemiologic, clinical criteria for the diagnosis of 1° or 2° APS, serologic- or coagulation-based tests, and major categories of vascular pathologic involvement with cross-reference to photomicrographs comprise Table 28.1. Eleven of the 18 patients had 1° APS, the remaining 7 had 2° APS due primarily to SLE. Eleven were white females (age range, 5 days–67 years); 3 were white males (age range, 23–45 years), and 4 were black females (age range, 26–50 years). Hematoxylin and eosin (H&E) stains were used except where specified: Vierhoeff van Gieson (VVG) for collagen and elastic tissue; Masson's trichrome for elastic tissue (fibrin red to blue-grey); Mallory's phosphotungstic acid hematoxylin (PTAH) for fibrin (purple); modified Giemsa (MG) for cells and bacteria (blue); and glial fibrillary acidic protein (GFAP) immunoperoxidase (brown); in selected skin or renal biopsies, and routine FA techniques for immunoglobulins G, M, A, and complement components C3 or C4 where specified [4–6].

As there are no systematic reviews or randomized control trials, most of the articles identified by re-performing the prior comprehensive Medline literature review (cross-referencing APS, aPL, lupus coagulation inhibitor, and vascular pathology categories) were reviewed for APS diagnostic criteria, EIA and coagulation-based

Table 28.1. Clinical, serologic, and pathologic findings in 18 antiphospholipid syndrome patients. 📖

Patient	1−	2−	aPL	LA	RT	RFL	TMA	EC/Fi	PV	FA	Other	Figure
1− 19y/o WF	+		CL, PE	+	CVA REN	+	+	+	+	IgG,C3	LR	28.1(A), 28.7(A,C)
2− 23y/o WM	+		CL		PTE REN DVT PVD	n.a	+	+	−	−	LR	28.1(B), 28.7(E), 28.6(A–C,F), 28.8(E), 28.9(E)
3− 67y/o WF	+		CL, PS, PE	+	VOD PTE DVT	+	+	+	−	−	Skin Ulcer	28.1(C), 28.3(D)
4− 44y/o WF	+		PS, PE	+	VOD DVT SKIN	n.a	+	+	−	−	Skin Ulcer Pap.	28.1(D), 28.2(D)
5− 45y/o WM	+		C		VOD	n.a	+	+	−	−	Dig. Inf.	28.1(E)
6− 53y/o WM	+		PE	+	VOD DVT SKIN	n.a	+	+	+	−	LR, Skin Ulcer	28.1(F), 28.2(C), 28.3(A)
7− 28y/o BF		+	CL	−	SKIN DVT	+	+	+	+	IgG C3	Skin Nod.	28.2(A)
8− 44y/o WF	+		PE	−	SKIN VOD PTE	−	+	+	+	IgG	Bulla. Calci.	28.2(B,E), 28.4(A–F)
9− 38y/o WF		+	PS, PE	+	PUL HEM DVT CVA	+	+	+	−	+	Skin ulcer	28.2(F), 28.6(E)
10− 53y/o WF	+		PE	+	SKIN DVT	+	+	+	+	−	Skin Nod, Gran.	28.3(B,E)
11 −38y/o WF		+	CL, PS	+	CVA TCP SKIN	+	+	−I	−	−	Skin ulcer, Calci.	28.3(C,F)
12 −50y/o BF		+	CL, PS	−	CVA AIHA REN	+	+	+	−	IgG C3	LR	28.7(B), 28.8(B), 28.9(A–D,F)
13 −33y/o WF		+	CL	+	CVA TCP REN VOD	+	+	−	−	IgG C3	GI Inf.	28.7(D), 28.8(A,D), 28.9(B)
14− 29y/o BF		+	CL, PE	+	SKIN REN DVT	+	+	+	−	IgG C3	LR	28.7(F)
15− 29y/o WF	+		PE	−	PUL. HEM. AIHA TCP	+	+	+	−	−	Capill	28.6(D)

Table 28.1. Continued

Patient	1−	2−	aPL	LA	RT	RFL	TMA	EC/Fi	PV	FA	Other	Figure
16− 5d/o WF	+		PS, PE	−	CVA VOD AMI	+	+	+	−	−	Mat. 1−, Heart Tx	28.5(A–F)
17− 5d/o WF	+		CL, PE	+	VOD TCP	+	+	+	−	−	Mat. 1−, Dig. Inf.	28.8(C,F)
18− 29y/o BF		+	CL, PT	+	VOD TCP REN	−	+	+	+	−	GI Inf. TMA	28.10(A–F)

W = white; B = black; F = female; M = male; 1−= primary APS; 2−= secondary APS; aPL = antiphospholipid antibody specificity; CL = cardiolipin; PS = phosphatidylserine; PE = phosphatidylethanolamine; LA = lupus anticoagulant [activated partial thromboplastin time (aPTT) and dilute Russell viper venom time (DRVVT)]; PT = antiprothrombin antibody; RT = recurrent thromboses; CVA = cerebrovascular accident; PTE = pulmonary thromboembolism; REN = renal thrombotic microangiopathy; DVT = deep venous thromboses; PVD = peripheral venous disease; VOD = vasocclusive disease, nonatherosclerotic, large vessels; SKIN = skin infarction/nodule/ulcer/papule; PUL HEM = pulmonary hemorrhage; TCP = thrombocytopenia; AIHA = autoimmune hemolytic anemia; AMI = acute myocardial infarction; LR = livedo reticularis, Heart tx = heart transplant; RFL = recurrent fetal loss; TMA = thrombotic microangiopathy; EC/Fi = endothelial cell hyperplasia/fibrin or fibrin thrombi; PV = perivasculitis, lymphocytic (where specified); FA = fluorescent antibody studies (skin vessels or glomeruli); Dig. Inf. = digital infarction; Bulla = bullous skin disease; Calci. = calciphylaxis; Gran.= granuloma (3 or greater nuclei per giant cell); GI Inf. = gastrointestinal infarction; Capill = capillaritis; Lymph = lymphocytic; MΦ = monocytic/macrophagic; Mat. 1− = maternal primary APS; n.a. = not applicable.

aPL tests, description and photomicrography for review of major components of APS pathology (thrombotic microangiopathy, endothelial cell swelling/fibrin deposition, pervasculitis, vasculitis, or necrosis). In some instances FA studies for immunoglobulin and complement deposition were available. Tables 28.1–28.6 summarize these major pathologic findings grouped by vessel site, APS classification, major pathologic findings, aPL and LA results, and the references from the literature arranged chronologically. Sixty original color slides from 18 patients were analyzed and digitally scanned to make composite Figures 28.1–28.10 (G. A. McCarty, Indiana University APS Database, IUMC Photography Department, and Matrix Digital Photography, Inc., Indianapolis IN).

Characteristic Macrovascular Pathologic Findings in APS

The hallmark lesion suggesting APS in all its forms is livedo reticularis, which can be evanescent, intermittent, or sustained, often overlooked by physicians in recorded physical exams, yet patients and family members often describe its presence as mottling, blotching, or "giraffe skin," and clearly identify it when presented with photographs. Figure 28.1 shows in 1° APS patients classic distributions over the thigh [Fig. 28.1(A)], elbow [Fig 28.1(B)], or accompanied by cutaneous necrosis [Fig. 28.1(C)] in patients 1–3. Livedo and digital infarctions as seen in patient 5 [Fig. 28.1(E)] are a highly specific combination for APS. That pyodermatous necrotic papules, and nodules of varying sizes also occur is increasingly recognized, as

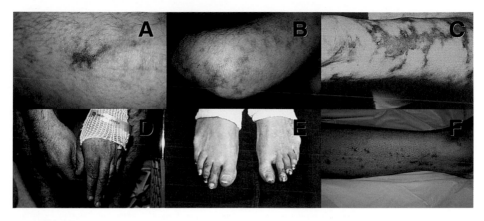

Figure 28.1. Macrovascular cutaneous pathology. (A) Livedo, thigh, patient 1. (B) Livedo, elbow, patient 2. (C) Livedo and necrosis, arm, patient 3. (D) Erythematous papules, livedo, healing ulcerations, hands, and peripheral venous thromboses, legs, patient 4. (E) Livedo and digital infarctions, patient 5. (F) Pyodermatous necrotic papules with infarction and thrombocytopenic bruising, leg, patient 6. (G. A. McCarty, Indiana University APS Database, IUMC Photography Department, and Matrix Digital Photography, Inc., Indianapolis, IN.)

exemplified by patient 6 [Fig. 28.1(F)], with bruising due to concomitant severe thrombocytopenia [18–20].

Cutaneous Vascular Pathology

At the microvascular level, the first major detailed cutaneous pathologic studies were H&E micrographs showing TMA from patients with 2° APS with LA in the setting of SLE, and subsequently in 2 patients with 1° APS [14, 18, 20]. Next to TMA, which was noted in all these patients in some vessels, endothelial cell changes including variable hypertrophy, positive staining for fibrin in vessel walls, and varying degrees of intra-luminal occlusion due to fibrin thrombi [patient 3, Fig. 28.3(D); patients 6 and 11, Fig. 28.3(A,C); Figs. 28.2, 28.3; patient 8, Fig. 28.4(A,D)]. Because of the short duration of these skin lesions from time of onset to biopsy, necrosis, fibrin staining, perivasculitis, and TMA were noted in many patients, rather than the endothelial cell fibrointimal "cushion" lesions that likely represent a combination of initial vascular injury and response to thrombosis, with reparative attempts at recanalization, and are of myointimal cell origin [1–6]. Because the first case of true vasculitis co-existent in a patient with SLE, APS, and multiple specificity aPLs, other secondary cases have been identified; however, patient 6 with 1°APS [Fig. 28.2(C), 28.3(A)] had a distinctive lymphocytic vascular infiltrate with oblitera-tion in a skin vessel not located underneath a skin ulcer, where this finding could occur due to an infection rather than a true vasculitis [12, 14, 27]. Patients 7 and 8 [Fig 28.2(A,B)] had nodular skin infiltrates mimicking a panniculitis [24]. Skin necrosis and ulcerations occur in all forms of APS with usual serologies by Harris criteria [21, 22–34]; patients 3, 4, and 7 [Figs. 28.1(D), Fig. 28.2(A), respectively] had antibodies to negative phospholipids, while patients 4 and 6 [Figs. 28.2(C), Fig 28.3(A)] notably had antibodies to PE. Widespread cutaneous necrosis is now rec-

Table 28.2. Cutaneous vascular pathology. 📖

1° APS	2° APS	TMA	EC/Fi	PV	VASC	NEC	aPL	LA+	Ref.
	+	+						+	14
+	+					+		+	18
+	+					+		+	20
	+ (HIV)					+	+	−	21
+						+			22
	+ (RA)								23
+		+		+ Lymphs	+ Lymphs	+	+		12
	+ (RA)				+ Nodule	+			24
+	+	+	+	+ MΦ			+		25
+×5	+×3	+	+		+×1 LCV		+×3	+×5	27
+		+	+				+β2gp		28
	+	+				+	+		29
	+		+				+		30
+		+					+	+	31
	+	+				Calci.		+	32
+		+					+		33
	+					+	+		34
+		+	+	+			CL, PE	+	Patient 1
+		+	+			+	CL		Patient 2
+		+	+			+	CL, PS	+	Patient 3
+		+	+			+	PS, PE	+	Patient 4
+							CL		Patient 5
+		+	+	+	+ Lymphs	+	PE	+	Patient 6
	+		+			+	CL		Patient 7
+		+	+	+ Pannic.			CL		Patient 8
+		+	+	+	+	Calci.	PE		Patient 9
	+	+	+			Calci.	PS, PE	+	Patient 10
+		+	+	+ Lymphs		Gran.	PE		Patient 11

ognized as a reason to prompt an APS workup. Calciphylaxis was noted in a patient with 2° APS and LA with uremia; 2 patients with 1° APS [patient 9, Fig. 28.2(F); patient 11 Fig. 28.3(C)] and 1 with 2° APS [patient 10, Fig. 28.3(B,F)] exhibited this finding [32, 34]. The first known report of a giant cell response in a central vessel was a novel finding in patient 10 [Fig. 28.3(E)], who presented with lower extremity nodules suggestive of a panniculitis but with no obvious drug or infectious etiology. Patient 8 with 1° APS had both classical livedo with coalescence, and skin necrosis, bullous lesions, and obliterated vessel markings [Figs. 28.2(B,E), 28.4(A,C)] in the setting of only antibodies to PE, and an overwhelming catastrophic syndrome with severe calciphylaxis. Patient 9 with 2° APS due to SLE presented with necrotic skin ulcers, calciphylaxis, and bullous lesions in the setting of pulmonary hemorrhage, and had antibodies to PE and PS [Figs. 28.2(F), Fig. 28.6(E)]. Thus, a growing panoply of cutaneous microvascular lesions comprise APS with varying macrovascular presentations.

Cardiovascular Pathology

Major advances in the understanding of the vasculopathy of APS was made when the first peripheral vascular photomicrographs of a femoral and an anterior tibial

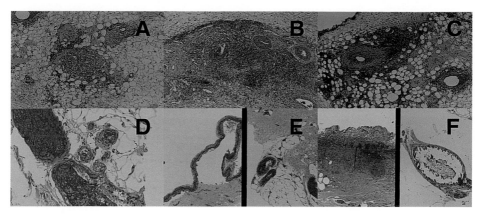

Figure 28.2. Cutaneous vascular pathology. (A) Lymphocytic nodular panniculitis (center), perivasculitis (upper left), lymphocytic perivasculitis with panvasculitis through small vessel wall (upper right), patient 7. (B) Lymphocytic epidermal and subdermal infiltrate (center and right), fibrin thrombi and early perivasculitis (left lower vessel), panvasculitis with red cells in lumen (right central vessel), and two normal vessels (above, right), patient 8. (C) Lymphocytic pervasculitis and panvasculitis with normal lumen (left) and mild perivasculitis with early fibrinoid change (right), patient 6. (D) Fibrin thrombi in multiple vessels with varying degrees of luminal occlusion, patient 4. (E) Bullous changes (left), fibrin thrombi and fibrinoid vessel changes (right), patient 8. (F) Pyodermatous skin ulcer above fibrin thrombi in several vessels (left) and bullous changes with early calciphylaxis, patient 9 (courtesy of Dr. Antoinette Hood). (G. A. McCarty, Indiana University APS Database, IUMC Photography Department, and Matrix Digital Photography, Inc., Indianapolis, IN.)

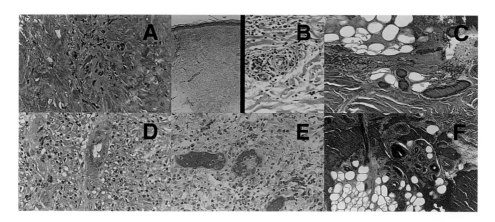

Figure 28.3. Cutaneous vascular pathology. (A) Vascular occlusion and obliteration of vascular markings, deep dermis, patient 6. (B) lymphocytic dermal infiltrate (left), small vessel perivasculitis and panvasculitis (right), patient 10. (C) Multiple fibrin thrombi in deep dermal vessels, patient 11. (D) Fibrin in dermal vessel wall, patient 3 (courtesy of Antoinette Hood). (E) Multiple fibrin thrombi and single area of giant cell formation central vessel (> 3 nuclei), patient 10 (courtesy of Dr. William Caro). (F) Multiple fibrin thrombi in deep dermal vessels with hemorrhage, fibrin thrombi, and several vessels with calciphylaxis, patient 11. (G. A. McCarty, Indiana University APS Database, IUMC Photography Department, and Matrix Digital Photography, Inc., Indianapolis, IN.)

Table 28.3. Comparative data. 📖

1° APS	2° APS	TMA	EC/Fi	PV	VASC	NEC	aPL	LA+	Ref.
+			+				+		11
	+	+	+	+ MΦ			+		12
+		+	+				CL		35
+		+	+				+		36
	+		+				+		37
+		+	+				CL	+	38
+ ×6		+ ×1	+ ×5				CL		39
+ ×8		+	+ ×13	+ MΦ		Calci.	CL, PS		40
	+	+	+				+		41
+			+				+		42
+		+	+	+	+	Calci	PS		Patient 8
+		+	+			+	PS, PE		Patient 16

artery were published in 2 patients with positive classical serologies, although the interpretation at the time was controversial [11, 12; reviewed in 4, 6–8]. The concept of intimal hyperplastic change in the femoral artery versus simple adherent thrombosis was exemplified by this first report, with a mild focal acute inflammatory infiltrate, whereas a mononuclear vasculitis was demonstrable in the tibial artery [4, 11, 12]. In subsequent cases of peripheral vessels, TMA in varying degrees is noted, along with endothelial cell changes and fibrin staining most commonly [11, 12, 35, 37, 38]. Table 28.3 presents comparative data; most cases are valvulopathies occurring in both 1° and 2° APS, with antibodies to classical aPLs, most commonly aCL, but also LA and PS [36–42]. In one case, a mononuclear/macrophage cellular

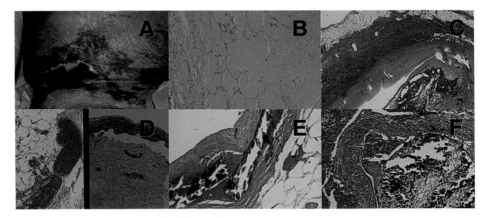

Figure 28.4. Skin, pulmonary, and coronary vascular pathology in catastrophic APS, patient 8. (A) Skin necrosis, superficial thrombosis, and coalescent livedo. (B) Pulminary arteriolar vessels with fibrin and red cells, extensive alveolar hemorrhage (WG). (C) Skin arteriole with obliterated vessel markings, adherent old calcified thrombus, and mild subdermal lymphocytic infiltrate. (D) Fibrin thrombi in multiple dermal vessels, subcutaneous edema (left) and superficial bulla above thrombosed vessels (right). (E) Coronary vein with adherent old thrombi with calciphylaxis. (F) Pulmonary arteriolar thrombi with calcified old thrombi and calciphylaxis eroding through vessel wall (lower left) causing fatal exsanguinations (courtesy of Dr. Darrell Davidson). (G. A. McCarty, Indiana University APS Database, IUMC Photography Department, and Matrix Digital Photography, Inc., Indianapolis, IN.) 📖

infiltrate was noted on the valve, and in another case, calciphylaxis [39, 40]. Platelet–fibrin surface deposition as sources of peripheral emboli, valvulitis with scarring and hypertrophy, and in rare instances calcific changes, are noted [40a]. While mitral valve involvement has been previously the sine qua non, other recent studies point out the growing awareness of aortic involvement and attendant risks for cerebrovascular embolization accruing over time [39a, 40a]. Patient 8 had significant coronary vein thromboses with adherent thrombi and calciphylactic changes at postmortem exam, and calciphylaxis was also noted segmentally in several heart valves [Fig. 28.4(E)], her death was caused by erosion of a calcified thrombus and calciphylaxis in a pulmonary arteriole causing a fatal exanguination despite being intubated on an intensive care unit; this patient made antibodies to only PE. Patient 16 was born with significant global livedo reticularis, thrombocytopenia, neonatal small vessel cerebrovascular infarcts in 3 territories, destruction of several heart valves with APS-related valvulopathy, and underwent open heart surgery at age 3 days for valvuloplasty complicated by an intra-operative myocardial infarction. Despite the maternal history of prior infertility, thrombocytopenia for the third trimester, and a DVT just prior to labor, maternal APS was not diagnosed prior to birth. Antibodies to PE were defined in both mother and infant when she was 3 days old. At 15 days, a successful heart transplantation was performed, and she remains alive to date, with only growth retardation due to chronic steroid therapy; 3 female family members have APS, and 2 who have been examined serologically have only antibodies to PE. Figure 28.5(A,B) shows her heart with intramyocardial hemorrhage and infarction, and a minimal polymorphonuclear perivascular infiltrate in the area of the acute myocardial infaction. Figure 28.5(C,D) documents TMA in the infarcted left anterior descending coronary, and necrotic

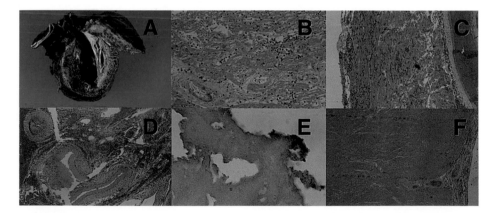

Figure 28.5. Cardiovascular pathology in neonatal APS requiring cardiac transplantation, patient 16. (A) Left ventricle hypertrophy with visible intra-myocardial hemorrhage and infarction. (B) Intra-myocardial small vessel with minimal polymorphonuclear perivascular infiltrate and dense infiltrate in an area of early necrosis and hemorrhage. (C) Left anterior descending coronary artery with thrombotic microangiopathy and transmural myocardial infarction. (D) Necrotic left anterior descending coronary artery and circumflex branch with thrombotic microangiopathy in small branches. (E) Aortic valve with fibrin thrombi, valvulitis, and early calcification. (F) Epicardial surface vessels with thrombotic microangiopathy above transmural myocardial infarction (courtesy of Dr. Mary M. Davis). (G. A. McCarty, Indiana University APS Database, IUMC Photography Department, and Matrix Digital Photography, Inc., Indianapolis, IN.) 📖

Table 28.4. Pulmonary vascular pathology. 📖

1° APS	2° APS	TMA	EC/Fi	PV	VASC	NEC	aPL	LA+	Ref.
	+	Capill.	+				CL	+	43
	+	+					+		44
	+	+	+				+		45
+		+	+			+	CL		Patient 2
+		+	+	+ Pann.			CL		Patient 8
+		+	+	+	+	Calci.	PE		Patient 9
+		Capill.	+				PE		Patient 15

branches with TMA in smaller distal vessels: epicardial vessels with TMA over the area of the acute myocardial infarction are seen in Fig. 28.5(F). Figure 28.5(E) shows the aortic valve with classic fibrin thrombi, valvulitis, and early calcification.

Pulmonary Vascular Pathology

Arterial and venous TMA occurs in the lungs of patients with APS, as well as capillaritis and pulmonary alveolar hemorrhage, but these latter entities are often go undiagnosed or are attributed to pneumonitis of infectious etiologies, and occur in both adult and pediatric patients [Table 28.4; Figs. 28.4(B), 28.6(A,F)] [43–45]. Septal capillary fibrin in concert with neutrophilic infiltration of the septa is characteristic but often capillaritis is often not considered on initial pathologic reading of these biopsies, which are often obtained bronchoscopically for the differentiation of bacterial versus pneumocystis pneumonitis so tissue sampling is limited, and prominent hemorrhage can obscure vascular detail such as TMA. That inflammatory cell infiltrate "spillage" in tissue spaces can occur has been cited above due to capillary structural differences(e.g., lack of a limiting basement membrane). Most of the published cases had classic antibodies to aCL and LA. Patient 15 had extensive pulmonary hemorrhage [Fig. 28.4(B)] with antibodies to PE, TCP/AIHA, infertility, and asymptomatic small vessel ischemic disease of the central nervous system (CNS). Patient 2 had undiagnosed TMA causing recurrent pulmonary emboli misdiagnosed as asthma throughout childhood, and at death in his 20s had pathologic evidence of old and new PTE and significant microvascular pulmonary hypertension [Fig. 28.6(A)] [4–6]. Figure 28.6(B,C) show both significant TMA and increased collagenous changed in a pulmonary arteriole, and recanalization processes in other areas of the lungs; resolution of TMA but residual fibrous strands are exemplified in Figure 28.6(F) that likely lead to chronic schistocytosis prominent in this patient in his later years. Patient 8 [Fig. 28.4(B)] had alveolar hemorrhage. Patient 9 had SLE and APS with antibodies to both PE and PS, and a classic pulmonary arteriole with fibrin staining is noted in Fig. 28.6(E), and similar changes with more alveolar capillary infiltrate "spillage" is noted in patient 15 [Fig. 28.6(D)]. An excellent review of the lung in APS is available [45a].

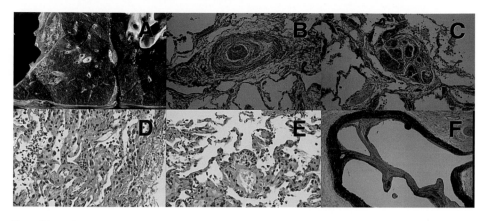

Figure 28.6. Pulmonaru vascular pathology. (A) Pulmonary arteriolar hypertrophy, fresh and recanalized thromboses, edema, and hemorrhage, patient 2. (B) Pulmonary arteriole with increased concentric intimal fibrosis in situ thrombosis (MT), patient 2. (C) Pulmonary arteriole with organizing thrombosis and early recanalization (VVG), patient 2. (D) Pulmonary capillaritis with inflammatory cells "spilling" into alveolar spaces (far left), patient 15. (E) Pulmonary arteriole with fibrinous walls and intra-luminal fibrin (center), patient 9. (F) Pulmonary arteriole with fibrous web residual of recanalization of old thrombi (VVG), patient 2 (courtesy of Dr. Michael Hugheson). (G. A. McCarty, Indiana University APS Database, IUMC Photography Department, and Matrix Digital Photography, Inc., Indianapolis, IN.)

Renal Vascular Pathology

The first reports of renovascular pathology involved patients with recurrent thrombosis and LA [6–8, reviewed in 10, 46, 47]. Renovascular lesions involve afferent arterioles and terminal branches of inter-lobular arteries, often without eliciting a cellular infiltrate or disruption of internal elastic laminae, but the deposition of hyaline material beneath the endothelium, which is immunoglobulin in nature by previously published electron microscopic studies, has also been noted [6–8, 10, 46, 47]. Table 28.5 collates the vascular pathology, clinical setting of APS independent of type of glomerulonephritis by WHO classification, as clinical renal disease is discussed elsewhere in this book; TMA is characteristic in all cases, as well as endothelial cell hyperplasia and fibrin staining. The earliest reports cite thrombotic thrombocytopenic and/or purpuric presentations which brought patients to early renal biopsy; the first 4 cases were patients with classical serologies, TMA, and SLE [46, 47]. Series of patients have subsequently been identified, with 1° and 2° APS, and a continuing prevalence of antibodies to aCL and/or LA [35, 50, 52–56, 58, 59]. Perivasculitis or vasculitis occurred infrequently, primarily in patients with 2° APS, but one case report documents a patient with 1 °APS [51, 52, 57]. Patients 2, 7, and 12–14 all had 2° APS and antibodies to aCL; additionally, patients 12 and 14 had antibodies to PS, and PE and LA, respectively. Patient 1 with 1°APS exhibited concentric renal arteriolar hypertrophy with a mild perivascular infiltrate but no true panvascular infiltrate, and normal tubules [Fig. 28.7(A)]; hyalinized thickened capillary loops with mild proliferative changes are shown in Figure 28.7(C) and she had antibodies to aCL and PE. Patient 2 showed glomerular capillary loop hypertrophy with eccentric intimal hyperplasia in an extraglomerular vessel [Fig. 28.7(E)].

Table 28.5. Renovascular pathology. 📖

1° APS	2° APS	TMA	EC/Fi	PV	VASC	NEC	aPL	LA+	Ref.
	+×3	+					+		46
	+	+						+	47
+×5	+×5	+	+	+			CL×4	+×3	48, 49
+		+	+				CL		50
+×1	+×5				+		Cl×3		51
+		+	+				CL		35
+×5			+				CL×4	+×5	52
	+×4	+	+	+	+		+		53
+×5		+	+				CL×4	+×1	54
+		+	+				CL		55
	+×3	+	+				CL		56
+		+	+		+	+	CL		57
	+×14	+	+				CL×13		58
	+×8	+					CL×3	+×5	59
	+	+	+	+			CL, PS		Patient 1
+		+	+			+	CL		Patient 2
	+		+			+	CL		Patient 7
	+	+	+				CL, PS		Patient 12
	+	+					CL		Patient 13
	+	+	+				CL, PE	+	Patient 14

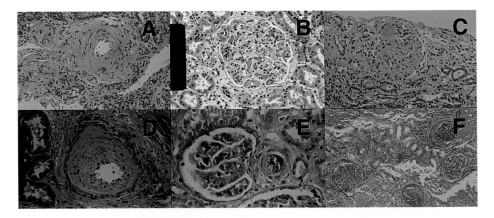

Figure 28.7. Renovascular pathology. (A) Concentric renal arteriolar hypertrophy with mild perivascular, but not panvascular, inflammatory infiltrate and normal tubules (top), patient 1. (B) Glomerular capillary loop small thromboses are scattered through the upper left and mid lower quadrants, patient 12. (C) Hyalinized, thickened glomerular capillary loop present superiorly with few inflammatory cells, arteriolar thickening, and proliferation; glomerular ischemia, patient 1. (D) Concentric renal arteriolar hypertrophy, patient 13. (E) Glomerular capillary loop hypertrophy with eccentric intimal hyperplasia in extraglomerular vessel, patient 2. (F) Renal arteriolar hypertrophy, crescentic glomerulopathy with varying degrees of capillary loop hypertrophy, hyalinization, and fibrosis, patient 14. (courtesy of Dr. Moo-Nahm Yum). (G. A. McCarty, Indiana University APS Database, IUMC Photography Department, and Matrix Digital Photography, Inc., Indianapolis, IN.) 📖

Patient 12 had small glomerular capillary loop thromboses and antibodies to aCL and PS [Fig. 27.7(B)]. Patient 13 showed concentric arteriolar hypertrophy [Fig. 27.7(D)], and patient 14 had crescentic glomerulopathy with varying degrees of hyalinization and fibrosis, and antibodies to aCL and PE [Fig. 28.7(F)]. Expected frequencies of IgG and/or C3 by FA studies were noted relative to lupus nephritis classification in some cases (data not shown). Fibrin, erythrocytes, and erythrocyte fragments are often components of a thickened media and effacement with hyaline material is common. The renovascular pathology of APS likely represents the culmination of endothelial cell effector functions in regulation of response to immune injury of various types in recent reviews [2, 10, 53]. A distinctive form of endothelial injury resulting in a novel glomerular basement membrane wrinkling and reduplication by silver staining, which was on electron microscopy shown to be accompanied by a new, straighter, thin membrane adjacent to the endothelium was described, which was not always associated with TMA in these primary APS patients [2, 60].

Cerebrovascular and Muscular Vascular Pathology

Early studies associated small vessel cerebrovascular ischemic lesions, usually of a multiple territory nature causing multi-infarct dementia, classical antibodies to aCL, and co-existent cardiac sources of microemboli due to APS valvulopathy [61, 62–64]. A true TMA with vasculitis was noted in 2 cases, 1 with a monocytic/macrophagic perivascultis in a patient with 1° APS, and co-existent intimal hyperplasia, and a transmural lymphocytic infiltrate consistent with true vasculitis in another patient with 1°APS, also with antibodies to aCL. This is the CNS equivalent

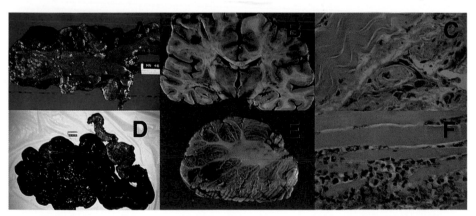

Figure 28.8. Mesenteric, cerebrovascular, and muscular vascular pathology. (A) Mesenteric arterial thrombosis present and distinct from proximal artherosclerosis, patient 13 (courtesy of Dr. Michael Hughson). (B) Multi-territory cerebral meningeal, gray, and white matter small vessel ischemic disease of varying ages, patient X. (C) Muscle arteriolar thrombosis and muscle fiber necrosis in left forearm, patient 17. (D) Intestinal ischemia due to mesenteric thrombosis in (A), patient 13. (E) Multiple areas of cerebellar small vessel ischemic disease, patient X. (F) Muscle necrosis with acute inflammatory infiltrate from small vessel thrombosis in (C), patient 17 (courtesy of Dr. Mary M. Davis). (G. A. McCarty, Indiana University APS Database, IUMC Photography Department, and Matrix Digital Photography, Inc., Indianapolis, IN.)

Table 28.6. Cerebrovascular and musculovascular pathology.

1° APS	2° APS	TMA	EC/Fi	PV	VASC	NEC	aPL	LA+	Ref.
+		+	+				+		13
+	+	+	+	+ MΦ			+		25
	+	+	+				+		41
+		+	+				CL		62
	+	+	+						63
	+	+	+		+				64
+		+	+	+			CL, PE	+	Patient 1
+		+	+			+	CL		Patient 2
	+	+	+				CL, PS		Patient 12
	+	+	+				CL	+	Patient 13
+		+	+			+	CL, PE	+	Patient 17

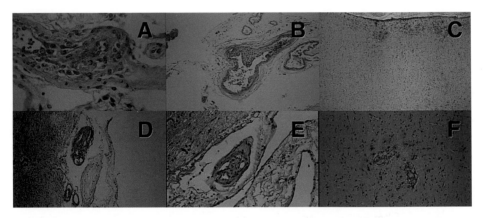

Figure 28.9. Cerebrovascular pathology. (A) Cerebral arteriolar endothelial cell edema and mitotic figure with intimal hyperplasia, fibrin, and major luminal occlusion, patient 12. (B) Intimal fibrous proliferation extending intra-luminally in cortical arteriole, patient 13. (C) Cortical infarct confined to cortical ribbon (GFAP), patient 12. (D) Meningeal arteriolar intimal hyperplasia with thrombotic microaniopathy and recanalization, patient 12. (E) Meningeal arteriolar intimal hyperplasia in vessel not overlying a cortical infarct, patient 2. (F) Deep cerebral cortical vessels with fibrous webs and thrombotic microangiopathy with recanalization, patient 12 (courtesy of Dr. Michael Hughson). (G. A. McCarty, Indiana University APS Database, IUMC Photography Department, and Matrix Digital Photography, Inc., Indianapolis, IN.)

of the previously described reactive angioendotheliomatosis described in our studies and by others [6–8, 19]. Three of the 4 patients here had 1°APS [patient 1, Fig. 28.9(A); patient 2, Figs. 28.8(E), 28.9(E); and patient 17, Fig. 28.8(C,F)] with antibodies to aCL, or aCL and PE (patients 1 and 17). Patient 1 [Fig. 28.9(A)] additionally had significant endothelial cell swelling and the novel finding of a mitotic figure, with almost complete obliteration of vascular lumen, and a mild periadventitial cellular infiltrate. Patient 12 [Figs. 28.8(B), 28.9(C,D,F)] showed a wide variety of TMA with varying webs of recanalization in several sites in both grey and white matter vessels. Special stains showed cortical ribbon infarction proceeding downwards from cortical meningeal arterioles. Patients 12, 13, and 2 also showed similar lesions in areas not underlying a cortical meningeal infarct [Fig. 28.9(A,B,E), respectively]. TMA characterized all the reports and significant endothelial cell changes were apparent [13, 25, 41, 61–64].

Intra-luminal platelet deposition in cerebral vasculopathy is important, and only recently have CNS lesions been identified with characteristic TMA changes in murine models of APS [65, 66]. Two patients have recently been seen at IUMC with multiple isotype aPLs to PE whose review of nerve biopsies previously read as normal were shown to have classic TMA in arterioles (data not shown); their diagnoses were chronic demyelinating immunologic peripheral neuropathy (CDIP) but they both have multiple criteria for 1° APS [31]. Patient 17 [Fig. 28.8(C,F)] is a neonate with unilateral cutaneous gangrene and 4 digital infarctions requiring amputation due to maternal APS that was not recognized despite maternal–fetal TCP and LR; muscular infarction due to TMA and subsequent necrosis is depicted from hand muscle biopsy, but the digital arteries were not examined distally. Both her mother and this baby girl had antibodies to aCL, PE, and LA.

Vascular Pathology in Other Organs

Isolated reports of TMA and endothelial cell changes with and without fibrin staining have been reported in other organs; an arterial occlusion in APS causing large bowel infarction similar to the gross aortic/mesenteric arterial occlusive disease as shown in patient 13 [Fig. 28.8(A,D)] who had SLE and APS, and died of bowel gangrene; a patient with 1° APS and giant ulcerations with a lymphocytic infiltrate in involved areas near an ulceration, but also around vessels not underlying an ulcer [67–69]. A 26-year-old black patient with known SLE presented to our institution with nausea, vomiting, diarrhea, and increasing abdominal discomfort during a period of lupus disease quiescence, but a prior history of Class IV nephritis previously successfully treated with steroids, immunosuppressives, and hemodialysis. Thrombosis of her shunts was attributed to dialysis; additional history suggested migranous headaches, but she had no recurrent fetal losses. Due to a change in her abdominal computed tomography (CT) scan suggesting jejunal wall edema but not increasing pain, she was taken to surgery before an IV steroid trial, and Figure 27.10(A–F) shows her jejunal vascular pathology. She had a spectrum of reactive angioendotheliomatosis, fibrin thrombi, acute inflammatory perivasculitis, and vessel wall involvement in areas of hemorrhage due to her lupus enteritis, and some early foamy cell changes suggesting the possibility of early atheromatous disease. She had no clinicoserologic disease activity, making systemic vasculitis unlikely and was on maintenance steroids and off immunosuppressives and hemodialysis with stable proteinuria. In vessels not shown, she had arteriolar thickening but no discrete plaques [5]. TMA was present in varying stages in areas clearly not related to the margins of her surgery, and retrospectively she had shortened aPTTs consistent with anti-prothrombin antibodies and concurrent aCL [70, 71]. Adrenal insufficiency due to vessel thrombosis, hemorrhage, and eventual atrophy with antibodies to aCL primarily are becoming increasing recognized in APS patients presenting with fatigue and weakness, and a high index of suspicion is needed for appropriate diagnosis: high resolution CT is diagnostic so laparoscopy is often avoided [72]; bladder infarction in a patient with criteria for 1°APS and antibodies to aCL [73], and lastly, pituitary vascular infarction resulting in a maternal death due to TMA and antibodies to aCL [74].

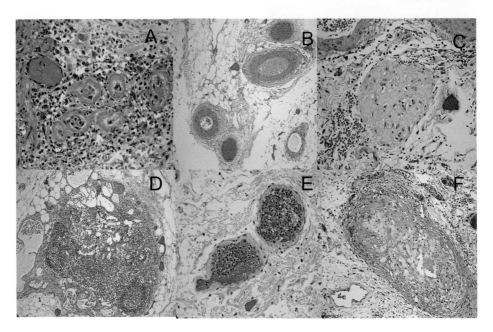

Figure 28.10. Jejunal vascular pathology. (A) Mucosal ischemic necrosis and inflammation with fibro-inflammatory debris and intra-mucosal fibrin deposition, sub-mucosal edema, and congestion is present, along with fibrin thrombi and fibrinoid necrosis of small vessels. (B) No apparent vasculitis in vessels outside of areas of hemorrhage. (C, D) Vasculopathy due to lupus enteritis and APS. (E, F) Endothelial cell intimal edema, hyperplasia, with vaso-occlusion due to foamy cells suggestive of atheromatous changes (no lipid stains done). No ulcerated atheromatous plaque was found in serial sections. Reactive endotheliomatosis is present (courtesy of Dr. Nancy S. Miller).

Prospectus

The spectra of vascular pathology in APS likely reflects the time course of initial versus chronic vascular injury, host response to immunologic perturbance, and the continual adjustment from a prothrombotic to nonthrombotic milieu of endothelial cells and platelets [reviewed in 1, 3, 5, 9, 75, 76]. Platelet activation, generation of platelet and endothelial cell microparticles due to vascular injury TMA has been considered to be the hallmark pathologic finding for APS [75]. aPLs circulate systemically yet cause antibody-mediated thrombosis only at certain times in certain vessels, which is the concept of the "systemic defect–local phenotype" paradox that has been recently elucidated from the cerebro-vascular standpoint in that there are locally determinative variables that result in a procoagulant or anticoagulant phenotype [reviewed in 76]. That vasculitis and perivasculitis can occur with APS, even in primary forms, or where autoantibodies are directed to phospholipids other than cardiolipin, is apparent in these cases and from the literature; however, tight correlation with levels of aPLs at the time of investigation is not always demonstrable, and might likely reflect the finding that antibodies to phospholipids are enriched in circulating immune complexes found in APS patients [77]. That aPLs are present on the average approx 3 years prior to the first thrombotic event and thus are contributing to cumulative vascular damage has elegantly demonstrated in a well-powered longitudinal study of SLE and APS patients using gold-standard testing

[78]. Because endothelial cell phenotypes differ, and there is an emerging concept that anti-endothelial cell antibodies as being directed against microvascular versus macrovascular endothelia, more studies into the longitudinal evaluation of endothelins, adhesion molecules, and monocyte-tissue factor expression upregulation also likely contribute to the ultimate expressions of immune mediated vascular injury, thrombosis, inflammation, and repair, but at least in treated APS pregnancies, evidence of globally elevated endothelial cell activation markers did not define disease [80, 81]. In in vivo thrombosis and microcirculation models testing patient-derived monoclonal aCLs, increased leukocyte adhesion to endothelial cells was noted versus controls, and there was enhanced expression of VCAM-1 [82]. Thus, there is a theoretic basis for involvement of inflammatory cells in APS related pathology that is not merely due to immune complex mechanisms. Human monoclonal aPLs have been shown by functional assays using atomic force microscopy to disrupt the protective annexin A5 shield on phospholipids bilayers in one laboratory [83]. Monocyte chemoattractant protein-1 are induced by aPLs on human vascular endothelial cells incubated with IgG–APS or monoclonal aCL, and the serum levels correlated with IgG aCL titers in 75 SLE patients; downregulation of mRNA expression was noted with steroid treatment [84]. Recent attempts at characterizing the upstream events in endothelial cell signaling using anti–$â_2$-glycoprotein I on human microvascular endothelial cells cleverly made as dominant-negative constructs of Delta TRAF2, TRAF6, MyD88 showed that anti–$â_2$-glycoprotein I react with antigens associated with members of the TLR/IL-1 receptor family on the endothelial surface and directly induce activation [85]. These exciting findings offer future diagnostic and possibly therapeutic avenues, and hopefully will lead to the development of better characterization of local endothelial cell phenotypes that might be exploited for more specific diagnostic pathology. That aPLs have a role in atherogenesis via interactions with oxidized low-density lipoprotein, and the modulation of aPL atherogenic potential via statins with attendant decrease in vaso-occlusive disease morbidity and mortality in SLE and APS are emerging areas [86, 87]. The saga of new aPLs such as anti-prothrombin associated with enhanced endothelial cell binding challenges our thinking as this aPL shortens not prolongs coagulation times [88]. A recent review of the multiple mechanisms by which aPLs cause vasculopathy is offered [89]. Future histopathology in APS should benefit from new phenotypic and molecular/biomarkers for further characterization and understanding of microvascular events as knowledge progresses.

References

1. Hunt BJ, Khamashta MA. Antiphospholipid antibodies and the endothelium. Curr Rheumatol Rep 2000;2:252–255.
2. Halevy D, Radhakrishnan J, Markowitz G, Appel G. Thrombotic microangiopathies. Crit Care Clin 2003;18:309–320.
3. Raschi E, Testoni C, Borghi MO, Fineschi S, Meroni PL. Endothelium activation in the antiphospholipid antibody syndrome. Biomed Pharmacother 2003;57:282–286.
4. Lie JT. Vasculopathy of the antiphospholipid syndromes revisited: thrombosis is the culprit and vasculitis the consort. Lupus 1996;368:71.
5. Sherer Y, Shoenfeld Y. Antiphospholipid antibody syndrome, antiphospholipid antibodies and atherosclerosis. Curr Atheroscler Rep 2001;3:328–333.
6. Hughson MD, Nadasdy T, McCarty GA, Sholer C, Min KW, Silva F. Renal thrombotic microangiopathy in patients with systemic lupus erythematosus and the antiphospholipid syndrome. Am J Kid Dis 1992;20:150–158.

7. Hughson MD, McCarty GA, Sholer CM, Brumback RA. Thrombotic cerebral arteriopathy in patients with the antiphospholipid syndrome. Mod Pathol 1993;6:644–653.
8. Hughson MD, McCarty GA, Brumback RA. Spectrum of vascular pathology affecting patients with the antiphospholipid syndrome. Hum Pathol 1995;26:716–724.
9. Pierangeli SS, Harris EN. Probing antiphospholipid antibody-mediated thrombosis-the interplay between anticardiolipin and antiendothelial cell antibodies. Lupus 2003;12:539–545.
10. Tektonidou MG, Sotsiou F, Nakopoulou L, Vlachoyiannopoulos PG, Moutsoupoulos HM. Antiphospholipid antibody syndrome nephropathy in patients with systemic lupus erythematosus and antiphospholipid antibodies. Arthritis Rheum 2004;50:2569–2579.
11. Alarcon-Segovia D, Cardiel MH, Reyes E, et al. Antiphospholipid arterial vasculopathy. J Rheum 1989;16:762–767.
12. Goldberger E, Elder RC, Schwartz RA, Phillips PE . Vasculitis in the antiphospholipid syndrome. A cause of ischemia responding to corticosteroids. Arthritis Rheum 1992;35:569–572.
13. Westerman EM, Miles JM, Backonja M, Sundstrom WR. Neuropathologic findings in multi-infarct dementia associated with anticardiolipin antibody. Evidence for endothelial injury as the primary event. Arthritis Rheum 1992;35:1038–1041.
14. Winklemann RK, Alegre VA . Histopathologic and immunofluorescence study of skin lesions associated with circulating lupus anticoagulant. J Am Acad Dermatol 1988;19:117–124.
15. Wilson WA, Gharavi AE, Koike T, et al. International concensus statement on preliminary criteria for definite antiphospholipid antibody syndrome: report of an international workshop. Arthritis Rheum 1999;42:1309–1311.
16. Brandt JT, Triplett DA, Alving B, Scharrer I, on behalf of the Subcommittee on Lupus Anticoagulant/Antiphospholipid Antibody Section of the Scientific and Standardization Committee of the International Society for Thrombosis and Haemostasis. Criteria for the diagnosis of lupus anticoagulant: an update. Thromb Haemost 1995;74:1185–1190.
17. McIntyre JA, Wagenknecht DR, Waxman DW. Frequency and specificities of antiphospholipid antibodies in volunteer blood donors. Immunobiology 2003;207:59–63.
18. Frances C, Tribout B, Boisnic S. Cutaneous necrosis associated with the lupus anticoagulant. Dermatologica 1989;178:194–201.
19. Creamer D, Black MM, Colange E. Reactive angioendotheliomatosis in association with antiphospholipid antibody syndrome. J Am Acad Dermatol 2000;42:903–906.
20. Dodd HJ, Sarkany I, O'Shaughnessy D. Widespread cutaneous necrosis associated with the lupus anticoagulant. Clin Exp Dermatol 1985;10:581–586.
21. Smith KJ, Skelton HG, James WD, et al. Cutaneous histopathologic findings in 'antiphospholipid syndrome': correlation with disease, including human immundeficiency virus disease. Arch Dermatol 1990;126:1176–1183.
22. O'Neill A, Gatenby PA, McGaw B, Painter DM, McKenzie PR. Widespread cutaneous necrosis associated with cardiolipin antibodies. J Am Acad Dermatol 1990;22:356–359.
23. Wolf P, Soyes HP, Aver Grunbach P. Widespread cutaneous necrosis in a patient with rheumatoid arthritis associated with anticardiolipin. Arch Dermatol 1991;127:1739–1740.
24. Elkayam O, Yaron M, Brasoush E, Carpi D. Rheumatoid nodules in a patient with primary antiphosphlipid antibody syndrome (Hughes' Syndrome). Lupus 1998;7:488–491.
25. Macucci M, Dotti MT, Battistini S, et al. Primary antiphospholipid syndrome: two case reports, one with histological examination of skin, peripheral nerve and muscle. Acta Neurol 1994;16:87–96.
26. Lalova A, Popov I, Dourmishev A, Baleva M, Nikolov K. Dramatic vasculopathy in a patient with antiphospholipid syndrome [letter]. Acta Derm Venerol 1996; 76:406
27. Abernethy ML, McGuinn JL, Callen JP. Widespread cutaneous necrosis as the initial manifestation of the antiphospholipid antibody syndrome. J Rheumatol 1995;22:1380–1383.
28. Katayama I, Nishioka K, Otoyama K. Clinical analysis of anti-cardiolipin.beta 2 glycoprotein 1 antibody positive patients in anti-phospholipid syndrome. J Dermatol Sci 1995;9:215–220
29. Frances C, Piette JC. Cutaneous manifestation of Hughes syndrome occurring in the context of lupus erythematosus. Lupus 1997;6:139–144.
30. van Genderen PJ, Michiels JJ. Erythromelagia: a pathogomonic microvascular thrombotic complication in essential thrombocythemia and polycythemia vera. Semin Thromb Hemost 1997;23:357–363.
31. McCarty GA. Indiana Antiphospholipid Antibody Database, unpublished data.
32. Coates T, Kirkland GS, Dymock RB, et al. Cutaneous necrosis from calcific uremic arteriolopathy. Am J Kidney Dis 1998;32:384–391.
33. Grone HJ . Systemic lupus erythematosus and antiphospholipid syndrome. Pathologe 1996;17:405–416.

34. Hill VA, Whittaker SJ, Hunt BJ, Liddell K, Spittle, MF, Smith NP. Cutaneous necrosis associated with the antiphospholipid syndrome and mycosis fungoides. Br J Dermatol 1994;130:92–96.
35. Kniaz D, Eisenberg GM, Elrad H, Johnson CA, Valaitis J, Bregman H. Postpartum hemolytic uremic syndrome associated with antiphospholipid antibodies. Am J Nephrol 1992;12:126–128.
36. Alvarez-Blanco A, Egurbide-Arberas MV, Aguirre-Errasti C. Severe valvular heart disease in a patient with primary antiphospholipid syndrome. Lupus 1994;3:433–434.
37. Trent K, Neustater BR, Lottenberg R. Chronic relapsing thrombotic thrombocytopenic purpura and antiphospholipid antibodies: a report of two cases. Am J Hematol 1997;54:155–159.
38. Hohlfeld J, Schneider M, Hein R, et al. Thrombosis of terminal aorta, deep vein thrombosis, recurrent fetal loss, and antiphospholipid antibodies. Case report. Vasa 1996;25:194–199.
39. Garcia-Torres R, Amigo MC, de la Rosa A, Moron A, Reyes PA. Valvular heart disease in primary antiphospholipid syndrome (PAPS): clinical and morphological findings. Lupus 1996;5:56–61.
39a. Lev S, Shoenfeld Y. Cardial valvulopathy in the antiphospholipid antibody syndrome. Clin Rev Allergy Immunol 2002;23:341–348.
40. Ziporen L, Goldberg L, Arad M, et al. Libman-Sacks endocarditis in the antiphospholipid syndrome immunopathologic findings in deformed heart valves. Lupus 1996;5:196–205.
40a. Eiken PW, Edwards WD, Tazelaar HD, McBane RD, Zekr KJ. Surgical pathology of nonbacterial thrombotic endocarditis in 30 patients, 1985-2000. Mayo Clin Proc 2001;76:1204–1212.
41. Borowska-Lehman J, Bakowska A, Michowska M, Rzepko R, Izycka E, Chrostowski L. Antiphospholipid syndrome in systemic lupus erythematosus – immunomorphological study of the central nervous system; case report. Folica Neuropathol 1995;33:231–233.
42. Hojnik M, George J, Ziporen L, Shoenfeld Y. Heart valve involvement Libman-Sacks endocarditis) in the antiphospholipid syndrome. Circulation 1996;93:1579–1587.
42a. Reshetniak TM, Kotel'nikova GP, Fomicheva OA, et al. Cardiological aspects of the antiphospholipid antibody syndrome. Part I. Valvular lesions in the primary and secondary antiphospholipid antibody syndrome and systemic lupus erythematosus. Kardiologiia 2002;42:38–43.
43. Asherson RA, Cervera R. Antiphospholipid antibodies and the lung [editorial]. J Rheumatol 1995;22:62–66.
44. Falcini F, Taccetti G, Ermini M, Trapani S, Matucci Cerinic M. Catastrophic antiphospholipid antibody syndrome in pediatric systemic lupus erythematosus. J Rheumatol 1997;24:389–392.
45. Yokoi T, Tomita Y, Fukaya M, Ichihara S, Kakudo K, Takahashi Y. Pulmonary hypertension associated with SLE: predominantly thrombotic arteriopathy accompanied by plexiform lesions. Arch Pathol Lab Med 1998;122:467–470.
45a. Espinoza G, Cervera R, Font J, Asherson RA. The lung in antiphospholipid antibody syndrome. Ann Rheum Dis 2003;61:195–198.
46. D'Agati V, Kunis C, William G, et al. Anticardiolipin and renal disease-a report of three cases. J Am Soc Nephrol 1980;1:777–784.
47. Kleinknecht D, Bobrie G, Meyer O, Noël LH, Callard P, Ramdane M. Recurrent thrombosis and renal vascular disease in patients with a lupus anticoagulant. Nephrol Dial Transplant 1989;4:854–858.
48. Asherson RA, Hughes GRV, Derksen RHWM. Renal infarction associated with antiphospholipid antibodies in systemic lupus erythematosus and 'lupus like' disease. J Urol 1988;140:1028.
49. Asherson RA, Cervera R, Piette JC, et al. Catastrophic antiphospholipid antibody syndrome: clinical and laboratory features of 50 patients. Medicine (Baltimore) 1998;77:195–207.
50. Legerton CW, Leaker B, McGregor A, et al. Insidious loss of renal function in patients with anticardiolipin antibodies and the absence of overt nephritis. Br J Rheumatol 1991;30:422–425.
51. Cacoub P, Wechsler B, Piette JC, et al. Malignant hypertension in antiphospholipid syndrome without overt lupus nephritis. Clin Exp Rheum 1993;11:479–485.
52. Mandreoli M, Zucchelli P. Renal vascular disease in patients with primary antiphospholipid antibodies. Nephrol Dial Transplant 1993;8:1277–1280.
53. Appel GB, Pirani CL, D'Agati V. Renal vascular complications of systemic lupus erythematosus [editorial]. J Am Soc Nephrol 4:1499–1515.
54. Amigo MC, Garcia-Torres R, Robles M, Bochicchio T, Reyes PA . Renal involvement in primary antiphospholipid syndrome. J Rheumatol 1992;19:1181–1185.
55. Petras T, Rudolph B, Filler G, et al. An adolescent with acute renal failure, thrombocytopenia, and femoral vein thrombosis. Nephrol Dial Transplant 1998;13:480–483.
56. Strief W, Monagle P, South M, Leaker M, Andrew M. Arterial thrombosis in children. J Pediatrics 1999;134:110–112.
57. Almeshari K, Alfurayh, Akhtar M. Primary antiphospholipid syndrome and self-limited renal vasculitis during pregnancy: case report and review of the literature. Am J Kidney Dis 1994;24:505–508.

58. Bhandari S, Harnden P, Brownjohn AM, Turney JH. Association of anticardiolipin antibodies with intra-glomerular thrombi and renal dysfunction in lupus nephritis. QJM 1998;91:401–409.
59. Lelievre G, Vanhille P. Renal thrombotic microangiopathy in SLE: clinical correlations and long term renal survival. Nephrol Dial Transplant 1998;13:298–304.
60. Griffiths MH, Papadaki L, Neild GH. The renal pathology of primary antiphospholipid antibody syndrome: a distinctive form of endothelial injury. QJM 2000;93:457–467.
61. Coull BM, Bourdette DN, Goodnight SH, Briley DP, Hart R. Multiple cerebral infarctions and dementia associated with anticardiolipin antibodies. Stroke 1987;18:1107–1112.
62. Fulham MJ, Gatenby P, Ruck RR. Focal cerebral ischemia and antiphospholipid antibodies: a case for cardiac embolism. Acta Neurol Scand 1994;90:417–423.
63. Futrell N, Asherson RA, Lie JT. Probable antiphospholipid syndrome with recanalization of occluded blood vessels mimicking proliferative vasculopathy. Clin Exp Rheum 1994;12:230–231.
64. Belmont HM, Abramson SB, Lie JT. Pathology and pathogenesis of vascular injury in systemic lupus erythematosus. Interaction of inflammatory cells and activated endothelium. Arthritis Rheum 1996;39:9–22.
65. Ellison D, Gatter K, Heryet A, Esiri M. Intramural platelet deposition in cerebral vasculopathy of systemic lupus erythematosus. J Clin Pathol 1993;46:37–40.
66. Olguin-Ortega L, Jara LJ, Becerra M, et al. Neurological involvement as a poor prognostic factor in catastrophic antiphospholipid antibody syndrome: autopsy findings in 12 cases. Lupus 2003;12:93–98.
67. Asherson R, Morgan S, Harris E, et al. Arterial occlusion causing large bowel infarction: a reflection of clotting diathesis in SLE. Clin Rheumatol 1986;5:102–106.
68. Kallman DR, Khan A, Romain PL, Nompleggi DJ. Giant gastric ulceration associated with antiphospholipid antibody syndrome. Am J Gastroenterol 1996;91:1244–1247.
69. Dessailloud R, Papo T, Vaneecloo S, Gamblin C, Vanhille P, Piette JC. Acalculous ischemic gallbladder necrosis in the catastrophic antiphospholipid syndrome. Arthritis Rheum 1998;41:1318–1320.
70. Ahmed N, Miller NS, Bagati R, Weinstein A, Jelinek JS, McCarty GA. Abdominal pain in a young woman with systemic lupus erythematosus – a paradigm shift from the 1980s to 2004? Proceedings of the DC Rheumatism Society Fellows' Forum, Washington Hospital Center/Georgetown University Division of Rheumatology and Immunology, 2004.
71. Sanchez-Guerrero J, Reyes E, Alarcon-Segovia D. Primary antiphospholipid antibody syndrome as a cause of intestinal infarction. J Rheumatol 1992;19:623–627.
72. Espinosa G, Santos E, Cervera R, et al. Adrenal involvement in the antiphospholipid antibody syndrome: clinical and immunologic characteristics of 86 patients. Medicine (Baltimore) 2003;82:106–118.
73. Brooks MD, Fletcher MS, Melcher DH. Venous thrombosis of the bladder associated with antiphospholipid syndrome. J R Soc Med 1994;87:633–634.
74. Bendon RW, Wilson J, Getahun B, van der Bel-Kahn J. A maternal death due to thrombotic disease associated with anticardiolipin antibody. Arch Pathol Lab Med 1987;111:370–373.
75. Giron-Gonzalez JA. Platelet and endothelial cell activation are requisites for the development of antiphospholipid antibody syndrome. Ann Rheum Dis 2004;63:600–601.
76. Connor P, Hunt BJ. Cerebral haemostasis and antiphospholiipid antibodies. Lupus 2003;12:929–934.
77. Arfors L, Lefvert VK. Enrichment of antibodies against phospholipids in circulating immune complexes (CIC) in the anti-phospholipid syndrome (APLS). Clin Exp Immunol 1996;108:47–51.
78. McClain MT, Arbuckle MR, Heinlen LD, et al. The prevalence, onset, and clinical significance of antiphospholipid antibodies prior to diagnosis of systemic lupus erythematosus. Arthritis Rheum 2004;50:1226–1232.
79. Miret C, Cervera R, Reverter JC, et al. Antiphospholipid syndrome without antiphospholipid antibodies at the time of the thrombotic event: transient 'seronegative' antiphospholipid syndrome? Clin Exp Rheumatol 1997;15:541–544.
80. Shoenfeld Y. Classification of anti-endothelial cell antibodies into antibodies against microvascular and macrovascular endothelial cells: the pathogenic and diagnostic implications. Cleve Clin J Med 2002;69(suppl 2):SII65–SII67.
81. Stone S, Hunt BJ, Seed PT, Parmara K, Khamashta MA, Poston L. Longitudinal evaluation of markers of endothelial cell dysfunction and hemostatis in treated antiphospholipid antibody syndrome and in health pregnancy. Am J Obstet Gynecol 2003;188:454–460.
82. Pierangeli SS, Liu X, Espinola R, et al. Functional analyses of patient-derived IgG monoclonal anticardiolipin antibodies using in vivo thrombosis and in vivo microcirculation models. Thromb Haemost 2000;84:388–395.

83. Rand JR, Wu XX, Quinn AS, et al. Human monoclonal antiphospholipid antibodies disrupt the annexin A5 anticoagulant crystal shield on phospholipids bilayers; evidence from atomic force microscopy and functional assay. Am J Pathol 2003;163:1193–2000.
84. Cho CS, Cho ML, Chen PP, et al. Antiphospholipid antibodies induce monocyte chemoattractant protein-1 in endothelial cells. J Immunol 2002;168:4209–4218.
85. Raschi E, Testoni C, Bosisio D, et al. Role of the MyD88 transduction signaling pathway in endothelial activation by antiphospholipid antibodies. Blood 2003;109:3495–3500.
86. Matsurra E, Kpbayashi K, Koike T, Shoenfeld Y, Khamashta MA, Hughes GR. Oxidized low density lipoprotein as a risk factor for thrombosis in antiphospholipid antibody syndrome. Lupus 2003;12:550–554.
87. Merrill JT. The antiphospholipid ntibody syndrome and atherosclerosis: clue to pathogenesis. Curr Rheumatol Rep 2003;5:401–406.
88. Zhao Y, Rumold R, Zhu M, et al. An IgG antiprothrombin antibody enhances prothrombin binding to damaged endothelial cells and shortens plasma coagulation times. Arthritis Rheum 1999;42:2132–2138.
89. Mackworth-Young CG. Antiphospholipid syndrome: multiple mechanisms. Clin Exp Immunol 2004;136:393–401.

29 Placental Pathology in Antiphospholipid Syndrome

Ann L. Parke

Introduction

Autoimmune disease, both organ and non–organ specific is associated with increased fetal wastage and/or infertility [1–3]. Fetal wastage was one of the earliest clinical features recognized as part of antiphospholipid syndrome (APS) [4–6] and even though the pathogenesis of APS fetal loss is not completely understood, it appears to be a consequence of placental failure as fetal abnormalities are rarely found. Failure to complete pregnancy successfully is one of several criteria used to define APS [7] .

Both early recurrent and late unexplained pregnancy failure are now recognized as clinical features of APS. Ware Branch has suggested that fetal wastage should be divided into pre-embryonal, embryonal, and fetal (more than 10 weeks' gestation), and has concluded that more than 70% of fetal wastage (more than 10 weeks' gestation) occurs in women with APS [8]. Fetal wastage in normal women who happen to have antibodies to negatively charged phospholipids is about 10% [9], but women with APS can expect a fetal loss rate of 80% [10]. Many of these women will experience recurrent fetal wastage with some of them never successfully completing pregnancy [11]. Other obstetric problems that occur in patients with APS include prematurity and pre-term delivery (less than 36 weeks' gestation) as well as intra-uterine growth restriction (IUGR) and hypertension including pre-eclampsia and toxemia of pregnancy [11–13].

For pregnancy to proceed normally the placenta must be allowed to develop and grow appropriately so that an adequate blood supply is available to support and promote the growth of the developing fetus. Failure of the normal uterine physiological changes to occur and the development of intra-placental pathology will ensure placental insufficiency and the features that accompany a failing placenta, that is, intra-uterine growth retardation, pre-term delivery (prior to 36 weeks' gestation), pre-eclampsia, and toxemia of pregnancy. All of these clinical features occur more frequently in APS than in normal pregnancies [11–13], although a recent study of women with a previous history of pre-eclampsia did not find aPL more frequently in those women who developed recurrent pre-eclampsia in a subsequent pregnancy [14].

These clinical associations as well as the recurrent fetal loss suggest that there may be multiple pathologies that complicate and disrupt pregnancy in patients with phospholipid antibodies. This chapter will describe the known pathological changes that have been described in the placentas of patients with APS, and will discuss the potential mechanisms that may contribute to this pathology.

Antiphospholipid Syndrome

The basic pathological process found in APS is that of a bland thrombosis in both the arterial and venous systems [15]. Even though this syndrome is almost certainly an antibody mediated process, thrombosis is the primary pathology. Animal studies reproducing human disease using passive immunization with aPL-positive immunoglobulin [16, 17] and active immunization with β_2-glycoprotein I [18, 19] suggest that these antibodies are directly involved in the thrombotic process.

The precise pathogenesis of the thrombotic diathesis associated with aPL remains unknown. It is now known that certain proteins are required as co-factors for the binding of antibody to negatively charged phospholipid and that some of these protein co-factors are natural anticoagulants [20, 21] or components of the coagulation cascade [22]. The recognition that some aPL require a protein co-factor to augment binding to phospholipid antibodies has helped explain some features [20–22]. However, as it is apparent that these antibodies are a family of antibodies [23] and that the required proteins can also vary [20–22], it would seem that one explanation for the thrombotic diathesis probably will not suffice. A full discussion of the potential prothrombotic mechanisms in aPL is presented in other chapters in this book and will not be presented here.

Approximately 50% of patients with APS who have experienced a clinical thrombosis will re-thrombose [24, 25], and several retrospective studies have suggested that the only way to prevent re-thrombosis in APS patients is to treat these patients with high dose, life long anticoagulation [25, 26], although a recent study has suggested that international normalized ratios (INRs) less than 3 may be adequate [27]. Some patients have persistent aPL for many years and yet they only develop clinical thrombotic events when they are exposed to certain pathological or physiological events. This has lead to the concept that a "second hit phenomenon" is needed in these patients. We feel that it is extremely important to identify specific known triggers for specific patients (Table 29.1). One of these known triggers is pregnancy and the postpartum period, a complication which makes pregnancy a rather dangerous time for patients with APS. Some patients only thrombose when they are pregnant, or during the postpartum period [29], whereas others will re-thrombose recurrently. Seventy percent of those that re-thrombose do so on the same side of the vascular tree [25, 26].

Table 29.1. Triggers for thrombosis in antiphospholipid antibody syndrome patients.

Pregnancy and postpartum state

Oral contraceptives

Lupus flares in patients who also have SLE

Infection

Elective surgical procedures

Invasive vascular studies, i.e., cardiac catherization

The factors that determine whether women with aPL will have a problem successfully completing pregnancy are not clear. Previous studies have determined that previous fetal losses and aPL predict poor fetal outcome in lupus patients [30]. Our study, which addressed the prevalence of aPL in women with recurrent fetal wastage, normal mothers, and women who had never been pregnant, showed that women with more than 1 positive test for aPL are more likely to experience fetal wastage especially if they have high liters of IgG aCL [31]. Others have shown that antibodies to high levels of IgG aCL and a lupus anticoagulant (LA) are also predictors of problems with pregnancy [13, 32].

Uterine Physiological Changes of Pregnancy

Many physiological changes must occur to allow the fetal semi-allograph to persist and grow [33]. Implantation of the blastocyst begins at the end of the first week and is completed by the end of the second week. Hertig estimated that only 58% of implanted blastocysts survived to the end of the week 2 [34] and spontaneous abortions continue with chromosomal abnormalities accounting for at least 61% of these losses [35].

Part of the implantation process involves syncytiotrophoblast invasion and erosion of maternal endometrial blood vessels, resulting in the development of a utero-placental circulation. Exactly how the invading trophoblast induces these changes in the maternal vasculature is not well understood, but the uterine spiral arteries develop changes in the endothelium with disruption of the smooth muscle layers and endovascular trophoblast can be found in the lumen of these arteries [36, 37]. Ultimately, the trophoblast become incorporated into the wall of the vessel which has now become a thin walled dilated vascular channel that ensures an adequate blood supply for the developing fetus. The lack of muscle in these modified arteries means that these vessels no longer respond to maternal vasoactive stimuli, thereby ensuring a continues blood flow to the fetus [38].

These vascular changes have been termed "physiological change" and "lack of physiological change" or "decidual vasculopathy" has been found to be a significant placental feature in certain diseases, for example, toxemia of pregnancy, intra-uterine growth retardation, pre-eclampsia, and eclampsia [39–41].

Placental Pathology

Placental Pathology in Systemic Lupus Erythematosus

Fetal wastage is increased in patients who have systemic lupus erythematosus (SLE) [42, 43] and it has been determined that disease activity at the time of conception or throughout pregnancy is one of the most important factors contributing to the observed increase in fetal losses [42, 43]. This is so much of a problem that we advise our patients to plan for months ahead prior to conception and prefer that they have an inactive disease for approximately 6 months before attempting to become pregnant. SLE can also flare during pregnancy [44, 45] and it is our policy in SLE patients who become pregnant on anti-malarial drugs, for example, hydroxy-

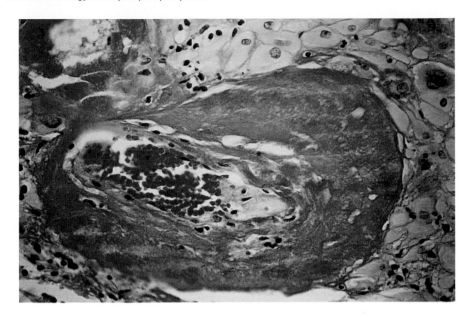

Figure 29.1. Decidual vessel showing fibrinoid necrosis. 📖

chloroquine, to maintain these medications, as it has been determined that stopping anti-malarial drugs can provoke a flare of disease [46, 47] and therefore put the pregnancy at risk.

The pathological changes found in the placenta of SLE patients reflect the inflammation of the underlying disease, with deposition of antibodies and immunoglobulin in various parts of the placenta, including the trophoblast and the trophoblast basement membranes [48]. Lupus placentas are small, and demonstrate placental infarction, decidual vessel thrombosis, atherosis of uterine vessels (Fig. 29.1), chronic villitis and intervillisitis (Fig. 29.2), and lack of physiological change [49, 50]. A prospective study by Hanly et al determined that lupus placentas were smaller than normal and that low placental weight correlated with active SLE, LA, thrombocytopenia, and hypocomplementemia. Fetal loss was not always associated with reduced placental weight, but did correlate with the presence of a circulating anticoagulant [49].

An earlier study by Abramowsky et al demonstrated a vasculopathy in decidual vessels that included fibrinoid necrosis, subintimal edema, necrotic breakdown of the vessel wall, and an infiltrate of cells with foamy cytoplasm, so-called atherosis [50]. Similar changes have been found in the placentas from patients with eclampsia, diabetes, and maternal hypertension [51]. In Abramowsky's study, this decidual vasculopathy correlated with late fetal death [50].

Placental Pathology in APS

Human Studies

Out et al studied placentas from patients who had experienced intra-uterine death, some of whom had APS. These authors determined that in addition to areas of gross

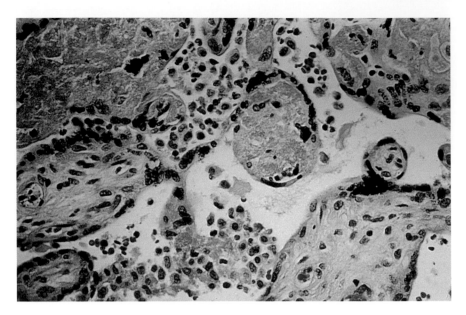

Figure 29.2. Placenta showing villitis and inter-villusitis. 📖

infarction that there was microscopic evidence of extensive villous ischemia in areas of villous parenchyma that did not appear to be grossly infarcted. They also determined that so-called APS placental pathology could be found in patients that did not have APS [52].

A recent study of 39 pregnancies occurring in 28 aPL-positive women determined that excessive perivillous coagulation, avascular terminal villi and chronic villitis, and utero-placental vasculitis were more common in patients with APS that were being treated compared to patients who just had aPL antibodies but did not have APS [53]. Multi-focal utero-placental thromboses were a significant feature in both treated and untreated patients with APS [53–55].

In those SLE patients who also have APS, thrombosis and placental infarction may be very extensive. This combination of inflammatory and thrombotic pathologies contributes to the spectrum of obstetric problems seen in these patients including pre-term birth, intra-uterine growth restriction, fetal wastage, and pre-eclampsia [11–13].

University of Connecticut Experience

At the University of Connecticut Health Center, it has been our policy to examine all placentas obtained from patients with SLE and patients with APS, and in multi-parous patients to obtain the placentas from previous pregnancies. This practice has given us vital information that has been used to determine treatment regimes in subsequent pregnancies.

In order to examine these placentas, we have divided placental pathology into 3 main categories [56].

1. Coagulation abnormalities: This category includes evidence of utero-placental vascular thrombosis, excessive perivillous deposition of fibrin, and intra-placental thrombosis in chorionic or fetal stem vessels.
2. Utero-placental vascular pathology and secondary villous damage: This category includes lack of physiological change in the spiral vessels, fibrinoid necrosis, and atherosis of the decidual vessels as well as utero-placental vasculitis. Lesions considered to be a consequence of utero-placental vascular pathology include abruption and infarction, fibrosis, and hypovascularity of villi. Also included are syncytiotrophoblast knotting and cytotrophoblast proliferation.
3. Intra-placental vascular lesions including either thrombotic, vasculitic, atrophic, or hyperplastic lesions in the chorionic vessels, fetal stem vessels, and the capillaries of the terminal villi.

Using these pathological categories we concluded that:

1. Thrombosis and infarction occur frequently in patients with APS (Fig. 29.3).
2. Treatment with anticoagulants, anti-inflammatory agents, and other therapeutic agents was not able to completely prevent pathological changes in patients with APS.
3. The pathological changes identified in one pregnancy generally would be repeated in subsequent pregnancies in these patients with APS.
4. Some aPL patients who do not meet criteria for SLE also have placental vasculitis as well as the more usual thrombotic pathology associated with APS.

These findings suggest that even in treated APS patients who successfully complete pregnancy, the pregnancies are still abnormal as indicated by the persistence of pathological changes found in these placentas. It is our impression that even though these treated pregnancies may result in a live infant, the pathological

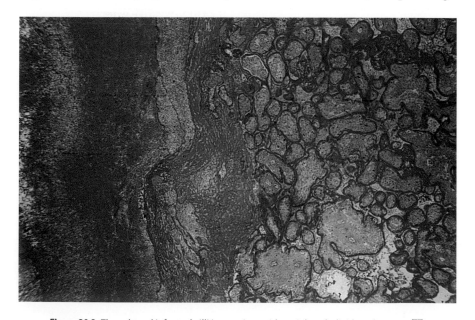

Figure 29.3. Thrombosed infracted villi in a patient with antiphospholipid syndrome. 📖

processes are slowed down so that gestation can progress to the point where a viable baby may be obtained. These placental studies also demonstrate the need for examination of previous placentas in these aPL patients as the original pathological changes will be repeated in subsequent pregnancies, and suggest that in some patients anticoagulation alone may be insufficient therapy to ensure a successful pregnancy.

Potential Mechanisms for APS Placental Pathology

Defective Placentation

β_2-glycoprotein I (apolipoprotein H) is the most studied of the protein co-factors. This protein is a natural anticoagulant that inhibits platelet aggregation and inhibits protein S binding to its binding protein C4Bp [57]. Several authors have suggested that abnormalities of the protein C and protein S anticoagulant system may contribute to the thrombotic diathesis known to be associated with aPL [58, 59]. In our report we determined that some aPL patients have low levels of free protein S that was not a consequence of antibodies to protein S or its binding protein [58]. These low levels fell even further when patients became pregnant, a possible explanation for the association of thrombosis with pregnancy that is well described in aPL patients.

β_2-glycoprotein I binds to endothelial cells and therefore may modulate endothelial cell function [60]. A recent study has shown that aPL can activate endothelial cells by binding to β_2-glycoprotein I expressed on endothelial cell membrane [61]. Previous studies have demonstrated that sera from APS patients can modulate prostacyclin production from endothelial cells [62, 63] and others have suggested a cross-reactivity between aPL and anti-endothlial cell antibodies [64, 65]. Anti–β_2-glycoprotein I antibodies have been demonstrated to react with trophoblast cell membranes and endothelial cell membranes in the placental villi of placentas from aPL patients [66, 67].

Recent studies have confirmed these findings and have demonstrated that aPL, both β_2-glycoprotein I 1–dependent and β_2 –glycoprotein I 2–independent, will bind to trophoblast [68]. This binding increased with time and became maximal after 72 hours of incubation at a time when syncytium formation is occurring and exposure of phosphatidyl serine increased. aPL binding also inhibited trophoblast invasiveness, measured using a Matrigel invasion assay, and reduced production of human chorionic gonadotropin (HCG) from the cultured trophoblast cells [68]. Previous studies had also demonstrated that affinity purified aPL could bind to normal term placenta in a variety of places including trophoblast micro villous surface and stromal and peri-vascular regions, and bind to a variety of placental proteins [69]. HCG release from cultured trophoblast cells, in response to gonadotrophin releasing hormone (GnRH), is impaired in the presence of aPL sera [70] and other in vitro studies have reported that aPL may affect cytotrophoblast by impairing fusion to syncytical cells [71]. All of this work would suggest that aPL can directly affect placental development demonstrating that defective placentation as well as placental thrombosis and infarction may contribute to the fetal wastage seen in patients with APS.

Annexins

Annexins are a family of proteins and have been determined to have a variety of origins and a variety of functions and previous studies have demonstrated that many members of this family inhibit phospholipase A2 and influence coagulation pathways [72]. Annexin V is also known as a placental anticoagulant protein 1. This annexin is also found in blood vessels, but is present in greatest amounts in the placenta [73, 74].

Annexin V avidly binds to anionic phospholipids and thereby interferes with the formation of thrombin by preventing the binding of activated Xa and prothombin [75, 76]. Some studies have shown that annexin V and aPL compete for phospholipid binding [77, 78], and it has been proposed that this could be a mechanism that contributes to placental failure in patients with aPL.

In normal pregnancy, large amounts of annexin V are expressed on the apical surfaces of micro villi of syncytotrophoblasts [79], probably in response to the phosphatidyl serine that is also expressed on these apical membranes. Annexin V clusters on exposed phospholipid [80] and forms a crystalline array, like a protective shield, over the exposed phospholipids [81, 82] and in this manner annexin V protects these surfaces from normal coagulation processes. Annexin V is required to maintain placental integrity in the mouse model, and treatment with annexin V antibodies results in placental infarction and fetal wastage [83].

Rand et al postulated that as aPL and annexin compete for binding to phospholipids, the presence of aPL could lead to disruption and displacement of the protective annexin V shield [84]. These authors in fact have demonstrated that the amount of annexin V expressed on apical membranes of syncytiotrophoblasts is reduced in placentas from APS patients compared to normal placentas [85] . In vitro co-culturing of placental villi from normal pregnancies with IgG fractions from APS patients, aPL IgG, or monoclonal aPL antibodies resulted in a reduced expression of annexin V on these normal placental villi [86].

Complement Activation

There is now evidence that complement activation contributes to aPL pregnancy failure. Previous observations have show that mice deficient in Crry, a complement regulatory protein that blocks activation of C3 and C4 [87], fail to complete pregnancy successfully [88]. The Crry –/– embryos are surrounded by activated C3 fragments and polymorpho nuclear leukocytes. Additional proof that this fetal wastage is due to complement activation is provided by the observation that in Crry–/–C3–/– hybrid strains complete pregnancy successfully [88]. To demonstrate that complement activation contributes to aPL fetal wastage, Holers et al produced a murine model of aPL induced pregnancy loss by injecting pregnant mice with human IgG that contained aPL. Pregnancy loss in this mouse model was prevented by a Crry–Ig, a C3 convertase inhibitor that blocks activation of C3 by both classical and alternate pathways [89]. Additional experiments revealed that aPL injected into complement deficient pregnant mice did not produce the same fetal wastage that occurred in normal mice injected with human aPL. Placental studies have revealed focal necrosis, inflammation, C3, and human IgG deposition in aPL treated mice which was not found in mice that also received that Crry–Ig [89].

Complement activation usually results in inflammation and, as the thrombotic diatheses found in aPL syndrome is typically a blood non-inflammatory thrombosis, it suggests that the complement activation is responsible for pregnancy failure by promoting other pathological changes.

Summary

It has become increasingly evident that there are a multitude of mechanisms whereby aPL can prevent normal placental development and can cause significant placental pathology. Placental thrombosis and infarction is only part of the story. Analyzing previous placentas has been helpful as patients appear to repeat the same pathological process in subsequent pregnancies, making it possible to tailor make a therapeutic regime for individual patients. Only those patients that demonstrate significant inflammation should be exposed to corticosteroids, particularly as our studies demonstrated the most significant change in placental pathology occurred in patients who had had active SLE in one pregnancy and inactive SLE in a subsequent pregnancy [54]. Anticoagulation does help some aPL patients successfully complete pregnancy [90, 91], and should be used in any aPL patient that has sustained a late fetal loss, that is, more than 10 weeks' gestation, and who wishes to attempt another pregnancy, but it is evident that some patients still do not successfully complete pregnancy even when fully anticoagulated throughout pregnancy. We use hydroxychloroquine in some of these patients hoping for the additive benefit of its antiplatelet effects as well as its anti-inflammatory properties.

Unfortunately it is still impossible to predict which patients will develop problems unless they have failed previous pregnancies [30]. We have seen patients with consistently high titers of IgG aPL who successfully completed every pregnancy and never developed a clinical thrombosis, failing to make criteria for APS. With the recent realization that some APS patients may be "sero-negative" and not produce the usual spectrum of aPL laboratory tests but complain of the usual aPL clinical complaints [92], the situation becomes even more complicated.

References

1. Roussex RG, Kaider BD, Price DE, et al. Laboratory evaluation of women experiencing reproductive failure. Am J Reprod Immunol 1996;35:415–420.
2. Fraga M, Mintz G, Orozeo J, et al. Sterility and fertility rates, fetal wastage and maternal morbidity in SLE. J Rheumatol 1974;1:293–298.
3. Kaplan J. Fetal wastage in patients with rheumatoid arthritis. J Rheumatol 1986:13:875–877.
4. Alarcon-Segovia D, Perez-Vasquez ME, Villa AR, et al. Preliminary classification criteria for the antiphospholipid syndrome within systemic lupus erythematosus. Semin Arthritis Rheum 1992;21:275–285.
5. Asherson RA, Cervera R, Piette C, Shoenfeld Y. The antiphospholipid syndrome: history, definition, classification, and differential diagnosis. In: The antiphospholipid syndrome. 1996:3–12.
6. Nilsson IM, Astedt B, Hedner U, et al. Intrauterine death and circulating anticoagulant "antithromboplastin." Act Med Scand 1975;197:153–159.
7. Wilson A, Gharavi AE, Koike T, et al. International consensus statement on preliminary classification criteria for definite antiphospholipid syndrome. Arthritis Rheum 1999;42:1309–1311.
8. Branch WD. Thoughts on the mechanism of pregnancy loss associated with antiphospholipid syndrome. Lupus 1994;3:275–280.

9. Harris EN, Spinnato JA. Should anticardiolipin tests be performed in otherwise healthy pregnant women? Am J Obstet Gynecol 1991;165:1272–1277.

10. Perez MC, Wilson WA, Brown HL, et al. Anticardiolipin antibodies in unselected pregnant women in relationship to fetal outcome. J Perinatol 1991;11:33–36.

11. Branch DW, Silver RM, Blackwell JC, et al. Outcomes of treated pregnancies in women with antiphospholipid syndrome: an update of the Utah experience. Obstet Gynecol 1992;80:614–620.

12. Lubbe WF, Butler WS, Palmer SJ, et al. Fetal survival after prednisone suppression of maternal lupus anticoagulant. Lancet 1983;1361–1363.

13. Out H, Bruinse HW, Christiaens GCML, et al. A prospective controlled multicenter study on the obstetric risks of pregnant women with antiphospholipid antibodies. Am J Obstet Gynecol 1992;167:26–32.

14. Branch DW, Porter TF, Rittenhouse L, et al. Antiphospholipid antibodies in women at risk for preeclampsia Am J Obstet Gynecol 2001;184:823–834.

15. Lie JT. Vasculitis in the antiphospholipid syndrome: culprit or consort? J Rheumatol 1994;21:397–399.

16. Branch DW, Dudley DJ, Mitchell MD, et al. Immunoglobulin G factions from patients with antiphospholipid antibodies cause fetal death in BALB/c mice: a model for autoimmune fetal loss. Am J Obstet Gynecol 1990;163:210–216.

17. Blank M, Cohen J, Toder V, et al. Induction of antiphospholipid syndrome by passive transfer of anticardiolipin antibodies. Proc Nat Acad Sci U S A 1991;88:3069–3073.

18. Gharavi AE, Sammaritano LR, Wen J, et al. Induction of antiphospholipid autoantibodies by immunization with B2 glycoprotein I (apolipoprotein H). J Clin Invest 1992;90:1105–1109.

19. Blank M, Faden D, Tincani A, et al. Immunization with anticardiolipin cofactor (beta 2-glycoprotein I) induces experimental antiphospholipid syndrome in naive mice. J Autoimmunity 1994;7:441–445.

20. McNeil HD, Simpson RJ, Chesterman CN, et al. Antiphospholipid antibodies are directed against a complex antigen that included a lipid-binding inhibitor of coagulation: beta-2- glucoprotein I (apolipoprotein H). Proc Nati Acad Sci U S A 1990;87:4120–4124.

21. Galli M, Confurius P, Massau C, et al. Anticardiolipin antibodies (ACA) directed not to cardiolipin but to a plasma protein cofactor. Lancet 1990;335:1544–1547.

22. Galli M, Barbui T. Prothrombin as cofactor for antiphospholipids. Lupus 1998;7(suppl 2):S37–S40.

23. Parke A, Maier D, Hakim C, et al. Subclinical autoimmune disease and recurrent spontaneous abortion. J Rheumatol 1986;13:1178–1160.

24. McNeil HP, Hunt JE, Krilis SA. Antiphospholipid antibodies – new insights into their specificity and clinical importance. Scand J Immunol 1992;36:647–652.

25. Khamashta M, et al. The management of thrombosis in the antiphospholipid antibody syndrome. N Engl J Med 1995;332:993–997.

26. Rosove MH, Brewer P. Antiphospholipid thrombosis: clinical course after the first thrombotic event in 70 patients. Ann Intern Med 1992;17:303–308.

27. Crowther MA, Ginsberg JS, Julian J, et al. A Comparison of two intensities of warfarin for the prevention of recurrent thrombosis in patients with antiphospholipid antibody syndrome. N Engl J Med 2003;349;1133 1138.

28. Lockshin MD. New perspectives in the study and treatment of antiphospholipid syndrome. In: The antiphospholipid syndrome. Boca Raton, FL: CRC Press; 1996:323–329.

29. Parke AL. Antiphospholipid antibody syndromes. Rheum Dis Clin North Am 1989;15:275.

30. Ramsey-Goldman R, Kutzer JE, Kuller LH, et al. Previous pregnancy outcome is an important determinant of subsequent pregnancy outcome in women with systemic lupus erythematosus. Am J Reprod Immunol 1992;28:195–198.

31. Parke AL, Wilson D, Maier D. The prevalence of antiphospholipid antibodies in habitual aborters compared to normal women and women who have never been pregnant. Arthritis Rheum 1991;34:1231–1235.

32. Maclean MA, et al. The prevalence of lupus anticoagulant and anticardiolipin antibodies in women with a history of first trimester miscarriages. Br J Obstet Gynecol 1994;101:103–106.

33. Panigel M. Anatomy and morphology clinic in obstetrics and gynecology. In: The human placenta. 1986:421.

34. Hertig AT. The overall problem in man. In: Benirschke K, ed. Comparative aspects of reproductive failure. New York: Springer-Verlag; 1986.

35. Boue J, Boue A, Lazar P. Retrospective and prospective epidemiological studies of 1500 karyotyped spontaneous abortions Teratology 1975;12:11.

36. Kam EPY, Gardner L, Loke YW, et al. The role of trophoblast in the physiological change in decidual spiral arteries. Human Reprod 1999;14:2131–2138.

37. Pijnenborg R, Trophoblast invasion and placentation in the human; morphological aspects. Trophoblast Res 1990;4:33–47.
38. Moll W, Kunzel W, Herberger J. Hemodynamic implications of hemochorial placentation. Eur J Obstet Gynecol Biol 1975;5:67–74.
39. Brosens I, Robertson WB, Dixon HG. The role of the spiral arteries in the pathogenesis of preeclampsia. Obstet Gynecol A 1972;1:177–191.
40 Pijnenborg R, Bland JM, Robertson WB. The pattern of interstitial trophoblastic invasion of the myometrium in early human pregnancy. Placenta 1981;2:303–315.
41 Pijnenborg R, Anthony J, Davey DA, et al. Placental bed spiral arteries in the hypertensive disorders of pregnancy. Br J Obstet Gynaecol 1991;98:648–655.
42. Zurier RB, et al. Systemic lupus erythematosus: management during pregnancy. Obstet Gynecol 1978;51:178–180.
43. Mintz G, et al. Prospective study of pregnancy in systemic lupus erythematosus: results of a multi-disciplinary approach. J Rheumatol 1986;13:732–739.
44. Petri M, Howard D, Repke J. Frequency of lupus flare in pregnancy. Arthritis Rheum 1991;34:1538–1545.
45. Hayslett JP. Effect of pregnancy in patients with SLE. Am J Kidney Dis 1982;2:223–228.
46. Rudnicki RD, Gresham GE, Rothfield NF. The efficacy of antimalarials in systemic lupus erythematosus. J Rheumatol 1975;2:323–330.
47. The Canadian Hydroxychloroquine Study Group. A randomized study of the effect of withdrawing hydroxychloroquine sulfate in systemic lupus erythematosus. N Engl J Med 1991; 342:150–154.
48. Grennan DM, et al. Immunological studies of the placenta in systemic lupus erythematosis. Ann Rheum Dis 1978;37:129–134.
49. Hanly JG, Gladman DD, Rose TH, et al. Lupus pregnancy, a prospective study of placental changes. Arthritis Rheum 1998;31:358–366.
50. Abramowsky CR, Vegas ME, Swinehart G, et al. Decidual vasculopathy of the placenta in systemic lupus erythematosus. N Engl J Med 1980:303:668–670.
51. Khong TY, Pearce JM, Robertson WB. Acute atherosis in preeclampsia: maternal determinants and fetal outcome in the presence of the lesions. Am J Obstet Gynecol 1987;157:360.
52. Out HJ, Kooijman CD, Bruinse HW, et al. Histopathological findings in placentas from patients with intrauterine fetal death and antiphospholipid antibodies. Eur J Obstet Gynecol Reprod Biol 1991;41:179.
53. Salafia CM, Cowchock FS. Placental pathology and antiphospholipid: a descriptive study. Am J Perinatol 1997;14:435–441.
54. Salafia CM, Parke AL. Placental pathology in systemic lupus erythematosus and phospholipid antibody syndrome. Clin Rheum Dis 1997;23:85–97.
55. Rosove MH, Tabsh K, Wasserstrum N, et al. Heparin therapy for pregnant women with lupus anticoagulant or anticardiolipin antibodies. Obstet Gynecol 1990;75:660–634.
56. Lowell DM, Kaplan C, Salafia CM, College of American Pathologists Conference XIX on the Examination of the Placenta. Report on the working group on the definition of structural changes associated with abnormal function in the maternal/fetal/placental unit in the second and third trimester. Arch Path Lab Med 1991;1:647.
57. Schousboe I. B2 glycoprotein-1: a plasma inhibitor of the contact activation of the intrinsic blood coagulation pathway. Blood 1985;66:1086–1091.
58. Parke AL, Weinstein RE, Bona RD, et al. The thrombotic diathesis associated with the presence of phospholipid antibodies may be due to low levels of free protein S. Am J Med 1992;93:49–56.
59. Atsumi T, Khamasta MA, Ames PR, et al. Effect of ft glycoprotein-1 and human monoclonal anti-cardiolipin antibody on the protein-S/C4b-binding protein system. Lupus 1997;6:358–364.
60. Meroni PL, Del Papa N, Beltrami B, et al. Modulation of endothelial cell function by antiphospholipid antibodies. Lupus 1996:5:448–450.
61. Meroni PL, Raschi E, Camera M, et al. Endothelial activation by aPL: a potential pathogenetic mechanism for the clinical manifestations of the syndrome. J Autoimmun 2000;15:337–340.
62. Carreras LO, Defreyn G, Machin SJ, et al. Arterial thrombosis, intrauterine death and "lupus" anticoagulant: detection of immunoglobulin interfering with prostacyclin formation. Lancet 1981;i:244–246.
63. Carreras LO, Vermylen J. Lupus anticoagulant and thrombosis. Possible role of inhibition of prostacyclin formation. Thromb Haemost 1982;48:38–40.
64. Del Papa N, et al. Endothelial cells as a target for antiphospholipid antibodies; role of anti B2 glycoprotein-1 antibodies. Am J Reprod Immunol 1997;38:212–217.

65. Del Papa N, et al. Relationship between antiphospholipid and antiendothelial antibodies III: B2 gly-coprotein-1 mediates the antibody binding to endothelial membranes and induces the expression of adhesion molecules. Clin Exp Rheumatol 1995;13:179–186.
66. McIntyre JA. Immune recognition at the maternal-fetal interface: overview. Am J Reprod Immunol 1992;28:127–131.
67. La Rosa, et al. β2 Glycoprotein-1 and placental anticoagulant protein-1 in placentae from patients with antiphospholipid syndrome. J Rheumatol 1994;21:1684–1698.
68. Di Simone N, Del Papa N, Raschi E, et al. Antiphospholipid antibodies affect trophoblast gonadotropin secretion and invasiveness by binding directly and through adhered B2-glycoprotein 1. Arthritis Rheum 2000;42:140–150.
69. Donohoe S, Kingdom JCP, Mackie IJ. Affinity purified human antiphospholipid antibodies bind normal term placenta. Lupus 1999;8:525–531.
70. Di Simone N, De Carolis S, Lanzone, et al. In vitro effect of antiphospholipid antibody-containing sera on basal and gonadotrophin releasing hormone dependent human chorionic gonadotrophin release by cultured trophoblast cells. Placenta 1995;16:75–83.
71. Katsuragawa H, Rote NS, Inoue T, et al. Monoclonal antiphosphatidylserine antibody reactivity against human first-trimester placental trophoblasts Am J Obstet Gynecol. 1995;172:1592.
72. Rand JH. "Annexinopathies" – a new class of diseases. N Eng J Med 1999;340:1035–1036.
73. Reutelingsperger CP, Kop JM, Hornstra G, et al. Purification and characterization of a novel protein from bovine aorta that inhibits coagulation. Inhibition of the phospholipid-dependent factor Xa cat-alyzed prothrombin activation, through a high-affinity binding of the anticoagulant to the phospho-lipids. Eur J Biochem 1988;173:171–178.
74. Tait JF, Sakata M, McMullen BA, et al. Placental anticogulant proteins isolation and comparative characterization of four members of the lipocortin family. Biochemistry 1988;27:6268–6276.
75. Tait JF, Gibson D, Kujikawa D. Phospholipid binding properties of human placental anticoagulant protein I, a member of the lipocortin family. Biol Chem 1989;264:7944–7949.
76. Conodo S, Naguchi M, Funakoshi T, et al. Inhibition of human factor VIIa tissue factor activity by placental anticoagulant protein. Thromb Res 1987;48:449–459.
77. Sammaritano LR, Gharavi AE, Soberano C, et al. Phospholipid binding of antiphospholipid antibod-ies and placental anticoagulant protein J Clin Immun 1992;12:27–35.
78. Calandri C, Rand JH, Anticardiolipin antibodies block placental anticoagulant protein activity. Clin Res 1990;38:427.
79. Lockwood CJ, Rand JII, The immunobiology and obstetrical consequences of antiphospholipid anti-bodies. Obstet Gynecol Surv 1994;49:432–441.
80. Andree HAM, Hermens WT, Hemker HC, et al. Displacement of factor Va by annexin V. In: Andree, ed. Phospholipid binding and anticoagulant action of Aanexin VHAM. Maastricht, The Netherlands: Universitaire Pers Maastricht; 1992:73–85.
81. Voges d, Berendes R, Burger A, et al. Three dimensional structure of membrane bound annexin V. A correlative electron microscopy X ray crystallography study. J Mol Biol 1994;238:199–213.
82. Mosser G, Ravanat C, Freyssinet JM, et al. Sub domain structure of lipid bound annexin V resolved by electron image analysis. J Mol Biol 1991;217:241–245.
83. Wang X, Campos B, Kaetzel MA, et al. Annexin V is critical in the maintenance of murine placental integrity. Am J Obstet Gynecol 1999;108;1008–1016.
84. Rand JH. Antiphospholipid antibody mediated disruption of the annexin V antithrombotic shield: a thrombotic genie mechanism of antiphospholipid syndrome. J Autoimmun 2000;15:107–113.
85. Rand JH, et al. Reduction of annexin-V (placental anticoagulant protein-I) on placental villi of women with antiphospholipid antibodies and recurrent spontaneous abortion. Am J Obstet Gynecol 1994;171:1566–1572.
86. Rand JH, Wu XX, Guller S, et al. Antiphospholipid immunoglobulin G antibodies reduce annexin-V levels on syncytiotrophoblast apical membranes and in culture media of placental villi. Am J Obstet Gynecol 1997;177:918–920.
87. Rehrig S, Fleming SD, Anderson J, et al. Complement inhibitor, complement receptor 1 related gene/protein y-lg attenuates intestinal damage after the onset of mesenleric ischemia/reperfusion injury in mice. J Immunol 2001;167:5921–5927.
88. Xu C, Mao D, Holers VM, et al. A critical role for the murine complement regulator Crry in fetal maternal tolerance. Science 2000;287:498–501.
89. Holers VM, Girardi G, Mo L, et al. Complement C3 activation is required for antiphospholipid anti-body induced fetal loss. J Exp Med 2002;178:66–76.

90. Rai R, Cohen H, Dave M, et al. Randomized controlled trial of aspirin and aspirin plus heparin in pregnant women with recurrent miscarriage associated with phospholipid antibodies (or antiphospholipid antibodies). Br Med J 1997;314:253–257.
91. Kutteh MD. Antiphospholipid antibody-associated recurrent pregnancy loss: treatment with heparin and low-dose aspirin is superior to low-dose aspirin alone. Am J Obstet Gynecol 1996;174:1584–1589.
92. Hughes GVR, Khamashta MA. Seronegative antiphopholipid syndrome. Ann Rheum Dis 2003;62:1127.

30 Antiphospholipid Syndrome – Experimental Models: Insight into Etiology, Pathogenesis, and Treatments

Miri Blank, Ilan Krause, and Yehuda Shoenfeld

Classical antiphospholipid syndrome (APS) – Hughes syndrome – is characterized by the presence of antiphospholipid antibodies (aPL) which bind phospholipid target molecules mainly *via* β_2-glycoprotein I (β_2-GPI), and/or lupus anticoagulant (LA) associated with recurrent fetal loss, thromboembolic phenomena, and thrombocytopenia [1–4]. Recently, accumulated evidence suggest that APS is a *systemic* autoimmune disease, associated not exclusively with coagulation failure or recurrent fetal loss but with many diverse clinical manifestations involving different organs such as the heart, the brain, the adrenal, and the skin [4–6]. Several animal models of APS have been used to address the mechanisms involved in the pathogenesis, etiology, and novel treatments. The animal models resembling APS manifestations entail: (1) MRL/lpr [7, 8] or (NZWxBxSB)F1 mice [9] which develop APS features on a genetic background; (2) passive transfer of aPL intravenously [10–13], intraperitoneally [13], or intrathecally into naive mice [14]; (3) Active immunization with aPL by idiotypic manipulation (e.g., a model based on Jerne's theory of the idiotypic network [15, 16]. Immunization of naive mice with an autoantibody (Ab1) results in generation of anti-idiotypic antibody (i.e., Ab2) followed by generation of mouse-anti-anti-idiotipic antibodies (i.e., Ab3). Ab3 may simulate Ab1 in its biological properties. The generation of Ab3 is followed by the emergence of the full-blown serological, immunohistochemical, and clinical manifestations of the respective autoimmune disease [17–20]; (4) immunization of naive mice with the autoantigen such as β_2-GPI or its synthetic derivatives [8, 21]; (5) β_2-GPI knockout mice [22]; (6) mice deficient in complement C3 [12], ICAM-I, P-selectin [23], E-selectin [24], apo-E [25], low-density lipoprotein (LDL)-receptor knockout mice [26], and SCID mice [27].

Based on studies conducted in these APS animal models, in the current chapter we will address the following topics: Reproductive failure caused by diverse autoantibodies such as direct binding aPL [e.g., cardiolipin (CL), phosphatidylserine ((PS), antibodies directed to β_2-GPI, β_2-GPI/PL, annexin V, and prothrombin]. Therapeutic approaches and mechanisms involving in modulating fetal loss in APS experimental models will be presented as well [7–55]; thrombosis caused by aPL or anti-prothrombin and its immunomodulation [55–63]; the origin of aPL and the infectious etiology of APS [64–74]; aPL involvement in the pathogenesis of brain heart and kidney [75–88]; athrosclerosisi and aPL [89–93].

Reproductive Failure and Experimental APS

An experimental model of APS was induced in naive mice by passive transfer of human polyclonal IgG fraction derived from a patient with primary APS, or a mouse aCL/β_2-GPI dependent monoclonal antibodies (mAbs) [10, 28]. The aCL/β_2-GPI were injected at different stages of pregnancy, resulting in lower fecundity rate, increased absorption index of embryos (the equivalent of human fetal loss), lower number of embryos per pregnancy, and lower mean weights of embryos and placenta. The above findings were accompanied by a prolonged activated partial thromboplastin time (aPTT) and thrombocytopenia [10, 28]. The passive transfer model was confirmed by other groups addressing different pathogenic properties of aPL such as mouse decidual necrosis [11] or placental thrombosis associated with the fetal loss [12].

Induction of mouse anti-β_2-GPI by immunization with β_2-GPI [8, 21] or by idiotypic manipulation [17–20], resulted in elevated percentage of fetal resorption, deposition of anti–CL/β_2-GPI on the affected placenta and the other experimental APS findings as described for passive transfer [10, 28].

The importance of the β_2-GPI molecule in supporting the outcome of normal pregnancy was shown previously by oral tolerance induction to β_2-GPI resulting in prevention of fetal loss [29] and recently in β_2-GPI knock out mice [22, 30]. In a serial of studies, Krilis et al [22, 30], showed the physiological requirement for functional β_2-GPI in pregnancy by evaluating reproductive outcomes in β_2-GPI–deficient mice. The study showed that although mice lacking β_2-GPI are fertile, functional β_2-GPI is essential for optimal implantation and placental morphogenesis [22, 30].

We investigated the pathogenic part in the aCL/β_2-GPI immunoglobulins responsible for the elevated fetal loss in naive mice [31]. In the past, we were able to isolate mouse monoclonal pathogenic aCL/β_2-GPI which cause reproductive failure and aCL/β_2-GPI mAbs which were not related to fetal loss from experimental APS and lupus models [18]. In order to clarify which part of the aCL/β_2-GPI Ig molecule has the pathogenic potential, we constructed and expressed several single chain Fv (scFv) of aCL/β_2-GPI, exchanging heavy and light chains between the Ig which caused fetal loss and the Ig which was not associated with reproductive failure [31]. All the expressed scFv$_s$ showed the same antigen binding properties as the original mAbs. Replacement of the fetal loss related Ig VH domain, with the non–fetal loss related VH, decreased the binding and avidity of the scFv to CL/β_2-GPI and completely abrogated the anticoagulant activity. Exchanging the pathogenic aCL/β_2-GPI VH with anti-DNA VH resulted in a shift from aCL/β_2-GPI to anti-DNA binding of the scFv. Replacement of the pathogenic aCL/β_2-GPI VL with a non-pathogenic VL, did not affect the avidity of the scFv for CL/β_2-GPI nor its anticoagulant activity. BALB/c mice were immunized with either aCL/β_2-GPI scFv$_s$, or scFv resulting from the replacement of the heavy and the light chains. The mice which were immunized with scFv$_s$ developed the same clinical manifestations, as the mice immunized with the original mAbs (elevated titers of mouse aCL/β_2-GPI , associated with LA activity, thrombocytopenia, and high percentage of fetal resorptions). Immunization with a non-pathogenic aCL/β_2-GPI–scFv did not lead to any clinical findings. Replacement of heavy/light chains between the pathogenic fetal loss related and non-fetal loss related Abs point to the importance of the heavy chain variable domains in the pathogenic potential of aCL/β_2-GPI associated with fetal loss [31].

The mechanism of pathogenicity provoked by anti–β_2-GPI was further analyzed in vivo by Salmon et al [12, 32], proposing the requirement of Complement C3 activation. Employing the anti–β_2-GPI passive transfer model, and the C3 complement deficiency mice, they proved that anti–β_2-GPI activate complement in the placenta, generating split products that mediate placental injury and lead to fetal loss and growth retardation [12, 32]. This group found that inhibition of the complement cascade in vivo, using the C3-convertase inhibitor complement receptor 1–related gene/protein y(Crry)-Ig, blocks fetal loss and growth retardation. Furthermore, mice deficient in complement C3 were resistant to fetal injury induced by anti–β_2-GPI. The data showed that the complement inhibitor Crry-Ig protects mice from the effects of human anti–β_2-GPI. The author suggest that in vivo complement activation is required for anti–β_2-GPI antibody–induced fetal loss and growth retardation.

Recently, anti–β_2-GPI with prothrombotic properties induced intrauterine death in naive mice put forward the thrombogenic mechanism as additional explanation for reproductive failure in experimental APS [33].

Although aCL/β_2-GPI was extensively studied in the context of fetal loss in different APS experimental models, other aPL were addressed as well.

A significantly higher rate of fetal resorptions and a reduction in fetal and placental weight associated with placental necrosis was shown also in naive mice infused with β_2-GPI–independent human aCL IgG mAbs [34].

Normally, the cell membrane bilayer is asymmetric with anionic phospholipids, particularly phosphatidylserine (PS), being sequestered in the inner leaflet through the action of aminophospholipid translocase. The presence of PS in the outer leaflet of the membrane occurs in 2 major instances: (a) During the early stage of the apoptosis process a disruption of lipid asymmetry leads to exposure of PS on the outer surface of the plasma membrane; (b) Placental trophoblast is the main organ in which PS is highly exposed on the outer leaflet of the membrane. The PS is a pregnancy supportive molecule, expressed on the trophoblast surface during differentiation and invasion of the extracellular matrix [35]. aPS either passively infused [36] or induced in naive mice by idiotypic manipulation [37], resulted in elevated levels of fetal resorptions, thrombocytopenia, and prolonged coagulation time.

During embryonic and placental differentiation, a disruption of the lipid asymmetry occurs, leading to exposure of PS on the outer surface during the apoptotic processes accompanying the trophoblast differentiation. Blockage of PS by hinders syncytium formation, thus enforcing apoptosis [38].

Evidence suggests that aPS are particularly pathogenic to the trophoblast. This pathogenicity could be explained by more than one mechanism, for example: (a) Shading the PS on the trophoblast cells interferes with signaling which leads to reduction in hCG production and invasion of the extracellular matrix to form the syncytiotrophoblast [39]; (b) Prevention of annexin V binding to PS which was shown to restrict intra-uterine growth [40]. As was demonstrated in vitro in a choriocarcinoma model of trophoblast differentiation, this annexin V removal can facilitate the binding of prothrombin to the trophoblast surface and increase thrombosis at the maternal–fetal interface [41].

Exposure of first trimester rat embryos to aPS mAbs in an ex vivo system caused enhanced apoptotic processes in the yolk sac, resulting in inhibition of the yolk sac growth and increase in apoptotic events of giant cells in the ectoplacental cone [42]. In vitro studies on the direct effect of aPS on human placenta showed that aPL, which are β_2-GPI–independent, or directed against β_2-GPI, decreased gonadotropin secretion and the invasiveness of the trophoblast cells to the substrate in an ex vivo human placental model [43]. Other studies have shown a strong cytotoxic reaction against mouse trophoblast upon exposure to sera of women with recurrent spontaneous abortions that have high titers of aPS [43]. Moreover, aPS was shown to be one of the main causes for implantation failure [44].

Annexin V (36 kD) is a calcium-dependent phosphatydilserine binding protein that exhibits anticoagulant activity on binding to PS exposed on the activated surfaces of endothelial cells and platelets. It inhibits the activation of factor X and prothrombin in the blood coagulation cascade. When PS is exposed on the surfaces of endothelial cells and platelets, annexin V is thought to prevent concentration of coagulant factors in PS-rich domains on cell surfaces and to amplify the coagulation response. The placenta is rich with annexin V (250 mg/10 kg placenta). Annexin V is localized on the microvillous surface of the syncytiotrophoblast because it binds to the PS expressed on the external layer of the trophoblast plasma membrane. The binding of annexin V to PS was postulated to protect the integrity of the placenta by creating the antithrombotic shield. Annexin V is decreased on placental trophoblasts and on endothelial cells in APS associated with pregnancy loss and with thrombosis [45]. The presence of pathogenic IgG anti-annexin V/PS is a risk factor for reproductive failures associated with early pregnancy loss or implantation failures [46].

A direct proof for the pathogenicity of anti–annexin V Abs came from studies in which anti–annexin V antibodies infusion caused fetal loss and placental thrombosis in the pregnant BALB/c mice [47]. Focal necrosis and fibrosis were present in the decidua of placentas from embryos that were significantly smaller than the normal embryos in the same uterus. Thus, replacing annexin V by aPS Abs for binding the phospholipid membranes, or neutralization of annexin V by anti–annexin V Abs, can interfere with 3 normal functions of the placenta: (a) Inhibition of intercellular fusion of the trophoblast; (b) a decrease in trophoblast hormone production; or (c) retardation in trophoblast invasion.

Recently, aPL mAb, annexin V dependent, induced fetal loss by passive transfer to naive mice [48]. Its variable regions contained mainly 3 replacement mutations. To clarify the role of these mutations in the pathogenicity of the antibody, the aPL/annexin V dependent, were reverted in vitro to the germline configuration. The resulting "germline" antibody reacted with multiple self-antigens, only partially lost its reactivity against PL, but was no more dependent on annexin V, and more importantly was no more pathogenic. This study illustrated that the in vivo antigen driven maturation process of natural autoreactive B cells can be responsible for pathogenicity.

The importance of T cells role in induction of experimental fetal loss on APS background was proven by an induction of fetal loss by bone marrow transplantation from APS mice into naive mice [49]. A whole-population or T cell-depleted bone marrow cells from mice with experimental primary APS were infused into total body irradiated naive BALB/c recipient [49]. BM cells (in the presence of T cells) had the potential to induce experimental APS in naive mice, which resulted in high serum titers of aPL, an increased number of antibody forming cells specific for phospholipids associated with clinical features of primary APS. T cell depleted BM cells did not transfer the disease, pointing to the important role of T cells in the development and transfer of experimental primary APS.

Therapeutic Interventions in aPL Related Fetal Loss

Anti-thrombotic Treatments

Aspirin has significant antithrombotic properties, and regimens using aspirin were suggested to be effective in protecting against fetal loss associated with APS. Employing the model of passively induced APS it was found that aspirin treatment, especially in low doses, significantly improved pregnancy outcome [49]. This was manifested by fewer fetal resorptions and higher mean embryo weights. In a later study it was shown that treatment of APS mice with thromboxane receptor antagonist caused significant reduction in fetal resorption rate, as well as increase in platelet count and decrease in aPTT. Anticoagulation with heparin has already been used to prevent fetal loss in pregnant women with APS. A potentially better preparation for use in pregnancy is low-molecular-weight heparin (LMWH). Comparing the effectiveness of LMWH with regular heparin in the prevention of fetal resorption in mice with experimental APS, it was found that although heparin treatment decreased the degree of fetal loss, LMWH was much more effective in this respect [summarized in 50].

Bone Marrow Transplantation

APS mice which were transfused with BM cells (T cell depleted) from syngeneic naive mice had reduced titers of aPL, which were related to depletion of antibody forming cells in vivo, and reduced proliferative response of lymph node cells to aCL mAbs. The recipients showed improvement in clinical parameters manifested also by a reduced percentage of pregnancy loss following syngeneic BMT treatment [50].

Oral Tolerance

Systemic tolerance to various Ags can be achieved by feeding with pathogenic proteins. Feeding of BALB/c mice with low-dose β_2-GPI at certain time points of experimental APS development, had different effect on disease improvement [29]. The serological and clinical markers of experimental APS were prevented when the mice received orally β_2-GPI before disease induction upon immunization with the autoantigen. The treated group was characterized by low titers of serum anti-β_2-GPI and aCL in the sera, lack of fetal resorptions, low incidence of thrombocytopenia, and normal values of aPTT. β_2-GPI given at an early stage of the disease reduced the clinical manifestations. However, administration of β_2-GPI 70 days post-immunization, had a less significant effect on disease expression. Tolerized mice exhibited diminished T lymphocyte proliferation response to β_2-GPI in comparison to β_2-GPI–immunized mice fed with Ovalbumin (OVA). When non-tolerant β_2-GPI–primed T lymphocytes were mixed with CD8$^+$ T cells from the tolerized mice, a significant inhibition of proliferation upon exposure to β_2-GPI was observed. The induction of suppression was β_2-GPI -specific and antigen driven, as well as transforming growth factor β (TGF-β) mediated. The β_2-GPI specific response of T lymphocytes from the β_2-GPI fed mice was reversed by anti–TGF-β Abs. The tolerance was adoptively transferred by CD8$^+$ T cells from the tolerized mice into naive mice. Those CD8$^+$ cells were MHC class I restricted, found to secrete TGF-β, and had no cytolytic activity. Oral administration of β_2-GPI suppressed priming of CTLs in the recipient mice. Finally, β_2-GPI–induced oral tolerance has an immunomodulating effect in experimental APS, demonstrating the importance of β_2-GPI in the pathogenesis of the disease [29].

Intravenous immunoglobulins (IVIg) contain a wide spectrum of anti-idiotypes associated with a variety of autoimmune diseases. Since part of these anti-idiotypes may bear an internal image of the eliciting antigen, IVIg might be suitable for induction of oral tolerance. Therefore, we attempted to induce tolerance in an experimental model of APS by oral administration of IVIg [51]. Experimental APS was induced by active immunization with β_2-GPI. Naive mice were fed with IVIg, as a whole molecule, F(ab)$_2$ or Fc fragments. In a parallel set of studies, mice were fed with anti–β_2-GPI–specific anti-idiotypic IVIg [IVIg(αId)]. Feeding was performed before APS induction, at early or late stages of the disease. Significantly diminished humoral response was noted in the groups of mice tolerized with IVIg either as a whole molecule or with IVIg-F(ab)$_2$ fragments, accompanied by a significant attenuation of clinical manifestations. The maximal effect was achieved in the mice tolerized before disease induction, resulting in a disappearance of autoantibodies and normalization of clinical parameters. A significant improvement in the serological and clinical parameters was also noted in mice fed at an early stage of experimental APS. Abrogation of T lymphocyte proliferation to β_2-GPI was detected in the mice fed with IVIg prior to β_2-GPI immunization, mediated by TGF-β1 and IL-10 secretion. The effect of IVIg feeding was non-specific because similar inhibition of T-cell proliferation was observed in IVIg-fed mice immunized with OVA. The tolerance induced by IVIg feeding could be adoptively transferred to syngeneic mice by CD8$^+$ cells, which were found to secrete high levels of TGF-β1 and IL-10. Similar inhibitory effect was observed for anti-OVA levels in OVA-immunized mice. The same set of studies, conducted with anti–β_2-GPI–specific anti-idiotypic IVIg resulted in tolerance induction that was specific for β_2-GPI immunized mice, pointing to idiotype–anti-idiotype reactions mediating the tolerance induced by IVIg. Hence, IVIg induced oral tolerance has a non-specific immunomodulatory effect in experimental APS, mediated by TGF-β1 and IL-10-secreting CD8$^+$ cells. Our results point to a possible application of IVIg in the induction of oral tolerance against various autoimmune diseases.

β_2-GPI Related Synthetic Peptides

Using a peptide phage display library, we identified 3 hexapeptides that react specifically with the anti–β_2-GPI mAbs ILA-1, ILA-3, and H-3, which cause endothelial cell activation and induce experimental APS [52]. Treatment of APS mice with the synthetic peptides, neutralized the pathogenic anti–β_2-GPI Abs endothelial cell activation manifested by prevention of adhesion molecules expression such as ICAM-I, P-selectin, E-selectin, and inhibition of monocyte adherence to endothelial cells [52]. The specific anti–β_2-GPI biological function neutralization by synthetic peptides was further proven by prevention of fetal loss and coagulation in a mouse APS model [51]. Moreover, in vivo subjection of β_2-GPI related synthetic peptides as monvalent or as branched peptides as tetravalent or octavalent, to APS mice, improved the fetal loss, most prominent in the group treated with branched octavalent form of the β_2-GPI synthetic peptide [50]. Multivalent β_2-GPI–related peptide treatment in rat immunized with the peptide, induced B cell tolerance of an anti-peptide immune response [53].

Immunomodulation by Abs

Administration of specific anti-idiotypic Abs to aCL/β_2-GPI was found to be effective, resulting in attenuation of clinical and serological manifestation of experimental APS [50]. The anti-idiotypic treatment was associated with a shift from Th2 to Th1 immune response, characterize by a rise in the level of Th1-related cytokines in the sera of the treated mice and decrease in Th2-related cytokines. Furthermore, elevation in the number of IL-2 and IFN-γ secreting cells (Th1) and elimination of the IL-4 and IL-6 secreting cells (Th2), was noticed in the APS treated mice, supporting the role of Th1 cytokines in suppression of idiotypic-induced APS manifestations. Intravenous immunoglobulins (IVIg) have been reported to be effective in treating several autoimmune diseases. Treatment of APS mice with IVIg resulted in a complete clinical, serological, and pathological remission, including fetal loss. Inhibition studies pointed to the presence of anti-idiotypic activity to aCL/β_2-GPI in the IVIG preparation [50]. Furthermore, in a set of preliminary experiments, a fraction of IVIg specific for anti–β_2-GPI Abs (anti-anti-β_2-GPI anti-idotypic IVIg), was subjected to naive mice induced by passive transfer of human anti–β_2-GPI Abs, resulted in prevention of fetal loss and other APS manifestations (in preparation).

Similarly, treatment with anti–CD4 mAbs prevented the appearance of clinical manifestations of experimental APS manifested by pregnancy loss, especially when the Abs were administered early in the course of the disease [50].

Interleukin-3

Treatment of pregnant mice with murine recombinant IL-3 resulted in abrogation of fetal loss, as well as by normal platelet count [50]. Ciprofloxacin, a potent antibiotic agent of the quinolone family, which enhances production of IL-3 in irradiated mice, was found to prevent pregnancy loss, as well as other clinical manifestations of APS [summarized in 50]. The effect was probably mediated *via* increased IL-3 and GM-CSF expressions, manifested by elevated levels of IL-3 in the sera and increased IL-3 mRNA transcription in splenocytes. GM-CSF increased expression was documented by elevated titers in the sera and enhanced number of colony forming cells in the bone marrow.

Bromocriptine

Bromocriptine (BRC), which inhibits the secretion of prolactin and has immunoregulatory properties [50], was found to suppress experimental APS, leading to a marked reduction of autoAbs level accompanied by disappearance of clinical and pathological manifestations of the disease. The effect of BRC was mediated through the induction of natural nonspecific CD8 suppressor cells [49]. This effect was related to enhancement of IL-3 expression because high level of the cytokine was found in the sera of ciprofloxacin treated mice, compared to control group.

TNF-α DNA Vaccination

TNF-α is an immunomodulatory cytokine predominantly produced by Th1 cells as well as mononuclear phagocytes, B cells, and natural killer cells. Although its complete biological function is not clear, its proinflammatory and prothrombotic actions are well recognized, pointing to its potential role in the pathogenesis of APS manifestations. Thus, inhibition of TNF-α activity may effectively attenuate or even prevent the development of experimental APS. We introduced naked DNA encoding TNF-α to BALB/c mice with experimental APS, which resulted in the generation of immunological memory to its gene product, associated with elevated circulating anti–TNF-α Abs [54]. Enriched IgG fraction of the mouse anti–TNF-α was biologically active because it prevented endothelial cell activation by TNF-α, for example, inhibition of monocyte adhesion to activated endothelial cells (HUVEC). Mice immunized with β_2-GPI, vaccinated with TNF-α DNA at an early stage of the disease, showed decreased titers of circulating anti–β_2-GPI Abs as compared to the group of mice vaccinated with a control naked DNA. The reduction of aPL production was followed by amelioration of the fetal loss, increased platelet count to normal values as well as normalization of the prolonged aPTT. APS mice which were introduced to the TNF-α DNA vector at a later stage of the disease development, showed less improvement in their clinical manifestations. This study suggests a way in which a DNA vaccine can be employed for induction of a protective immunity in experimental APS.

Omega-3 (ω-3) Diet

The immunomodulatory potential of a diet enriched with ω-3 polyunsaturated fatty acids derived from linseed oil, was analyzed in naive mice with experimental APS provoked by active immunization with anti–β_2-GPI mAb [55]. Downregulation of the disease severity was noticed in the ω-3 treated mice, shown by reduced cellular and humoral activities like T cell response to the idiotype, mouse anti–β_2-GPI production on the single cell level and circulating autoantibodies. Fetal loss and other clinical manifestations of APS were improved in the ù-3 fed APS mice [54]. Several mechanisms were addressed in the literature explaining the beneficial effect of ω-3 in autoimmune state: (a) as the concentration of dietary ω-3 increases, a concomitant decrease of ω-6 metabolites take place. This is consequent to the inhibition of the prostaglandin synthetase complex and due to the reduced amount of arachidonic acid available as a substrate. (b) Alteration in the plasma-membrane viscosity. (c) Ability to reduce platelet adhesiveness and aggregation. (d) Immunomodulate cytokine production such s IL-1, TNF-α on the level of mRNA and protein synthesis.

Thrombosis Caused by aPL or Anti-prothrombin and Immunomodulation

aPL and Thrombus Formation

Pierangeli et al [56–58] employed a mouse model of induced venous thrombosis to elucidate the thrombogenic role of aPL in vivo. The model allows continuous and quantitative monitoring of focally induced, non-occlusive mural thrombus of a mouse femoral vein. The animal is anesthetized, femoral vein minimally mobilized, and subjected to a standardized "pinch" injury to induce thrombosis. The vessel is trans-illuminated using acrylic optical fibers connected to a light source, and clot formation and dissolution are visualized by a standard surgical microscope equipped with a video camera, video recorder, and computer assisted analysis system.

Employing this model, CD1 mice were intraperitoneally injected with either immunoglobulins derived from APS patients or healthy controls, while monitoring the size and dynamics of thrombus formation or disappearance [56, 57]. It was found that Ig from APS patients, or affinity purified aCL of IgG and IgM isotypes enhanced significantly the thrombus area and the mean disappearance time, indicating that aCL play a role in thrombus formation. To investigate whether the thrombogenic effect of aPL is due to their aPL or their anti–β_2-GPI activity, mice were injected with either aCL or anti–β_2-GPI Abs [59]. It was shown that the size of the thrombus in animals injected with murine aCL was larger than that in control groups, while there was no difference in thrombus kinetics between anti–β_2-GPI injected mice and controls, indicating that murine aCL, but not anti–β_2-GPI Abs, were thrombogenic in vivo [59]. Trying to decipher the mechanisms involved in this aPL–thrombus formation, the contribution of adhesion molecules to thrombus formation was addresses in mice [23, 24]. The dynamics of thrombus formation and the number of adhering leukocytes were studied in ICAM-1-deficient [ICAM-I(-/-)] mice or ICAM-I-/P-selectin-deficient [ICAM-I(-/-)/P-selectin(-/-)] mice treated with affinity-purified aPL IgG-APS or with control IgG and compared with wild-type mice treated in a similar fashion [23]. The data indicate that ICAM-I, P-selectin, and VCAM-I expression are important in thrombotic complications by aPL [23]. Infusion of the mice with anti–VCAM-I antibodies significantly reversed the enhanced adhesion of leukocytes and thrombus size in mice treated with aPL IgG-APS. Furthermore, aPL increased significantly the number of adhering leukocytes to endothelial cells in vivo in C57BL/6 J mice when compared to IgG-NHS treated mice [24]. This effect was abrogated in E-selectin–deficient mice. This enhancement in thrombus size by aPL antibodies was abrogated in E-selectin–deficient mice treated with aPL [24].

Therapeutic Interventions in aPL Related Thrombus Formation

This ex vivo "pinch"–thrombus formation model was used as a tool to test diverse therapeutic modalities.

Hydroxychloroquine

The anti-malarial drug hydroxychloroquine has been used successfully in prevention of post-operative thrombosis and in treatment of patients with SLE or APS. Mice treated with hydroxychloroquine had significantly smaller thrombi that persisted for a shorter period of time compared with animals treated with placebo [60]. In order to explore the mechanism involved in this antithrombotic activity, the effects of hydroxychloroquine on activation of platelets by aPL in the presence of a thrombin agonist was studied. Human platelets were exposed in vitro to aPL in the presence of thrombin agonist receptor peptide (TRAP). The changes in the expression of GPIIb/IIIa (CD41a) and GPIIIa (CD61) on platelet membrane were used as indicators of platelet activation. The effects of aPL and TRAP on expression of platelet surface markers of activation was completely abrogated by hydroxychloroquine in a dose-dependent fashion [60].

Treatment with IVIg

The potential mechanisms of action of IVIg in the same model has also been examined [61]. Mice infused with human aCL enriched IgG fraction were treated with

IVIg, saline, or OVA. IVIg treatment inhibited aCL induced endothelial cell activation and enhancement of thrombosis in mice passively infused with human aCL, associated with a decrease in aPL levels. Similarly, IVIg lowered aPL levels and inhibited thrombogenesis in mice immunized with β_2-GPI. It was also shown that blockade of stimulatory Fc gammaR on inflammatory cells is not necessary for this effect. The mechanism of action of IVIg is more likely saturation of the IgG transport receptor, leading to accelerated catabolism of pathogenic aPL.

Treatment with Synthetic β_2-GPI Related Peptide

Recently, one of the β_2-GPI derived peptide – NTLKTPRVGGC (named peptide A), showed previously to inhibit fetal loss [52], reversed thrombus formation in mouse APS model [62]. CD1 mice were injected with affinity purified aPL or with control IgG-NHS twice intraperitoneally. Seventy hours after the first injection, and 30 min before the surgical procedure (induction of experimental thrombus), mice were infused IV in each group with either peptide A or with a scrambled form of peptide A. The femoral vein of the anesthetized mice were dissected to examine the dynamics of an induced thrombus in treated and control mice. The mean aCL titer of mice injected with aPL was 60 G phospholipid (GPL) units. Mice treated with aPL and infused with a control scrambled form of peptide A produced significantly larger thrombi when compared to mice treated with IgG-NHS and peptide scA (2466 ± 462 ìm² vs. 772.5 ± 626.4 ìm²). Treatment with peptide A significantly decreased thrombus size in mice injected with aPL antibodies (1063 ± 890 ìm² compared to 2466 ± 462 ìm²). This may have important implications in designing new modalities of prevention and/or treatment of thrombosis in APS.

Anti-prothrombin and Thrombus Formation

The role of anti-prothrombin Abs in inducing thrombosis and other clinical manifestations of APS was evaluated [63]. Thrombosis was studied in a novel ex vivo model in which the aorta was sutured for 1 minute and the presence or absence of visible thrombus was qualitatively evaluated. Mice were immunized with either prothrombin, β_2-GPI, or β_2-GPI followed by prothrombin. The groups immunized with β_2-GPI or β_2-GPI/prothrombin, but not with prothrombin alone, developed prolonged aPTT, thrombocytopenia, and increased fetal resorption rate. All prothrombin-immunized mice as well as most β_2-GPI/prothrombin–immunized mice developed visible thrombus within the aorta. Some β_2-GPI–immunized mice developed very mild thrombus.

Origin of aPL and the Infectious Etiology of APS

The β_2-GPI molecule is an ubiquitous molecules. Several pathways were proposed to explain the generation of anti-β_2-GPI Abs: (A) Exposure of hidden epitopes or neoepitopes as adducts of oxidized phospholipid associated proteins, including β_2-GPI molecule [64, 65]. (B) Oxidized form of β_2-GPI undergo conformational changes presenting neoepitopes which may induce anti-β_2-GPI Abs [64, 65]. (C) Presentation of β_2-GPI molecules on apoptotic cells via binding to phosphatidylserine, could induce B cells with immunoglobulin receptors for apoptotic cells and DNA which are positively selected and could cause generation of anti-β_2-GPI in the appropriate condition [66, 67]. Infusion of BALB/c mice with β_2-GPI–bound apoptotic cells, induced the generation of mouse aPL/β_2-GPI, suggesting that cell-bound β_2-GPI is the true immunogen for production of aPL. The induced aPL reacted with murine, as well as bovine β_2-GPI, suggesting that heterologous β_2-GPI bound to apoptotic cells can break tolerance and induce auto-antibodies reactive with autologous β_2-GPI. This phenomenon was later proven in naïve mice immunized with human β_2-GPI generated Abs reactive with human, bovine, and murine β_2-GPI [68]. The loss of tolerance to mouse β_2-GPI was attributable to the high interspecies homology of β_2-GPI. (D) During the last years, the infectious origin of APS was proven to be one of the explanations for generation of anti–β_2-GPI Abs by sharing molecular mimicry with common bacteria or with CMV derived synthetic peptide [69–74].

Previously, using a hexapeptide phage display library, we identified 3 hexapeptides that react specifically with the anti–β_2-GPI mAbs , which cause endothelial cell activation and induce experimental APS [52]. All the 3 peptides specifically inhibit both in vitro and in vivo the biological functions of the corresponding anti–β_2-GPI mAbs. These peptides were capable of preventing fetal loss in experimental model of APS [52] and 1 of the peptide (peptide A) inhibited thrombus formation in animal model [62]. Using the Swiss Protein database revealed high homology between the hexapeptide LKTPRV and TLRVYK with different bacteriae and viruses [69, 70]. We hypothesized that molecular mimicry between structures on the β_2-GPI molecule and pathogen may induce APS [71, 72]. Thus, prepared bacterial relevant particles from *Pseudomonas aeroginosa*, *Haemophilus influenzae*, *Streptococcus pneumonia*, *Shigella dysenteriae*, *Neisseria gonorrhoeae*, and from the yeast *Candida albicans*. Naive mice were immunized, in the hind footpads, with the pathogen particles. Anti-TLRVYK Abs were affinity purified on a peptide column, bound β_2-GPI, and infused into naive mice. Only the mice which were infused with mouse antibodies derived from mice immunized with *Haemophilus influenzae* or with *Neisseria gonorrhoeae* directed to the peptide TLRVYK had the potential to induce clinical manifestations which resembles experimental APS (e.g., thrombocytopenia, prolonged aPTT, and elevated percentage of fetal loss). We hypothesize, in the current case, that the mechanism of pathogenic anti-generation is induced by epitope mimicry. B cells, present mimicking epitopes of bacteria or virus to T cells *via* a MHC class II pathway. These B cells produce antibodies with specificity for the instigating epitope that cross-react with host β_2-GPI as a native molecule or in a complex with platelets or endothelial cells, expressing the mimicked self epitope in the context of MHC class I and, depending on the appropriate secondary signaling, a pathogenic autoreactivity develop. In parallel, Pierangeli et al [33, 73, 74] have shown that antibodies generated by immunization with TIFI, a 15 amino acid peptide from CMV virus that shares similarity with GDKV (a peptide found in the Vth domain of β_2-GPI), has thrombogenic effects and induces endothelial cell activation and pregnancy loss in vivo.

aPL Involvement in the Pathogenesis of Brain, Heart, and Kidney

Brain

When the specific organs derived from MRL/lpr mice were analyzed, the mice showed significant vasculopathy in the central nervous system, including vascular occlusions and perivascular infiltrates in the choroid plexus was observed [75]. Hence, the MRL/lpr mice were suggested as a model for neurological complication of APS [76]. These mice were treated with S-farnesylthiosalicylic acid (FTS), a synthetic substance that detaches Ras from the inner cell membrane and induces its rapid degradation, leading to modulation of Ras activation, and the autoimmune lymphocyte downregulation. Subjection of Ras inhibitor (FTS), resulted in 50% decrease in splenocyte proliferation in the presence of β_2-GPI, reduced levels of circulating anti–β_2-GPI Abs and normalized the grip strength [77].

Naive mice showed neurological impairment upon induction of aPL [78–80]. APS-mice induced by idiotypic manipulation with aPL were significantly impaired neurologically and performed several reflexes less accurately compared to the controls, including placing reflex, postural reflex, and grip test [78]. These APS mice also exhibited hyperactive behavior in an open field, which tests spatial behavior, and displayed impaired motor coordination on a rotating bar [78]. Electron microscope evaluation of cerebral tissue revealed pathological changes in the microvessels. T Thrombotic occlusion of capillaries in combination with mild inflammation was the main finding and may underlie the neurological defects displayed by mice with APS [79]. Naive mice immunized with β_2-GPI showed hyperacivity as defined by number of rears and number of stairs climbed by the immunized mice in comparison to control mice [80]. Intrathecal subjection of anti–β_2-GPI Abs purified from APS patients into naive mice, resulted in deposition of the Abs in the hippocampus and cerebral cortex, associated with neurological disfunction [81].

Heart

Deposits of anti–β_2-GPI were documented in deformed valves obtained from patients with primary and secondary APS [82]. Such deposits were suggested to be involved in the pathogenesis of valvular lesions in Libman–Sacks endocarditis [83, 84]. Recently, an association of Libman–Sacks endocarditis to infection was proposed based on β_2-GPI related synthetic peptide studies [85]. The hearts had thickened valves in 68% of MRL-*lpr/lpr* mice, however the aPL deposition in the affected mice had no association with any of the antibodies tested [86].

Kidney

Systemic APS include renal manifestations such as intra-renal vascular lesions, glomerular capillary thrombosis, renal artery occlusions, renal vein thrombosis, end-stage renal failure, and hemodialysis are associated with systemic APS [4–6, 87]. We showed in SCID mice the role of aPL as possible inducers of renal damage [27]. Isolated PBLs from an APS patient accompanied by renal involvement, manifested as membranous nephropathy, as proven by a renal biopsy were subjected to SCID mice. The mice transfused with PBL from the affected patient, exemplified aPL following a renal lesion consistent with the human membranous nephropathy lesion was precipitated.

Atherosclerosis and aPL

Atherosclerosis is considered analogous to chronic inflammatory diseases. During the last years the involvement of aPL in atherosclerosis was well established.

Table 30.1. gLessons from antiphospholipid syndrome experimental models.

Pathology	Clinical complication	Autoantibody involved	Reference
Reproductive failure	Fetal loss, embryo and placenta small for date, low fecundity	Anti–CL/β$_2$-GPI Anti–β$_2$-GPI	10–13, 17–20, 27, 62, 28, 29
		Anti–phosphatidylserine (aPS)	36, 37
		Anti–β$_2$-GPI related peptides mimetics of bacteria	71
	Intrauterian fetal death	Anti–CMV derived peptide	33
	Placental necrosis	aCL β$_2$-GPI independent	12
	Decidual necrosis	Total IgG with aPL activity	11
	Fetal loss, placental thrombosis, decidual necrosis	Anti–annexin V	47, 48
Thrombosis	Anti–CL/β$_2$-GPI, aCL, anti–β$_2$-GPI, anti–β$_2$-GPI-related synthetic peptides, Thrombus formation ex vivo	anti–prothrombin	23–25, 56–62, 73, 74 63
CNS involvement	Neurological impairment (e.g., hyperactivity in an open field, impaired motor coordination) Thrombotic occlusion of brains' capillaries	Total IgG with aPL activity, anti–CL/β$_2$-GPI, anti–β2-GPI	75–81
Heart affliction	Vale thickening in MRL/lpr/lpr mice	Not defined	86
Kidney manifestations	Membranous nephropathy lesions in SCID mice	aPL producing human PBLs	27
Atherosclerosis	Fatty streak formation, CD4 infiltration into aortic sinus	Anti–CL/β$_2$-GPI, aCL, anti–β$_2$-GPI	25, 26, 88–90
Etiology and mechanisms			
The infectious origin of APS		aPL/β$_2$-GPI can induce fetal loss by molecular mimicry between the β$_2$-GPI and bacteria or tetanus toxoid.	71, 72
		CMV derived peptide which share structural similarity with β$_2$-GPI, induce thrombus formation, activates endothelial cells in vivo and cause intrauterine death.	33, 73, 74
Apoptotic cells as inducers of aPL		Propagation of aPL by circulating apoptotic thymocytes/β$_2$-GPI.	66, 67
aPL pathogenicity based on structural characteristics		The heavy chain CDRs variable regions contribute to the aPL binding properties, anticoagulant activity and fetal loss.	31
		The aPL/annexin V binding characteristics and fetal loss activity, relates to 3 mutations in the variable region.	48
aPL and complement dysregulation		anti–β$_2$-GPI activate complement in the placenta, generating split products that mediate placental injury and lead to fetal loss and growth retardation.	12, 32

Table 30.1. Continued

Pathology	Clinical complication	Autoantibody involved	Reference
aPL prothrombotic properties		aPL induced adhesion molecule expression such as ICAM-I, E-selectin, P-selectin following enhancement in thrombus formation.	23, 24
PS disturb placental differentiation		aPS enhance apoptosis in rat embryo yolk sac	42
β_2-GPI support normal pregnancy		Physiological requirement for functional β_2-GPI for successful pregnancy	22, 30
β_2-GPI is the autoantigen in exp.APS		Immunization with β_2-GPI induce generation of anti–β_2-GPI, fetal loss, prolonged coagulation and thrombocytopenia. Feeding with β_2-GPI cause tolerance and prevent the disease.	21, 29
		Fetal loss, anticoagulant activity, thrombocytopenia were transferred by bone marrow (BM) transplantation and not by T cell depleted BM cells.	49
T cells aPL/β2GPI specific can transfer the pathogenic properties of APS.		Adoptive transfer of T cells from β_2-GPI immunized mice, enhanced early atherosclerosis in LDL-receptor deficient mice	26

Treatments:
therapeutic modalities in experimental models

		Therapeutic effects in target organs	
Antithrombotics and anticoagulants	Aspirin, thromboxane receptor antagonist, LMWH	Improved pregnancy outcome, fewer fetal resorptions, and higher mean embryo weights.	50
Bone marrow transplantation		Reduced titers of aPL, reduced percentage of pregnancy loss.	50
Immunomodulation by Abs	anti-idiotypic Abs Anti-CD4 mAbs, IVIg	Complete clinical, serological, and pathological remission, including . fetal loss	50, 61
		Attenuation of clinical and serological manifestation of experimental APS, associated with a shift from Th2 to Th1 immune response.	
		Inhibition of aCL-induced endothelial cell activation and of thrombogenesis i n mice infused with aPL	50
Specific aPL targeting with synthetic peptide	β_2-GPI–related synthetic peptides	Monovalent β_2-GPI related peptides prevented fetal loss and enhanced coagulation in mice passively infused with aPL.	52
		Reversion of thrombus formation	62
Specific B cell targeting with branched synthetic peptides	β_2-GPI–related peptides	Branched octapeptides inhibited aPL production, fetal loss, and prolonged coagulation innaive mice induced for generation of aPL.	50
		Multivalent peptides cause reduction in anti-peptide generation in rat immunized with the specific β_2-GPI–related peptides.	53

Table 30.1. Continued

Therapeutic modalities in experimental models	Therapeutic effects in target organs involved	Reference
Cytokines	IL-3,	Abrogation of fetal loss, normalization of platelet count.	50
	Ciprofloxacin (enhances IL-3 secretion)		
Bromocriptine		Marked reduction of autoAbs levels, disappearance of clinical and pathological manifestations of the disease.	50
Oral tolerance	β2GPI, IVIg	Low titers of anti–β_2-GPI and aCL, lack of fetal resorptions, low incidence of thrombocytopenia and normal values of aPTT.	29, 51
β_2-GPI-related synthetic peptides		Neutralization of pathogenic anti–β_2-GPI-induced endothelial cell activation. Prevention of fetal loss and coagulation. Reversion of thrombus formation.	50, 52, 53, 62
TNF-α DNA Vaccination		Decreased titers of anti–β_2-GPI, followed by amelioration of the fetal loss, increased platelet count to normal values and normalization of aPTT.	54
Omega-3 diet		Downregulation of disease, shown by reduced cellular and humoral activities. Fetal loss and other clinical manifestations of APS were improved.	55
Hydroxychloroquine		Anti-thrombotic effect: smaller thrombi that persisted for a shorter period of time.	
FTS		Neurological improvement- decrease in splenocyte proliferation to β_2-GPI, reduced levels of circulating anti–β_2-GPI Abs and normalization of grip strength.	60 77

β_2-GPI = β_2-glycoprotein; aCL = anticardiolipin.

Immunization of mice prone to develop atherosclerosis such as LDL-receptor deficient (LDL-RD) mice with β_2-GPI resulted in the production of high titers of anti-β_2-GPI accompanied with accelerated early atherosclerosis [88]. In addition, mouse aCL induced by idiotypic manipulation with human aCL from an APS patient enhance atherogenesis in LDL-RD mice and imply that these antibodies may play a role in atherosclerosis development in patients with APS [89]. Furthermore, adoptive transfer of β_2-GPI-reactive T cells from LDL-RD immunized mice to LDL-RD mice, enhanced fatty streak formation in the later studied group [26]. Oral administration of β_2-GPI suppressed atherogenesis in the LDL-RD mice [26]. Oral tolerance was also capable of reducing reactivity to oxidized LDL in mice immunized against oxLDL. IL-4 and IL-10 production was upregulated in lymph node cells of β_2-GPI–tolerant mice immunized against β_2-GPI, upon priming with the respective protein [90]. The pro-atherogenic activity of anti–β_2-GPI was demonstrated in the apo-E-deficient mice. Accelerated atherosclerosis accompanied by infiltration of CD4 lymphocytes into aortic sinus in the ?β_2-GPI immunized mice was documented [25].

Conclusions

The tool of animal models paved us the way to better understand the involvement of aPL in the different pathogenic conditions accompanying the classical Hughes syndrome. Furthermore, the mechanisms leading to the pathogenesis of the disease could be better understand as well as the origin of the disease. All of that may give us tools for studying new therapeutic approaches for treatments.

In the Table 30.1, we summarize the conclusions achieved in analyzing APS following employment of animal experimental models.

References

1. Hughes GRV, Harris EN, Gharavi AE. The anti-cardiolipin syndrome. J Rheumatol 1986;13:486–489.
2. Asherson RA, Cervera R, Piette JC, Shoenfeld Y. Milestones in the antiphospholipid syndrome. In: Asherson RA, Cervera R, Piette JC, Shoenfeld Y, eds. The antiphospholipid syndrome II – autoimmune thrombosis. Amsterdam: Elsevier; 2002.
3. Galli M, Comfurious P, Massen C, et al. Anti-cardiolipin antibodies (ACA) directed not to cardiolipin but to a plasma protein cofactor. Lancet 1990;335:1544–1547.
4. Shoenfeld Y. Systemic antiphospholipid syndrome. Lupus 2003;12:497–498.
5. Cervera R, Piette JC, Font J, et al. Euro-Phospholipid Project Group. Antiphospholipid syndrome: clinical and immunologic manifestations and patterns of disease expression in a cohort of 1,000 patients. Arthritis Rheum 2002;46:1019–1027.
6. Asherson RA, Cervera R. Unusual manifestations of the antiphospholipid syndrome. Clin Rev Allergy Immunol 2003;25:61–78.
7. Gharavi AE, Mellors RC, Elkon KB. IgG anti-cardiolipin antibodies in murine lupus. Clin Exp Immunol 1989;78:233–238.
8. Aron AL, Cuellar ML, Brey RL, et al. Early onset of autoimmunity in MRL/++ mice following immunization with beta 2 glycoprotein I. Clin Exp Immunol 1995;101:78–81.
9. Hashimoto Y, Kawamura M, Ichikawa K, et al. Anticardiolipin antibodies in NZW x BXSB F1 mice. A model of antiphospholipid syndrome. J Immunol 1992;149:1063–1068.
10. Blank M, Cohen J, Toder V, Shoenfeld Y. Induction of anti-phospholipid syndrome in naive mice with mouse lupus monoclonal and human polyclonal anti-cardiolipin antibodies. Proc Natl Acad Sci U S A 1991;88:3069–3073.

11. Piona A, La Rosa L, Tincani A, et al. Placental thrombosis and fetal loss after passive transfer of mouse lupus monoclonal or human polyclonal anti-cardiolipin Abs in pregnant naive BALB/c mice. Scand J Immunol 1995;41:427–432.
12. Holers VM, Girardi G, Mo L, et al. Complement C3 activation is required for antiphospholipid antibody-induced fetal loss. J Exp Med 2002;195:211–220.
13. Branch DW, Dudley DJ, Mitchell MD, et al. Immunoglobulin G fractions from patients with antiphospholipid Abs cause fetal death in BALB/c mice: a model for autoimmune fetal loss. Am J Obstet Gynecol 1990;163:210–216.
14. Shoenfeld Y, Nahum A, Korczyn AD, et al. Neuronal-binding antibodies from patients with antiphospholipid syndrome induce cognitive deficits following intrathecal passive transfer. Lupus 2003;12:436–442.
15. Jerne NK. Towards a network theory of the immune system. Ann Immunol 1974;125c:373–389.
16. Jerne NK, Roland J, Cazenave PA. Recurrent idiotopes and internal images. EMBO J 1982;1:243–247.
17. Bakimer R, Fishman P, Blank M, Sredni B, Djaldetti M, Shoenfeld Y. Induction of primary antiphospholipid syndrome in mice by immunization with a human monoclonal anticardiolipin antibody (H-3). J Clin Invest 1992;89:1558–1563.
18. Blank M, Krause I, Ben-Bassat M, Shoenfeld Y. Induction of experimental anti-phospholipid syndrome associated with SLE following immunization with human monoclonal pathogenic anti-DNA idiotype. J Autoimmun 1992;5:495–509.
19. Shoenfeld Y. Idiotypic induction of autoimmunity: a new aspect of the idiotypic network. FASEB J 1994;8:1296–1301.
20. Shoenfeld Y. The idiotypic network in autoimmunity: Abs that bind Abs that bind Abs. Nat Med 2004;10:17–18.
21. Blank M, Faden D, Tincani A, et al. Immunization with cardiolipin cofactor (beta-2-glycoprotein I) induces experimental antiphospholipid syndrome in naive mice. J Autoimmun 1994;7:441–455.
22. Robertson SA, Roberts CT, van Beijering E, et al. Effect of beta2-glycoprotein I null mutation on reproductive outcome and antiphospholipid antibody-mediated pregnancy pathology in mice. Mol Hum Reprod 2004;10:409–416.
23. Pierangeli SS, Espinola RG, Liu X, Harris NE. Thrombogenic effects of antiphospholipid antibodies are mediated by intercellular cell adhesion molecule-1, vascular cell adhesion molecule-1, and P-selectin. Circ Res 2001;88:245–250.
24. Espinola RG, Liu X, Colden-Stanfield M, Hall J, Harris EN, Pierangeli SS. E-Selectin mediates pathogenic effects of antiphospholipid antibodies. Thromb Haemost 2003;1:843–848.
25. George J, Shoenfeld Y, Harats D. The involvement of beta2-glycoprotein I (beta2-GPI) in human and murine atherosclerosis. J Autoimmun 1999;13:57–60.
26. George J, Harats D, Gilburd B, et al. Adoptive transfer of beta(2)-glycoprotein I-reactive lymphocytes enhances early atherosclerosis in LDL receptor-deficient mice Circulation 2000;102:1822–1827.
27. Levy Y, Ziporen L, Gilburd B, et al. Membranous nephropathy in primary antiphospholipid syndrome: description of a case and induction of renal injury in SCID mice. Hum Antibodies Hybridomas 1996;7:91–96.
28. George J, Blank M, Levy Y, et al. Differential effects of anti-beta2-glycoprotein I antibodies on endothelial cells and on the manifestations of experimental antiphospholipid syndrome. Circulation 1998;97:900–906.
29. Blank M, George J, Barak V, Tincani A, Koike T, Shoenfeld Y. Oral tolerance to low dose beta 2-glycoprotein I: immunomodulation of experimental antiphospholipid syndrome. J Immunol 1998;161:5303–5312.
30. Miyakis S, Robertson SA, Krilis SA. Beta-2 glycoprotein I and its role in antiphospholipid syndrome-lessons from knockout mice. Clin Immunol 2004;112:136–143.
31. Blank M, Waisman A, Mozes E, Shoenfeld Y. Characteristics and pathogenic role of anti-beta2-glycoprotein I single-chain Fv domains: induction of experimental antiphospholipid syndrome. Int Immunol 1999;11:1917–1926.
32. Salmon JE, Girardi G, Holers VM. Activation of complement mediates antiphospholipid antibody-induced pregnancy loss. Lupus 2003;12:535–538.
33. Gharavi AE, Vega-Ostertag M, Espinola RG, et al. Intrauterine fetal death in mice caused by cytomegalovirus-derived peptide induced aPL antibodies. Lupus 2004;13:17–23.
34. Ikematsu W, Luan FL, La Rosa L, et al. Human anticardiolipin monoclonal autoAbs cause placental necrosis and fetal loss in BALB/c mice. Arthritis Rheum 1998;41:1026–1039.
35. Morrish DW, Dakour J, Li H. Life and death in the placenta: new peptides and genes regulating human syncytiotrophoblast and extravillous cytotrophoblast lineage formation and renewal. Curr Protein Pept Sci 2001;2:245–259.

36. Blank M, Tincani A, Shoenfeld Y. Induction of antiphospholipid syndrome in naive mice with purified IgG anti-phosphatidylserine antibodies. J Rheumatol 1994;21:100–104.
37. Yodfat O, Blank M, Krause I, Shoenfeld Y. The pathogenic role of anti-phosphatidylserine antibodies: active immunization with the antibodies leads to the induction of antiphospholipid syndrome. Clin Immunol Immunopathol 1996;78:14–20.
38. Levy R, DM Nelson. To be, or not to be, that is the question. Apoptosis in human trophoblast. Placenta 2000;21:1–13.
39. Shurtz-Swirsky R, Inbar O, Blank M, et al. *In vitro* effect of anticardiolipin autoantibodies upon total and pulsatile placental hCG secretion during early pregnancy. Am J Reprod Immunol 1993;29:206–210.
40. Sugimura M, Kobayashi T, Shu F, Kanayama N, Terao T. Annexin V inhibits phosphatidylserine-induced intrauterine growth restriction in mice. Placenta 1999;20:555–560.
41. Vogt E, Ng AK, Rote NS. Antiphosphatidylserine antibody removes annexin-V and facilitates the binding of prothrombin at the surface of a choriocarcinoma model of trophoblast differentiation. Am J Obstet Gynecol 1997;177:964–972.
42. Matalon ST, Shoenfeld Y, Blank M, Yacobi S, von Landenberg P, Ornoy A. Antiphosphatidylserine antibodies affect rat yolk sacs in culture: a mechanism for fetal loss in antiphospholipid syndrome. Am J Reprod Immunol 2004;51:144–151.
43. Di Simone N, Meroni PL, de Papa N, et al. Antiphospholipid antibodies affect trophoblast gonadotropin secretion and invasiveness by binding directly and through adhered beta 2 glycoprotein I. Arthritis Rheum 2000;43:140–150.
44. McIntyre JA. Antiphospholipid antibodies in implantation failures. Am J Reprod Immunol 2003;49:221–229.
45. Rand JH, Wu XX, Guller S, et al. Reduction of annexin-V (placental anticoagulant protein-I) on placental villi of women with aPL Abs and recurrent spontaneous abortion. Am J Obstet Gynecol 1994;171:1566–1572.
46. Matsubayashi H, Arai T, Izumi S, Sugi T, McIntyre JA, Makino T. Anti-annexin V antibodies in patients with early pregnancy loss or implantation failure. Fertil Steril 2001;76:694–699.
47. Wang X, Campos B, Kaetzel MA, Dedman JR. Annexin V is critical in the maintenance of murine placental integrity. Am J Obstet Gynecol 1999;180:1008–1016.
48. Lieby P, Poindron V, Roussi S, et al. Pathogenic antiphospholipid antibody: an antigen selected needle in a haystack. Blood 2004;104:1711–1715.
49. Blank M, Krause I, Lanir N, Shoenfeld Y. Transfer of experimental antiphospholipid syndrome by bone marrow cell transplantation. The importance of the T cell. Arthritis Rheum 1995;38:115–122.
50. Blank M, Krause I, Shoenfeld Y. The contribution of experimental models to our understanding of etiology, pathogenesis and novel therapies in the antiphospholipid syndrome. In: Khamashta MA, ed. Hughes syndrome – antiphospholipid syndrome. London: Springer; 2000:379–388.
51. Krause I, Blank M, Sherer Y, Gilburd B, Kvapil F, Shoenfeld Y. Induction of oral tolerance in experimental antiphospholipid syndrome by feeding with polyclonal immunoglobulins. Eur J Immunol 2002;32:3414–3424.
52. Blank M, Shoenfeld Y, Cabilly S, Heldman Y, Fridkin M, Katchalski-Katzir E. Prevention of experimental antiphospholipid syndrome and endothelial cell activation by synthetic peptides. Proc Natl Acad Sci U S A 1999;96:5164–5168.
53. Jones DS, Coutts SM, Gamino CA, et al. Multivalent thioether-peptide conjugates: B cell tolerance of an anti-peptide immune response. Bioconjug Chem 1999;10:480–488.
54. Blank M, Krause I, Wildbaum G, Karin N, Shoenfeld Y. TNFalpha DNA vaccination prevents clinical manifestations of experimental antiphospholipid syndrome. Lupus 2003;12:546–549.
55. Reifen R, Amital H, Blank M, et al. Linseed oil suppresses the anti-beta-2-glycoprotein-I in experimental antiphospholipid syndrome. J Autoimmun 2000;15:381–385.
56. Pierangeli SS, Harris EN. Antiphospholipid antibodies in an in vivo thrombosis model in mice. Lupus 1994;3:247–251.
57. Pierangeli SS, Liu XW, Barker JH, Anderson G, Harris EN. Induction of thrombosis in a mouse model by IgG, IgM and IgA immunoglobulins from patients with the antiphospholipid syndrome. Thromb Haemost 1995;74:1361–1367.
58. Pierangeli SS, EN Harris. In vivo models of thrombosis for the antiphospholipid syndrome. Lupus 1996;5:451–455.
59. Gharavi AE, Pierangeli SS, Gharavi AE, et al. Thrombogenic properties of antiphospholipid antibodies do not depend on their binding to beta2 glycoprotein 1 (beta2GP1) alone. Lupus 1998;7:341–346.
60. Edwards MH, Pierangeli SS, Liu X, Barker JH, Anderson G, Harris EN. Hydroxychloroquine reverses thrombogenic properties of antiphospholipid antibodies in mice. Circulation 1997;96:4380–4384.

61. Pierangeli SS, Espinola R, Liu X, Harris EN, Salmon JE. Identification of an Fc gamma receptor-independent mechanism by which intravenous immunoglobulin ameliorates antiphospholipid antibody-induced thrombogenic phenotype. Arthritis Rheum 2001;44:876–883.
62. Pierangeli SS, Blank M, Liu X, et al. A peptide that shares similarity with bacterial antigens reverses thrombogenic properties of antiphospholipid antibodies in vivo. J Autoimmun 2004;22:217–225.
63. Haj Yahja S, Sherer Y, Blank M, Kaetsu H, Smolinsky A, Shoenfeld Y. Anti-prothrombin antibodies cause thrombosis in a novel qualitative ex-vivo animal model. Lupus 2003;12:364–369.
64. Matsuura E, Igarashi Y, Yasuda T, Triplett DA, Koike T. Anticardiolipin antibodies recognize beta 2-glycoprotein I structure altered by interacting with an oxygen modified solid phase surface. J Exp Med 1984;179:457–462.
65. Horkko S, Miller E, Branch DW, Palinski W, Witztum JL. The epitopes for some antiphospholipid antibodies are adducts of oxidized phospholipid and beta2 glycoprotein 1 (and other proteins), Proc Nat Acad Sci U S A 1997;94:10356–10361.
66. Levine JS, Koh JS, Subang R, Rauch J. Apoptotic cells as immunogen and antigen in the antiphospholipid syndrome. Exp Mol Pathol 1999;66:82–98.
67. Levine JS, Subang R, Koh JS, Rauch J. Induction of anti-phospholipid autoantibodies by beta2-glycoprotein I bound to apoptotic thymocytes. J Autoimmun 1998;11:413–424.
68. Tincani A, Gilburd B, Abu-Shakra M, et al. Immunization of naive BALB/c mice with human beta2-glycoprotein I breaks tolerance to the murine molecule. Arthritis Rheum 2002;46:1399–1404.
69. Blank M, Y Shoenfeld. Beta-2-glycoprotein-I, infections, antiphospholipid syndrome and therapeutic considerations. Clin Immunol 2004;112:190–199.
70. Blank M, Asherson RA, Cervera R, Shoenfeld Y. Antiphospholipid syndrome infectious origin. J Clin Immunol 2004;24:12–23.
71. Blank M, Krause I, Fridkin M, et al. Bacterial induction of autoantibodies to $\beta_2$glycoprotein I accounts for the infectious etiology of antiphospholipid syndrome. J Clin Invest 2002;106:797–804.
72. Shoenfeld Y. Etiology and pathogenetic mechanisms of the anti-phospholipid syndrome unraveled. Trends Immunol 2003;24:2–4.
73. Gharavi AE, Pierangeli SS, Colden M , Liu X, Espinola RG, Harris EN. GDKV-induced antiphospholipid antibodies enhance thrombosis and activate endothelial cells in vivo and in vitro. J Immunol 1999;163:2922–2927.
74. Gharavi AE, Pierangeli SS, Espinola RG, Liu X, Colden-Stanfield M, Harris EN. Antiphospholipid antibodies induced in mice by immunization with a cytomegalovirus-derived peptide cause thrombosis and activation of endothelial cells *in vivo*. Arthritis Rheum 2002;46:545–552.
75. Smith HR, Hansen CL, Rose R, Canoso RT. Autoimmune MRL-lpr/lpr mice are an animal model for the secondary antiphospholipid syndrome. J Rheumatol 1990;17:911–915.
76. Hess DC. Models for central nervous system complications of antiphospholipid syndrome. Lupus 1994;3:253–257.
77. Katzav A, Kloog Y, Korczyn AD, et al. Treatment of MRL/lpr mice, a genetic autoimmune model, with the Ras inhibitor, farnesylthiosalicylate (FTS). Clin Exp Immunol 2001;126:570–577.
78. Ziporen L, Shoenfeld Y, Levy Y, Korczyn AD. Neurological dysfunction and hyperactive behavior associated with antiphospholipid antibodies. A mouse model. J Clin Invest 1997;100:613–619.
79. Ziporen L, Polak Charcon S, Korczyn D, et al. Neurological dysfunction associated with antiphospholipid syndrome: histopathological brain findings of thrombotic changes in a mouse model. Clin Dev Immunol 2004;11:67–75.
80. Katzav A, Pick CG, Korczyn AD, et al. Hyperactivity in a mouse model of the antiphospholipid syndrome. Lupus 2001;7:494–499.
81. Shoenfeld Y, Nahum A, Korczyn AD, et al. Neuronal-binding antibodies from patients with antiphospholipid syndrome induce cognitive deficits following intrathecal passive transfer. Lupus 2003;12:436–442.
82. Ziporen L, Goldberg I, Arad M, et al. Libman-Sacks endocarditis in the antiphospholipid syndrome: immunopathologic findings in deformed heart valves. Lupus 1996;5:196–205.
83. Libman E, Sacks BA. Hitherto undescribed from of valvular and mural endocarditis. Arch Intern Med 1924;33:701–737.
84. Asherson RA, Hughes GRV. The expanding spectrum of Libman Sacks endocarditis; the role of antiphospholipid antibodies. Clin Exp Rheumatol 1989;7:225–228.
85. Blank M, Shani A, Goldberg I, et al. Libman-Sacks endocarditis associated with antiphospholipid syndrome and infection . Thromb Res 2004. In press.
86. Vianna JL, Trotter S, Khamashta MA, Chikte S, Olsen E, Hughes GR.The heart and antiphospholipid antibodies in MRL-lpr/lpr mice. Lupus 1992;1:1357–1361.

87. Nzerue CM, Hewan-Lowe K, Pierangeli SS, Harris EN. "Black swan in the kidney": renal involve-ment in the antiphospholipid antibody syndrome. Kidney Int 2002;62:733–744.
88. George J, Afek A, Gilburd B, et al. . Induction of early atherosclerosis in LDL-receptor-deficient mice immunized with beta2-glycoprotein I. Circulation 1998;98:1108–1115.
89. George J, Afek A, Gilburd B, et al. Atherosclerosis in LDL-receptor knockout mice is accelerated by immunization with anticardiolipin antibodies. Lupus 1997;6:723–729.
90. George J, Yacov N, Breitbart E, et al. Suppression of early atherosclerosis in LDL-receptor deficient mice by oral tolerance with beta 2-glycoprotein I. Cardiovasc Res 2004;62:603–609.

31 Antiphospholipid Antibody–Induced Pregnancy Loss and Thrombosis

Guillermina Girardi and Jane E. Salmon

Antiphospholipid (aPL) antibodies are a family of autoantibodies that exhibit a broad range of target specificities and affinities, all recognizing various combinations of phospholipids, phospholipid binding proteins, or both. The first aPL antibody, a complement fixing antibody that reacted with extracts from bovine hearts, was detected in patients with syphilis in 1906 [1]. The relevant antigen was later identified as cardiolipin, a mitochondrial phospholipid [2]. The presence of aPL antibodies in serum has been associated with arterial and venous thrombosis and recurrent pregnancy loss [3–7], but the pathogenic mechanisms mediating these events are unknown. Several hypotheses have been proposed to explain the cellular and molecular mechanisms by which aPL antibodies induce thrombosis and fetal loss. There are reports that aPL antibodies activate endothelial cells, monocytes, and platelets [8–10]. In vivo and in vitro studies have shown that exposure to aPL antibodies induces activation of endothelial cells and a prothrombotic phenotype, as assessed by upregulation of the expression of adhesion molecules, secretion of cytokines, and the metabolism of prostacyclins [8, 10, 11]. aPL antibodies recognize β_2-glycoprotein I bound to resting endothelial cells, although the basis for the interaction of β_2-glycoprotein I with viable endothelial cells remains unclear [12, 13]. As β_2-glycoprotein I is considered a natural anticoagulant [14], some authors propose that aPL antibodies interfere with or modulate the function of phospholipid binding proteins involved in the regulation of coagulation, activate platelets, or induce monocytes to express tissue factor [9]. That endothelial cell, monocyte, and platelet activation are associated with aPL antibodies and thrombophilia, and that these cell phenotypes may also occur as a consequence of complement activation products, suggested a role for complement activation in aPL antibody–induced tissue damage.

The Complement System

Complement is part of the innate immune system and provides one of the main effector arms of host defense. Complement was first identified as a heat labile principle in serum that "complemented" antibodies in the killing of bacteria. We now know that complement is a system of more than 30 proteins in plasma and on cell surfaces that act in concert to protect the host against invading organisms, initiates inflammation, and tissue injury [15].

There are 3 pathways of complement activation: the classical, mannose binding lectin, and alternative pathways (Fig. 31.1). These 3 initiation pathways converge at the point of cleavage of the third component of complement (C3) and the steps leading to the cleavage of C3 are amplifying cascades of enzymes, analogous to those in coagulation. The classical pathway is activated when natural or elicited antibodies bind to antigen and unleash potent effectors associated with humoral responses in immune mediated tissue damage. Activation of the classical pathway is initiated by the binding of the C1 complex to antibodies complexed to antigens on cell or bacterial surfaces. C1s first cleaves C4, which binds covalently to the cell (or bacterial) surface, and then cleaves C2, leading to the formation of a C4b2a enzyme complex, the C3 convertase of the classical pathway. Activation of the classical pathway by natural antibody plays a major role in the response to neoepitopes unmasked on ischemic endothelium, and thus may be involved in reperfusion injury [16]. In addition, the classical pathway is activated through the action of

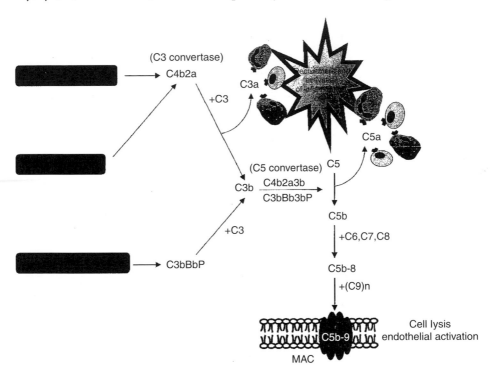

Figure 31.1. Proposed mechanism for the pathogenic effects of aPL antibodies on tissue injury. First, aPL antibodies are preferentially targeted to the placenta where they activate complement via the classical pathway. The complement cascade is initiated; C3 and subsequently C5 are activated. C5a is generated and attracts and activates neutrophils, monocytes, and platelets, and stimulates the release of inflammatory mediators, including reactive oxidants, proteolytic enzymes, chemokines, cytokines, and complement factors. Complement activation is amplified by the alternative pathway. This results in further influx of inflammatory cells and ultimately fetal injury. Depending on the extent of Damage, either death in utero or fetal growth restriction ensues. PMN-neutrophil; MF-monocyte–macrophage. (Adapted from Girardi G, et al Complement C5a receptors and neutrophils mediate fetal injury in the antiphospholipid syndrome. J Clin Invest 2003;112:1652, with copyright permission from the Journal of Clinical Investigation.

C-reactive protein (CRP) and serum amyloid P as they bind nuclear constituents released from necrotic or dying cells, or directly when apoptotic bodies derived from cells bind C1q [17, 18]. Activation of the mannose binding lectin pathway is triggered by binding of the complex of mannose binding lectin and the serine proteases, mannose binding lectin – associated proteases 1 and 2 (MASP1 and MASP2, respectively). MASP2 acts in a manner similar to C1s to lead to the formation of the C3 convertase enzyme. MASP1 may also be able to cleave C3 directly. Alternative pathway activation mechanisms differ in that they are initiated by the binding of spontaneously activated complement components to the surface of pathogens. Under normal physiologic conditions, C3 undergoes low-grade spontaneous hydrolysis. This pathway is antibody independent and is triggered by the activity of factor B, factor D, and properdin. Triggering of the alternative pathway is initiated by the covalent binding of a small amount of C3b to hydroxyl groups on cell surface carbohydrates and proteins and is activated by low-grade cleavage of C3 in plasma. This C3b binds factor B, a protein homologous to C2, to form a C3bB complex. Factor D cleaves factor B bound to C3b to form the alternative pathway C3 complex C3bBb. Properdin (P) binds to and stabilizes this enzyme complex.

Convergence of the 3 complement activation pathways on the C3 protein results in a common pathway of effector functions. The initial step is generation of the fragments C3a and C3b. C3a, an anaphylatoxin that binds to receptors on leukocytes and other cells, causes activation and release of inflammatory mediators (reviewed in [19]). C3b and its further sequential cleavage fragments, iC3b and C3d, are ligands for complement receptors 1 and 2 (CR1 and CR2) and the β_2 integrins, CD11b/CD18 and CD11c/CD18, present on a variety of inflammatory and immune accessory cells (reviewed in [20, 21]). C3b is covalently bound to the site of complement activation and then binds to C4b or C3b in the convertase enzymes of the classical (C4b2a3b) and alternative (C3bBb3bP) pathways, respectively, forming C5 convertase enzymes. This C3b acts as an acceptor site for C5, which is cleaved by C5 convertase to C5b and anaphylatoxin C5a. C5a is a potent soluble inflammatory anaphylatoxic and chemotactic molecule that promotes recruitment and activation of neutrophils and monocytes and mediates endothelial cell activation through its receptor, C5a receptor (C5aR [CD88]), a member of the heptahelical 7 transmembrane spanning protein family [22, 23]. Binding of C5b to the target initiates the non-enzymatic assembly of the C5b-9 membrane attack complex (MAC). MAC is a pore forming lipophilic complex that can destroy cells by permeabilization of the membranes and act as an ion channel that triggers cell activation. Insertion of C5b-9 MAC causes erythrocyte lysis through changes in intracellular osmolarity, while C5b-9 MAC damages nucleated cells primarily by activating specific signaling pathways through the interaction of the membrane associated MAC proteins with heterotrimeric G proteins [24, 25].

Because activated complement fragments have the capacity to bind and damage self tissues, it is imperative that autologous bystander cells be protected from the deleterious effects of complement. To avoid the potentially deleterious activities of complement acting on self tissues, the activation of the complement cascade is tightly controlled by membrane and soluble regulatory proteins. C3 is an important site of such complement regulation. Inhibition of C3 activation blocks the generation of most mediators of inflammation and tissue injury along the complement pathway. Two membrane bound proteins regulate the activation of C3 on the surface of host cells [26, 27]. Decay accelerating factor (DAF) and membrane cofactor protein (MCP) are expressed on most human cells and inactivate C3 convertases, thus limiting all 3 initiating pathways. DAF inhibits the assembly and accelerates the decay of the C3 convertase enzymes that activate C3 and amplify the classical and alternative complement pathways. MCP is a co-factor for factor I mediated degradation and inactivation of C3b and C4b [28]. A third protein, CD59, also membrane anchored, prevents assembly of C5b-9 MAC. CD59 inhibits both the insertion and polymerization of C9, blocking the MAC formation and thus preventing the terminal effector functions of complement [24]. The MAC is also inhibited by S protein and clusterin. There are also soluble complement inhibitors, including C1 inhibitor (inhibits C1r and C1s) and factor H and C4 binding protein (inhibitors of C3 and C4, respectively) [29].

Complement and Pregnancy Loss

Recent murine studies underscore the importance of complement regulation in fetal control of maternal processes that mediate tissue damage. In mice, Crry is a membrane bound intrinsic complement regulatory protein with function similar to MCP and DAF. Crry blocks C3 and C4 activation on self membranes, inhibiting the classical and alternative pathway C3 convertases [30]. The absolute necessity for appropriate complement inhibition in a normal pregnancy has been demonstrated by the finding that Crry deficiency in utero leads to progressive embryonic lethality [31]. Importantly, $Crry^{-/-}$ embryos are completely rescued from this 100% lethality and live pups are born at a normal Mendelian frequency when the $Crry^{+/-}$ parents are inter-crossed with $C3^{-/-}$ mice to generate $C3^{-/-}$, $Crry^{-/-}$ embryos, suggesting that the $Crry^{-/-}$ embryos die in utero due to their inability to suppress complement activation and tissue damage mediated by C3. Based on these findings, we proposed that aPL antibodies activate complement within decidual tissue, overwhelm the normally adequate inhibitory mechanisms described above, and induce inflammation and fetal damage.

To examine the role of complement in aPL antibody–induced pregnancy loss, we used a murine model of antiphospholipid syndrome (APS) induced by passive transfer of human aPL antibodies (aPL–IgG). Using this model, we observed that aPL–IgG induces complement activation and that by blocking this activation we can prevent fetal loss and growth restriction [32, 33]. In our studies, we found that F(ab´)2 fragments of aPL–IgG do not mediate fetal injury, indicating that the Fc portion of IgG is necessary for aPL antibody–mediated injury [32]. Do aPL antibodies initiate inflammation and fetal demise by cross-linking stimulatory Fcg receptors (FcγRs) expressed on monocytes, neutrophils, platelets, or mast cells, or by activating the classical pathway of complement? When we examined the effects of aPL–IgG in mice with a targeted deletion of the common γ subunit that lack stimulatory Fc receptors ($Fc\gamma^{-/-}$), we found that they were not protected from poor pregnancy outcomes after passive transfer of aPL–IgG. Thus, aPL–IgG initiates fetal damage in the absence of activating FcγRs. Yet, the Fc portion of aPL–IgG is required, supporting a role for activation of the classical pathway in fetal injury. Indeed, mice lacking C4 were protected.

To further study the role of complement in aPL antibody–induced pregnancy loss, we inhibited C3 activation with Crry-Ig, an exogenously administered inhibitor of C3 activation. Crry–IgG prevented aPL–IgG induced complement deposition within the deciduas and protected mice from pregnancy complications. We observed similar results when C3-deficient mice were treated with aPL–IgG; there was no pregnancy loss or growth restriction [33]. While the nature of the antigens recognized by aPL antibodies is clearly important, complement activation seems to be the major effector mechanism by which these antibodies mediate tissue injury.

Complement components downstream from C3 are involved in aPL antibody-induced tissue injury [32]. Blockade of C5 activation with anti-C5 monoclonal antibodies, as well as experiments in C5-deficient mice, indicate that C5 split products are required for pregnancy complications in APS. In fact, the pro-inflammatory sequelae of C5a–C5aR interactions and the recruitment of neutrophils are critical intermediates linking pathogenic aPL antibodies to fetal damage. After aPL–IgG treatment, embryos die surrounded by massive leukocyte infiltration. C5a, a potent anaphylatoxin that recruits and activates neutrophils by interacting with C5aR, plays an important role in aPL–IgG induced tissue injury. Absence of C5aR or blockade of C5aR with specific antagonist peptides protects mice from pregnancy complications of aPL–IgG treatment [32]. Activation of complement is amplified by the alternative pathway, evidenced by the protection afforded by factor B deficiency or treatment with anti-factor B monoclonal antibodies [32, 34]. Neutrophil depletion with monoclonal antibodies also prevented aPL–IgG induced embryo injury, confirming the importance of inflammation in this model [32].

We propose the following mechanism for the pathogenic effects of aPL antibodies on tissue injury (Fig. 31.2). First, aPL are preferentially targeted to the placenta where they activate complement via the classical pathway. C3 and subsequently C5 are activated. C5a is generated and attracts and activates neutrophils, monocytes, and mast cells, and stimulates the release of inflammatory mediators, including reactive oxidants, proteolytic enzymes, chemokines, and cytokines. Proteases secreted by inflammatory cells, particularly neutrophils, can also increase C5a generation by directly cleaving C5 [35], leading to autocrine and paracrine stimulation and further recruitment of leukocytes.

Complement and Thrombosis

Complement activation and thrombophilia are linked in inflammatory diseases. Using an in vivo microcirculation model, we showed that aPL–IgG antibodies induce endothelial cell activation, and enhanced and accelerated thrombus formation in the presence of a vascular injury [11, 36, 37]. The average size of injury-induced thrombi in mice treated with aPL–IgG was 5 times greater than that of mice treated with IgG from healthy individuals. Administration of Crry–Ig significantly decreased aPL–IgG induced enhancement of thrombosis, resulting in values near those of the controls [32]. Thus, complement activation also appears to play a central role in aPL antibody–induced thrombophilia.

But how does complement activation cause a prothrombotic phenotype? Complement fragments (such as C3a or C5a) can directly activate endothelial cells by binding to cell surface receptors or indirectly activate endothelial cells by binding to receptors on neighboring phagocytes or platelets; complement split products may thereby induce a prothrombotic phenotype [38, 39]. C5a–C5aR interactions can trigger thrombosis. In a rat model of antibody mediated thrombotic glomerulonephritis, C5aR blockade prevents thrombus formation and leukocyte

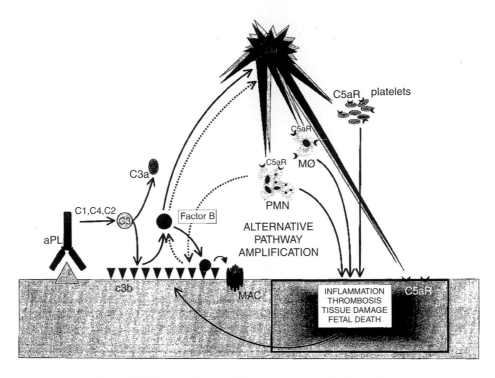

Figure 31.2. Schematic diagram of the 3 complement activation pathways.

accumulation and, similar to our findings, depletion of neutrophils prevents glomerular thrombosis, despite the presence of C3 and MAC [40]. C5a also recruits and stimulates other inflammatory cells, such as mast cells, monocytes, macrophages, and eosinophils. Enzymes in eosinophil granules function as powerful procoagulants [41]. C5a stimulates production of plasminogen activator inhibitor-1 in human mast cells and basophils which may be triggers of thrombosis [42]. Mast cells also release tumor necrosis factor α (TNF-α) stored in granules upon stimulation by C5aR, and TNF-α induces tissue factor expression on endothelial cells and monocytes [43]. Finally, C5a can directly induce release of tissue factor on endothelial cells, demonstrating an important aspect of interrelationship between the inflammatory and coagulation cascades [44]. It is therefore not surprising that in C5 deficient mice, aPL–IgG did not cause thrombophilia [45].

Formation of C5b-9 MAC involves the sequential assembly of the 5 terminal complement proteins into a heteropolymeric complex. MAC can activate pro-inflammatory and prothrombotic signaling pathways through the interaction of membrane associated MAC proteins with heterotrimeric G proteins [24, 46]. The insertion of MAC into the membrane causes considerable perturbation of the lipid bilayer. MAC may cause tissue necrosis by lysing cells. However, most nucleated cells are resistant to lysis and non-lethal effects of the MAC which trigger cell activation are likely to be more important to pathology [44, 47]. MAC activation is regulated by CD59, which interferes with its assembly and generation of the MAC pore.

CD59 has been shown to protect glomerular endothelium from thrombosis, whereas blockade of CD59 with a monoclonal antibody was associated with C5b-9 formation in glomeruli and increased platelet and fibrin deposition [48]. Mice express 2 CD59 genes (mCd59a and mCd59b); mCd59b knockout mice present a strong phenotype characterized by hemolytic anemia, platelet activation, and thrombophilia [49].

Although the cause of tissue injury in APS is likely multifactoral, complement activation is an absolute requirement for 2 of the most deleterious phenotypic outcomes in this condition. Blockade of complement is effective in preventing fetal injury and thrombosis in experimental models of APS and may have therapeutic implications in patients. Complement inhibitors are now being tested in patients with inflammatory, ischemic, and autoimmune diseases. Identifying the complement components involved in aPL antibody–induced pregnancy complications in patients may define targets for interventions that prevent, arrest, or modify APS.

References

1. Wassermann A, Neisser A, Bruck C. Eine serodiagnostiche Reaktion bei Syphilis. Deutsche Med Wochenschr 1906;32:745–746.
2. Pangborn MC. A new serologically active phospholipid from beef heart. Proc Soc Exp Biol Med 1941;48:484–486.
3. Asherson RA, et al. The "primary" antiphospholipid syndrome: major clinical and serological features. Medicine (Baltimore) 1989;68:366–374.
4. Lockshin MD. Antiphospholipid antibody and antiphospholipid antibody syndrome. Curr Opin Rheumatol 1991;3:797–802.
5. Lockwood CJ, Rand JH. The immunobiology and obstetrical consequences of antiphospholipid antibodies. Obstet Gynecol Surv 1994;49:432–441.
6. Sammaritano LR, Gharavi AE, Lockshin MD. Antiphospholipid antibody syndrome: immunologic and clinical aspects. Semin Arthritis Rheum 1990;20:81–96.
7. Shapiro SS. The lupus anticoagulant/antiphospholipid syndrome. Annu Rev Med 1996;47:533–553.
8. Del Papa N, et al. Endothelial cells as target for antiphospholipid antibodies. Human polyclonal and monoclonal anti-beta 2-glycoprotein I antibodies react in vitro with endothelial cells through adherent beta 2-glycoprotein I and induce endothelial activation. Arthritis Rheum 1997;40:551–561.
9. Roubey RA. Tissue factor pathway and the antiphospholipid syndrome. J Autoimmun 2000;15:217–220.
10. Simantov R, et al. Activation of cultured vascular endothelial cells by antiphospholipid antibodies. J Clin Invest 1995;96:2211–2219.
11. Pierangeli SS, et al. Antiphospholipid antibodies from antiphospholipid syndrome patients activate endothelial cells in vitro and in vivo. Circulation 1999;99:1997–2002.
12. Ma K, et al. High affinity binding of beta 2-glycoprotein I to human endothelial cells is mediated by annexin II. J Biol Chem 2000;275:15541–15548.
13. Meroni PL, et al. Beta2-glycoprotein I as a "cofactor" for anti-phospholipid reactivity with endothelial cells. Lupus 1998;7(suppl 2):S44–S47.
14. Kandiah DA, Krilis SA. Beta 2-glycoprotein I. Lupus 1994;3:207–212.
15. Walport MJ. Complement. First of two parts. N Engl J Med 2001;344:1058–1066.
16. Weiser MR, et al. Reperfusion injury of ischemic skeletal muscle is mediated by natural antibody and complement. J Exp Med 1996;183:2343–2348.
17. Korb LC, Ahearn JM. C1q binds directly and specifically to surface blebs of apoptotic human keratinocytes: complement deficiency and systemic lupus erythematosus revisited. J Immunol 1997;158:4525–4528.
18. Mevorach D, et al. Complement-dependent clearance of apoptotic cells by human macrophages. J Exp Med 1998;188:2313–2320.
19. Hugli TE. Structure and function of C3a anaphylatoxin. Curr Top Microbiol Immunol 1990;153:181–208.
20. Brown EJ. Complement receptors and phagocytosis. Curr Opin Immunol 1991;3:76–82.
21. Holers VM. In: Rich R, ed. Complement, principles and practices of clinical immunology. St. Louis, MO: Mosby, 1995:363.

22. Gerard NP, Gerard C. The chemotactic receptor for human C5a anaphylatoxin. Nature 1991;349:614–617.
23. Wetsel RA. Structure, function and cellular expression of complement anaphylatoxin receptors. Curr Opin Immunol 1995;7:48–53.
24. Morgan BP, Meri S. Membrane proteins that protect against complement lysis. Semin Immunopathol 1994;15:369–396.
25. Shin ML, Rus HG, Nicolescu FI. Membrane attack by complement: assembly and biology of terminal complement complexes. Biomembranes 1996;4:123–149.
26. Hourcade D, Holers VM, Atkinson JP. The regulators of complement activation (RCA) gene cluster. Adv Immunol 1989;45:381–416.
27. Lublin DM, Atkinson JP. Decay-accelerating factor and membrane cofactor protein. Curr Top Microbiol Immunol 1989;153:123–145.
28. Oglesby TJ, et al. Membrane cofactor protein (CD46) protects cells from complement-mediated attack by an intrinsic mechanism. J Exp Med 1992;175:1547–1551.
29. Holers VM. Complement as a regulatory and effector pathway in human diseases. In: Lambris JD, Holers VM, eds. Therapeutic interventions in the complement system. Totowa, NJ: Humana Press: 2000;1–32.
30. Kim YU, et al. Mouse complement regulatory protein Crry/p65 uses the specific mechanisms of both human decay-accelerating factor and membrane cofactor protein. J Exp Med 1995;181:151–159.
31. Xu C, et al. A critical role for murine complement regulator crry in fetomaternal tolerance. Science 2000;287:498–501.
32. Girardi G, et al. Complement C5a receptors and neutrophils mediate fetal injury in the antiphospho-lipid syndrome. J Clin Invest 2003;112:1644–1654.
33. Holers VM et al. Complement C3 activation is required for antiphospholipid antibody-induced fetal loss. J Exp Med 2002;195:211–220.
34. Thurman T, et al. A novel inhibitor of the alternative pathway of complement protects mice from fetal injury in the antiphopsholipid syndrome. Mol Immunol 2004;41:318.
35 Huber-Lang M, et al. Generation of C5a by phagocytic cells. Am J Pathol 2002;161:1849–1859.
36. Pierangeli SS, et al. Effect of human IgG antiphospholipid antibodies on an in vivo thrombosis model in mice. Thromb Haemost 1994;71:670–674.
37. Pierangeli SS, et al. Induction of thrombosis in a mouse model by IgG, IgM and IgA immunoglobu-lins from patients with the antiphospholipid syndrome. Thromb Haemost 1995;74:1361–1367.
38. Benzaquen LR, Nicholson-Weller A, Halperin JA. Terminal complement proteins C5b–9 release basic fibroblast growth factor and platelet-derived growth factor from endothelial cells. J Exp Med 1994;179:985–992.
39. Hattori R, et al. Complement proteins C5b–9 induce secretion of high molecular weight multimers of endothelial von Willebrand factor and translocation of granule membrane protein GMP-140 to the cell surface. J Biol Chem 1989;264:9053–9060.
40. Kondo C, et al. The role of C5a in the development of thrombotic glomerulonephritis in rats. Clin Exp Immunol 2001;124:323–329.
41. Samoszuk M, Corwin M, Hazen SL. Effects of human mast cell tryptase and eosinophil granule pro-teins on the kinetics of blood clotting. Am J Hematol 2003;73:18–25.
42. Wojta J, et al. C5a stimulates production of plasminogen activator inhibitor-1 in human mast cells and basophils. Blood 2002;100:517–523.
43. Shebuski RJ, Kilgore KS. Role of inflammatory mediators in thrombogenesis. J Pharmacol Exp Ther 2002;300:729–735.
44. Ikeda K, et al. C5a induces tissue factor activity on endothelial cells. Thromb Haemost 1997;77:394–398.
45. Pierangeli SS, et al. Complement C5 Activation is required for antiphospholipid antibody-induced thrombofilia. Arthritis Rheum 2003;48:S163.
46. Shin ML, et al. Membrane factors responsible for homologous species restriction of complement-mediated lysis: evidence for a factor other than DAF operating at the stage of C8 and C9. J Immunol 1986;136:1777–1782.
47. Morgan BP. Complement membrane attack on nucleated cells: resistance, recovery and non-lethal effects. Biochem J 1989;264:1–14.
48. Nangaku M, et al. CD59 protects glomerular endothelial cells from immune-mediated thrombotic microangiopathy in rats. J Am Soc Nephrol 1998;9:590–597.
49. Qin X, et al. Deficiency of the mouse complement regulatory protein mCd59b results in spontaneous hemolytic anemia with platelet activation and progressive male infertility. Immunity 2003;18:217–227.

32 Mechanism of Thrombosis in Antiphospholipid Syndrome: Binding to Platelets

Joan-Carles Reverter and Dolors Tàssies

Introduction

Antiphospholipid antibodies (aPL) are related to thrombosis in the antiphospholipid syndrome (APS) [1, 2] and numerous pathophysiological mechanisms have been suggested involving cellular effects, plasma coagulation regulatory proteins, and fibrinolysis [3, 4]: aPL may act as blocking agents directly inhibiting antigen enzymatic or co-factor function of hemostasis; may bind fluid-phase antigens of hemostasis involved proteins and then decrease plasma antigen levels by clearance of immune complexes; may form immune complexes with their antigens that may be deposited in blood vessels causing inflammation and tissue injury; may cause dysregulation of antigen–phospholipid binding due to cross-linking of membrane bound antigens; and may trigger cell mediated events by cross-linking of antigen bound to cell surfaces or cell surface receptors [3, 4]. Moreover, several characteristics of the aPL, such as the concentration, class/subclass, affinity or charge, and several characteristics of the antigens, as the concentration, size, location or charge, may influence which of the theoretical autoantibody actions will occur in vivo [3].

Among the cellular mechanisms supposed to be involved, platelets have been considered as one of the most promising potential target for circulating aPL that may cause antibody mediated thrombosis as a part of the clinical spectrum of the autoimmune disorder of the APS. In the present chapter we will focus on the interactions that involve aPL binding to platelet membrane or platelet membrane bound antigens.

Platelets as Target for aPL

Platelets play a central role in primary hemostasis involving platelet adhesion to the injured blood vessel wall, followed by platelet activation, granule release, shape change, and rearrangement of the outer membrane phospholipids and proteins, transforming them into a highly efficient procoagulant surface [5]. In addition, thrombocytopenia is also a clinical manifestation of APS. For these reasons platelets itself have been considered as a potential target for aPL and this fact has been extended to thrombotic mechanisms [3].

Several facts support platelets as the target for aPL. Studies performed in the aggregometer or in flowing conditions and the evaluation of platelet activation markers in vitro and in vivo in patients with the APS are used as demonstration.

Activation and spontaneous aggregation of platelets was reported in aggregometric studies to be caused directly by aPL in early reports [6, 7]. Other authors did not find this ability of aPL to initiate platelet activation [8, 9] or report inhibition of aggregation caused by aPL [10]. However, the most realistic interpretation is that in the aggregometric studies aPL may cooperate in platelet activation by making platelets more reactive to the action of weak or low-dose agonists [8, 11–13]. A calcium independent platelet aggregation (thromboagglutination) has also been found in patients with APS [14].

Other studies performed using flowing systems that simulate physiological conditions [15, 16] demonstrated, in both systemic lupus erythematosus (SLE) patients and in primary APS patients, increased formation of platelet thrombi when small amounts of patients' plasmas or purified immunoglobulins with anticardiolipin activity were added to normal blood, but this increase only occurs when plasma or immunoglobulins from patients with thrombotic history was employed. Similar results were obtained in the same system when the experiments were performed using human monoclonal anticardiolipin (anti–β_2-glycoprotein I) antibodies [17], and the β_2-glycoprotein–dependence of this phenomenon has been evidenced [18]. Additionally, dimers of β_2-glycoprotein I, that mimic effects of β_2-glycoprotein I–anti–β_2-glycoprotein I antibody complexes, have been found to increase platelet adhesion and thrombus formation in a flow system but not increased aggregation in an aggregometer [19].

Several studies have been performed to identify platelet activation markers in patients with APS. Some of them investigate the eicosanoid regulation in these patients showing inhibition of prostacyclin synthesis [20–22] and/or increased platelet thromboxane production [13, 22–24]. These results were found in in vitro experiments and in vivo in patients with the APS. However, these results have not been found by others [25]. More recently, anticardiolipin–β_2-glycoprotein I complexes have been found to induce platelet overactivity resulting in excessive production of thromboxane A2, presumably by decreased platelet cyclic AMP activity, causing increased platelet aggregation [26].

Looking for more direct markers of platelet activation, other authors have found an increase of the CD62p (P-selectin), an integral protein found in the α-granules, on platelet surface [27, 28] and/or the soluble CD62 [29, 30], loss from the activated platelet membranes to the plasma, in patients with APS, but not all the authors found the same results [31, 32]. Moreover, platelet CD63 expression, a lysosomal granule protein exposed after platelet activation, has been found increased in primary APS patients [30], but not in all the studies [28]. PAC-1, an antibody that detects the conformational change of the platelet membrane glycoprotein IIb–IIIa complex that occurs when the platelet is activated and probably a more sensitive index of platelet activation than degranulation proteins, binding has been also reported significantly increased in patients with primary APS [30]. In these patients, a significantly increased number of circulating platelet microparticles have been found [33], supporting an increased platelet activation in vivo, but these results have not been confirmed by others [30]. Annexin V binding to platelets, which indicates phosphatidyl serine exposure on the outer leaflet of the membranes during platelet activation, measured by flow cytometry has been reported as increased in a series of patients with SLE with thrombosis [34], most of them with aPL, but has been found normal in primary APS [30]. In several studies, increased platelet–leukocyte complexes, generated after platelet activation or as an inflammatory feature of autoimmune disease, have been found in APS patients [30, 35]. Finally, β-thromboglobulin, another platelet activation marker, has been evaluated in vitro or in vivo in few studies with discrepant results [34, 36, 37].

The interaction of aPL with platelets can occur in at least three different ways. First, immunoglobulins may bind through the Fab terminus with specific platelet antigens (or with other antigens deposed on platelets) in a classical antigen–antibody reaction; second, immune complexes may bind to platelets via Fcγ receptor (FcγR); and third, aPL, as other immunoglobulins, may bind to platelets in a nonspecific manner by mechanisms not well characterized but probably related to platelet membrane injuries [38]. The last mechanism, non-specific binding, does not seem to have a pathophysiological role in APS-related thrombosis.

Binding of aPL to Phospholipids on Platelet Membrane

Normal platelet membranes have a clear phospholipid asymmetry. The outer leaflet of the phospholipid bilayer is rich in choline-phospholipids, whereas amino-phospholipids are located in the inner leaflet [39]. Then, in resting platelets phosphatidyl serine is predominantly located in the cytoplasmic leaflet of the platelet membranes, but platelets undergoing activation lose their physiological phospholipid asymmetry and increase the exposure of anionic phospholipids, mainly phosphatidyl serine, on the external cell membrane [40]. During platelet activation a fast transbilayer movement of phospholipids (flip-flop) is produced [39]. In addition, during platelet activation exposure of anionic phospholipids is accompanied by shedding of procoagulant microvesicles [41]. The extent of the platelet membrane phospholipid expression depends on the type of platelet activator, being calcium-ionophore the most potent, followed in order of potency by the complement complex C5b-9, collagen plus thrombin, collagen, and thrombin [39]. ADP and epinephrine are very weak activators considering the induction of the phospholipid flip-flop.

Some studies have demonstrated that aPL may bind to platelet surface, and this binding is higher on activated or damaged platelets than in resting ones [16, 37, 42]. In addition, several agonists, like collagen, may be more able to activate platelets in a way that makes them reactive to aPL than others, like ADP [16]. These results agree with the differential expression of phospholipids during platelet activation.

APL with lupus anticoagulant (LA) activity also bind to platelets and to platelet-derived microvesicles at least in part by membrane-bound prothrombin [43]. However, it has been reported that LA antibodies can bind to activated platelets in absence of any plasma component, but it can not be excluded that the required cofactor may be released from the platelet granules [43].

Membranes from activated platelets are an important source of negatively charged phospholipids to provide a catalytic surface for interacting coagulation factors [43]. The ability of platelets to support tenase and prothrombinase activity (and also protein C activity) correlates with the extent to the platelet membrane phospholipid asymmetry [39]. By binding to phospholipid surface, aPL may interfere in the protrombinase activity by hampering the assembly of the prothrombin activating complex (factors Xa and Va, phospholipid and calcium) on the platelet procoagulant surface by reducing the binding of prothrombin to a otherwise normal prothrombinase complex [44]. The binding of aPL (or at least some of them with LA activity) to phospholipids causes a decrease in the peak amount of prothrombinase activity that has been attributed to both deficient formation of the complex and to poor prothrombin binding [44]. This effect may be inhibited by the presence of phospholipids depending more on their amount than on their nature and no specific platelet product could be identified as responsible [44]. These effects inhibiting the coagulation pathway may explain the results observed in vitro with LA, but in vivo aPL cause thrombosis and not bleeding. However, we can suppose that aPL may interfere with the protein C pathway inhibiting their phospholipid dependent reactions that occurs on platelet surfaces in the same way in which they act in the prothrombinase reaction [3, 45]. Then, these actions in the regulatory protein C system may lead to a decreased of its physiological anticoagulant activity. It has been suggested that these antibodies that alter protein C pathway may be associated with venous thrombosis.

Role of Phospholipid-binding Proteins: β_2-glycoprotein I

It is now known that aPL are in fact directed against phospholipid-binding proteins eventually bound to phospholipids exposed on surfaces [3]. The main protein associated to the anticardiolipin antibodies activity is the β_2-glycoprotein I bound to phospholipids [46–48] and then anticardiolipin antibodies bind directly to these protein immobilized on irradiated surfaces [49] constituting the actual epitope of anticardiolipin antibodies. β_2-glycoprotein I and other phospholipid-binding protein could be considered a mechanism to protect the organism from excessive coagulation leading by negatively charged phospholipids exposed on platelet (or other cells) membranes during cell activation or apoptosis [3].

β_2-glycoprotein I is a highly glycosylated single chain protein present in plasma that avidly binds to negatively charged phospholipids as cardiolipin, phosphatidyl serine, or phosphatidyl inositol [50] through their highly positively charged amino acid sequence Cys281–Cys288 [51] located in the fifth domain [52], whereas the possible epitope for anticardiolipin antibodies binding seems to be located in the fourth domain [53]. Mutations in the fifth domain of β_2-glycoprotein I have been described affecting the binding to phospholipids in patients with APS and SLE [54, 55].

The affinity of β_2-glycoprotein I for phospholipid surfaces highly depends on their phospholipid composition. In physiological conditions, β_2-glycoprotein I may inhibit phospholipid dependent hemostasis reactions, but due to its low affinity for phospholipids [51, 56], β_2-glycoprotein I is by itself only a weak anticoagulant. However, aPL (or at least aPL with LA activity) may enhance the affinity of β_2-glycoprotein I to phospholipids and, then, β_2-glycoprotein I may become a real competitor to phospholipid dependent hemostasis reactions. Using artificial bilayer membranes with physiological phosphatidyl serine concentration and purified human aPL with LA activity, a high-affinity interaction was identified in the binding of aPL–β_2-glycoprotein I complexes to phospholipids due to the bivalent interactions between antibodies and lipid bound β_2-glycoprotein I [56].

It has been demonstrated [37] that human anticardiolipin antibodies only can bind to activated platelets but not to resting platelets and this binding was in a β_2-glycoprotein I–dependent way. Moreover, it has been demonstrated [18], using reconstituted blood in flowing systems that simulate physiological conditions β_2-glycoprotein, that the β_2-glycoprotein dependence of the increased platelet–vessel wall interaction induced by human monoclonal anti–β_2-glycoprotein I antibodies obtained from patients with APS. In addition, it has been reported [8] that murine monoclonal antibodies against β_2-glycoprotein I with LA activity potentiate the effect of sub-threshold concentrations of aggregation agonists (ADP or adrenaline) but requiring the presence of β_2-glycoprotein I.

The reason why aPL with anti–β_2-glycoprotein I activity bind to β_2-glycoprotein I bound to platelets but not to free β_2-glycoprotein 1 in plasma needs to be answered. At physiological concentrations of β_2-glycoprotein I, aPL binding to β_2-glycoprotein I in the fluid phase is weak [57]. This fact is due to a low intrinsic affinity of the antibodies to β_2-glycoprotein I. Clustering or a high density of immobilized antigen, as may occur in the surface of activated platelets, allows bivalent or multivalent antibody binding and then aPL may act locally [3, 57]. In addition, conformational changes induced in β_2-glycoprotein I by its binding to negatively charged surfaces causing the expression of neo-epitopes (or the expression of cryptic epitopes) have been suggested [58, 59] and aPL could be directed against this neo-epitopes (or cryptic epitopes) but not to free β_2-glycoprotein I. For these reasons aPL need the presence of platelet surfaces to exert their actions through their anti–β_2-glycoprotein I activity.

In this scenario [60], β_2-glycoprotein I may form a small amount of monovalent complexes in the fluid phase, and both monovalent complexes and free β_2-glycoprotein I bind to negatively charged phospholipids on cellular surfaces, such as activated platelet membranes, with low affinity [51, 60]. APL can bind then to β_2-glycoprotein I bound to membrane phospholipids forming new monovalent aPL–phospholipid complexes [60]. In the platelet membrane, monovalent complexes have a high mobility because its binding to phospholipids is based to ionic interactions and, due to this mobility and depending of aPL–β_2-glycoprotein 1 density, bivalent stable complexes may form [60]. Such bivalent complexes have high affinity for phospholipids and may interfere with both anticoagulant and pro-coagulant reactions [51]. APL also could potentiate the inhibitory activity of β_2-glycoprotein I in coagulation by cross-linking membrane-bound β_2-glycoprotein I and by enhancing the avidity of the β_2-glycoprotein I–phospholipid interaction [3]. In addition, aPL, in experimental studies using human polyclonal purified antibodies, may enhance β_2-glycoprotein I binding to negatively charged phospholipid surfaces [56].

Interaction of aPL with the Platelet Fcγ Receptor IIA

It has been demonstrated that both Fab and Fc fragments of the aPL are essentials for the effect of murine monoclonal antibodies against β_2-glycoprotein I increasing platelet aggregation by weak agonists [8]. This effect is dependent on the action of the FcγR IIA, as it could be blocked by inhibitory monoclonal antibodies [8].

There are 3 families of FcγR molecules (RI, RII, and RIII) [61], each containing several allelic variants. The only FcγR molecules present on platelets are the FcγRIIA [62]. The FcγRIIA (CD32) is present on platelets, neutrophils, and monocytes, and has weak affinity for the Fc portion of monomeric IgG, but high affinity for the Fc portion of IgG contained in immune complexes or to IgG bound to an antigen on the platelet surface [63]. Activation of the FcγRIIA causes platelet activation and granule release. This receptor reacts best with murine IgG subclasses 1 and 2b and to human IgG subclasses 1 and 3 [64]. Human subclass IgG2 reacts weakly with the receptor.

A common functional polymorphism of the FcγRIIA gene has been described [62, 65]. The two allelic forms differ by a single base substitution in the codon for amino acid 131 that causes an Arginine (Arg) to Histidine (His) amino acid change. This polymorphism plays a particular role in the expression of IgG2 mediated antibody responses. The His 131 allele is essential for handling IgG2 immune complexes and reacts much more efficiently to subclass 2 of human IgG than the Arg 131 allele [65].

The most interesting proposal to relate anti–β_2-glycoprotein I activity, aPL platelet binding, and platelet activation leading to thrombosis suppose a pathogenic scenario very similar to these proposed for heparin induced thrombocytopenia [64, 66] involving the FcγRIIA. In this hypothesis, small initial platelet activation is produced by physiological or pathological conditions resulting in the expression of phospholipids on the platelet surface. Then, the binding of β_2-glycoprotein I (or in a lesser extent other phospholipid binding proteins) to these phospholipids may occur. APL subsequently may bind to the formed β_2-glycoprotein I–phospholipid complexes, and, then, interact by their Fc portion with the platelet surface FcγRIIA. Through these interaction platelets may be activated and a vicious circle of cellular activation may be created finally ending in a thrombotic event. Then, in the APS, as probably in a similar way in much other situations, thrombosis seems to be a two hit phenomenon. Autoantibodies, the first hit, are continually present in the circulation, but need a local trigger, the second hit, to produce hemostasis dysregulation leading to a thrombotic event in a particular localization [4]. Thrombosis would require this second hit, so explaining why patients with persistent plasma antibodies have thrombosis only occasionally and in absence of vascular immunoglobulin deposits [64].

Activation of the FcγRIIA by the aPL bound to β_2-glycoprotein I cause platelet activation and thromboxane A2 generation [64]. Activation of FcγRIIA produces intracellular ionic calcium flux, an increase of phosphatidyl inositol metabolism and also a rapid phosphorylation of tyrosine residues on a number of molecules [38]. Then, the action of the FcγRIIA activated by β_2-glycoprotein I bound aPL may constitute the second hit to thrombosis in these patients.

Some other indirect evidences supporting this mechanism, the activation of FcγRIIA by antibodies after their binding to β_2-glycoprotein I, have been highlighted [64]. The need of an initial "triggering" activation to start the process is congruent with the high degree of recurrence of thrombotic events in the same arterial or venous territory [67]. This fact is compatible with a local trigger causing slight activation that can be followed by a secondary amplification due to aPL [64].

However, there are several reasons that do not permit this model to explain all the effects of aPL in thrombosis. First, anti–β_2-glycoprotein I antibodies in autoimmune patients are mainly restricted to the IgG2 subclass [68] and IgG2 subclass antibodies can not efficiently react with the FcγRIIA if the mutation His–His in the position 131 of FcγRIIA is not present. It may be suggested that patients with the form His 131 of the polymorphism may be at greater risk to develop thrombosis by this platelet activation mechanism via FcγRIIA [64], similarly as it has been reported in heparin induced thrombocytopenia [69]. However, this hypothesis has not been sustained by epidemiological studies and no increased frequency of the His 131 form of this polymorphism has been found in patients with the APS [70], and in a recent meta-analysis a complex genetic background underlying the relationship between the FcγRIIA-R/H131 polymorphism and the APS has been suggested [71]. An alternative explanation to the platelet activation by IgG2 subclass aPL via the FcγRIIA is that activated platelet express increased number of FcγRIIA up to 50% [72] and, by this way, the first "triggering" event may improve IgG2 subclass aPL interactions with platelets in Arg–Arg FcγRIIA R/H131 genotype.

Second, the proposed schema of FcγRIIA activation may not explain the prothrombotic action of IgM aPL. For this reason, an alternative hypothesis considering the activation of complement by aPL after their attachment to protein–phospholipid complexes on platelet surfaces has been suggested [64], as it will be discussed latter.

Third, in a thrombosis model in hamster, F(ab)2 fragments of an anti–β_2-glycoprotein I antibody were equally able to promote thrombus formation [73].

In addition, using an in vivo thrombosis model in mice, it has been suggested [74] that the thrombogenic effect of aPL passively administered is not dependent on their anti–β_2-glycoprotein I activity alone.

Finally, it has been reported an additive effect of LA and anticardiolipin antibodies that may directly activate platelets [75] and this effect could not be attributed to the FcγRIIA because separately anticardiolipin antibodies and LA fractions did not activate platelets.

A calcium-independent mechanism for the initiation of thrombus formation in APS has been proposed [14]. In this model aPL bind specifically to platelet membrane phospholipids under slow shear flow and, then, antibodies cross bridges to an adjacent platelet containing phosphlipid–β_2-glycoprotein I complexes. This results in thromboagglutination followed by release of granules, recruitment of platelets, and fibrin formation.

Complement Activation

As mentioned previously, the aPL bound to platelet membranes may also exert their action through the activation of complement. Some authors have reported decreased levels of serum complement in patients with aPL [76] although others did not confirm this data [77]. Moreover, increased levels of inactivated terminal membrane attack complex of complement (C5b-9) were found in patients with aPL and cerebral ischemia [78]. C3 activation seems to be essential for antiphospholipid antibody induced thrombophilia and fetal loss in a mouse model [79]. Additionally, complement-fixing anticardiolipin antibodies have been found in patients with aPL and had been related to thrombotic manifestations [49]. These data support the possible role of complement activation in the pathophysiology of APS.

It is known that C5b-9 causes platelet activation [80–82], and it has been demonstrated complement activation by aPL bound to cardiolipin liposomes when these aPL were obtained from APS patients but not when were obtained from syphilis patients [83]. Then, the complement generated in presence of aPL bound to negatively charged phospholipids may cause platelet activation and, eventually, platelet destruction [84].

Considering this scenario, the double hit hypothesis suggested for the FcγRIIA mediated activation [66] can also be applied to the complement mediated platelet activation in the APS. First, an initial activation of platelets is needed (provided by local events as small vascular lesions). Then, negatively charged phospholipids are exposed in a small extent on the platelet surface and aPL may bind to these exposed phospholipids or to proteins bound to these phospholipids. APL fixed in the platelet surface may induce complement activation in an Fc independent manner causing more platelet activation [84]. In addition, C5b-9 action may increase the transbilayer migration of phosphatidyl serine in the platelet membrane [85] causing increased binding of aPL and, then, C5b-9 activation, and platelet activation.

Other Platelet Receptors for aPL

The ability of aPL to bind to platelets through different epitopes, like CD36 [86] or the glycoprotein IIIa [87] has been reported, and these special bindings have been related to thrombotic phenomena and/or to platelet activation. However, the mechanism of platelet activation in these peculiar aPL binding sites is not known. Recently [19], it has been suggested that dimeric β_2-glycoprotein I may bind apoER2', the splice variant that constitutes the only member of the low-density lipoproteins present in platelets, which results in a slight platelet activation and, then, aPL may bind to these exposed phospholipids or phospholipids–β_2-glycoprotein I complexes.

Conclusion

Platelets are a potential target for circulating aPL that may cause antibody mediated thrombosis. In vitro studies performed in the aggregometer or in flowing conditions and the evaluation of platelet activation markers in vitro and in vivo in patients with the APS demonstrated the ability of aPL to interact with platelets and promote their function. The most reliable explanation for the prothrombotic action of aPL in platelets includes, first, previous platelet activation and the binding of them to platelet membrane phospholipid bound proteins, mainly β_2-glycoprotein I. Then, in a second step, aPL may act activating platelets, via FcγRIIA or complement C5-9 formation. However, several points of this suggested mechanism of action of aPL on thrombus formation are not clearly established and further studies on the interaction between platelet and aPL are needed.

References

1. Hughes GRV, Harris EN, Gharavi AE. The anticardiolipin syndrome. J Rheumatol 1986;13:486–489.
2. Love PE, Santoro SA. Antiphospholipid antibodies: anticardiolipin and the lupus anticoagulant in systemic lupus erythematosus (SLE) and in non-SLE disorders. Ann Intern Med 1990;112:682–698.

3. Roubey RAS. Immunology of the antiphospholipid antibody syndrome. Arthritis Rheum 1996;39:1444–1454.
4. Roubey RAS. Mechanisms of autoantibody-mediated thrombosis. Lupus 1998;7(suppl 2):S114–S119.
5. Machin SJ. Platelets and antiphospholipid antibodies. Lupus 1996;5:386–387.
6. Lin YL, Wang CT. Activation of human platelets by the rabbit anticardiolipin antibodies. Blood 1992;80:3135–3143.
7. Wiener HM, Vardinon N, Yust I. Platelet antibody binding and spontaneous aggregation in 21 lupus anticoagulant patients. Vox Sang 1991;61:111–121.
8. Arvieux J, Roussel B, Pouzol P, et al. Platelet activating properties of murine monoclonal antibodies to β_2-glycoprotein I. Thromb Haemost 1993;70:336–341.
9. Ford I, Urbaniak S, Greaves M. IgG from patients with antiphospholipid syndrome binds to platelets without induction of platelet activation. Br J Haematol 1998;102:841–849.
10. Ostfeld I, Dadosh-Goffer N, Borokowski S, et al. Lupus anticoagulant antibodies inhibit collagen-induced adhesion and aggregation of human platelets in vitro. J Clin Immunol 1992;12:415–423.
11. Campbell AL, Pierangeli SS, Wellhausen S, et al. Comparison of the effects of anticardiolipin antibodies from patients with the antiphospholipid syndrome and with syphilis on platelet activation. Thromb Haemost 1995;73:529–534.
12. Ichikawa Y, Kobayashi N, Kawada T, et al. Reactivities of antiphospholipid antibodies to blood cells and their effect on platelet aggregations in vitro. Clin Exp Rheumatol 1990;8:461–465.
13. Martinuzzo ME, Maclouf J, Carreras LO, et al. Antiphospholipid antibodies enhance thrombin-induced platelet activation and tromboxane fromation. Thromb Haemost 1993;70:667–671.
14. Wiener MH, Burke M, Fried M, et al. Thromboagglutination by anticardiolipin antibody complex in the antiphospholipid syndrome. A possible mechanisms of immune-mediated thrombosis. Thromb Res 2001;103:193–199.
15. Escolar G, Font J, Reverter JC, et al. Plasma from systemic lupus erythematosus patients with antiphospholipid antibodies promotes platelet aggregation: studies in a perfusion system. Arterioscler Thromb 1992;12:196–200.
16. Reverter JC, Tàssies D, Escolar G, et al. Effect of plasma from patients with primary antiphospholipid syndrome on platelet function in a collagen rich perfusion system. Thromb Haemost 1995;73:132–137.
17. Reverter JC, Tàssies D, Font J, et al. Effect of human monoclonal anticardiolipin antibodies on platelet function and on tissue factor expression on monocytes. Arthritis Rheum 1998;41:1420–1427.
18. Font J, Espinosa G, Tassies D, et al. Effects of beta2-glycoprotein I and monoclonal anticardiolipin antibodies in platelet interaction with subendothelium under flow conditions. Arthritis Rheum 2002;46:3283–3289.
19. Lutters BCH, Derksen RHW, Tekelenburg WL, et al. Dimers of $\beta2$-glycoprotein I increase platelet deposition to collagen via interaction with phospholipids and the apolipoprotein E receptor 2'. J Biol Chem 2003;278:33831–33838.
20. Carreras LO, Defreyn G, Machin SJ, et al. Recurrent arterial thrombosis, repeated intrauterine death and "lupus" anticoagulant: detection of immunoglobulin interfering with prostacyclin formation. Lancet 1981;i:244–246.
21. Carreras LO, Vermylen JG, Deman R, et al . "Lupus" anticoagulant and thrombosis -possible role of inhibition of prostacyclin formation. Thromb Haemost 1982;48:28–40.
22. Lellouche F, Martinuzzo M, Said P, et al. Imbalance of thromboxane/ prostacyclin biosynthesis in patients with lupus anticoagulant. Blood 1991;78:2894–2899.
23. Forastiero R, Martinuzzo M, Carreras LO, et al. Anti-β-2-glycoprotein I antibodies and platelet activation in patients with antiphospholipid antibodies: association with increased excretion of platelet-derived thromboxane urinary metabolites. Thromb Haemost 1998;79:42–45.
24. Maclouf J, Lellouche F, Martinuzzo M, et al. Increased production of platelet derived thromboxane in patients with lupus anticoagulants. Agents Actions suppl 1992;37:27–33.
25. Rustin MHA, Bull HA, Machin SJ. Effects of the lupus anticoagulant in patients with systemic lupus erythematosus on endothelial cell prostacyclin release and procoagulant activity. J Invest Dermatol 1988;90:744–748.
26. Opara R, Robbins DL, Ziboh VA. Cyclic-AMP agonists inhibit antiphospholipid /beta2-glycoprotein I induced synthesis of human platelet thromboxane A2 in vitro. J Rheumatol 2003;30:55–59.
27. Emmi L, Bergamini C, Spinelli A, et al. Possible pathogenetic role of activated platelets in the primary antiphospholipid syndrome involving the central nervous system. Ann N Y Acad Sci 1997;823:188–200.
28. Fanelli A, Bergamini C, Rapi S, et al. Flow cytometric detection of circulating activated platelets in primary antiphospholipid syndrome. Correlation with thrombocytopenia and anticardiolipin antibodies. Lupus 1997;6:261–267.

29. Joseph JE, Donohoe S, Harrison P, et al. Platelet activation and turnover in the primary antiphospholipid syndrome. Lupus 1998;7:333–340.
30. Joseph JE, Harrison P, Mackie IJ, et al. Increased circulation platelet-leucocyte complexes and platelet activation in patients with antophospholipic syndrome, systemic lupus erythematosus and rheumatoid arthritis. Br J Haematol 2001;115:451–459.
31. Out HJ, de Groot P, van Vliet M, et al. Antibodies to platelets in patients with antiphospholipid antibodies. Blood 1991;77:2655–2659.
32. Shechter Y, Tal Y, Greenberg A, et al. Platelet activation in patients with antiphospholipid syndrome. Blood Coag Fibrinol 1998;9:653–657.
33. Galli M, Grassi A, Barbui T. Platelet-derived microvesicles in the antiphospholipid syndrome. Thromb Haemost 1993;69:541.
34. Ekdahl KN, Bengtsson AA, Andersson J, et al. Thrombotic disease in systemic lupus erythematosus is associated with a maintained systemic platelet activation. Br J Haematol 2004;125:74–78.
35. Specker C, Perniok A, Brauckmann U, et al. Detection of cerebral microemboli in APS-introducing a novel investigation method and implications of analogies with carotid artery disease. Lupus 1998;7(suppl 2):S75–S80.
36. Galli M, Cortelazzo S, Viero P, et al. Interaction between platelets and lupus anticoagulant. Eur J Haematol 1988;41:88–94.
37. Shi W, Chong BH, Chesterman CN. β-2-glycoprotein is a requirement for anticardiolipin antibodies binding to activated platelets: differences with lupus anticoagulants. Blood 1993;81:1255–1262.
38. Chong BH, Brighton TC, Chesterman CN. Antiphospholipid antibodies and platelets. Semin Thromb Hemost 1995;21:76–84.
39. Bevers EM, Comfurius P, Dekkers DWC, et al. Regulatory mechanisms of transmembrane phospholipid distributions and pathophysiological implications of transbilayer lipid scrambling. Lupus 1998;7(suppl 2):S126–S131.
40. Schroit AJ, Zwaal RFA. Transbilayer movement of phospholipid in red cell and platelet membranes. Biochim Biophys Acta 1991;1071:313–329.
41. Sims PJ, Wiedmer T, Esmon CT, et al. Assembly of the platelet prothrombinase complex is linked to vesiculation of the platelet plasma membrane. Studies in Scott's syndrome: an isolated defect in procoagulant activity. J Biol Chem 1989;264:17049–17057.
42. Khamashta MA, Harris EN, Gharavi AE, et al. Immune mediated mechanism for thrombosis: Antiphospholipid antibody binding to platelet membranes. Ann Rheum Dis 1988;47:849–854.
43. Galli M, Bevers EM, Comfurius P, et al. Effect of antiphospholipid antibodies on procoagulant activity of activated platelets and platelet-derived microvesicles. Br J Haematol 1993;83:466–472.
44. Galli M, Béguin S, Lindhout T, et al. Inhibition of phospholipid and platelet-dependent prothrombinase activity in the plasma of patients with lupus anticoagulant. Br J Haematol 1989;72:549–555.
45. Galli M, Ruggeri L, Barbui T. Differential effects of anti-β-2-glycoprotein I and anti-prothrombin antibodies on the anticoagulant activity of activated protein C. Blood 1998;91:1999–2004.
46. Galli M, Comfurius P, Maassen C, et al. Anticardiolipin antibodies (ACA) directed not to cardiolipin but to a plasma protein cofactor. Lancet 1990;335:1544–1547.
47. Matsuura E, Igarashi Y, Fujimoto M, et al. Anticardiolipin cofactors and diferential diagnoses of autoimmune diseases. Lancet 1990;336:177–178.
48. McNeil HP, Simpson RJ, Chesterman CN, et al. Anti-phospholipid antibodies are directed against a complex antigen that includes a lipid-binding inhibitor of coagulation: β₂-glycoprotein I (apolipoprotein H). Proc Natl Acad Sci U S A 1990;87:4120–4124.
49. Munakata Y, Saito T, Matsuda K, et al. Detection of complement-fixing antiphospholipid antibodies in association with thrombosis. Thromb Haemost 2000;83:728–731.
50. Wurm H. Beta 2-glycoprotein I (apolipoprotein H) interactions with phospholipid vesicles. Int J Biochem 1984;16:511–515.
51. Arnout J, Vermylen J. Mechanism of action of β-2-glycoprotein I-dependent lupus anticoagulants. Lupus 1998;7(suppl 2):S23–S28.
52. Hunt JE, Krilis S. The fifth domain of β-2-glycoprotein I contains a phospholipid binding site (Cys281-Cys288) and a region recognized by anticardiolipin antibodies. J Immunol 1994;152:653–659.
53. Igarashi M, Matsuura E, Igarashi Y, et al. Human β-2-glycoprotein I as an anticardiolipin cofactor determined using deleted mutans expressed by a Baculovirus system. Blood 1996;87:3262–3270.
54. Gushiken FC, Arnett FC, Ahn C, et al. Polymorphism of β2-glycoprotein I at codons 306 and 316 in patients with systemic lupus erythematosus and antiphospholipid syndrome. Arthritis Rheum 1999;42:1189–1193.

55. Gushiken FC, Arnett FC, Thiagarajan P. Primary antiphospholipid antibody syndrome with mutations in the phospholipid binding domain of beta (2)-glycoprotein I. Am J Hematol 2000;65:160–165.
56. Willems GM, Janssen MP, Pelsers MMAL, et al. Role of divalency in the high-affinity binding of anticardiolipin antibody-beta-2-glycoprotein I complexes to lipid membranes. Biochemistry 1996;35:13833–13842.
57. Roubey RAS, Eisenberg RA, Harper MF, et al. "Anti-cardiolipin" autoantibodies recognize β2-glycoprotein I in the absence of phospholipid: Importance of antigen density and bivalent binding. J Immunol 1995;154:954–960.
58. Matsuura E, Igarashi Y, Yasuda T, et al. Anticardiolipin antibodies recognize β_2-glycoprotein I structure altered by interacting with an oxygen modified solid phase surface. J Exp Med 1994;179:457–462.
59. Wagenknecht DR, McIntyre JA. Changes in beta-2-glycoprotein I antigenicity induced by phospholipid binding. Thromb Haemost 1993;69:361–365.
60. Arnout J, Wittelvrongel C, Vanrusselt M, et al. Beta-2-glycoprotein I dependent lupus anticoagulants form stable divalent antibody-beta-2-glycoprotein I complexes on phospholipid surfaces.
61. Thromb Haemost 1998;79:79–86.61. van de Winkel JGJ, Capel PJA. Human IgG Fc receptor heterogeneity. Immunol Today 1993;14:215–221.
62. Anderson CL, Chacko GW, Osborne JM, et al. The Fc receptor for immunoglobulin G (Fc gamma RII) on human platelets. Semin Thromb Hemost 1995;21:1–9.
63. De Reys S, Blom C, Lepoudre B, et al. Human platelet aggregation by murine monoclonal antibodies is subtype-dependent. Blood 1993;81:1792–1800.
64. Vermylen J, Hoylaerts MF, Arnout J. Antibody-mediated thrombosis. Thromb Haemost 1997;78:420–426.
65. Warmerdam PAM, van de Winkel JGJ, Vlug A, et al. A single amino acid in the second Ig-like domain of the Fc gamma RII is critical for human IgG2 binding. J Immunol 1991;147:1338–1343.
66. Arnout J. The pathogenesis of the antiphospholipid syndrome: a hypotesis based on parallelisms with heparin-induced thrombocytopenia. Thromb Haemost 1996;75:536–541.
67. Khamashta MA, Cuadrado MJ, Mujic F, et al. The management of thrombosis in the antiphospholipid-antibody syndrome. N Engl J Med 1995;332:993–997.
68. Arvieux J, Roussel B, Ponard D, et al. IgG2 subclass restriction of anti beta-2-glycoprotein I antibodies in autoimmune patients. Clin Exp Immunol 1994;95:310–315.
69. Carlsson LE, Santoso S, Baurichter G, et al. Heparin-induced thrombocytopenia: new insights into the impact of the FcγRIIa-R-H131 polymorphism. Blood 1998;92:1526–1531.
70. Atsumi T, Caliz R, Amengual O, et al. Fc gamma Receptor IIA H/R131 polymorphism in patients with the antiphospholipid syndrome. Thromb Haemost 1998;79:924–927.
71. Karassa FB, Bijl M, Davies KA, et al. Role of the Fcγ receptor IIA polymorphism in the antiphospholipid syndrome: an international meta-analysis. Arthritis Rheum 2003;48:1930–1938.
72. McCrae KR, Shattil SJ, Cines DB. Platelet activation induces increased Fc gamma receptor expression. J Immunol 1990;144:3920–3927.
73. Jankowski M, Vreys I, Wittevrongel C, et al. Thrombogenicity of beta 2-glycoprotein I-dependent antiphospholipid antibodies in a photochemically induced thrombosis model in the hamster. Blood 2003;101:157–162.
74. Gharavi AE, Pierangeli SS, Gharavi EE, et al. Thrombogenic properties of antiphospholipid antibodies do not depend on their binding to β-2- glycoprotein I (β2GPI) alone. Lupus 1998;7:341–346.
75. Nojima J, Suehisa E, Kuratsune H, et al. Platelet activation induced by combined effects of anticardiolipin and lupus anticoagulant IgG antibodies in patients with systemic lupus erythematosus. Thromb Haemost 1999;81:436–441.
76. Shibata S, Sasaki T, Hirabayashi Y, et al. Risk factors in the pregnancy of patients with systemic lupus erythematosus: association of hypocomplementaemia with poor prognosis. Ann Rheum Dis 1992;51:619–623.
77. Hess DC, Sheppard JC, Adams RJ. Increased immunoglobulin binding to cerebral endothelium in patients with antiphospholipid antibodies. Stroke 1993;24:994–999.
78. Davis WD, Brey RL. Antiphospholipid antibodies and complement activation in patients with cerebral ischemia. Clin Exp Rheumatol 1992;10:455–460.
79. Salmon JE, Girardi G, Holers VM. Complement activation as a mediator of antiphospholipid antibody induced pregnancy loss and thrombosis. Ann Rheum Dis 2002;61(suppl II):ii46–ii50.
80. Rinder CS, Rinder HM, Smith BR, et al. Blockade of C5a and C5b-9 generation inhibits leukocyte and platelet activation during extracorporeal circulation. J Clin Invest 1995;96:1564–1572.
81. Solum NO, Rubach-Dahlberg E, Pedersen TM, et al. Complement-mediated permeabilization of platelets by monoclonal antibodies to CD9: inhibition by leupeptin, and effects on the GPI-acting-binding protein system. Thromb Res 1994;75:437–452.

82. Wiedmer T, Hall SE, Ortel TL, et al. Complement-induced vesiculation and exposure of membrane prothrombinase sites in platelets of paroxysmal nocturnal hemoglobinuria. Blood 1993; 82:1192–1196.
83. Santiago MB, Gaburo N, de Oliveira RM, et al. Complement activation by anticardiolipin antibodies. Ann Rheum Dis 1991;50:249–250.
84. Stewart MW, Etches WS, Gordon PA. Antiphospholipid antibody-dependent C5b-9 formation. Br J Haematol 1997;96:451–457.
85. Chang CP, Zhao J, Wiedmer T, et al. Contribution of platelet microparticle formation and granule secretion to the transmembrane migration of phosphatidylserine. J Biol Chem 1993;268:7171–7178.
86. Rock G, Chauhan K, Jamieson GA, et al. Anti-CD36 antibodies in patients with lupus anticoagulant and thrombotic complications. Br J Haematol 1994;88:878–880.
87. Tokita S, Arai M, Yamamoto M, et al. Specific cross-reaction of IgG antiphospholipid antibody with platelet glycoprotein IIIA. Thromb Haemost 1996;75:168–174.

33 Interaction of Antiphospholipid Antibodies with Endothelial Cells

Pier Luigi Meroni, Elena Raschi, Cinzia Testoni, Arianna Parisio, Maria Gerosa, and Maria Orietta Borghi

Anti-phospholipid Antibody Reactivity with Endothelial Cells

Antiphospholipid antibodies (aPL) are the formal laboratory diagnostic tools for the antiphospholipid syndrome (APS) and important players in its pathogenesis at the same time [1]. Different pathogenic mechanisms have been reported, suggesting that aPL can cause thrombosis or fetal loss in several ways [2].

Owing to its emerging role in hemostasis, inflammation, and immune response regulation, endothelium has been deeply investigated as one of the "most likely" target for aPL. Perturbed endothelium actually displays a procoagulant phenotype that might be pivotal in sustaining the APS vasculopathy [3].

The first report that found a relationship between aPL and endothelial cells (EC) showed that lupus anticoagulant (LA)-positive plasmas suppressed prostacyclin (PGI_2) release by vascular endothelium and the consequent unbalance between endothelial prostacyclin $(PGI)_2$ and platelet thromboxane (TXA_2) was suggested to support the in vivo thrombotic diathesis [4].

Since the first report by Carreras and Vermylen, several authors clearly demonstrated the aPL reactivity with EC and the antibody ability to affect endothelium functions in different in vitro experimental models (Table 33.1).

Interestingly, a direct EC involvement is also evident in some in vivo experimental models of aPL induced thrombosis. Pierangeli et al demonstrated that passive infu-

Table 33.1. Pleiotropic effect of aPL on endothelial cells.

- Induction of a pro-adhesive and a pro-inflammatory phenotype [5–11]
- Tissue factor upregulation [12–15, Vega-Ostertag et al, submitted]
- Interaction with the protein C/S system [16–20]
- Annexin V displacement from the endothelial cell membrane [21]
- Interaction with the eicosanoid metabolism: inhibition of PGI_2 synthesis [4]
- Induction of pre-proET-1 synthesis [22]
- Induction of apoptosis [23]
- Interaction with the late endosomes [24]

PGI_2 = prostacyclin 2; ET-1 = endothelin-1.

sion of aPL in naive mice might increase the leukocyte adherence to the vessel walls of the cremaster muscle microcirculation [25]. The same group also reported that E-selectin expression – the adhesion molecule specific for EC – is essential for the clot formation in their experimental pinch model after the passive infusion of aPL [26]. We have recently described an additional experimental in vivo model, in which the infusion of IgG fractions with strong anti–β_2-glycoprotein I (β_2-GPI) activity, but not control IgG, can induce leukocyte aggregation and endothelial adhesion in the mesenteric rat microcirculation when small amounts of lipopolysaccharide (LPS) are also injected at the same time (Fischetti et al, submitted).

β_2-GPI as the Main aPL Antigenic Target on EC

Several authors described the presence of an anti-endothelial binding activity in sera from both primary and secondary APS, however such a reactivity was not always related to anti-cardiolipin (aCL) or LA activity [27–32]. On the other hand, APS sera were found to react with constitutive EC membrane components whose exact nature was not identified [33].

β_2-GPI – the major plasma protein co-factor for aPL – was then found to represent the bridge for targeting circulating aPL to EC membranes [5–8, 10].

In fact, sera positive for aCL (and anti–β_2-GPI) antibodies displayed anti-endothelial cell activity only when the cells were grown in the presence of bovine serum. Cell starvation in serum-free medium abolished the reactivity that was in turn restored after the addition of purified human β_2-GPI. It was suggested that the fetal calf serum of the culturing media could be the source of β_2-GPI. The molecule, in fact, is apparently able to adhere to EC monolayers and then to be recognized by anti–β_2-GPI antibodies cross-reacting with β_2-GPI of different species, including the bovine one [34]. Studies carried out with affinity purified polyclonal IgG fractions as well as with human IgM anti–β_2-GPI monoclonal antibodies supported the hypothesis [8].

As a whole these findings suggest that most of the reactivity against EC in sera of APS patients is sustained by antibodies that recognize β_2-GPI, but autoantibodies directed against constitutive EC membrane proteins can be also detectable.

Endothelium is a heterogenic tissue that displays phenotypic and functional differences depending on the anatomical localization [3]. Such a heterogeneity has been claimed to explain why thrombotic events are generally episodic and often localized, being frequently determined by local/regional pathologic processes besides systemic risk factors. Anti–β_2-GPI antibodies have been found to recognize β_2-GPI on EC monolayers obtained from both large venous vessels and from the microcirculation, in line with the widespread anatomical distribution of thrombosis in APS [35]. However, a reactivity with brain and dermal microvascular EC higher than that with human umbilical cord vein EC (HUVEC) has been recently reported.

Altogether these data suggest that although β_2-GPI endothelial expression is apparently shared in common by the whole endothelium, different binding/expression characteristics on definite anatomical sites could be responsible for some of the APS clinical manifestations (i.e., the high frequency of skin and central nervous system involvement).

Endothelial Cell Receptor(s) for β_2-GPI

It has been demonstrated that plasma proteins can adhere to in vitro unfixed EC monolayer cultures, so endothelial adhesion of β_2-GPI might be simply the result of a phenomenon common to many other plasma proteins [36, Meroni et al, personal communication].

However, a relatively more specific endothelial binding was described: β_2-GPI binds to EC membranes through the highly positively charged amino acid sequence located in the fifth domain of β_2-GPI that was previously reported to be the putative "PL-binding site" in CL-coated plates [9]. Actually, synthetic β_2-GPI molecules mutated at the PL-binding site lost their binding activity to CL-coated plates as well as to EC monolayers. In addition, synthetic peptides, spanning the amino acid sequence of the PL-binding site, were able to bind EC and to be recognized by specific autoantibodies. β_2-GPI adhesion through the highly cationic PL-binding site suggests that a corresponding negatively charged structure on EC membranes should be involved. Heparan sulphate (HS) – the major proteoglycan of the vascular endothelium – was suggested to represent the most likely candidate [37]. Actually, EC treatment with heparitinase I, an enzyme able to cleave specifically the α-N-acetyl-D-glucosaminidic linkage in HS, could affect the binding in a dose dependent manner, but not completely [35]. These findings suggested that endothelial structures other than HS might be also responsible for the co-factor adhesion.

Because β_2-GPI is a glycoprotein able to bind and transport lipids, cell membrane receptors for lipoproteins could be the structures naturally involved in its cell binding. Interestingly, β_2-GPI has been suggested to display an EC viability maintaining factor activity, which could be related to its ability to supply lipids for energy production and membrane synthesis [38].

In this regard, it has been reported that megalin – an endocytic component of the low-density lipoprotein receptor (LDL-R) family expressed on placenta, kidney and other tissues – might behave as a β_2-GPI receptor [39]. However, Cao et al failed to demonstrate any megalin–mRNA expression in both human vein and arterial umbilical EC [40]. A further indirect evidence that megalin is not an endothelial receptor for β_2-GPI turns out from the observation that the presence of EDTA buffer did not affect the binding that is, by definition, Ca^{++} ion-dependent (Meroni et al, personal communication).

It has recently been reported that β_2-GPI can bind to another component of the LDL-R family: the apolipoprotein E receptor-2 (ApoER2) [41]. In fact, apoER2 was found to mediate the β_2-GPI binding to platelets. Because apoER2 is expressed on EC also, it might be an additional EC membrane receptor for β_2-GPI [42].

Furthermore, annexin II, an EC receptor for tissue plasminogen activator (t-PA) [43–45] was shown to be able to bind β_2-GPI with an affinity that was even much higher than that displayed by β_2-GPI for phospholipid (PL) micelle preparations [46].

Altogether these findings do support the idea that β_2-GPI adhesion to EC might take place via different mechanisms, spanning from a simple non-specific adhesion as many other plasma proteins, to electric charge interaction between the cationic PL-binding site and anionic cell membrane structure, to the binding to LDL-R family components or to annexin II (Fig. 33.1).

Finally, it is still open the question whether β_2-GPI is synthetized by EC themselves and then exposed on the cell membrane. While, in fact, one group found β_2-GPI in HUVEC both at protein and at mRNA level [47], these results were not confirmed by others [48]. In any case, it is not clear why cells able to synthesize a protein are apparently unable to re-express the same molecule once it has been displaced from the surface level by starvation in serum-free medium.

Although the nature of the endothelial receptor(s) for β_2-GPI is still under investigation, the above-mentioned findings do support the fact that β_2-GPI can be

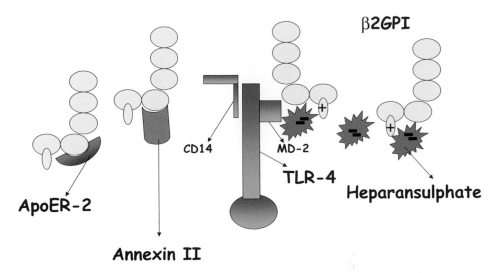

Figure 33.1. Potential endothelial cell membrane receptors for β_2-GPI: heparansulphate, toll- like receptor (TLR)-4, annexin II, and apolipoprotein E receptor-2 (ApoER2).

expressed on EC membranes in a manner that offers suitable epitopes for circulating anti–β_2-GPI antibodies.

Is β_2-GPI Expressed on Endothelium also In Vivo?

Several groups reported the in vitro expression of β_2-GPI on EC derived from umbilical cord vein, and we also found that primary human brain and skin EC monolayers might express β_2-GPI on their surface [35]. However few data are available on whether or not such an expression takes also place in the tissues in vivo.

In fact, while anti-human β_2-GPI antisera can clearly stain endothelium in trophoblast vessels, we did not find a comparable endothelial staining in skin biopsies obtained from normal donors or patients affected by inflammatory disorders [Meroni et al, personal communication]. In addition, immuno-histological studies on human atherosclerotic plaques revealed that β_2-GPI was abundantly expressed within the sub-endothelial regions and intimal-medial borders only [49]. On the other hand, β_2-GPI-dependent aPL are able to induce endothelial perturbation in in vivo experimental animal models suggesting that the reactivity of the antibodies with the co-factor should take place [25].

It is possible that the amount of β_2-GPI expressed on the endothelium in vivo is too small to be detectable by the common immuno-histological techniques, at variance with what is taking place in placenta. In any case, further studies are needed to confirm whether or not β_2-GPI is expressed on EC in vivo.

Pleiotropic Effect of aPL on Endothelial Functions

In Vitro

aPL not only react with EC but, once bound, are able to modulate several cell functions that can play a role in supporting the procoagulant diathesis. If perturbed, endothelium itself displays a pro-inflammatory and procoagulant phenotype and might also have a "gong effect" on other cell types, such as leukocytes and platelets. Due in fact to the interplay between endothelium and these cells, EC activation might in turn trigger their procoagulant effect [50]. For example, adhering leukocytes activated by pro-inflammatory cytokines as well as by the adhesion itself express a procoagulant phenotype [51]. Such a series of events might play a key role in the thrombophilic state of APS.

Actually, there is a sound evidence in the literature for the ability of aPL to affect EC functions in different in vitro experimental models (Table 33.1).

Most, if not all, of the aPL functional effects on endothelium have been the object of previous reviews and they will not be taken into consideration any more in the present chapter.

However, it should be pointed out that the aPL ability to activate EC in vitro was mainly evaluated by using HUVEC monolayers. We have recently been able to demonstrate that primary cultures of human brain and skin EC can also be activated by aPL to upregulate adhesion molecule expression as well as the secretion of pro-inflammatory cytokines [35]. This finding does support the idea that the phenomenon is apparently common to the whole endothelium.

In Vivo

The ability of aPL to affect the endothelium has been addressed in few in vivo APS animal models [25, 52, 53, Fischetti et al, submitted].

Passive infusion of aPL was shown to be able to increase white blood cell (WBC) adherence to cremaster muscle vessel walls in an apparent direct manner, suggesting that the antibodies might activate the endothelium favoring the appearance of a pro-adhesive phenotype in vivo as reported in vitro [25]. The increase in WBC adherence was inhibited or completely abrogated in mice deficient for adhesion molecule expression (ICAM-1, P-selectin, E-selectin) or in mice pretreated with blocking anti-VCAM-1 antibodies [52]. Interestingly, the fact that the effect was abrogated in E-selectin deficient mice strongly supports a pivotal role of the endothelium because of the selective expression of E-selectin on EC [26].

Other experimental models have been reported, in which aPL passive infusion displayed a thrombophilic activity only if an additional thrombogenic stimulus was applied, accordingly to the "two hit hypothesis" [2].

In the model reported by Pierangeli et al, a mechanical trauma to the femoral vein was required to induce the thrombus formation. The infusion of aPL was then found to be able to increase the clot size and such an effect was inhibited or abrogated in mice deficient for adhesion molecules (ICAM-1, P-selectin, and E-selectin) or treated with blocking anti-VCAM-1 antibodies [52]. Once again these findings indirectly support an endothelial perturbation.

Fischetti et al have recently reported a model in which the infusion of β_2-GPI–dependent aPL IgG in naive rats induced the formation of large clots in the mesenteric microcirculation if a preliminary endothelial activation mediated by the intra-peritoneal injection of small amounts of LPS tooks place. The thrombus formation was found to be associated with an increased WBC adhesion to the mesenteric vessel walls, but the study did not directly address whether or not an endothelium perturbation did occur (Fischetti et al, submitted).

Finally, Jankowski et al showed that a β_2-GPI–dependent LA-positive murine monoclonal antibody was effective in increasing the carotid artery thrombus formation in a photochemically induced thrombosis model in the hamster. The model complies with the concept of the two hit hypothesis and was shown to be mediated by the F(ab)$_2$ antibody fragments. Immunohistochemical analysis of the arterial thrombus revealed antibody deposition mainly bound to platelets but no clear endothelial involvement [53].

Do APS Patients Display an Endothelial Perturbation In Vivo?

The question whether an endothelial perturbation comparable to that detectable in in vitro studies might be also detectable in vivo in APS patients is still matter of debate.

While some studies reported increased plasma levels of single soluble adhesion molecule isoforms or endothelial derived microparticles in APS patients, others did not confirm these findings [54–58].

These data are actually in contrast with the clear demonstration that the aPL thrombogenic effect is closely mediated by adhesion molecule expression in a murine experimental model [52].

On the other hand, immuno-histological evaluation of tissues affected by aPL-related thrombotic lesions did not reveal any clear signs of endothelial activation with the only exception of the increased EC expression of $\alpha 3\beta 1$ integrin in biopsies taken from patients affected by the APS-related heart valvulopathy [59].

We have recently investigated several indirect in vivo parameters of endothelial dysfunction in aPL-positive patients: soluble adhesion molecules (sEselectin, sICAM-1, sVCAM-1), soluble thrombomodulin (sTM), von Willebrand factor (vWF), and t-PA evaluated by solid-phase assays. Plasma levels of soluble adhesion molecule, as well as levels of sTM, vWF, and t-PA have been actually reported to be increased in different disorders characterized by the presence of an endothelial perturbation [60, 61]. These parameters have been investigated in patients with APS both primary and secondary to non-active systemic lupus erythematosus (SLE) (ECLAM score ≤ 2) to avoid any potential variables related to the immune-mediated inflammation sustained by the lupus disease itself. In addition a series of patients was also investigated for: (i) the presence of circulating EC identified by flow cytometry and (ii) the brachial artery flow mediated dilation (FMV) at rest, during reactive hyperemia and after glyceryl nitrate. High levels of circulating EC have been actually reported in patients suffering from disorders characterized by an endothelial damage sustained by systemic immune mediated inflammation such as in patients suffering from ANCA-associated vasculitis or by ischaemic processes [62]. On the other hand, an impaired endothelial dependent FMV was also reported in comparable conditions [63].

Plasma levels of soluble adhesion molecules sTM and t-PA did not differ in APS patients in comparison with controls. On the contrary, significant increased vWF titers were found in APS patients. No significant difference between patients and controls was found regarding the number of circulating EC as well as the brachial artery FMV (Meroni et al, submitted).

As a whole these findings suggest that aPL per se are not able to support a full-blown endothelial perturbation in vivo. This finding is in line with the two hit hypothesis and with the results reported in the experimental animal models in which the infusion of aPL does not induce clot formation or a strong endothelial activation in uninjured vessels unless a mechanical trauma or an inflammatory trigger is also applied [25, 53, Fischetti et al, submitted]. Since Pierangeli et al reported that aPL infusion is directly able to increase WBC adherence to the vessel walls in the cremaster muscle microcirculation [25], it is possible that the endothelial activation taking place in this experimental model might be at higher level than that spontaneously occurring in APS patients. In other words, the endothelial perturbation could take place in patients but at a level that cannot be detectable by using the indirect plasma parameters commonly available.

Mechanisms of EC Activation by aPL

Taking into account the hypothesis that β_2-GPI and anti–β_2-GPI antibodies play a major role in EC perturbation, it has been suggested that the cell activation is likely the consequence of the cross-link of the co-factor complexed with its receptor(s) by the antibodies. The eventual result is the intracellular signaling with gene activation for pro-inflammatory cytokine and adhesion molecule synthesis [64].

Translocation of nuclear factor-κB (NF-κB) from the cytoplasm to the nucleus was reported to be involved in in vitro EC activation mediated by aPL (and particularly by anti–β_2-GPI antibodies) by three different groups [64–66, Vega-Ostertag et al, submitted]. More recently, Pierangeli et al have demonstrated that EC activated by aPL also displayed increased phosphorylation of p38 mitogen activated protein kinase (MAPK) and the use of specific inhibitors was found to block cell activation (Vega-Ostertag et al, submitted).

Interestingly, NF-κB and p38 MAPK inhibitors did not display a complete abrogation of the endothelial activation by aPL when used independently, so suggesting that none of the pathways – per se – might be completely responsible for the whole gene activation (Fig. 33.2).

However, the upstream signaling steps have been only partially characterized. Our group has showed that both human monoclonal IgM as well as polyclonal anti–β_2-GPI IgG antibodies trigger an endothelial signaling cascade comparable to that activated by LPS or interleukin (IL)-1 and involving TRAF6 and MyD88 [67]. We also found that anti–β_2-GPI antibodies and LPS induce a comparable phosphorylation of the IL-1 receptor-activated kinase (IRAK) – the first kinase recruited by the IL-1R/Toll Like Receptor (TLR) superfamily, but not by other receptors. These findings raised the possibility that one of the signaling cascades triggered by aPL is associated to TLRs [67].

Toll-like receptors are a key component of the innate immune response able to recognize specific microbial products, including LPS, bacterial lipoproteins, pepti-

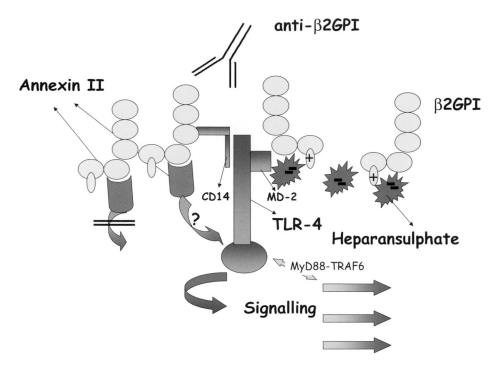

Figure 33.2. Endothelial cell activation by anti–β_2-GPI antibodies. Cell activation has been found to be associated with NF-κB nuclear translocation as well as with p38 MAPK phosphorylation. Upstream signaling was found to be dependent on MyD88 and TRAF6 suggesting the involvement of TLRs. It has been hypothesized that β_2-GPI adhered to heparansulphate structures might interact with TLR-4 owing to its homology with infectious agents – the natural ligands of TRL-4. A similar interaction was also suggested for β_2-GPI bound to annexin II. TLR-4 might in fact represent the unknown "adaptor" protein required by annexin II to signal the cells.

doglycan, and bacterial DNA [68, 69]. All the members of the Toll family are type I transmembrane proteins with an extracellular leucine rich repeat (LRR) domain and an intracellular signaling domain known as TIR domain; such a common structure makes them efficient membrane receptors able to drive a prompt inflammatory response after their interaction with the specific ligands [68, 69]. As mediators of the innate immunity TLRs are widely expressed in both lymphoid and non-lymphoid tissues, including in particular EC, that express significant amount of TLR-4 [68, 69].

Anti–β_2-GPI antibodies were shown to recognize β_2-GPI peptides displaying a molecular mimicry with common bacteria and viruses, both at the level of aminoacid sequence and conformational structure [70, 71]. Such a homology was thought to represent the rationale for the possible infectious origin of the syndrome [72]. Because common microbial structures do represent the natural ligands for TLRs, we speculate that β_2-GPI might in turn interact with TLRs and that anti–β_2-GPI antibodies recognizing the molecule might cross-link it together with TLRs, eventually triggering the inflammatory cascade.

Such a possibility likely appears to have a major role particularly during the "thrombotic storm" in the so-called catastrophic variant of APS. On the other hand, lot of experimental evidence and preliminary clinical reports have suggested a close association between aPL and accelerated atherosclerosis [73]. The widely accepted prominent role of EC in the earliest events of the atherosclerotic process as well as the recent finding of TLR increased expression in the plaques [74–76] offer an additional possible mechanism through which aPL (and particularly anti–β_2-GPI antibodies) may be involved in atherosclerosis.

Finally, the possibility that anti–β_2-GPI antibodies activate EC through the interaction with membrane receptors able to drive an inflammatory response might explain the apparent paradox in annexin II studies. It has been actually reported that annexin II might be a high affinity EC receptor for β_2-GPI and that anti–β_2-GPI antibodies as well as bivalent specific anti-annexin II antibodies induce a comparable EC activation. However, annexin II is known as a non-transmembrane protein and it has been suggested to require a yet unknown "adaptor" protein to signal the cells [44]. We speculate that TLR-4 involvement could represent the cell membrane structure responsible for EC signaling transduction (Fig. 33.2).

Conclusions

The ability of aPL to interact with the endothelium is still an attractive potential mechanism to explain the APS vasculopathy. However, the experimental evidence for such a pathogenic mechanism is mainly from in vitro models and more in vivo studies are necessary.

Understanding the events in EC perturbation by aPL might be useful in designing new therapeutical modalities or in supporting current therapeutical approaches. This is the case for the recent demonstration of the efficacy of statins in inhibiting EC activation by aPL in vitro that was reproduced also in in vivo experimental models [2, 77].

Finally, it is still open the question how local anatomical and/or functional factors might be important in conditioning the susceptibility of the endothelium to activation/damage by aPL.

Acknowledgments

The present study was supported by Ricerca Corrente 2004 IRCCS Istituto Auxologico Italiano (to PLM).

Reference List

1. Levine JS, Branch DW, Rauch J. The antiphospholipid syndrome. N Engl J Med 2002;346:752–763.
2. Meroni PL, Riboldi P. Pathogenic mechanisms mediating antiphospholipid syndrome. Curr Opin Rheumatol 2001;13:377–382.
3. Cines DB, Pollak ES, Buck CA, et al. Endothelial cells in physiology and in the pathophysiology of vascular disorders. Blood 1998;91:3527–3561.
4. Carreras LO, Vermylen JG. Lupus anticoagulant and thrombosis: possible role of inhibition of prostacyclin formation. Thromb Haemost 1992;48:38–40.

5. Del Papa N, Guidali L, Spatola L, et al. Relationship between anti-phospholipid and anti-endothelial antibodies III: β2-glycoprotein I mediates the antibody binding to endothelial membranes and induces the expression of adhesion molecules. Clin Exp Rheumatol 1995;13:179–186.
6. Simantov R, LaSala JM, Lo SK, et al. Activation of cultured vascular endothelial cells by antiphospholipid antibodies. J Clin Invest 1995;96:2211–2219.
7. Le Tonqueze M, Salozhin K, Dueymes M, et al. Role of β2-glycoprotein I in the anti-phospholipid antibody binding to endothelial cells. Lupus 1995;4:179–186.
8. Del Papa N, Guidali L, Sala A, et al. Endothelial cell as target for antiphospholipid antibodies. Arthritis Rheum 1997;40:551–561.
9. Del Papa N, Sheng YH, Raschi E, et al. Human β2-glycoprotein I binds to endothelial cells through a cluster of lysine residues that are critical for anionic phospholipid binding and offers epitopes for anti-β2-glycoprotein I antibodies. J Immunol 1998;160:5572–5578.
10. George J, Blank M, Levy Y, et al. Differential effects of anti-beta 2 glycoprotein I antibodies on endothelial cells and on the manifestations of experimental antiphospholipid syndrome. Circulation 1998;97:900–906.
11. Cho CS, Cho ML, Chen PP, et al. Antiphospholipid antibodies induce monocyte chemoattractant protein-1 in endothelial cells. J Immunol 2002;168:4209–4215.
12. Hasselaar P, Derksen RH, Oosting JD, et al. Synergistic effect of low doses of tumor necrosis factor and sera from patients with systemic lupus erythematosus on expression of procoagulant activity by cultured endothelial cells. Thromb Haemost 1989;62:654–660.
13. Branch DW, Rodgers G. Induction of endothelial cell tissue factor activity by sera from patients with antiphospholipid syndrome: a possible mechanism of thrombosis. Am J Obstet Gynecol 1993;168:206–210.
14. Kornberg A, Renaudineau Y, Blank M, et al. Anti-beta 2-glycoprotein I antibodies and anti-endothelial cell antibodies induce tissue factor in endothelial cells. Isr Med Assoc J 2000;2(suppl):27–31.
15. Ferrara DE, Swerlick R, Casper K, et al. Fluvastatin inhibits upregulation of tissue factor expression by antiphospholipid antibodies on endothelial cells. Thromb Haemost 2004. In press.
16. Marciniak E, Romond EH. Impaired catalytic function of activated protein C: a new in vitro manifestation of lupus anticoagulant. Blood 1989;74:2426–2432.
17. Ruiz-Arguelles GJ, Ruiz-Arguelles A, Deleze M, et al. Acquired protein C deficiency in a patient with primary antiphospholipid syndrome. Relationship to reactivity of anticardiolipin antibody with thrombomodulin. J Rheumatol 1989;16:381–383.
18. Ieko M, Sawada KI, Koike T, et al. The putative mechanism of thrombosis in antiphospholipid syndrome: impairment of the protein C and the fibrinolytic systems by monoclonal anticardiolipin antibodies. Semin Thromb Hemost 1999;25:503–507.
19. de Groot PG, Derksen RHWM. The influence of antiphospholipid antibodies on the protein C pathway. In: Khamashta MA, ed. Hughes syndrome, antiphospholipid syndrome. London: Springer; 2000:307–316.
20. Esmon NL, Safa O, Smirnov MD, et al. Antiphospholipid antibodies and the protein C. J Autoimmun 2000;15:221–225.
21. Rand JH. Molecular pathogenesis of the antiphospholipid syndrome. Circ Res 2002;90:29–37.
22. Atsumi T, Khamashta MA, Haworth RS, et al. Arterial disease and thrombosis in the antiphospholipid syndrome: a pathogenic role for endothelin 1. Arthritis Rheum 1998;41:800–807.
23. Nakamura N, Ban T, Yamaji K, et al. Lupus anticoagulant autoantibody induces apoptosis in HUVEC: involvement of annexin V. Biochem Byophys Res Commun 1994;205:1488–1493.
24. Galve-de Rochemonteix B, Kobayashi T, Rosnoblet C, et al. Interaction of anti-phospholipid antibodies with late endosomes of human endothelial cells. Arterioscler Thromb Vasc Biol 2000;20:563–574.
25. Pierangeli SS, Gharavi AE, Harris N. Experimental thrombosis and antiphospholipid antibodies: new insights. J Autoimmun 2000;15:241–247.
26. Espinola RG, Liu X, Colden-Stanfield M, et al. E-Selectin mediates pathogenic effects of antiphospholipid antibodies. J Thromb Haemost 2003;1:843–848.
27. Vismara A, Meroni PL, Tincani A, et al. Antiphospholipid antibodies and endothelial cells. Clin Exp Immunol 1988;74:247–253.
28. Hasselaar P, Derksen RH, Blokzijl L, et al. Cross-reactivity of antibodies directed against cardiolipin, DNA, endothelial cells and blood platelets. Thromb Haemost 1990;63:69–173.
29. Le Roux G, Wautier MP, Guillevin L, et al. IgG binding to endothelial cells in systemic lupus erythematosus. Thromb Haemost 1986;56:144–146.
30. Rosenbaum J, Pottinger BE, Woo P, et al. Measurement and characterization of circulating anti-endothelial cell IgG in connective tissue diseases. Clin Exp Immunol 1998;72:450–456.

31. McCrae KR, DeMichele A, Samuels P, et al. Detection of endothelial cell reactive immunoglobulin in patients with anti-phospholipid antibodies. Br J Haematol 1991;79:595–605.
32. Del Papa N, Meroni PL, Tincani A, et al. Relationship between antiphospholipid and antiendothelial antibodies: further characterization of the reactivity on resting and cytokine-activated endothelial cells. Clin Exp Rheumatol 1992;10:37–42.
33. Del Papa N, Conforti G, Gambini D, et al. Characterization of the endothelial surface proteins recognized by anti-endothelial antibodies in primary and secondary autoimmune vasculitis. Clin Immunol Immunopathol 1994;70:211–216.
34. Tincani A, Spatola L, Prati E, et al. The anti-β2 glycoprotein I activity in human antiphospholipid syndrome sera is due to monoreactivity low-affinity autoantibodies directed to epitopes located on native β2 glycoprotein I and preserved during species' evolution. J Immunol 1996;157:5732–5738.
35. Meroni PL, Tincani A, Sepp N, et al. Endothelium and the brain in CNS lupus. Lupus 2003;12:919–928.
36. Revelen R, Bordron A, Dueymes M, et al. False positivity in a cyto-ELISA for anti-endothelial cell antibodies caused by heterophile antibodies to bovine serum proteins. Clin Chemistry 2000;46:273–278.
37. Harper L, Savage CO. Anti-heparin antibodies: part of the repertoire of anti-endothelial cell antibodies (AECA). Lupus 1998;7:68–72.
38. Cai G, Satoh T, Hoshi H. Purification and characterization of an endothelial cell-viability maintaining factor from fetal bovine serum. Biochim Biophys Acta 1995;1269:13–18.
39. Moestrup SK, Schousboe I, Jacobsen C, et al. β2-glycoprotein-I (apolipoprotein H) and β2-glycoprotein-I-phospholipid complex harbor a recognition site for the endocytic receptor megalin. J Clin Invest 1998;102:902–909.
40. Cao W, Atsumi T, Yamashita Y, et al. A possible binding of β2-glycoprotein I to megaline, an endocytic receptor on trophoblast. J Autoimmun 2000;15:A61.
41. Lutters BC, Derksen RH, Tekelenburg WL, et al. Dimers of beta 2-glycoprotein I increase platelet deposition to collagen via interaction with phospholipids and the apolipoprotein E receptor 2'. J Biol Chem 2003;278:33831–33838.
42. Sacre SM, Standard AK, Owen JS. Apolipoprotein E (apoE) isoforms differentially induce nitric oxide production in endothelial cells. FEBS Lett 2003;540:181–187.
43. Cesarman GM, Guevara CA, Hajjar KA. An endothelial cell receptor for plasminogen/tissue plasminogen activator (t-PA). II. Annexin II-mediated enhancement of t-PA-dependent plasminogen activation. J Biol Chem 1994;269:21198–21203.
44. Hajjar KA, Jacovina AT, Chacko J. An endothelial cell receptor for plasminogen/tissue plasminogen activator. I. Identity with annexin II. J Biol Chem 1994;269:21191–21197.
45. Hajjar KA, Mauri L, Jacovina AT, et al. Tissue plasminogen activator binding to the annexin II tail domain. Direct modulation by homocysteine. J Biol Chem 1998;273:9987–9993.
46. Ma K, Simantov R, Zhang JC, et al. High affinity binding of β2-glycoprotein I to human endothelial cells is mediated by Annexin II. J Biol Chem 2000;20:15541–15548.
47. Caronti B, Calderaro C, Alessandri C, et al. Beta2-glycoprotein I (beta2-GPI) mRNA is expressed by several cell types involved in anti-phospholipid syndrome-related tissue damage. Clin Exp Immunol 1999;115:214–219.
48. Alvarado-de la Barrera C, Bahena S, Llorente L, et al. Beta2-glycoprotein-I mRNA transcripts are expressed by hepatocytes but not by resting or activated human endothelial cells. Thromb Res 1998;90:239–243.
49. George J, Harats D, Gilburd B, et al. Immunolocalization of beta2-glycoprotein I (apolipoprotein H) to human atherosclerotic plaques: potential implications for lesion progression. Circulation 1999;99:2227–2230.
50. Nawrot P, Stern D. Endothelial cell procoagulant properties and the host response. Semin Thromb Hemost 1987;13:391–398.
51. Carlos TM, Harlam JM. Leukocyte-endothelial adhesion molecule. Blood 1994;84:2068–2101.
52. Pierangeli SS, Espinola RG, Liu X, et al. Thrombogenic effects of antiphospholipid antibodies are mediated by intercellular cell adhesion molecule-1, vascular adhesion molecule-1, and P-selectin. Circ Res 2001;88:245–250.
53. Jankowski M, Vreys I, Wittevrongel C, et al. Thrombogenicity of beta 2-glycoprotein I-dependent antiphospholipid antibodies in a photochemically induced thrombosis model in the hamster. Blood 2003;101:157–162.
54. Ferro D, Pittoni V, Quintarelli C, et al. Coexistence of anti-phospholipid antibodies and endothelial perturbation in systemic lupus erythematosus patients with ongoing prothrombotic state. Arthritis Rheum 1997;95:1425–1432.

55. Combes V, Simon AC, Grau GE, et al. In vitro generation of endothelial microparticles and possible prothrombotic activity in patients with lupus anticoagulant. J Clin Invest 1999;104:93–102.
56. Kaplanski G, Cacoub P, Farnarier C, et al. Increased soluble vascular cell adhesion molecule 1 concentrations in patients with primary or systemic lupus erythematosus-related antiphospholipid syndrome: correlations with the severity of thrombosis. Arthritis Rheum 2000;43:55–64.
57. Williams FMK, Parmar K, Hughes GRV, et al. Systemic endothelial cell markers in primary antiphospholipid syndrome. Thromb Haemost 2000;84:742–746.
58. Frijns CJM, Derksen RHWM, De Groot PG, et al. Lupus anticoagulant and history of thrombosis are not associated with persistent endothelial cell activation in systemic lupus erythematosus. Clin Exp Immunol 2001;125:149–154.
59. Afek A, Shoenfeld Y, Manor R, et al. Increased endothelial cell expression of alpha3beta1 integrin in cardiac valvulopathy in the primary (Hughes) and secondary antiphospholipid syndrome. Lupus 1999;8:502–507.
60. Boffa MC, Karmochkine M. Thrombomodulin: an overview and potential implications in vascular disorders. Lupus 1998;7(suppl 2):S120–S125.
61. Raitakari OT, Celermajer DS. Testing for endothelial dysfunctiom. Ann Med 2000;32:293–304.
62. Dignat-Gorge F, Sampol J. Circulating endothelial cells in vascular disorders: new insights into an old concept. Eur J Haematol 2000;65:215–220.
63. Faulx MD, Wright AT, Hoit BD. Detection of endothelial dysfunction with brachial artery ultrasound scanning. Am Heart J 2003;145:943–951.
64. Meroni PL, Raschi E, Testoni C, et al. Statins prevent endothelial cell activation induced by antiphospholipid (anti-β2 glycoprotein I) antibodies. Arthritis Rheum 2001;44:2870–2878.
65. Dunoyer-Geindre S, de Moerloose P, Galve-de Rochemonteix B, et al. NFkappaB is an essential intermediate in the activation of endothelial cells by anti-beta(2)-glycoprotein 1 antibodies. Thromb Haemost 2002;88:851–857.
66. Pierangeli SS, Vega-Ostertag M, Harris EN. Intracellular signaling triggered by antiphospholipid Antibodies in platelets and endothelial cells: a pathway to targeted therapies. Thromb Res 2004. In press.
67. Raschi E, Testoni C, Bosisio D, et al. Role of the MyD88 transduction signaling pathway in endothelial activation by anti-phospholipid antibodies. Blood 2003;101:3495–3500.
68. Medzhitov R. Toll-like receptors and innate immunity. Nat Rev Immunol 2001;1:135–145.
69. Lien E, Ingalls RR. Toll-like receptors. Crit Care Med 2002;30:S1–S11.
70. Gharavi AE, Pierangeli SS, Colden-Stanfield M, et al. GDKV-induced antiphospholipid antibodies enhance thrombosis and activate endothelial cells in vivo and in vitro. J Immunol 1999;163:2922–2927.
71. Blank M, Krause I, Fridkin M, et al. Bacterial induction of autoantibodies to β2-glycoprotein-1 accounts for the infectious etiology of antiphospholipid syndrome. J Clin Invest 2002;109:797–804.
72. Blank M, Asherson RA, Cervera R, et al. Antiphospholipid syndrome infectious origin. J Clin Immunol 2004;24:12–23.
73. George J, Haratz D, Shoenfeld Y. Accelerated atheroma, antiphospholipid antibodies, and the antiphospholipid syndrome. Rheum Dis Clin North Am 2001;27:603–610.
74. Ross R. Atherosclerosis an inflammatory disease. N Engl J Med 1999;340:115–126.
75. Xu XH, Shah PK, Faure E, et al. Toll-like receptor-4 is expressed by macrophages in murine and human lipid-rich atherosclerotic plaques and upregulated by oxidized LDL. Circulation 2001;104:3103–3108.
76. Edfeldt K, Swedenborg J, Hansson GK, et al. Expression of toll-like receptors in human atherosclerotic lesions: a possible pathway for plaque activation. Circulation 2002;105:1158–1161.
77. Ferrara DE, Liu X, Espinola RG, et al. Inhibition of the thrombogenic and inflammatory properties of antiphospholipid antibodies by fluvastatin in an in vivo animal model. Arthritis Rheum 2003;48:3272–3279.

34 The Influence of Antiphospholipid Antibodies on the Protein C Pathway

Philip G. de Groot and Ronald H. W. M. Derksen

Introduction

Blood coagulation is the mechanism that maintains the integrity of the high pressure closed circulatory system of blood. To prevent extravasations of the blood after injury, the hemostatic mechanism, which includes platelets, coagulation, and fibrinolytic proteins in plasma and endothelial cells, is activated. A platelet plug will be formed that prevents further blood loss. Subsequently, the coagulation cascade replaces the unstable platelet plug by the stable fibrin clot. An essential feature of the hemostatic reaction is that platelet deposition and fibrin formation is localized and limited to the immediate area of the injury. Therefore, it is essential that different natural anticoagulant mechanisms are operative to regulate coagulation. When the natural anticoagulant mechanisms do not function optimally, this will lead to thrombotic complications. One of the most important natural anticoagulant systems is the protein C pathway [1, 2]. The high number of patients that have been described with heterozygous protein C or protein S deficiency and familial thrombophilia highlight the clinical importance of the anticoagulant properties of protein C and protein S. Complete protein C deficiency represents a potentially lethal condition. Thrombotic complications can be controlled with protein C replacement therapy [3, 4].

Antiphospholipid antibodies (aPL) are a heterogeneous group of autoantibodies defined by 2 very distinct assay methods. One group, called lupus anticoagulant (LA), is defined as antibodies that inhibit in vitro phospholipid dependent coagulation assays. The second group, anticardiolipin antibodies (aCL), is defined by their ability to bind to negatively charged phospholipids in an enzyme-linked immunosorbent assay (ELISA) [5]. Paradoxically, the presence of aPL in plasma is a major risk factor for the development of arterial and venous thrombosis and is not associated with a bleeding diathesis, as would be expected when clotting times are prolonged [6].

The pathophysiology that underlies the relation between the aPL in plasma and the risk for thrombo-embolic complications is still unexplained [7] but an attractive hypothesis is that the aPL interfere with (one of) the natural anticoagulant pathways in the body. In this chapter we will discuss one of these possibilities: a link between aPL and the protein C system.

Protein C axis

In the early 1980s, a phospholipid dependent antithrombotic pathway was described that soon turned out to be one of the body's major defense mechanisms to uncontrolled coagulation. Vascular endothelium expresses a membrane bound receptor on its surface, thrombomodulin, which binds thrombin and thereby alters its substrate specificity. Thrombin bound to thrombomodulin is no longer able to activate platelets or to convert fibrinogen into fibrin, but it converts a vitamin K dependent protein, protein C, into activated protein C (APC) [8]. APC is a physiological anticoagulant via its potential to inactivate clotting factors Va and VIIIa, which results in inhibition of further thrombin formation (Fig. 34.1). Protein C activation by thrombin–thrombomodulin complex is further enhanced about 20-fold when protein C is bound to the endothelial cell protein C receptor (EPCR). Thrombomodulin also influences fibrinolysis. Thrombin bound to thrombomodulin activates TAFI (thrombin inducible fibrinolysis inhibitor, carboxypeptidase B). TAFI removes carboxyterminal lysine residues from fibrin, thereby preventing the binding of tissue plasminogen activator (tPA) and plasmin(ogen) to fibrin. TAFI thus reduces fibrinolysis. Activation of TAFI is thought essential for the stability of a fibrin clot [9].

The role of the protein C axis extends beyond hemostasis. Activated protein C has potent anti-inflammatory properties and administration of human activated protein C significantly decreases mortality in patients with severe sepsis [10]. Furthermore protein C has a role in cell survival and cell proliferation [11].

Protein C is a vitamin K dependent glycoprotein with a molecular weight of 62 kDa. In blood it circulates as an inactive zymogen, mostly in the form of a two chain molecule [12]. The thrombin–thrombomodulin complex activates protein C by

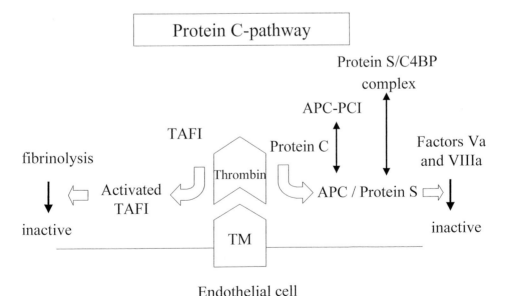

Figure 34.1. The protein C pathway.

splitting off a 12 amino acid activation peptide after cleavage at position Arg 169. The plasma concentration of protein C is 4 μg/mL (65 nM) and the circulating level of APC in healthy subjects is about 2.2 ng/mL [13]. The biological half-life of protein C is about 8 hours. In plasma, APC is neutralized by forming complexes with the APC inhibitor (PCI or PAI-3), α1-antiproteinase (α1-antitrypsin) and α2-macroglobulin. The inactivation of APC by PCI is accelerated by heparin [14].

Protein S, another vitamin K dependent protein, amplifies the activity of APC. Protein S is a single chain plasma glycoprotein with a molecular weight of 70 kDa [15]. The total plasma concentration of protein S is about 25 μg/mL (350 nM). The biological half-life of protein S is 42.5 hours. Protein S forms a 1:1 complex with APC on phospholipid surfaces. Two independent processes regulate the APC co-factor activity of protein S. First, protein S is cleaved by thrombin, resulting is a molecule that has lost its APC co-factor function [16]. The second inhibition of APC co-factor activity of protein S is the result of its ability to form a 1:1 complex with C4b binding protein (C4BP). Approximately 60% of plasma protein S circulates in complex with C4BP. Only the free form of protein S has APC co-factor activity [17]. The complex between protein S and C4BP arises by a non-covalent association between protein S and the β-chain of C4BP. About 80% of C4BP in the circulation is composed of 7 α-chains and 1 β-chain, joined together by inter-chain disulfide bridges in the C-terminal region. The remaining C4BP contains only α-chains. During acute-phase reactions the plasma levels of C4BP increases dramatically. However, due to the preferential synthesis of the α-chain, only β-chain-free C4BP is synthesized. As β-chain-free C4BP cannot bind protein S, the levels of free protein S remain stable during inflammation.

Thrombomodulin is an endothelial transmembrane protein consisting of a lectin domain, 6 EGF domains, a carbohydrate rich domain, a transmembrane domain, and a 36 amino acid long intracellular tail [18]. The thrombin-binding region is located in EGF domains 5 and 6 but for protein C activation, the presence of EGF domain 4 is also essential. Thrombomodulin expression is not restricted to the cell membrane. There also exists a soluble form in plasma. Plasma concentrations of soluble thrombomodulin are around 25 ng/mL. In many vascular disorders (including diabetes mellitus) soluble thrombomodulin levels are increased [19].

Endothelial cell protein C receptor is a transmembrane protein homologous to the major histocompatibility complex class 1 family members [20]. Human EPCR is palmitoylated on the terminal cysteine, suggesting that ECPR is located in the caveolae of the cells. Large vessel endothelial cells predominantly express EPCR. Its function is to concentrate protein C near the surface of the vessel wall and to increase APC formation through mass action effects. When APC is generated, it remains bound to EPCR for a short while. As long as APC is bound to EPCR, it cannot inactivate factors Va and VIIIa. However, it can cleave the protease activatable receptor PAR-1, initiating responses in PAR-1 bearing cells.

The discovery of the concept of activated protein C resistance followed by the explanation of the resistance by a mutation in clotting factor V further emphasizes the importance of the protein C-axis as an antithrombotic pathway [21, 22]. During blood coagulation factor V is converted into factor Va. Factor Va serves as a non-enzymatic co-factor in the prothrombinase complex. The presence of factor Va tremendously accelerates further thrombin formation [23]. Factor Va is inactivated by proteolytic degradation of its heavy chain by APC. The inactivation is a sequential event; the first cleavage takes place at Arg 506, followed by cleavages at Arg 306 and Arg 679. The first cleavage results in a partly inactivated form of factor Va with 30% residual activity, cleavage at Arg 306 results in a completely inactive molecule [24]. In 1993, Dahlback and co-workers described patients with thrombophilia whose plasma was resistant to APC [21]. With this APC resistance test large populations of thrombophilic patients could be characterized. In 1994, a point mutation in factor V gene was identified as the genetic risk factor that described the patients with APC resistance [22]. The point mutation is a GA transition of nucleotide 1691, which predicts the synthesis of a variant factor V molecule with an Arg506Gln mutation. Replacement of Arg 506 by Gln will prevent cleavage of factor Va by APC, which results in a delay in the inactivation of factor Va and thus in sustained thrombin formation.

Specificity of aPL

Research over the last 15 years has shown that the subset of aPL that are related to the risk for thrombo-embolic complications do not recognize phospholipids alone. In conventional aCL and LA assays the antibodies are primarily directed towards different phospholipid binding proteins, most notably β_2-glycoprotein I and prothrombin [25, 26]. Both β_2-glycoprotein I and prothrombin bind to negatively charged phospholipids. When bivalent complexes between 2 target molecules and 1 antibody molecule are formed, the affinity for a phospholipid surface of β_2-glycoprotein I and prothrombin increases about 100 times, which subsequently favors the binding of the complexes to phospholipids over the binding of other phospholipid binding proteins present in plasma, such as clotting factors [27].

New studies on the correlation between clinical manifestations and the presence of certain sub-populations of aPL suggested that specially those anti–β_2-glycoprotein I antibodies that are able to prolong clotting times are clinical relevant [28]. The recognition that β_2-glycoprotein I is the real target for aPL logically led to the deduction that the pathogenesis of thrombosis is the result of interference of anti–β_2-glycoprotein I antibodies with the biological function of β_2-glycoprotein I. Despite different types of functions related to β_2-glycoprotein I in in vitro assays, individuals with complete deficiency of β_2-glycoprotein I do not have an increased thrombotic risk [29]. Also knockout mice for β_2-glycoprtein I do not show an increased occurrence of thrombo-embolic complications [30]. Apparently β_2-glycoprotein I is not involved in regulation of pro-or antithrombotic pathways. However, in the presence of anti–β_2-glycoprotein I antibodies, the situation may be different. Due to the increased affinity of β_2-glycoprotein I antibody complexes for phospholipids, β_2-glycoprotein I may now be able to interfere with the function of proteins such as protein C and protein S, that only can express their biological activity in the presence of negatively charged phospholipids.

Whether anti–β_2-glycoprotein I antibodies are the only pathological subset of autoantibodies is not known. A large number of antibodies directed to other phospholipid binding proteins have been identified. The most interesting antibodies found are antibodies directed against prothrombin, protein C, protein S, and thrombomodulin, because the presence of these antibodies could be immediately linked to thrombo-embolic complications [31, 32].

aPL and the Protein C axis

The assembly of coagulation complexes on negatively charged phospholipid surfaces is a prerequisite for their activity: no exposure of anionic phospholipids, no binding, no activity. Prolongation of clotting times in coagulation assays by aPL is the result of competition between antibody–protein complexes and clotting factors for the available catalytic surface. Also, assembly of the APC–protein S complexes on anionic phospholipid surfaces is essential for the catalytic activity. Thus, it is logical to assume that when aPL inhibit the binding of the clotting factors, they also inhibit the binding of protein C and protein S and thereby their activity. Extensive investigations, however, have shown that there are more interactions between aPL, β_2-glycoprotein I, and proteins of the protein C system. Long before the discovery of the role of co-factors in the aPL syndrome, Canfield and Kisiel isolated an APC inhibitor with a N-terminal amino acid sequence identical to β_2-glycoprotein I [33]. This original and forgotten observation has been repeated and extended to characterize aPL/β_2-glycoprotein I as an inhibitor to the protein C system. The antiphospholipid antibodies and/or β_2-glycoprotein I can interfere with the protein C system in different ways [34].

1. The antibodies inhibit the formation of thrombin, the activator of protein C (the *thrombin paradox*)
2. The antibodies inhibit the activation of protein C via interference with thrombomodulin (*anti-thrombomodulin antibodies*).
3. The antibodies inhibit APC activity (*acquired APC resistance*). This can be achieved:
   (a) via inhibition of the assembly of the proteins on the anionic surface:
   (b) via direct inhibition of APC activity;
   (c) via antibodies against the cofactors Va and VIIIa.
4. The antibodies interfere with the level of protein C and/or S (*acquired protein C/S deficiency*).

The Thrombin Paradox

At first glance it is not easy to understand that inhibition of thrombin formation could cause thrombosis. In 1993, the group of Hanson et al made an interesting observation [35]. They infused 2 U/kg/min thrombin in baboons that were connected with an ex vivo thrombosis model. The low doses of thrombin reduced platelet deposition and fibrin incorporation in the ex vivo thrombus. Circulating APC levels increased significantly. This suggests that low doses of thrombin preferentially activate protein C. These and other observations have led to the development of the so-called thrombin paradox [36]: thrombin exerts both anti-and prothrombotic properties (Table 34.1) and, as a consequence, thrombin is the key factor in the regulation of hemostasis. When thrombin has so many different activities, its substrate specificity should be well regulated. One of the fundamental ideas on thrombin activity is that, due to the affinity of thrombin for its substrates and receptors, the concentration of the formed thrombin is one of the main factors that determine its substrate specificity (Fig. 34.2). When only low concentrations of

Table 34.1. Substrates for thrombin.

Substrate	Product	Activity
Fibrinogen	Fibrin	Prothrombotic
Factor V	Factor Va	Prothrombotic
Factor VIII	Factor VIIIa	Prothrombotic
Factor XI	Factor XIa	Prothrombotic
Platelets	Aggregation	Prothrombotic
Protein S	Inactivation	Prothrombotic
Protein C	APC	Antithrombotic
Endothelial cells	NO & PGI$_2$ production	Antithrombotic
Carboxypeptidase B (TAFI)	Activation	Antifibrinolytic
Urokinase	Inactivation	Antifibrinolytic
Factor XIII	Factor XIIIa	Antifibrinolytic

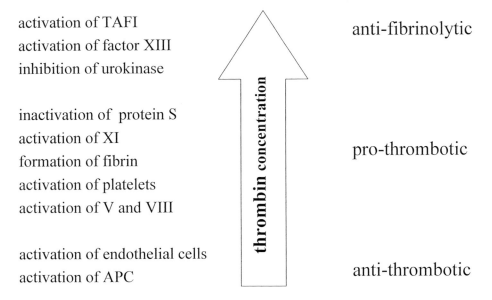

The thrombin paradox

activation of TAFI   anti-fibrinolytic
activation of factor XIII
inhibition of urokinase

inactivation of protein S
activation of XI   pro-thrombotic
formation of fibrin
activation of platelets
activation of V and VIII

activation of endothelial cells
activation of APC   anti-thrombotic

thrombin concentration

Figure 34.2. The thrombin paradox.

thrombin are formed protein C is preferentially activated and thrombin acts as an antithrombotic agent. However, when more thrombin is formed, fibrinogen is converted into fibrin and factors V and VIII are activated. Thrombin now expresses prothrombotic properties. When large amounts of thrombin are formed, TAFI and factor XIII are activated resulting in an antifibrinolytic response.

An attractive hypothesis to explain the prothrombotic action of aPL relies on its well-known inhibitory effect on thrombin formation. Low concentrations of APC circulate in normal individuals. This suggests a continuous activation of protein C and thus a continuous low-level formation of thrombin. It can be hypothesized that the presence of aPL inhibits this low-level thrombin formation and so decreases circulating APC levels. After damage of a vessel, there now will be insufficient circulating APC to prevent uncontrolled thrombin formation and a thrombus is formed. In this way aPL might shift the hemostatic balance to a more prothrombotic state. To test this hypothesis, we measured levels of APC in patients with SLE and related the levels to presence or absence of aPL. We found that levels of circulating APC were significantly lower in patients with systemic lupus erythematosus compared to normal controls, but, in contrast to what was expected, the lower levels of APC were not correlated with the presence of antiphospholipid antibodies or anti–β_2-glycoprotein I antibodies [37]. We did find a correlation between APC levels and levels of plasma prothromin and anti-prothrombin antibodies. Therefore, it can be speculated that the presence of antiprothrombin antibodies results in lower prothrombin levels and subsequently in lower circulating APC levels. Further studies are necessary to validate this hypothesis.

Anti–thrombomodulin or Anti–EPCR Antibodies

In 1983, Comp et al described in an abstract that 2 out of 7 IgGs isolated from LA-positive plasmas inhibited protein C activation by thrombin [38]. They claimed that the antibodies were directed towards thrombomodulin. Two French groups using purified thrombomodulin or endothelial cells as source of thrombomodulin extended these observations [39, 40]. However, other groups did not support these observations [41–43]. Potzsch et al tested IgGs of 46 different patients with LA and found only 2 cases with reduced rates of APC formation [44]. The contradictory results are not easy to explain. There is no doubt that in some patients antibodies towards thrombomodulin can be detected. Whether these antibodies always inhibit the functional activity of thrombomodulin is not known. Thrombomodulin activity is regulated by the phospholipid composition in which it is incorporated. Therefore, differences in assay conditions might explain the contradictory results. However, as the frequency of antithrombomodulin antibodies in the populations tested is very low, it cannot be a general mechanism that can explain the majority of the aPL-related thrombotic events. A few publications showed raised levels of thrombomodulin in the circulation of patients with the aPL syndrome [45]. Raised levels of thrombomodulin point to an altered endothelial cell metabolism of thrombomodulin, for example, an increased synthesis or a preferential secretion of newly synthesized molecules. It is not necessarily associated with a decreased expression of thrombomodulin on the endothelial cell surface. Moreover, circulating thrombomodulin might add to APC formation and be protective against thrombosis.

In a recent paper Hurtado et al [46] showed in a cohort of 43 patients with APS syndrome and in a cohort of 87 patients with a first episode of unexplained fetal death that the presence of anti-EPCR IgG and IgM are independent risk factors for fetal loss with odds ratios (OR) of 23.0 and 6.8, respectively. In this respect it is interesting to note that in women with unexplained fetal loss the presence of mutations in the EPCR gene are more prevalent [47] and that disruption of the EPCR gene in mice causes placental thrombosis and early embryonic lethality [48]. Most likely, EPCR plays a key role in preventing thrombosis at the maternal–embryonic interface and antibodies that inhibit EPCR activity might be a cause of the increased pregnancy morbidity in APS. More studies are necessary to follow this interesting lead.

Acquired APC Resistance

In a group of 175 patients with systemic lupus erythematosus (SLE), Fijnheer et al showed that hereditary APC resistance is not related to aPL [49]. However, a number of publications have shown that aPL inhibit the binding of protein C and protein S to negatively charged phospholipids, thereby inhibiting their activity [see 50–56]. The antibodies induce an "acquired APC resistance." Also in a cohort of pediatric patients a significant association between LA , acquired APC resistance, and thrombotic events was found [57]. Interestingly not all LA affect APC activity and the effects are not always seen in every test system [58]. Differences in test systems and/or the heterogeneity of the antibody population influences the outcome of the in vitro test systems. It is not clear whether the acquired APC resistance is due to the presence of anti-β_2-glycoprotein I antibodies [59, 60], anti-prothrombin antibodies [61, 62], anti-protein S antibodies [55], or by combinations of antibodies.

Smirnov et al showed that aPL require the phospholipid PE to have anti-APC activity [63]. When the assays were performed in the presence of PE, aPL inhibited APC activity more potently than prothrombinase activity. There are enough clinical data that show that a partial reduction of prothrombin activation is not sufficient to induce a bleeding diathesis in patients. However, a partial reduction of APC anticoagulant activity is a major thrombotic risk [64]. The observation that oxidation of PE enhances the anticoagulant activity of APC without influence on plasma clotting times [65] strengthens the hypothesis on an important role of PE because oxidative damage is believed to be involved in the genesis of the antiphospholipid syndrome. It has been shown that lipid peroxidation has been increased in patients with aPL [66].

In an elegant study, Mori et al showed that purified β_2-glycoprotein I inhibits the binding of protein C to phospholipids much better than the binding of prothrombin, resulting in a prothrombotic effect [67]. aPL recognize protein C only in the presence of β_2-glycoprotein I [68]. These results suggest that aPL-induced protein C dysfunction is mediated by β_2-glycoprotein I.

An interesting but insufficiently studied option is that patients may have autoantibodies directed against factor Va that protect this coagulation factor against inactivation by APC. Kalafatis et al [69] described a patient with such an autoantibody against factor V, almost complete APC resistance, and severe thrombotic manifestations. Whether these antibodies occur often in APS is not known.

Acquired Deficiencies of Protein C and/or Protein S

There are a number of publications describing acquired protein C or S deficiencies in isolated patients with aPL syndrome [see 70, 71]. Studies in larger populations of aPL- positive patients failed to show a correlation between decreased protein C plasma levels and the presence of aPL. In one study, a small but significant decrease of plasma protein S levels was found, although protein S levels in the aPL antibody group still were within the normal range [72]. Nojima et al [55] found a correlation between acquired APC resistance and anti-protein S antibodies and suggested a functional relationship, however, this observation was not confirmed in other studies.

Atsumi et al [73] made an interesting observation. They found that β_2-glycoprotein I down regulates the binding between protein S and C4Bp significantly and that aPL abolish the β_2-glycoprotein I inhibitory effect. Thus, aPL increase the affinity of protein S for C4Bp which may result in an acquired free protein S deficiency. These observations warrant further investigations.

In general, no decrease in protein C or protein S plasma levels were found in patients with aPL, but in some individual cases a combination of low levels of protein C or protein S in combination with the presence of aPL may be found. These cases are probably very susceptible for thrombotic complications

Concluding Remarks

aPL are a heterogeneous population of antibodies directed against different phospholipid binding proteins. It is not clear which mechanism is responsible for the thrombogenic activity of all aPL. There is, however, an attractive hypothesis that suggests that aPL selectively inhibit one of the dominant natural anticoagulant pathways, the protein C pathway. Most attention has been focused on the induction of an acquired APC resistance, probably due to interference of the antibodies with binding of protein C or S to negatively charged phospholipids It is questionable whether in aPL-related thrombosis, an acquired APC resistance is responsible for both arterial and venous events. Although exogenous APC could prevent arterial thrombosis in a number of animal models, deficiencies in the protein C axis are correlated with venous thrombosis and not with arterial thrombosis. A safe conclusion is that interference of the protein C pathway can explain a large part of the venous complications in patients with APS. The observations that suggest a correlation between antibodies against EPCR and pregnancy morbidity warrant further studies.

Acknowledgment

Our own studies described in this review were supported by grants from Dutch Organization of Scientific Research (Zon-MW grant no. 902-26-290) and the Netherlands Heart Foundation (grant no. 2003B074).

References

1. Esmon CT. The protein C anticoagulant pathway. Arterioscler Thromb 1992;12:135–145.
2. Dahlback B. Progress in the understanding of the protein C anticoagulant pathway. Int J Hematol 2004;79:109–116.
3. Gresele P, Momi S, Berrettini M, et al. Activated human protein C prevents thrombin induced thromboembolism in mice. J Clin Invest 1998;101:667–676.

4. Taylor FB, Chang A, Esmon CT, et al. Protein C prevents the coagulopathic and lethal effects of *Escherichia coli* infusion in the baboon. J Clin Invest 1987;9:918–925.
5. Hughes GRV. Hughes 'syndrome: the antiphospholipid syndrome. A historical view. Lupus 1998;7:S1–S7.
6. De Groot PG, Oosting JD, Derksen RHWM. Antiphospholipid antibodies: specificity and pathophysiology. Baillieres Clin Haematol 1993;6:691–709.
7. Arnout J, Vermylen J. Current status and implications of autoimmune antiphospholipid antibodies in relation to thrombotic disease. Thromb Haemost 2003;1:931–942.
8. Esmon CT, Owen WG. Identification of an endothelial cell cofactor for thrombin catalyzed activation of protein C. Proc Natl Acad Sci U S A 1981;78:2249–2252.
9. Bajzar L, Morser J, Nesheim ME. TAFI or plasma procarboxypeptidase B couples the coagulation and fibrinolytic cascades through the thrombin-thrombomodulin complex. J Biol Chem 1996;27:16603–16608.
10. Bernard GR, Vincent JL, Laterre PF, et al. Efficacy and safety of recombinant human activated protein C for severe sepsis. N Engl J Med 2001;344:699–709.
11. Mosnier LO, Gale AJ, Yegneswaran S, Griffin JH. Activated protein C variants with normal cytoprotective but reduced anticoagulant activity. Blood 2004. Epub ahead of print.
12. Lane DA, Mannucci PM, Bauer KA, et al. Inherited thrombophilia, part 1.Thromb Haemost 1996;76:651–662.
13. Gruber A, Griffin JH. Direct detection of activated protein C in blood from human subjects. Blood 1992;79:2340–2348.
14. Suzuki K, Nishioka J, Hashimoto S. Protein C inhibitor. Purification from human plasma and characterization. J Biol Chem 1983;258:163–168.
15. Di Scipio RG, Davie EW. Characterization of protein S, a γ-carboxyglutamic acid containing protein from bovine and human plasma. Biochemistry 1979;18:899–904.
16. Walker FJ. Regulation of vitamin K dependent protein S. Inactivation by thrombin. J Biol Chem 1984;259:10335–10339.
17. Dahlback B. Protein S and C4b-binding protein: components involved in the regulation of the protein C anticoagulant pathway. Thromb Haemost 1991;66:49–61.
18. Esmon CT, Owen WG. The discovery of thrombomodulin. Thromb Haemost 2004;2:209–213.
19. Lohi O, Urban S, Freeman M. Diverse substrate recognition mechanisms for rhomboids; thrombomodulin is cleaved by mammalian rhomboids. Curr Biol 2004;14:236–241.
20. Fukudome K, Esmon CT. Molecular cloning and expression of murine and bovine endothelial cell protein C/activated protein C receptor (EPCR). The structural and functional conservation in human, bovine, and murine EPCR. J Biol Chem 1995;270:5571–5577.
21. Dahlback B, Carlsson M, Svennson PJ. Familiar thrombophilia due to a previous unrecognized mechanism characterized by poor anticoagulant response to activated protein C: prediction of a cofactor to activated protein C. Proc Natl Acad Sci U S A 1993;90:1004–1008.
22. Bertina RM, Koeleman BPC, Koster T, et al. Mutation in blood coagulation factor V associated with resistance to activated protein C. Nature 1994;369:64–67.
23. Nicolaes GA, Dahlback B. Factor V and thrombotic disease: description of a janus-faced protein. Arterioscler Thromb Vasc Biol 2002;22:530–538.
24. Rosing J, Tans G. Coagulation factor V: an old star shines again. Thromb Haemost 1997; 78:427–433.
25. McNeil HP, Simpson RJ, Chesterman CN, Krilis SA. Anti-phospholipid antibodies are directed against a complex antigen that includes a lipid-binding inhibitor of coagulation: beta 2-glycoprotein I (apolipoprotein H). Proc Natl Acad Sci U S A 1990;87:4120–4124.
26. Bevers EM, Galli M, Barbui T, Comfurius P, Zwaal RF. Lupus anticoagulant IgG's (LA) are not directed to phospholipids only, but to a complex of lipid-bound human prothrombin. Thromb Haemost 1991;66:629–632.
27. Willems GM, Janssen MP, Pelsers MM, et al. Role of divalency in the high-affinity binding of anticardiolipin antibody-beta 2-glycoprotein I complexes to lipid membranes. Biochemistry 1996;35:13833–13842.
28. de Laat HB, Derksen RHWM, Urbanus RT, Roest M, de Groot PG. β₂-glycoprotein I dependent lupus anticoagulant highly correlates with thrombosis in the antiphospholipid syndrome. Blood 2004;105:1540–1545
29. Takeuchi R, Atsumi T, Ieko M, et al. Coagulation and fibrinolytic activities in 2 siblings with beta(2)-glycoprotein I deficiency. Blood 2000;96:1594–1595.
30. Sheng Y, Reddel SW, Herzog H, et al. Impaired thrombin generation in beta 2-glycoprotein I null mice. J Biol Chem 2001;276:13817–13821.

31. Oosting JD, Derksen RHWM, Bobbink IWG, Hackeng T, Bouma BN, de Groot PG. Antiphospholipid antibodies are directed to a combination of phospholipids with prothrombin, protein C or protein S. An explanation for their pathogenic mechanism? Blood 1993;81:2618–2625.

32. Oosting JD, Preissner KT, Derksen RHWM, de Groot PhG. Autoantibodies directed against the epidermal growth factor-like domains of thrombomodulin inhibit protein C activation in vitro. Br J Haematol 1993;85:761–768.

33. Canfield WM, Kisiel W. Evidence of normal functional levels of activated protein C inhibitor in combined Factor V/VIII deficiency disease. J Clin Invest 1982;70:1260–1272.

34. De Groot PG, Horbach DA, Derksen RHWM. Protein C and other cofactors involved in the binding of antiphospholipid antibodies. Relation to the pathogenesis of thrombosis. Lupus 1996;5:488–493.

35. Hanson SR, Griffin JH, Harker LA, Kelly AB, Esmon CT, Gruber A. Antithrombotic effects of thrombin-induced activation of endogenous protein C in primates. J Clin Invest 1993;92:2003–2012.

36. Griffin JH. Blood coagulation. The thrombin paradox. Nature 1995;378:337–338.

37. Simmelink MJA, Fernandez JA, Derksen RHWM, Griffin JH, de Groot PhG. Low levels of activated protein C in patients with systemic lupus erythematosus do not relate to lupus anticoagulants but to low levels of factor II. Br J Haematology 2002;117:676–684.

38. Comp PC, deBault LE, Esmon NL, Esmon CT. Human thrombomodulin is inhibited by IgG from two patients with non-specific anticoagulants [abstract]. Blood 1983;62:299.

39. Freyssinet JM, Wiesel ML, Gauchy J, Boneu B, Cazenave JP. An IgM lupus anticoagulant that neutralizes the enhancing effect of phospholipid on purified endothelial thrombomodulin activity – a mechanism for thrombosis. Thromb Haemost 1986;55:309–313.

40. Cariou R, Tobelem G, Bellucci S, et al. Effect of lupus anticoagulant on antithrombogenic properties of endothelial cells – inhibition of thrombomodulin-dependent protein C activation. Thromb Haemost 1988;60:54–58.

41. Oosting JD, Preissner KT, Derksen RHWM, de Groot PhG. Autoantibodies directed against the epidermal growth factor-like domains of thrombomodulin inhibit protein C activation in vitro. Br J Haematol 1993;85:761–768.

42. Schorer AE, Wickham NW, Watson KV. Lupus anticoagulant induces a selective defect in thrombin-mediated endothelial prostacyclin release and platelet aggregation. Br J Haematol 1989;71:399–407.

43. Keeling DM, Wilson AJ, Mackie IJ, Isenberg DA, Machin SJ. Role of beta 2-glycoprotein I and antiphospholipid antibodies in activation of protein C in vitro. J Clin Pathol 1993;46:908–911.

44. Potzsch B, Kawamura H, Preissner KT, Schmidt M, Seelig C, Muller-Berghaus G. Acquired protein C dysfunction but not decreased activity of thrombomodulin is a possible marker of thrombophilia in patients with lupus anticoagulant. J Lab Clin Med 1995;25:56–65.

45. Kawakami M, Kitani A, Hara M, et al. Plasma thrombomodulin and alpha 2-plasmin inhibitor-plasmin complex are elevated in active systemic lupus erythematosus. J Rheumatol 1992;19:1704–1709.

46. Hurtado V, Montes R, Gris JC, et al. Autoantibodies against EPCR are found in antiphospholipid syndrome and are a risk factor for foetal death. Blood 2004;104:1369–1374.

47. Franchi F, Biguzzi E, Cetin I, et al. Mutations in the thrombomodulin and endothelial protein C receptor genes in women with late fetal loss. Br J Haematol 2001;114:641–646.

48. Gu JM, Crawley JT, Ferrell G, et al. Disruption of the endothelial cell protein C receptor gene in mice causes placental thrombosis and early embryonic lethality. J Biol Chem 2002;277:43335–43343.

49. Fijnheer R, Horbach DA, Donders RCJM, et al. Factor V Leiden, antiphospholipid antibodies and thrombosis in systemic lupus erythematosus. Thromb Haemost 1996;76:514–517.

50. Malia RG, Kitchen S, Greaves M, Preston FE. Inhibition of activated protein C and its cofactor protein S by antiphospholipid antibodies. Br J Haematol 1990;76:101–107.

51. Marciniak E, Romond EH. Impaired catalytic function of activated protein C: a new in vitro manifestation of lupus anticoagulant. Blood 1989;74:2426–2432.

52. Borrell M, Sala N, de Castellarnau C, Lopez S, Gari M, Fontcuberta J. Immunoglobulin fractions isolated from patients with antiphospholipid antibodies prevent the inactivation of factor Va by activated protein C on human endothelial cells. Thromb Haemost 1992;68:268–272.

53. Amer L, Kisiel W, Searles RP, Williams RC Jr. Impairment of the protein C anticoagulant pathway in a patient with systemic lupus erythematosus, anticardiolipin antibodies and thrombosis. Thromb Res 1990;57:247–258.

54. Munoz-Rodriguez FJ, Reverter JC, Font J, et al. Clinical significance of acquired activated protein C resistance in patients with systemic lupus erythematosus. Lupus 2002;11:730–735.

55. Nojima J, Kuratsune H, Suehisa E, et al. Acquired activated protein C resistance associated with anti-protein S antibody as a strong risk factor for DVT in non-SLE patients. Thromb Haemost 2002;8:716–722.

56. Galli M, Duca F, Ruggeri L, Finazzi G, Negri B, Moia M. Congenital resistance to activated protein C in patients with lupus anticoagulants: evaluation of two functional assays. Thromb Haemost 1998;80:246–249.
57. Male C, Mitchell L, Julian J, Vegh P, et al. Acquired activated protein C resistance is associated with lupus anticoagulants and thrombotic events in pediatric patients with systemic lupus erythematosus. Blood 2001;97:844–849.
58. Gennari LC, Blanco AN, Alberto MF, Grosso SH, Peirano AA, Lazzari MA. Antiphospholipid antibodies impact the protein C (PC) pathway behavior. Am J Hematol 2002;71:128–130.
59. Galli M, Ruggeri L, Barbui T. Differential effects of anti-beta2-glycoprotein I and antiprothrombin antibodies on the anticoagulant activity of activated protein C. Blood 1998;91:1999–2004.
60. Izumi T, Pound ML, Su Z, Iverson GM, Ortel TL. Anti-beta(2)-glycoprotein I antibody-mediated inhibition of activated protein C requires binding of beta(2)-glycoprotein I to phospholipids. Thromb Haemost 2002;88:620–626.
61. Nojima J, Kuratsune H, Suehisa E, et al. Acquired activated protein C resistance is associated with the co-existence of anti-prothrombin antibodies and lupus anticoagulant activity in patients with systemic lupus erythematosus. Br J Haematol 2002;118:577–583.
62. Horbach DA, van Oort E, Derksen RHWM, de Groot PG. Anti-prothrombin antibodies with LAC activity inhibits tenase, prothrombinase and protein C activity by increasing the affinity of prothrombin for phospholipids. Lupus 1998;7:S209.
63. Smirnov MD, Triplett DT, Comp PC, Esmon NL, Esmon CT. On the role of phosphatidylethanolamine in the inhibition of activated protein C activity by antiphospholipid antibodies. J Clin Invest 1995;95:309–316.
64. Esmon NL, Smirnov MD, Esmon CT. Thrombogenic mechanisms of antiphospholipid antibodies. Thromb Haemost 1997;78:79–82.
65. Safa O, Hensley K, Smirnov MD, Esmon CT, Esmon NL. Lipid oxidation enhances the function of activated protein C. J Biol Chem 2001;276:1829–1836.
66. Pratico D, Ferro D, Iuliano L, et al. Ongoing prothrombotic state in patients with antiphospholipid antibodies: a role for increased lipid peroxidation. Blood 1999;93:3401–3407.
67. Mori T, Takeya H, Nishioka, Gabazza EC, Suzuki K. b2-glycoprotein I modulates the anticoagulant activity of protein C on the phospholipid surface. Thromb Haemost 1996;75:49–55.
68. Atsuma T, Khamashta MA, Amengual O, et al. Binding of anti-cardiolipin antibodies to protein C via β2-glycoprotein I: a possible mechanism in the inhibitory effect of antiphospholipid antibodies on the protein C system. Clin Exp Immunol 1998;112:325–333.
69. Kalafatis M, Simioni P, Tormene D, Beck DO, Luni S, Girolami A. Isolation and characterization of an antifactor V antibody causing activated protein C resistance from a patient with severe thrombotic manifestations. Blood 2002;99:3985–3992.
70. Harrison RL, Alperin JB. Concurrent protein C deficiency and lupus anticoagulant. Am J Hematol 1992;40:33–37.
71. Parke AL, Weinstein RE, Bona R, et al. The thrombotic diathesis associated with the presence of phospholipid antibodies may be due to low levels of free protein S. Am J Med 1992;93:49–56.
72. Hasselaar P, Derksen RHWM, Blokzijl L, et al. Risk factors for thrombosis in lupus patients. Ann Rheum Dis 1989;48:933–940.
73. Atsumi T, Khamashta MA, Ames PRJ, Ichikawa K, Koike T, Hughes GRV. Effect of 2 β-glycoprotein I and human monoclonal anticardiolipin antibody on the protein S/C4b-binding protein system. Lupus 1997;6:358–364.

35 Contribution of Tissue Factor to the Pathogenesis of Thrombosis in Patients with Antiphospholipid Syndrome

Chary López-Pedrera, Francisco Velasco, and Maria J. Cuadrado

Introduction

Antiphospholipid syndrome (APS) is an acquired autoimmune disorder of unknown etiology. The syndrome is defined by the association of arterial or venous thrombosis and/or pregnancy morbidity, in the presence of antiphospholipid antibodies (aPL), anticardiolipin antibodies (aCL), and lupus anticoagulant (LA) [1].

aPLs are a heterogeneous family of autoantibodies with diverse cross-reactivities whose origin and role have not been fully elucidated. It is now recognized that many of the autoantibodies associated with APS are directed against phospholipid binding plasma proteins, such as β_2-glycoprotein I (β_2-GPI) and prothrombin, or phospholipid–protein complexes [2], expressed on or bound to the surface of vascular endothelial cells, platelets, or monocytes [3].

β_2-GPI, a plasma protein bearing the major antigenic epitope for aPL, interacts with negatively charged phospholipids involved in the coagulation process, and has both procoagulant and anticoagulant properties. β_2-GPI suppresses the thrombomodulin–protein C system [4], factor XII activation, factor X activation, and prothrombinase activity. Antibodies against β_2-GPI may modify the properties of β_2-GPI and favor a prothrombotic state. However, individuals with β_2-GPI deficiency do not have a thrombotic tendency [5]; thus, aPL-associated thrombosis cannot be explained merely by β_2-GPI insufficiency.

Prothrombin, another plasma protein, is the second major target of aPL and the zymogen of the serine protease thrombin [6]. Thrombin is one of the most potent enzymes, and it catalyzes several reactions which may be important in blood coagulation. In this way, recent studies have demonstrated that anti-prothrombin antibodies with LA activity can inhibit coagulation reactions in a phospholipid and prothrombin dependent manner, by enhancing the intrinsic inhibitory effect of prothrombin itself [7]. Therefore, aPL may also modify prothrombin properties, ultimately leading to a thrombotic state.

Thrombosis is the key lesion of the APS [8]. Several non-exclusive mechanisms have been proposed to explain the involvement of aPL in the pathogenesis of thrombosis in APS, including the induction of tissue factor (TF) expression by endothelial cells and monocytes [9, 10]. This chapter focuses on the contribution of

TF to the pathogenesis of thrombosis in patients with APS and the intracellular mechanisms involved in TF expression.

TF Pathway and Thrombosis in APS

TF is a specific transmembrane single chain glycoprotein composed of 263 amino acids (47 kDa), that requires interaction with specific membrane phospholipids (PL) to become functionally active [11–13]. TF serves as both high-affinity receptor and enzyme activator for plasma FVII or FVIIa in initiating a localized procoagulant activity (PCA) on the anionic PL cell surface. TF is widely accepted to be the major initiator of in vivo coagulation [14]. It is also believed that TF has a key role in fibrin deposition in immunologic disorders, as well as in disseminated intra-vascular coagulation and clot formation in gram-negative bacterial sepsis, cancer, and inflammatory bowel disease [12, 13, 15]. TF is expressed on the surface of many cell types but, in the resting state, is normally absent from cells in contact with blood. However, TF can be induced, in vitro, to appear on endothelial cells and monocytes in a transcriptionally regulated manner by several physiologic or non-physiologic stimuli [16–18].

In APS patients, our recent in vivo studies have shown that patients with primary APS have increased expression of TF on the monocyte surface, along with increased mRNA-TF, TF antigen, and activity levels in peripheral blood mononuclear cells, where the source of TF is the monocyte [19–21]. Moreover, TF expression was found increased in APS patients with thrombosis when compared with those without and with healthy controls. TF expression in these patients was found to be further increased in those positive for IgG aCL, but not in those positive for IgM aCL of LA. In addition, TF expression in APS did not appear to be related to plasma levels of tumor necrosis factor α (TNF-α) and interleukin 1β (IL-1β), two inflammatory mediators that influence TF production, suggesting that inflammatory changes do not determine TF production in the steady state.

Recent evidence has suggested a role for the TF pathway in the pathogenesis of aPL-related thrombosis. Experimental data have shown that procoagulant activity in cultured EC and monocytes is induced by plasma from patients with APS and by purified aPL [22]. Furthermore, it has been demonstrated that antibodies against β_2-GPI induce the expression and activity of TF in vitro [10]. In addition, β_2-GPI expression on monocytes is significantly increased in patients with APS and correlate with TF expression, thus contributing to the maintenance of a persistent pro-thrombotic state [23].

Signal Transduction Mechanisms Associated with the Increased Expression of TF in Response to aPL

The mechanism(s) by which aPL induce TF expression is unknown. A potential role or Fcγ receptors (FcγR) in the pathogenesis of APS was suggested [24], but Pierangeli et al [25] showed in a murine model that these effects are not dependent on binding of antibody to FcγR. Rand and coworkers have proposed a thrombogenic mechanisms [26, 27] in which the high affinity of the aPL for anionic PL bound proteins on the cell surface may in itself explain the prothrombotic effects including TF expression. They suggest that annexin V has a physiologic role in inhibiting coagulation, by forming clusters that bind with high affinity to anionic PL on cell surfaces exposed to flowing blood, and thus fully shielding these surfaces from the assembly of the TF–FVIIa and other coagulation complexes. More recently, annexin II, a phospholipid binding protein, has been identified as an EC or monocyte surface molecule and might be involved in aPL mediated cellular signaling, playing a critical role in the upregulation of monocyte TF [28].

At a molecular level, it has been suggested that aPL may interact with specific cell surface receptors (proteins and/or lipids), inducing signals that have consequences downstream, that ultimately will result in upregulation of cell surface proteins (i.e., TF). In an in vitro recent study, Pierangeli et al [29] have shown that aPL induces activation of the nuclear factor kappa B (NFκB) in EC. In turn, NFκB activation leads to upregulation of gene transcription of adhesion molecules on EC and to initiation of various signal transduction pathways. In an in vivo recent study, our group has studied the activation of NFκB and the expression of its inhibitor IκBα in monocytes from patients with primary APS and their association with monocyte TF expression.

Our study, performed on purified monocytes from APS patients, showed both increased proteolysis of the cytoplasmic inhibitory protein IκBα and nuclear translocation and activation of the NFκB proteins p65 and p50, compared to controls. Moreover, NFκB activation was accompanied by an increased expression of TF in these patients. Furthermore, the analysis of the p38 and pERK MAP kinase activity, which have been demonstrated to be involved in the aPL induced upregulation of TF in endothelial cells [29], indicated that mean levels of phosphorylated forms of p38 and ERK1/2 MAP kinases were significantly higher in monocytes of APS patients compared to controls. In addition, Pearson's relational statistic indicated significant inverse correlation between levels of pp38 MAP kinase and IκBα ($P = 0.018$). Hence, increased levels of pp38 correlated with diminished levels of cytosolic IκBα expression. Thus, our data might suggest an implication of p38 MAP kinases in NFκB activation in monocytes of APS patients [30].

As an intermediate early gene in activated EC, TF is rapidly induced in response to pathophysiologically relevant stimuli such as cytokines and growth factors, including vascular endothelial growth factor (VEGF), in EC and monocytes [31]. VEGF is a critical regulator of angiogenesis that stimulates proliferation, migration, and proteolitic activity of EC. Although the mitogenic activity of VEGF is EC specific, recent reports indicate that VEGF is able to stimulate chemotaxis and TF production in monocytes [32]. Previous studies have demonstrated significantly higher levels of plasma VEGF in APS patients compared to control [33]. In a recent study by our group, and in order to elucidate the origin of this plasma VEGF, we measured VEGF expression in monocytes from APS patients by several methods, including real time polymerase chain reaction (RT-PCR), Western blot, immunocytochemistry, and flow cytometry. We found significantly higher levels of both mRNA and protein VEGF in monocytes from APS patients compared to controls, thus pointing to the monocytes as the possible source of this plasmatic VEGF. In addition, increased VEGF expression correlated positively with the levels of both mRNA and cell surface TF expression. VEGF stimulated activity in monocytes is mediated by the VEGF receptor Flt-1. Monocytes, in contrast to endothelium, express only this specific receptor, which functions as a mediator of monocyte recruitment and procoagulant activity [34]. In our study, VEGF-Flt-1 expression in monocytes from APS was found elevated in parallel with VEGF. Moreover, a positive correlation was found between the expression of this receptor and that of monocyte TF. Thus, increased VEGF activity could be responsible for TF overexpression in monocytes of APS patients [35].

Recent studies have suggested that p38 and ERK1/2 MAP kinases are two essential mediators of VEGF-induced endothelial TF [36]. Moreover, VEGF induced activation in monocytes and EC has been proved to be mediated by p38 MAP kinase pathway. Our group recently showed that phosphorylated forms of p38 and ERK1/2 were significantly increased in APS patients compared to controls (described in previous paragraphs). The increased ERK activity observed (which did not seem to be involved in NFkB activation) might play a role as a mediator of VEGF induced TF expression in monocytes of PAS patients, as suggested for EC [36]. Nevertheless, as p38 MAP kinase has also proved to be involved in both the upregulation of VEGF [37, 38] and the VEGF induced activation of TF expression, an additional and may be independent role for this kinase cannot be ruled out. Additional in vitro studies are required to evaluate this hypothesis.

TF and Therapeutic Intervention in APS

APS is associated with an increased risk of recurrent thrombosis [39], being thromboprophylaxis similar to that used in the general population. However, the contribution of TF to a prothrombotic state in this syndrome provides a renewed focus on antithrombotic therapies in current use (i.e., oral anticoagulation) and supports the need for antithrombotic strategies that more specifically target the activity of the TF–VIIa complex or the antibody mediated TF expression.

Oral anticoagulation reduces the availability of functional FVII and minimizes thrombotic risk, even if TF is highly expressed. Retrospective studies have strongly suggested the efficacy of high-intensity oral anticoagulation for the prevention of recurrent thrombosis in APS, but there is some debate regarding the duration of therapy. High recurrence rates have been seen after the cessation of anticoagulant therapy as well as in patients who were not receiving anticoagulants, suggesting that patients with APS require long-term treatment [39]. In patients with APS, monocyte TF expression and procoagulant activity remain high for years after the last thrombotic episode despite receiving oral anticoagulants [19]. Thrombotic complications should be expected if the intensity of anticoagulation drops below target values.

Strategies aimed to prevent antibody mediated TF overproduction or agents that could lower TF expression by other mechanisms must be identified. In this regard, the newly discovered anti-inflammatory, anticoagulant, antiproliferative, and immunoregulatory effects of statins are of great interest. These compounds are being tried as an additional therapeutic tool in the treatment of thrombosis in APS patients. Meroni et al [40] have recently described the effects of statins on EC activated in vitro by pro-inflammatory cytokines and/or by aPL (anti–β_2-GPI antibodies). Fluvastatin and simvastatin were found to be able to inhibit the induction of a pro-adhesive and pro-inflammatory phenotype in a specific manner because the addition of mevalonate reversed the inhibition.

Statins effects on coagulation process have also been described. Statins have antithrombotic properties although the mechanisms leading to this effect are still unclear. Undas et al [41] found that simvastatin treatment reduces blood clotting by decreasing rates of prothrombin activation, factor Va generation, fibrinogen cleavage, factor XIII activation, and increased rate of factor Va inactivation. Furthermore, impaired TF expression on cultured human macrophages and monocytes induced by statins has been demonstrated in vitro and has been attributed to the inhibition of the TF gene induction [42, 43]. If statins are able to reduce, in vivo, the TF expression in these patients, this could have an important impact in the future therapeutic approach of patients with aPL.

Conclusions

Increased TF expression may contribute to thrombosis in patients with APS. This effect might ultimately depend on antibody engagement of PL binding proteins on the monocyte and the EC surface, leading to signal transduction and altered cell activity. Understanding the intracellular mechanism(s) of aPL mediated TF activation may help to establish new therapeutic approaches to revert the prothrombotic state observed in APS patients.

Acknowledgements

This work was supported by grants from the Junta de Andalucia (exp. 171/03) and the Fondo de Investigación Sanitaria (FIS 01/0715 and 03/1033) of Spain.

References

1. Wilson WA, Garavi AE, Koike T, et al. International consensus statement on preliminary classification criteria for definite antiphospholipid syndrome. Arthritis Rheum 1999;42:1309–1311.
2. Roubey RAS. Immunology of the antiphospholipid antibody syndrome. Arthritis Rheum 1996;39:1444–1454.
3. Amengual O, Atsumi T, Khamashta MA. Tissue Factor in antiphospholipid syndrome: shifting the focus from coagulation to endothelium. Rheumatology 2003;42:1029–1031.
4. Ieko M, Ichikawa K, Tripplett D, et al. β2-glycoprotein I is necessary to inhibit protein C activity by monoclonal anticardiolipin antibodies. Arthritis Rheum 1999;42:167–174.
5. Takeuchi R, Atsumi T, Ieko M, et al. Coagulation and fibrinolytic activities in two siblings with β2-glycoprotein I deficiency. Blood 2000;96:1594–1595.
6. Permpikul P, Rao LVM, Rapaport SI. Functional and binding studies of the roles of prothrombin and β2-glycoprotein I in the expression of lupus anticoagulant activity. Blood 1994;83:2878–2892.
7. Simmelink MJA, Horbach DA, Derksen RHWM, et al. Complexes of anti-prothrombin antibodies and prothrombin cause lupus anticoagulant activity by competing with the binding of clotting factors for catalytic phospholipids surfaces. Br J Haematol 2001;113:621–629.
8. Khamashta MA, Asherson RA. Hughes syndrome: antiphospholipid antibodies move closer to thrombosis in 1994. Br J Rheumatol 1995;34:493–494.
9. Reverter J-C, Tassies D, Font J, et al., Effects of human monoclonal anticardiolipin antibodies on platelet function and on tissue factor expression on monocytes. Arthritis Rheum 1998;41:1420–1427.
10. Amengual O, Atsumi T, Khamashta MA, Hughes GRV. The role of the tissue factor pathway in the hypercoagulable state in patients with the antiphospholipid syndrome. Thromb Haemost 1998;79:276–281.
11. Nemerson Y, Gentry R. An ordered addition, essential activation model of the tissue factor pathway of coagulation: evidence for a conformational cage. Biochemistry 1986;25:4020–4033.

12. Nemerson Y. Tissue factor and hemostasis. Blood 1988;71:1–12.
13. Rodgers GM. Hemostatic properties of normal and perturbed vascular cells. FASEB J 1988;2:116–123.
14. Nemerson Y. The tissue factor pathway of blood coagulation. Semin Haematol 1992;29:170–176.
15. Weis JR, Pitas RE, Wilson BD, Rodgers GM. Oxidized low-density lipoprotein increases cultured human endothelial cell tissue factor activity and reduces protein C activation. FASEB J 1991;5:2459–2465.
16. Gregory SA, Morrissey JH, Edgington TS. Regulation of tissue factor gene expression in the monocyte procoagulant response to endotoxin. Mol Cell Biol 1989;9:2752–2755.
17. Mackman N. Regulation of the tissue factor gene. FASEB J 1995;9:883–889.
18. Courtney MA, Haidaris PJ, Marder VJ, Sporn LA. Tissue factor mRNA expression in the endothelium of an intact umbilical vein. Blood 1996;87:174–179.
19. Cuadrado MJ, López-Pedrera Ch, Khamashta MA, et al. Thrombosis in primary antiphospholipid syndrome. A pivotal role for monocyte tissue factor expression. Arthritis Rheum 1997;40:834–841.
20. Dobado-Berrios PM, Lopez-Pedrera Ch, Velasco F, et al. Increased levels of tissue factor mRNA in mononuclear blood cells of patients with primary antiphospholipid syndrome. Thromb Haemost 1999;82:1578–1582.
21. Dobado-Berrios PM, López-Pedrera Ch, Velasco F, et al. The role of tissue factor in the antiphospholipid syndrome. Arthritis Rheum 2001;44:2467–2476.
22. Kornberg A, Blank M, Kaufman S, Shoenfeld Y. Induction of tissue factor-like activity in monocytes by anti-cardiolipin antibodies. J Immunol 1994;153:1328–1332.
23. Conti F, Sorice M, Circella A, et al. Beta-2-glycoprotein I expression on monocytes is increased in anti-phospholipid antibody syndrome and correlates with tissue factor expression. Clin Exp Immunol 2003;132:509–516.
24. Arnout J. The pathogenesis of the antiphospholipid syndrome: a hypothesis based on parallelisms with heparin-induced thrombocytopenia. Thromb Haemost 1996;75:536–541.
25. Pierangeli S, Espinola R, Liu X, Harris E, Salmon J. Identification of an Fc gamma receptor independent mechanism by which intravenous immunoglobin ameliorates antiphospholipid antibody-induced thrombogenic phenotype. Arthritis Rheum 2001;44:876–883.
26. Rand JH, Wu X-X, Andree HAM, et al. Antiphospholipid antibodies accelerate plasma coagulation by inhibiting annexin-V binding to phospholipids: a "lupus procoagulant" phenomenon. Blood 1998;92:1652–1660.
27. Rand JH, Wu X-X, Andree HAM, et al. Pregnancy loss in the antiphospholipid syndrome: a possible thrombogenic mechanism. N Engl J Med 1997;337:154–160.
28. Zhou H, Roubey RAS. Annexin A2 and antiphospholipid-antibody induced upregulation of monocyte tissue factor. Arthritis Rheum 2002;46:S232.
29. Pierangeli SS, Ferrara DE, Harris EN, et al. Inhibitors of NFκB and p38 kinase abrogate TF up-regulation by anti-phospholipid antibodies. Thromb Haemost 2003.
30. Cuadrado MJ, Lopez-Pedrera Ch, Buendía P, et al. Regulation of NFkB activation in the antiphospholipid síndrome: involvement of ERK1/2 and p38 MAP kinase pathways. Arthritis Rheum 2004;33:S34.
31. Baddwin AS. The transcription factor NFκB and human disease. J Clin Invest 2001;107:3–6.
32. Chen J, Bierhaus A, Schiekofer S, et al. Tissue factor: a receptor involved in the control of cellular properties, including angiogenesis. Thromb Haemost 2001;86:334–345.
33. Williams FMK, Parmar K, Hughes GRV, et al. Systemic endothelial cell markers in primary antiphospholipid syndrome. Thromb Haemost 2000;84:742–746.
34. Clauss N, Weich H, Breier G, et al. The vascular endothelial growth factor receptor Flt-1 mediates biological activities. Implications for a functional role of placenta growth factor in monocyte activation and chemotaxis. J Biol Chem 1996;271:17629–17634.
35. Cuadrado MJ, Buendia P, Lopez-Pedrera Ch, et al. Increased tissue factor expression in monocytes from patients with antiphospholipid syndrome depends on NFkB activation. Arthritis Rheum 2003;48:S322.
36. Blum S, Issbrüker K, Willuweit A, et al. An inhibitory role of the phosphatidylinositol 3-kinase-signaling pathway in vascular endothelial growth factor-induced tissue factor expression. J Biol Chem 2001;276:33428–33434.
37. Itaya H, Imaizumi T, Yoshida H, et al. Expression of vascular endothelial growth factor in human monocyte/macrophages stimulated with lipopolysaccharide. Thromb Haemost 2001;85:171–176.
38. Jung YD, Liu W, Reinmuth N, et al. Vascular endothelial growth factor is upregulated by interleukin-1 beta in human vascular smooth muscle cells via the p38 mitogen-activated protein kinase pathway. Angiogenesis 2001;4:155–162.

39. Khamashta MA, Cuadrado MJ, Mujic F, Taub NA, Hunt BJ, Hughes GRV. The management of thrombosis in the antiphospholipid-antibody syndrome. N Engl J Med 1995;332:993–997.
40. Meroni PL, Raschi E, Testoni C, et al. Statins prevent endothelial cell activation induced by anti-phospholipid (anti-β2 glycoprotein I) antibodies: effect on the pro-adhesive and pro-inflammatory phenotype. Arthritis Rheum 2001;44:2870–2878.
41. Undas A, Brummel KE, Musial J, Mann KG, Szceklik A. Simvastatin depresses blood clotting by inhibiting activation of prothrombin, factor V and factor XIII and by enhancing factor Va inactivation. Circulation 2001;103:2248–2257.
42. Colli S, Eligni S, Lalli M, et al. Vastatins inhibit tissue factor in cultured human macrophages: a novel mechanism of protection against atherothrombosis. Arterioscler Thromb Vasc Biol 1997;17:265–272.
43. Ferro D, Basili S, Alessandri C, et al. Inhibition of tissue-factor-mediated thrombin generation by simvastatin. Atherosclerosis 2000;149:111–116.

36 Annexins in Antiphospholipid Syndrome

Jacob H. Rand and Xiao-Xuan Wu

Introduction

Annexin A5 is a potent anticoagulant protein that binds to anionic phospholipid containing bilayers with high affinity. The protein has potent anticoagulant properties that are a consequence of its forming two-dimensional crystals that shield the bilayers from being available for critical coagulation enzyme reactions. Autoantibodies against phospholipid binding proteins or against annexin A5 itself may disrupt the crystallization of the annexin A5 shield, expose anionic phospholipids (PL), and thereby make them available for phospholipid dependent coagulation reactions. This interference with annexin A5 crystallization may be a mechanism for pregnancy losses and thrombosis in antiphospholipid syndrome (APS) – a condition that is also known as the Hughes syndrome.

Anticoagulant Effect of Annexin A5

The various annexins were isolated from different tissues, characterized by different research groups, and given different names prior to their becoming recognized to be a homologous family of proteins in 1990 [1]. The family is composed of several thousand different proteins that have been identified in eukaryotic phyla [2]. Their canonical structure consists of repetitive homologous domains of about 70 amino acids, with almost all of the annexins having 4 of these domains. The unique amino terminal tails are thought to contribute to each of the protein's unique properties. The protein forms highly ordered two-dimensional crystalline arrays over the bilayers [3–5] [Fig. 36.1(A)]. The monomer of annexin A5 is a concave disk, with the phospholipid membrane binding domain and calcium binding domains located on the convex surface. These monomers assembles into large, slightly convex crystals on membranes that, when added to large spherical phospholipid vesicles, form planar facets that transform the vesicles into polyhedrons [6]. Annexin A5 appears to be synthesized ubiquitously, but is especially highly expressed by cells that serve a barrier function between tissues and an extracellular fluid [7], such as vascular endothelial cells, placental trophoblasts, proximal renal tubules, and bile ductules.

As mentioned above, the anticoagulant properties of annexin A5 result from its shielding phospholipids from availability for coagulation reactions. Phospholipids are critically required for the sequence of blood coagulation reactions from their

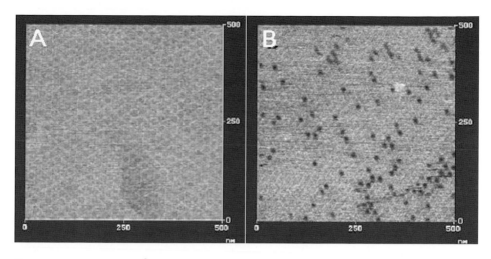

Figure 36.1. Crystal structure of annexin A5 and its disruption by monoclonal aPL. (A) An atomic force image of annexin A5 that has formed a highly ordered two-dimensional crystal over a phospholipid bilayer composed of 30% phosphatidylserine/70% phosphatidyl choline that was formed on a mica chip. (B) When an aPL mAb and β_2-glycoprotein I were added to the pre-formed annexin A5 crystal lattice on the bilayer, vacancy defects (small round dark holes) appeared, indicating disruptions in the crystal lattice. (Reprinted from Rand JH, et al. Human monoclonal antiphospholipid antibodies disrupt annexin a5 anticoagulant crystal shield on phospholipid bilayers: evidence from atomic force microscopy and functional assay. Am J Pathol 2003;163:1193–1200, with permission from the American Society for Investigative Pathology.)

initiation by the exposure of the transmembrane protein tissue factor (TF) through the reaction that generates thrombin. This requirement localizes coagulation reactions to sites of vascular injury. TF, in complex with adjacent phospholipids, binds circulating coagulation factor VII, which becomes activated to VIIa. The TF–phospholipids–VIIa complex then binds to, and then cleaves, each of its substrates – the zymogens, factor X, and factor IX – to generate their active enzyme forms, factors Xa and IXa. Each of these enzymes, in turn, cleaves its own substrate – factor II (also known as prothrombin) and factor X, respectively – through the enzyme–cofactor–substrate complexes that require also anionic phospholipids, in particular phosphatidylserine [8], for assembly. These are the factors Xa–Va–II complex (also known as "prothrombinase") that results in the generation of factor IIa (also known as thrombin), and the factors IXa–VIIIa–X complex (also known as "tenase") that augments the formation of factor Xa. The thrombin that is generated then cleaves fibrinogen to form fibrin, has a number of additional complex effects on coagulation proteins and anticoagulant proteins, and also triggers signaling events on platelets and other cells.

Role of Annexin A5 in Placental Trophoblasts and Vascular Endothelium

The role of annexin A5 in pregnancy has been recently reviewed [9]. Annexin A5 is highly expressed by placental trophoblasts, in an apparently constitutive manner

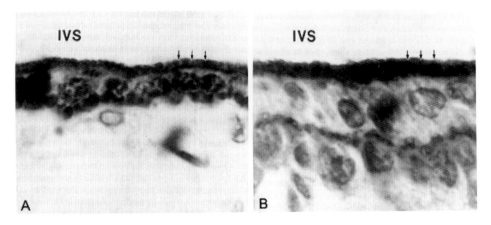

Figure 36.2. Immunohistochemical staining for annexin A5 in human term and first trimester placental chorionic villi. (A) Immunoreactivity of term placental villi incubated with affinity purified anti-human annexin A5 IgG. The brush border of the syncytiotrophoblast apical surface stains for immunoreactive annexin A5 (*arrows*). Note the dense immunostaining of vesicles present within the cytoplasm of the syncytiotrophoblast layer. IVS = intervillous space. Original; magnification, 400x. (B) Immunoreactivity of first trimester placental villi incubated with affinity purified anti-human annexin A5 IgG. Heavy immunostaining for annexin A5 localizes to the apical surface of the syncytiotrophoblast layer (*arrows*) as well as adjacent cytotrophoblasts. Original magnification, 1000x. (Reprinted with permission from Krikun G, et al. The expression of the placental anticoagulant protein, annexin V, by villous trophoblasts: immunolocalization and in vitro regulation. Placenta 1994;15:601–612, with permission from Elsevier.)

and is abundant on the apical surfaces of syncytiotrophoblasts (Fig. 36.2) [10], an anatomic position where it can to modulate blood fluidity in the maternal circulation through the intervillous space. The protein assembles on the apical membranes that express phosphatidylserine [11]. In an animal model, annexin A5 was shown to serve a thrombomodulatory role in the placental circulation where it was necessary for maintenance of placental integrity [12]; infusion of antibodies against annexin A5 resulted in placental infarction and pregnancy losses. Dissociation of annexin A5 from the surfaces of cultured human trophoblasts by treatment with EGTA exposes the unshielded apical membranes to circulating blood and accelerates coagulation of plasma exposed to the cells [13]. Pre-eclamptic placentas have decreased annexin A5 on their trophoblasts, and the degree of the decrease correlates with elevation of markers for activation of blood coagulation [14]. In an in vitro study, a monoclonal anti-annexin A5 antibody, bound to syncytialized trophoblasts, induced trophoblast apoptosis and significantly reduced gonadotrophin secretion [15].

Annexin A5 may also have a thrombomodulatory role in the systemic vasculature. The protein was isolated from bovine aortic intima as vascular anticoagulant-α [16]. It was immuno-localized to vascular endothelial cells [7] and was shown to be expressed in cultured human umbilical vein endothelial cells (HUVECs) [17]. Dissociation of the protein from the apical membranes of cultured HUVECs by aPL accelerated coagulation of plasma exposed to these cells [13].

Taken together, the available data support the hypothesis that annexin A5 plays a antithrombotic role on the apical surfaces of placental syncytiotrophoblasts that line the placental villi and face the maternal blood. It is also possible that annexin A5 may play a similar role in the systemic vasculature.

apL Antibody Mediated Targeting of the Annexin A5 Anticoagulant Shield

Reduced expression of immunohistochemically detectable annexin A5 on placental villi of patients with the APS has been reported [18], however, others did not find annexin A5 to be decreased in most [19] or all [20, 21] of the aPL placentas that they examined. Because both aPL and annexin A5 have affinity for anionic phospholipids, we proposed the possibility that aPL might interfere with annexin A5 binding to phospholipid membranes [13].

IgG fractions from APS patients reduce the quantity of annexin A5 on cultured placental villi [18, 22], trophoblasts (primary cultures of trophoblasts, as well as the BeWo cell line) [Fig. 36.3(A,B)], and cultured HUVECS [13], and platelets [23]. aPL IgGs also accelerate the coagulation of plasma which is incubated with cultured trophoblasta and endothelial cells following their exposure to the antibodies [13] [Fig. 36.3(C)]. A monoclonal antiphosphatidylserine antibody reduced the level of

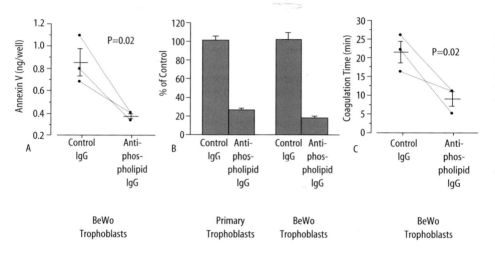

Figure 36.3. Effects of antiphospholipid IgG antibody on annexin A5 and plasma coagulation on trophoblasts. Cultured trophoblasts (from the BeWo cell line) grown to confluence were exposed to IgGs purified from sera with protein G–sepharose (final IgG concentrations: 2 mg/mL) from 3 patients and their controls for 2 hours at 4°C to inhibit the recycling of membranes and vesicles. Annexin A5 was then dissociated with buffer containing EGTA and measured by immunoassay. (All tests were performed in quadruplicate.) Panel A shows that the mean (± SE) level of annexin A5, indicated by the horizontal line and error bar, was significantly lower after exposure to antiphospholipid IgG than after exposure to control IgG (0.37 ± 0.02 vs. 0.85 ± 0.12 ng/well, $P = 0.02$). Panel B shows how antiphospholipid IgG affects annexin A5 levels on primary cultured trophoblasts and BeWo trophoblasts. (The data on the former were normalized for the DNA concentration, and both sets of data were normalized as percentages of the control values so that the two cell types could be shown together.) Annexin A5 levels on the surface of both types of trophoblasts were significantly reduced ($P < 0.001$ for both). Panel C shows the coagulation time of plasma added to BeWo trophoblasts exposed to preparations of IgG from the 3 patients for 2 hours at 4°C, as compared with controls. In these experiments, annexin A5 was not dissociated from the cells. The mean (± SE) coagulation time was significantly shorter in the antiphospholipid–IgG exposed trophoblasts than in the controls (8.7 ± 2.0 vs. 21.3 ± 2.9 minutes, $P = 0.02$). (Reprinted with permission from Rand JH, et al. Pregnancy loss in the antiphospholipid-antibody syndrome – a possible thrombogenic mechanism. N Engl J Med 1997;337:154–160, copyright © 1997 Masssachusetts Medical Society. All rights reserved.)

annexin A5 on cultured syncytialized BeWo trophoblasts and concurrently increased their binding of prothrombin [24].

The aPL antibody mediated reduction of annexin A5 does not require cellular membranes; displacement also occurs on artificial phospholipid bilayers. This has been demonstrated by the techniques of ellipsometry [23], measurements of protein levels [23, 25], coagulation assays [23], and, most recently, through atomic force microscopic imaging [4] [Fig. 36.1(B)]. IgG fractions of aPL displace annexin A5 in a β_2-glycoprotein I (β_2-GPI) dependent manner [23]; this displacement of annexin A5 results in acceleration of coagulation [23, 26]. Monoclonal murine [27] and human [28] aPL also displace annexin A5 and accelerate coagulation reactions. IgG fractions isolated from patients with the aPL reduce the binding of annexin A5 to phospholipid coated microtiter plates; this reduction of annexin A5 binding is dependent upon anti–β_2-GPI antibodies and correlates with clinical thrombosis [29]. One group was unable to find that aPL IgG antibodies reduce annexin A5 binding [30] or reduce annexin A5 mediated anticoagulant activity [31].

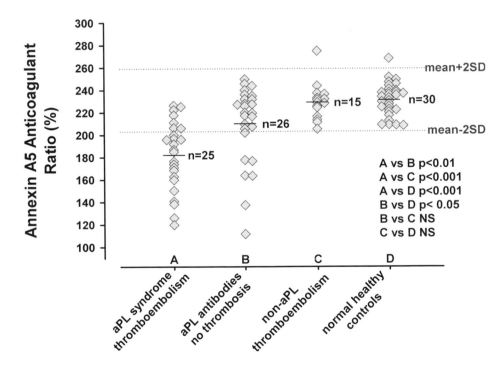

Figure 36.4. Annexin A5 resistance assays in APS, aPL without thrombosis, and in non-aPL thrombosis. The annexin A5 anticoagulant ratio for the aPL syndrome with thromboembolism group (A) was significantly decreased (mean ± SD, 182 ± 31%, n = 25) as compared to the aPL without thrombosis history group (B) (210 ± 35%, n = 26, $P < 0.01$), the non-aPL thromboembolism group (C) (229 ± 16%, n = 15, $P < 0.001$), and the normal healthy control group (D) (231 ± 14%, n = 30, $P < 0.001$). The ratio for the plasmas from the aPL without thrombosis history group (B) also significantly reduced as compared to the normal healthy control group (D) ($P < 0.05$). There were no significant differences in annexin A5 anticoagulant ratio for the non-aPL. (Reprinted from Rand JH, et al. Detection of antibody-mediated reduction of annexin A5 anticoagulant activity in plasmas of patients with the antiphospholipid syndrome. Blood 2004;104:2783–2790.)

Assays for annexin A5 binding and anticoagulant activity that could be applicable to clinical blood samples have recently been described [23, 25, 32, 33]. Plasmas of patients with thrombosis and aPL significantly reduced annexin A5 anticoagulant activity compared to plasmas of patients with genetic thrombophilias and normal healthy controls [32] (Fig. 36.4). This supports the concept that antibody mediated disruption of annexin A5 function may play a thrombogenic role in both the placental and systemic blood circulations.

A model for this mechanism for the aPL mediated acceleration of coagulation that we initially described in 1998 [23], and referred to as the lupus procoagulant

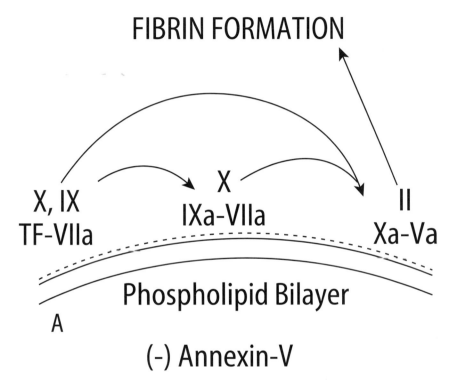

Figure 36.5. Proposed model for the "lupus anticoagulant effect" paradox and a "lupus procoagulant effect": (A) Anionic phospholipids (negative charges), when exposed on the apical surface of the cell membrane bilayer, serve as potent cofactors for the assembly of 3 different coagulation complexes: the tissue factor (TF)–VIIa complex, the IXa–VIIIa complex, and the Xa–Va complex, and thereby accelerate blood coagulation. The TF complexes yields factors IXa or factor Xa, the IXa complex yields factor Xa, and the Xa formed from both of these reactions is the active enzyme in the prothrombinase complex which yields factor IIa (thrombin), which in turn cleaves fibrinogen to form fibrin. (B) Annexin A5, in the absence of aPL, serves as a potent anticoagulant by forming a crystal lattice over the anionic phospholipid surface, shielding it from availability for assembly of the phospholipid dependent coagulation complexes. (C) In the absence of annexin A5, aPL antibody–β_2-GPI complexes can prolong the coagulation times, compared to control antibodies. This occurs via antibody recognition of domains I on the β_2-GPI, which results in dimers and pentamers of antibody–β_2-GPI complexes having high affinity for phospholipid via domain V. These high affinity complexes reduce the access of coagulation factors to anionic phospholipids. This may result in a "lupus anticoagulant" effect in conditions where there are limiting quantities of anionic phospholipids.

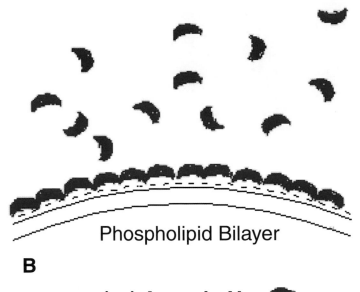

Phospholipid Bilayer

B

(+) Annexin-V

FIBRIN FORMATION

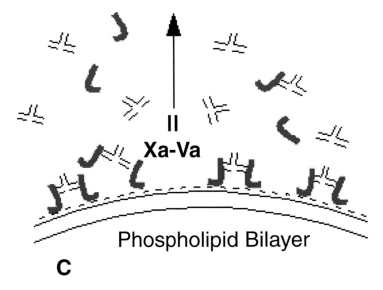

II

Xa-Va

Phospholipid Bilayer

C

(+) aPL

β2GPI

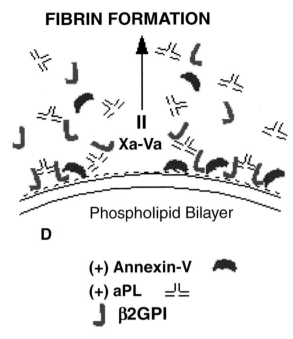

FIBRIN FORMATION

Xa-Va

Phospholipid Bilayer

D

(+) Annexin-V

(+) aPL

β2GPI

Figure 36.5. (continued) (D) In the presence of annexin A5, aPL, either directly or via interaction with protein–phospholipid cofactors, disrupt the ability of annexin A5 to form ordered crystals on the phospholipid surface. This results in a net increase of the amount of anionic phospholipid available for promoting coagulation reactions. The aPL–co-factor complexes expose significantly more phospholipids by disrupting the annexin A5 shield than they block by direct binding. This manifests in the net acceleration of coagulation in vitro, that is, a "lupus procoagulant effect" – and in thrombophilia in vivo. (Reprinted with permission from Rand JH. Molecular pathogenesis of the antiphospholipid syndrome. Circ Res 2002;90:29–37, copyright © 2002 Lippincott Williams & Wilkins.)

effect, is shown in Figure 36.5. This mechanism also offers a plausible explanation for the paradoxical association of the lupus anticoagulant effect with thrombosis rather than bleeding.

Antibodies Against Annexin A5 in Patients with APS

In addition to the effects of antibodies with aPL specificities described above, some patients with APS also have evidence for antibodies that are directed against annexin A5 itself. Antibodies against annexin A5 were reported to be increased in patients with recurrent miscarriages [34] and were reported [35] to be independent risk factors associated with pregnancy losses [36, 37]. An association with pregnancy loss was also reported in patients with systemic lupus erythematosus (SLE) [38]. In another of the studies, elevated anti-annexin A5 antibodies were associated with the presence of elevated aPL in patients with recurrent miscarriages, but were not an independent risk factor [34]. In one of the studies cited above [35], elevated anti-annexin A5 antibody levels were also associated with recurrent in vitro fertilization – embryo transfer (IVF-ET) failure. Another group, however, reported a low prevalence of anti-annexin A5 antibodies in patients with the aPL and recurrent spontaneous pregnancy losses [39]. No association was found between IgA anti-annexin A5 antibodies and pregnancy complications such as early recurrent spontaneous abortions and recurrent IVF–ET failures [40]; interestingly, although IgG anti-annexin A5 antibodies were associated with pregnancy complications in this study, they were found to be independent of aPL.

Antibodies against annexin A5 have also been reported to be increased in patients with thrombosis [41, 42]. However, there are conflicting data on this [38, 43, 44]. It is interesting to note that elevated antibodies against 2 other annexins – annexin A4 [42] and annexin A11 [45] – have also been reported to be associated with vascular thrombosis.

Conclusions

In conclusion, annexin A5 is a potent anticoagulant protein that forms an antithrombotic shield over anionic phospholipids containing bilayers. Autoantibodies may interfere with this shielding function via high affinity antibodies that recognize phospholipid binding proteins that are capable of interfering with the assembly of the annexin A5 shield on phospholipid surfaces or via direct recognition of annexin A5 functional epitopes by autoantibodies. Antibody mediated interference with the integrity of the two-dimensional annexin A5 crystal shield may be a mechanism for thrombosis and for pregnancy complications, including recurrent spontaneous pregnancy losses, in APS.

Acknowledgements

This work was supported in part by the National Institutes of Health/National Heart Lung and Blood Institute grant no. HL-61331.

References

1. Crumpton MJ, Dedman JR. Protein terminology tangle. Nature 1990;345:212.
2. Moss SE, Morgan RO. The annexins. Genome Biol 2004;5:219.
3. Mosser G, Ravanat C, Freyssinet JM, Brisson A. Sub-domain structure of lipid-bound annexin-V resolved by electron image analysis. J Mol Biol 1991;217:241–245.
4. Rand JH, Wu XX, Quinn AS, et al. Human monoclonal antiphospholipid antibodies disrupt the annexin a5 anticoagulant crystal shield on phospholipid bilayers: evidence from atomic force microscopy and functional assay. Am J Pathol 2003;163:1193–1200.
5. Voges D, Berendes R, Burger A, Demange P, Baumeister W, Huber R. Three-dimensional structure of membrane-bound annexin V. A correlative electron microscopy-X-ray crystallography study. J Mol Biol 1994;238:199–213.
6. Andree HAM, Stuart MC, Hermens WT, et al. Clustering of lipid-bound annexin V may explain its anticoagulant effect. J Biol Chem 1992;267:17907–17912.
7. van Heerde WL, Lap P, Schoormans S, de Groot PG, Reutelingsperger CPM, Vroom TM. Localization of annexin A5 in human tissues. Annexins 2004;1:56–62.
8. Lentz BR. Exposure of platelet membrane phosphatidylserine regulates blood coagulation. Prog Lipid Res 2003;42:423–438.

9. van Eerden P, Wu XX, Chazotte C, Rand JH. The role of annexins in pregnancy. Annexins 2004;1:90–98.
10. Krikun G, Lockwood CJ, Wu XX, et al. The expression of the placental anticoagulant protein, annexin V, by villous trophoblasts: immunolocalization and in vitro regulation. Placenta 1994;15:601–612.
11. Lyden TW, Vogt E, Ng AK, Johnson PM, Rote NS. Monoclonal antiphospholipid antibody reactivity against human placental trophoblast. J Reprod Immunol 1992;22:1–14.
12. Wang X, Campos B, Kaetzel MA, Dedman JR. Annexin V is critical in the maintenance of murine placental integrity. Am J Obstet Gynecol 1999;180:1008–1016.
13. Rand JH, Wu XX, Andree HA, et al. Pregnancy loss in the antiphospholipid-antibody syndrome – a possible thrombogenic mechanism. N Engl J Med 1997;337:154–160.
14. Shu F, Sugimura M, Kanayama N, Kobayashi H, Kobayashi T, Terao T. Immunohistochemical study of annexin V expression in placentae of preeclampsia. Gynecol Obstet Invest 2000;49:17–23.
15. Di Simone N, Castellani R, Caliandro D, Caruso A. Monoclonal anti-annexin V antibody inhibits trophoblast gonadotropin secretion and induces syncytiotrophoblast apoptosis. Biol Reprod 2001;65:1766–1770.
16. Reutelingsperger CP, Kop JM, Hornstra G, Hemker HC. Purification and characterization of a novel protein from bovine aorta that inhibits coagulation. Inhibition of the phospholipid- dependent factor-Xa-catalyzed prothrombin activation, through a high-affinity binding of the anticoagulant to the phospholipids. Eur J Biochem 1988;173:171–178.
17. Flaherty MJ, West S, Heimark RL, Fujikawa K, Tait JF. Placental anticoagulant protein-I: measurement in extracellular fluids and cells of the hemostatic system. J Lab Clin Med 1990;115:174–181.
18. Rand JH, Wu XX, Guller S, et al. Reduction of annexin-V (placental anticoagulant protein-I) on placental villi of women with antiphospholipid antibodies and recurrent spontaneous abortion. Am J Obstet Gynecol 1994;171:1566–1572.
19. Donohoe S, Kingdom JC, Mackie IJ, et al. Ontogeny of beta 2 glycoprotein I and annexin V in villous placenta of normal and antiphospholipid syndrome pregnancies. Thromb Haemost 2000;84:32–38.
20. La Rosa L, Meroni PL, Tincani A, et al. Beta 2 glycoprotein I and placental anticoagulant protein I in placentae from patients with antiphospholipid syndrome. J Rheumatol 1994;21:1684–1693.
21. Lakasing L, Campa JS, Poston R, Khamashta MA, Poston L. Normal expression of tissue factor, thrombomodulin, and annexin V in placentas from women with antiphospholipid syndrome. Am J Obstet Gynecol 1999;181:180–189.
22. Rand JH, Wu XX, Guller S, et al. Antiphospholipid immunoglobulin G antibodies reduce annexin-V levels on syncytiotrophoblast apical membranes and in culture media of placental villi. Am J Obstet Gynecol 1997;177:918–923.
23. Rand JH, Wu XX, Andree HAM, et al. Antiphospholipid antibodies accelerate plasma coagulation by inhibiting annexin-V binding to phospholipids: a "lupus procoagulant" phenomenon. Blood 1998;92:1652–1660.
24. Vogt E, Ng AK, Rote NS. Antiphosphatidylserine antibody removes annexin-V and facilitates the binding of prothrombin at the surface of a choriocarcinoma model of trophoblast differentiation. Am J Obstet Gynecol 1997;177:964–972.
25. Hanly JG, Smith SA. Anti-beta2-glycoprotein I autoantibodies, in vitro thrombin generation, and the antiphospholipid syndrome. J Rheumatol 2000;27:2152–2159.
26. Rand JH, Wu XX, Giesen P. A possible solution to the paradox of the "lupus anticoagulant": antiphospholipid antibodies accelerate thrombin generation by inhibiting annexin-V. Thromb Haemost 1999;82:1376–1377.
27. Rand JH, Wu XX, Giesen P, et al. Antiphospholipid antibodies reduce annexin-V and accelerate coagulation on cell membranes: mechanistic studies with a monoclonal antiphospholipid antibody. Thromb Haemost 1999;82(suppl):1531a.
28. Rand JH, Wu XX, Chen PP. Human monoclonal antiphospholipid antibodies displace annexin-V from phospholipid bilayers and accelerate thrombin generation. Blood 1999;94(suppl 1):623a.
29. Hanly JG, Smith SA. Anti-beta2-glycoprotein I (GPI) autoantibodies, annexin V binding and the anti-phospholipid syndrome. Clin Exp Immunol 2000;120:537–543.
30. Willems GM, Janssen MP, Comfurius P, Galli M, Zwaal RF, Bevers EM. Competition of annexin V and anticardiolipin antibodies for binding to phosphatidylserine containing membranes. Biochemistry 2000;39:1982–1989.
31. Bevers EM, Janssen MP, Willems GM, Zwaal FA. No evidence for enhanced thrombin formation through displacement of annexin V by antiphospholipid antibodies. Thromb Haemost 2000; 83:792–794.

32. Rand JH, Wu XX, Lapinski R, et al. Detection of antibody-mediated reduction of annexin A5 antico-agulant activity in plasmas of patients with the antiphospholipid syndrome. Blood 2004. Epub ahead of print.

33. Tomer A. Antiphospholipid antibody syndrome: rapid, sensitive, and specific flow cytometric assay for determination of anti-platelet phospholipid autoantibodies. J Lab Clin Med 2002;139:147–154.

34. Arnold J, Holmes Z, Pickering W, Farmer C, Regan L, Cohen H. Anti-beta 2 glycoprotein 1 and anti-annexin V antibodies in women with recurrent miscarriage. Br J Haematol 2001;113:911–914.

35. Matsubayashi H, Arai T, Izumi S, Sugi T, McIntyre JA, Makino T. Anti-annexin V antibodies in patients with early pregnancy loss or implantation failures. Fertil Steril 2001;76:694–699.

36. Gris JC, Perneger TV, Quere I, et al. . Antiphospholipid/antiprotein antibodies, hemostasis-related autoantibodies, and plasma homocysteine as risk factors for a first early pregnancy loss: a matched case-control study. Blood 2003;102:3504–3513.

37. Kristoffersen EK, Ulvestad E, Bjorge L, Aarli A, Matre R. Fc gamma-receptor activity of placental annexin II. Scand J Immunol 1994;40:237–242.

38. Nojima J, Kuratsune H, Suehisa E, et al. Association between the prevalence of antibodies to beta(2)-glycoprotein I, prothrombin, protein C, protein S, and annexin V in patients with systemic lupus erythematosus and thrombotic and thrombocytopenic complications. Clin Chem 2001;47:1008–1015.

39. Siaka C, Lambert M, Caron C, et al. Low prevalence of anti-annexin V antibodies in antiphospholipid syndrome with fetal loss. Rev Med Interne 1999;20:762–765.

40. Arai T, Matsubayashi H, Sugi T, et al. Anti-annexin A5 antibodies in reproductive failures in relation to antiphospholipid antibodies and phosphatidylserine. Am J Reprod Immunol 2003;50:202–208.

41. Lakos G, Kiss E, Regeczy N, et al. Antiprothrombin and antiannexin V antibodies imply risk of thrombosis in patients with systemic autoimmune diseases. J Rheumatol 2000;27:924–929.

42. Satoh A, Suzuki K, Takayama E, et al. Detection of anti-annexin IV and V antibodies in patients with antiphospholipid syndrome and systemic lupus erythematosus. J Rheumatol 1999;26:1715–1720.

43. Pasquier E, Amiral J, de Saint ML, Mottier D. A cross sectional study of antiphospholipid-protein antibodies in patients with venous thromboembolism. Thromb Haemost 2001;86:538–542.

44. Romisch J, Schuler E, Bastian B, et al. Annexins I to VI: quantitative determination in different human cell types and in plasma after myocardial infarction. Blood Coagul Fibrinolysis 1992;3:11–17.

45. Horlick KR, Ganjianpour M, Frost SC, Nick HS. Annexin-I regulation in response to suckling and rat mammary cell differentiation. Endocrinology 1991;128:1574–1579.

37 Plasminogen Activation, Fibrinolysis, and Cell Proteolytic Activity in Antiphospholipid Syndrome

Eduardo Anglés-Cano

Fibrinolysis and Extracellular Proteolysis in the Vascular Wall

The basic mechanism underlying fibrinolysis and pericellular proteolysis is the transformation of plasminogen into plasmin by tissue type or urokinase type plasminogen activators (u-PA, t-PA) on, respectively, fibrin or cell surfaces (Fig. 37.1). These plasminogen activators and a specific inhibitor (PAI-1) are synthesized and released by endothelial and smooth muscle cells, and by leukocytes infiltrating the vascular wall [1]. These cells also express receptors for plasminogen and u-PA (u-PAR/CD87) that allow their molecular assembly and efficient plasmin formation for pericellular proteolysis [2–4]. The latter includes extracellular matrix remodelling, cell migration, and proteolytic activation of metalloproteinases (collagenases) and growth factors. It has been well demonstrated that single chain u-PA (pro-urokinase) is the most important activator for pericellular proteolysis in the extravascular space. In contrast, fibrinolysis, the basic mechanism for clot dissolution in the intravascular space, is triggered by the assembly of circulating plasminogen and t-PA released from endothelial cells [5] (Fig. 37.1). However, recent studies suggest that pro-urokinase, which has no affinity for fibrin, may induce fibrin specific lysis by activating plasminogen bound to new binding sites unveiled by plasmin on degrading fibrin [6]. Furthermore, although endothelial t-PA is the main plasminogen activator in the intravascular space, it can also be synthesized by vascular smooth muscle cells and by neurons [7] and can locally favor the development of cell proteolytic activity that may participate in cell migration or in cell detachment induced apoptosis [8].

These mechanisms are regulated at the plasminogen activator level by PAI–1 present in plasma or released from cells in the vascular wall (Fig. 37.2). PAI–1 reacts with single chain and two chain t-PA and with two chain u-PA, but not with single chain u-PA. The second order rate constant for inhibition of these enzymes is in the order of 10^7 M^{-1} s^{-1}. A second type of inhibitor of plasminogen activators and plasmin, protease nexin-1, which also inhibits thrombin, has been identified in the

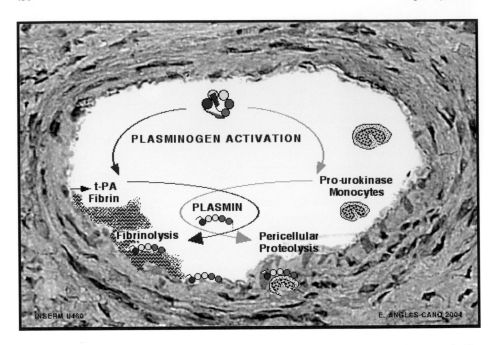

Figure 37.1. Fibrinolysis and extracellular proteolysis in the vascular wall. Cross-section of an arteriole. The endothelial cell lining is marked with a peroxidase labeled antibody directed against the tissue-type plasminogen activator (t-PA) [78]. Circulating plasminogen bound to fibrin and membrane proteins is transformed into plasmin either at the surface of fibrin by fibrin bound t-PA released from endothelial cells or by pro-urokinase bound to its cellular receptor. Plasmin formed in situ specifically degrades fibrin or participate in pericellular proteolytic activities. 📖

central nervous system and in the vascular wall, where it may play a role in the regulation of pericellular proteolysis [9–11].

Plasmin, once formed, remains bound to the cell membrane or to the surface of fibrin, a condition that prevents inhibition by α_2-antiplasmin. However, plasmin released into the circulation during fibrinolysis is rapidly inhibited by α_2-antiplasmin with a second order rate constant of 2 to 4×10^7 M^{-1}s^{-1}.

In conclusion, surface activation on fibrin and cells, and fluid phase inhibition in plasma and extracellular fluids, ensure the specificity of fibrinolysis, control the extent of fibrin degradation, and regulate important cellular proteolytic functions.

The activation of plasminogen may be abnormally inhibited, however. For instance, the atherogenic lipoprotein Lp(a) may interfere with fibrinolysis and pericellular proteolysis by its ability to compete with plasminogen for binding to fibrin and cell membranes [12]. The different population of autoantibodies observed in APS may disturb fibrinolysis and contribute thereby to vascular complications [13]. Thrombosis may therefore result from an impaired or insufficient fibrinolytic cellular response to vascular injury provoked by factors such as Lp(a) and autoantibodies. The relationship between auto-antibodies and the plasminogen activation system in APS is analyzed in this chapter.

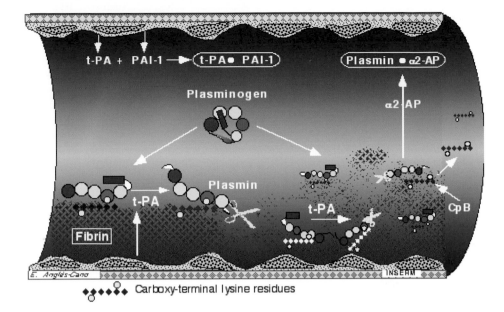

Figure 37.2. Acceleration of fibrinolysis by carboxy terminal lysine residues, and regulation by PAI-1 and α2-antiplasmin. Plasmin unveils new carboxy terminal lysine residues to which plasminogen bind [17]. Plasma carboxypeptidase B (CpB) may regulate fibrinolysis by cleaving these residues. 📖

Protein Interactions with Biological Surfaces: Beyond Fibrinolysis and Autoimmunity

Plasmin is a large spectrum proteolytic enzyme that cleaves lysyl and arginyl peptide bonds in a number of proteins. However, under physiological conditions its activity is specifically restricted to the lysis of fibrin, to extracellular matrix remodelling, and to the activation of growth factors and metalloproteinases. To develop these specialized and specific functions, plasmin must be generated at the surface of fibrin or cell membranes (Fig. 37.1). The surface dependence of this reaction is closely related to:

- The structural organization of proteins in functional domains.
- The structure of fibrin as an anchoring surface.
- The molecular assembly of proteins on cell membranes.

Functional Domains of Proteins

The glycoproteins of the plasminogen activation system are organized as an array of structural domains with functional autonomy [14]: the epidermal growth factor-like domain (EGF), the "finger" domain, the triple loop structures or "kringle" domains, and the serine proteinase region (Fig. 37.2). These domains govern the molecular assembly of proteins on fibrin and cell membranes. The EGF domain of pro-urokinase contains a sequence that is recognized by the u-PA receptor. The finger domain of t-PA allows its binding to fibrin. Plasminogen consists of 5 kringle domains; kringle 1 and 4 contain a substructure, the lysine-binding site, that binds to cells and fibrin. The plasminogen-like apolipoprotein apo(a) consists of a variable number of copies (10 to 40) of kringle 4, and single copies of kringle 5 and the serine–proteinase domain of plasminogen. Apo(a) is disulphide linked to the apo B100 of a low-density lipoprotein (LDL) to form Lp(a), a recognized cardiovascular risk factor lipoprotein [15]. Kringle 4 in plasminogen and the corresponding kringle 4 copies in apo(a) share binding properties to fibrin and cell surfaces. In contrast, the serine–proteinase domain of apo(a) cannot be cleaved by activators and remains in an inactive state. Apo(a) may therefore replace plasminogen on fibrin and cells and inhibit thereby fibrinolysis and extracellular proteolysis [12].

Fibrin as a Surface Anchoring Structure

The formation of fibrin unveils binding sites for t-PA and plasminogen that are buried in fibrinogen. Fibrinogen is a complex molecule composed of 3 pairs of polypeptide chains (Aα, Bβ, and γ), linked by disulphide bonds and organized in a trinodular structure [16]. The amino terminal regions form the central domain E that is linked to two globular D domains by a coiled coil connector region. The binding site for t-PA is most probably located in region D or in D dimers in a sequence that interacts with the finger domain of t-PA. Binding of plasminogen to fibrin is mediated by interactions between the lysine-binding sites of kringles 1 and 4 and lysine residues of fibrin. Binding of t-PA and plasminogen to fibrin results in a trimolecular complex with catalytic advantages. Plasmin thus formed cleaves lysyl bonds in fibrin and unveils new carboxy terminal lysine residues to which plasminogen may bind [17] (Fig. 37.2). Because plasminogen bound to carboxy terminal lysines of progressively degraded fibrin is readily transformed into plasmin by fibrin bound t-PA, this mechanism represents the most important pathway for the acceleration and amplification of fibrinolysis [18] (Fig. 37.2).

Protein Assembly on Receptors and in the Phospholipid Membrane

The phospholipid bilayer provides both a hydrophobic milieu and anionic charges for proteins engaged in interactions at the cell surface such as coagulation factors and β_2-glycoprotein I (β_2-GPI) [19]. The receptor for u-PA (uPAR) is attached to the phospholipid bilayer through a glycosyl–phosphatidyl–inositol anchor. Plasminogen and t-PA binds to "integral" membrane proteins: a receptor for t-PA (annexin II) [20] and a number of membrane proteins with exposed carboxy terminal lysine residues to which plasminogen binds [4]. As for the fibrin surface, degradation of membrane proteins by plasmin unveils new carboxy terminal lysine residues for plasminogen binding [4].

Protein Assembly and Neo-antigen Formation

The assembly of activators and plasminogen onto distinct binding sites of fibrin and cell surfaces results in conformational changes that are of physiological significance but also lead to exposure of domains or active sites (not constituted in the enzyme precursor) with unique antigenic properties. It has been proposed that these neo-epitopes may evoke an autoimmune response in patients with immuno-logical disorders [21]. Autoantibodies directed against an epitope exposed on fibrin bound t-PA in the sera of patients with scleroderma [22], systemic lupus erythe-matosis (SLE) [23], and primary pulmonary hypertension [24] have been described. Recently, antibodies directed against the active site of t-PA or plasmin that may inhibit fibrinolysis have also been described in patients with APS [25, 26]. These observations suggest that conformational changes of molecules upon binding to their ligands results in the expression of conformation induced neo-epitopes. This phenomenon is probably similar to the reactivity of antiphospholipid antibodies against β_2-GPI (or other proteins) bound to anionic phospholipid surfaces.

Endothelial Cell Dysfunction and Fibrinolysis in APS

Following the original description, 25 years ago, of impaired fibrinolysis associated with thrombosis and antiphospholipid antibodies in SLE [27], a number of reports confirmed these findings [28, 29]. Although these abnormalities were not found in one study [30], in several other studies it was further shown that the hypofibrinoly-sis detected in these patients is most probably a manifestation of endothelial cell dysfunction, as indicated by increased plasma levels of PAI-1 and t-PA antigens [31–34]. The t–PA thus detected circulates complexed to PAI-1 and is therefore inactive, a condition which explains why hypofibrinolysis is observed in the pres-ence of high t-PA antigenic levels. High levels of PAI-1 have been associated with an increased risk of thromboembolic disease and myocardial infarction [35]. These manifestations of endothelial cell dysfunction have been found in association with antibodies directed against endothelial cells, or with the presence of immune com-plexes, thus suggesting that endothelial cells are important sites of action for anti-bodies that have a role in the pathogenesis of thrombosis [36]. Of note, patients with primary pulmonary hypertension present signs of endothelial cell dysfunction (elevated PAI-1 and t-PA plasma antigens) [37] and may have antiphospholipid antibodies [38].

Similar manifestations of endothelial dysfunction have also been found in primary APS [39, 40], though at present there are no solid arguments to propose a direct association between aPL and impaired fibrinolysis in the thrombotic manifes-tation of APS [41–43]. It has been shown, however, that anti-endothelial cell anti-bodies in sera of patients with SLE and in patients with primary and secondary APS may alter the fibrinolytic activity of endothelial cells [44]. Antiphospholipid and anti-endothelial cell antibodies may co-exist in both primary and secondary APS [45]. Furthermore, cross-reaction between these antibodies has been demonstrated [46]. Antiphospholipid antibodies activate vascular endothelial cells and induce a procoagulant and pro-inflammatory phenotype both in vitro and in vivo as docu-mented by an increased expression of tissue factor, leukocyte adhesion molecules such as intercellular adhesion molecule-1, vascular cell adhesion molecule (VCAM)-1, and E-selectin [47–49], and the production of microparticles [50]. It is possible that such antibodies may induce the secretion of others markers of endothelial cell injury/activation such as t-PA and PAI-1. The increase levels of PAI–1 and t-PA·PAI-1 complexes may explain the low fibrinolytic activity in a similar fashion as in patients with SLE [27].

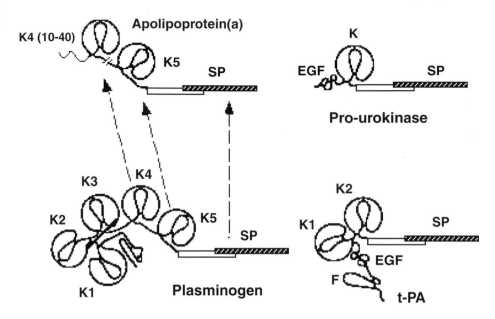

Figure 37.3. Domain structure of apo(a), plasminogen and its activators. Serine–proteinase (SP) region. Kringle (K), finger (F), and epidermal growth factor-like (EGF) domains. Apo(a) contains a variable number of a domain homologous to plasminogen kringle 4, and single copies of kringle 5 and the serine–proteinase region. 📖

β_2-GPI and Plasminogen Activation: New Insights

β_2-GPI, the major antigenic target for antiphospholipid antibodies, consist of a single polypeptide chain of 326 amino acids arranged in 5 contiguous domains (short consensus repeats or "Sushi domains"). Domain V differs from the first 4 domains in that it contains an aberrant carboxy terminal loop of 20 amino acids where the terminating Cys326 forms an extra disulfide bond with Cys288 (see Fig. 24.1). Although binding substructures for membrane phospholipids and heparin glycosaminoglycans are located in domain V [51–53], β_2-GPI may also interact with unique cell surface proteins, for example, high affinity binding to annexin II on endothelial cells [54]. This finding may be of biological relevance as annexin II also mediates the binding of t-PA and plasminogen to endothelial cells [20]. Finally, it has been recently shown that binding of β_2-GPI to coagulation factor XI inhibits its activation by thrombin [55].

In 1993, Hunt et al [56] reported the existence of a modified form of β_2-GPI cleaved between Lys317–Thr318 in the carboxy terminal tail of domain V. After cleavage, the 9 residues Thr318–Cys326 remains linked to domain V by disulfide bonding (Cys326–Cys288). Reduction of this disulfide bond liberates this peptide resulting in a slight decrease (approximately 1 kDa) of the molecular mass as compared to native β_2-GPI. This "clipped" form has lost its ability to bind negatively charged phospholipids and heparin, and to act as anticardiolipin co-factor [53, 57] (Table 37.1). Novel hydrophobic and electrostatic interactions appeared in domain V after cleavage, thus indicating that the integrity of the Lys317-Thr318 bond is nec-

Table 37.1. Proteolytic cleavage of β_2-glycoprotein I at Lys317–Thr318 by plasmin: consequences on its biological properties.

- No binding to negatively charged phospholipids [56]
- No binding to heparin [53]
- Inability to act as cardiolipin co-factor [57]
- Inability to bind LDLox [57]
- Specific binding to plasminogen [61]

essary to preserve the spatial array cluster of positively charged residues (mainly in the loop Cys281–Cys288) and the membrane insertion loop Ser311–Lys317 that are critical for phospholipid binding and anticardiolipin antibody activity [51, 52]. Finally, clipped β_2-GPI is also unable to inhibit the activation of coagulation factor XI by thrombin [55].

Using recombinant domain V and purified β_2-GPI it was shown that the Lys317–Thr318 proteolytic cleavage is produced by plasmin; in human plasma, cleavage of β_2-GPI occurs when α_2-plasmin inhibitor levels are decreased[58]. This proteolytic processing has also been demonstrated in vivo, as patients with an activated fibrinolytic system, that is, disseminated intravascular coagulation, thrombolytic therapy [59], leukaemia [60], ischemic stroke [61], have increased plasma levels of clipped β_2-GPI (Table 37.2). A correlation exist with the levels of plasmin-a_2–antiplasmin complexes, an in vitro marker of fibrinolytic activity. It is not clear if phospholipid bound β_2-GPI can still be cleaved by plasmin. However, because heparin greatly enhances the plasmin mediated cleavage of β_2-GPI and the heparin and phospholipid recognition sites in domain V are the same, it is possible that β_2-GPI bound to heparin-like glycosaminoglycans, to phospholipids, or to annexin II may be cleaved by plasmin formed on the cell membrane or on the extracellular matrix [53]. Taken altogether these data suggest that plasminogen activation may function as a mechanism of defence against antibody mediated thrombosis via plasmin mediated proteolytic cleavage of β_2-GPI.

Domain Interactions Between β_2-GPI and Kringle Domains in Plasminogen and apo(a)

Although most of the binding properties of β_2-GPI are lost after the plasmin mediated cleavage (Table 37.1), it has recently been described that clipped β_2-GPI specifically binds to plasminogen (Kd = 0.37 μM) and that this binding may inhibit plasmin formation [61]. However, the biological relevance of these findings remains to be demonstrated.

Recent clinical and experimental evidence suggest that Lp(a), the atherothrombogenic particle, may be implicated in the thrombotic complications of APS

Table 37.2. Proteolytic cleavage of β_2-glycoprotein I in vivo.

- Disseminated intravascular coagulation [59]
- Thrombolytic treatment [59]
- Leukemia [60]
- Lupus anticoagulant [60]

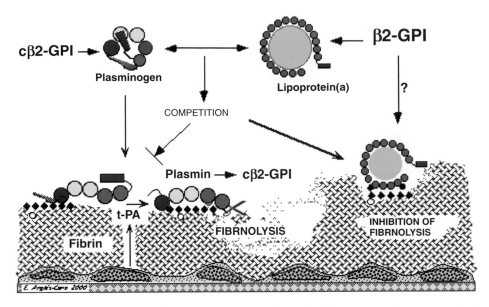

Figure 37.4. Lp(a) effects on fibrinolysis and interactions with β_2-GPI. Apo(a) the characteristic glycoprotein of Lp(a) shares structural homology with plasminogen and impairs its binding to cells and fibrin, thus inhibiting fibrinolysis and pericellular proteolysis [12]. β_2-GPI may be localized on these surfaces through interactions with apo(a) [73] and may be proteolyzed by plasmin [58, 59]. Plasmin cleaves β_2-GPI at Lys317–Thr318. Clipped β_2-GPI (cβ_2-GPI) binds specifically to plasminogen and may interfere with fibrinolysis [61]. 📖

(Fig. 37.4). The mechanism by which high Lp(a) levels may favor atherothrombosis is still a matter of debate but the fact that Lp(a) has both LDL- and plasminogen-like moieties suggest that Lp(a) may constitute a link between the processes of atherosclerosis and thrombosis. A number of experimental in vitro studies resulted in convincing evidence that Lp(a) binds to the fibrin surface and cell membranes and thereby competes with plasminogen so as to inhibit its activation [12]. Such unique behavior was attributed to the fibrin binding properties conferred by the kringle 4 repeats of apo(a) [62]. The levels of Lp(a) are under genetic control by the apo(a) gene and are not modified by current pharmacological means employed to decrease LDL. A few pathological conditions (acute phase reactions, nephrotic syndrome) may produce a transitory increase in Lp(a) levels. Increased levels of Lp(a) has also been reported in autoimmune diseases [63–65], including primary and secondary APS [66–72]. Because Lp(a) levels are genetically determined and no correlation between Lp(a) levels and aPL was found, the question remains as whether these patients had already a high Lp(a) before developing the autoimmune disease. The high Lp(a) levels observed in these patients may impair plasminogen binding and/or induce the secretion of PAI-1 by endothelial cells, two mechanism that may contribute to the thrombotic complications in APS as suggested by Atsumi et al [71]. However, the effect of high Lp(a) levels on plasminogen binding to fibrin or cells in these patients remains to be determined.

Besides being an additional factor for thrombosis, high Lp(a) levels in APS may be of importance within the context of recent data indicating that β_2-GPI may interact with distinct kringle 4 domains of apo(a) in a specific manner [73]. The interaction of apo(a) with β_2-GPI requires a sequence (181 amino acids) contained in domain II to IV. The interaction was demonstrated with apo(a) in both its free form and as a part of the Lp(a) particle. The role of this interaction remains unknown. However, it may be of pathophysiological relevance if in the presence of high Lp(a) levels, the β_2-GPI–Lp(a) complex could be the trigger of decreased fibrinolytic activity. Binding of the β_2-GPI–Lp(a) complex to fibrin and cells may also favor localization of β_2-GPI to these surfaces where it may be cleaved and inactivated by plasmin. The consequences of the proteolytic processing of β_2-GPI by plasmin are indicated in Table 37.1.

New Directions and Perspectives in Plasminogen Activation and APS

As new development arises in the field of plasminogen activation, new directions of research in the pathophysiology of the plasminogen activation system and antibody induced thrombosis deserve investigation. For instance, the concept that cells focus proteolytic activity at their surface is emphasized by recent data emerging in this

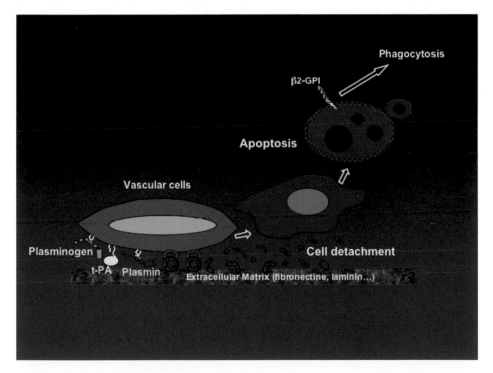

Figure 37.5. Plasminogen activation dependent cell detachment and apoptosis of vascular cells; β_2-GPI as cofactor for the clearance of apoptotic bodies. In this sequence of proteolytic reactions, plasminogen is activated by t-PA expressed by vascular smooth muscle cells; the plasmin formed in situ degrades extracellular matrix proteins (e.g., fibronectin, laminin) and promotes cell detachment and apoptosis. β_2-GPI bridges apoptotic bodies and phagocytic cells. Plasmin dependent cleavage of β_2-GPI could interfere with this process.

area. It has been recently shown that uncontrolled plasminogen activation on cells may result in unwanted cell death [8, 11] (Fig. 37.5). In these studies it was demonstrated that t-PA constitutively expressed by vascular smooth muscle cells and other adherent cells can generate plasmin on the cell surface and induce thereby the proteolysis of extracellular matrix proteins, for example, fibronectin and laminin, cell retraction, and, finally, cell detachment and apoptosis (Fig. 37.5). Apoptotic bodies are produced during this process, their uptake by phagocytes prevents, among other complications, the eventual role of exposed phosphatidyl serine in triggering thrombosis. A number of soluble molecules including β_2-GPI bridge the apoptotic target and phagocytes [74] (Fig. 37.5). Because plasmin produced on the cell surface may also be found on apoptotic bodies [75], the question arises as whether the proteolytic processing of β_2-GPI by plasmin may interfere with the clearance of apoptotic bodies.

The reported cross-reaction of aPL with oxidized LDL [76], a major atherosclerotic component, needs to be studied on Lp(a) in patients with primary and secondary APS. The fact that Lp(a) interferes with fibrinolysis, and decreases the fibrinolytic potential of endothelial cells, underscores the relevance of these studies.

It has recently been suggested that activated carboxipeptidase B, an exopeptidase present in plasma in a pro-enzyme form, may play a role in the downregulation of fibrinolysis by cleaving carboxy terminal lysine residues, the plasminogen binding sites unveiled by plasmin on fibrin [77] (Fig. 37.2). The study of downregulated fibrinolysis by the carboxypeptidase B pathway in patients with APS has not as yet been investigated.

References

1. Ellis V. Plasminogen activation at the cell surface. Curr Top Dev Biol 2003;54:263–312.
2. Kim J, Hajjar KA. Annexin II: a plasminogen-plasminogen activator co-receptor. Front Biosci 2002;7:d341-348.
3. Blasi F, Carmeliet P. uPAR: a versatile signalling orchestrator. Nat Rev Mol Cell Biol 2002;3:932–943.
4. Herren T, Swaisgood C, Plow EF. Regulation of plasminogen receptors. Front Biosci 2003;8:1–8.
5. Lijnen HR. Elements of the fibrinolytic system. Ann N Y Acad Sci 2001;936:226–236.
6. Fleury V, Lijnen HR, Angles-Cano E. Mechanism of the enhanced intrinsic activity of single-chain urokinase-type plasminogen activator during ongoing fibrinolysis. J Biol Chem 1993;268:18554–18559.
7. Tsirka SE. Tissue plasminogen activator as a modulator of neuronal survival and function. Biochem Soc Trans 2002;30:222–225.
8. Meilhac O, Ho-Tin-Noe B, Houard X, Philippe M, Michel JB, Angles-Cano E. Pericellular plasmin induces smooth muscle cell anoikis. FASEB J 2003;17:1301–1303.
9. Monard D. Cell-derived proteases and protease inhibitors as regulators of neurite outgrowth. Trends Neurosci 1988;11:541–544.
10. Choi BH, Suzuki M, Kim T, Wagner SL, Cunningham DD. Protease nexin-1. Localization in the human brain suggests a protective role against extravasated serine proteases. Am J Pathol 1990;137:741–747.
11. Rossignol P, Ho-Tin-Noe B, Vranckx R, et al. Protease nexin-1 inhibits plasminogen activation-induced apoptosis of adherent cells. J Biol Chem 2004;279:10346–10356.
12. de la Pena-Diaz A, Izaguirre-Avila R, Angles-Cano E. Lipoprotein Lp(a) and atherothrombotic disease. Arch Med Res 2000;31:353–359.
13. Kolev K, Gombas J, Varadi B, et al. Immunoglobulin G from patients with antiphospholipid syndrome impairs the fibrin dissolution with plasmin. Thromb Haemost 2002;87:502–508.
14. Tulinsky A. The structures of domains of blood proteins. Thromb Haemost 1991;66:16–31.

15. McLean JW, Tomlinson JE, Kuang WJ, et al. cDNA sequence of human apolipoprotein(a) is homologous to plasminogen. Nature 1987;330:132–137.
16. Mosesson MW, Siebenlist KR, Meh DA. The structure and biological features of fibrinogen and fibrin. Ann N Y Acad Sci 2001;936:11–30.
17. Fleury V, Angles-Cano E. Characterization of the binding of plasminogen to fibrin surfaces: the role of carboxy-terminal lysines. Biochemistry 1991;30:7630–7638.
18. Suenson E, Lutzen O, Thorsen S. Initial plasmin-degradation of fibrin as the basis of a positive feedback mechanism in fibrinolysis. Eur J Biochem 1984;140:513–522.
19. Zwaal RF, Schroit AJ. Pathophysiologic implications of membrane phospholipid asymmetry in blood cells. Blood. 1997;89:1121–1132.
20. Cesarman GM, Guevara CA, Hajjar KA. An endothelial cell receptor for plasminogen/tissue plasminogen activator (t-PA). II. Annexin II-mediated enhancement of t-PA-dependent plasminogen activation. J Biol Chem 1994;269:21198–21203.
21. von Muhlen CA, Chan EK, Angles-Cano E, Mamula MJ, Garcia-De La Torre I, Fritzler MJ. Advances in autoantibodies in SLE. Lupus 1998;7:507–514.
22. Fritzler MJ, Hart DA, Wilson D, et al. Antibodies to fibrin bound tissue type plasminogen activator in systemic sclerosis. J Rheumatol 1995;22:1688–1693.
23. Salazar-Paramo M, Garcia de la Torre I, Fritzler MJ, Loyau S, Angles-Cano E. Antibodies to fibrin-bound tissue-type plasminogen activator in systemic lupus erythematosus are associated with Raynaud's phenomenon and thrombosis. Lupus 1996;5:275–278.
24. Morse JH, Barst RJ, Fotino M, et al. Primary pulmonary hypertension, tissue plasminogen activator antibodies, and HLA-DQ7. Am J Respir Crit Care Med 1997;155:274–278.
25. Cugno M, Cabibbe M, Galli M, et al. Antibodies to tissue-type plasminogen activator (tPA) in patients with antiphospholipid syndrome: evidence of interaction between the antibodies and the catalytic domain of tPA in 2 patients. Blood 2004;103:2121–2126.
26. Yang CD, Hwang KK, Yan, et al. Identification of anti-plasmin antibodies in the antiphospholipid syndrome that inhibit degradation of fibrin. J Immunol 2004;172:5765–5773.
27. Angles-Cano E, Sultan Y, Clauvel JP. Predisposing factors to thrombosis in systemic lupus erythematosus: possible relation to endothelial cell damage. J Lab Clin Med 1979;94:312–323.
28. Glas-Greenwalt P, Kant KS, Allen C, Pollak VE. Fibrinolysis in health and disease: severe abnormalities in systemic lupus erythematosus. J Lab Clin Med 1984;104:962–976.
29. Awada H, Barlowatz-Meimon G, Dougados M, Maisonneuve P, Sultan Y, Amor B. Fibrinolysis abnormalities in systemic lupus erythematosus and their relation to vasculitis. J Lab Clin Med 1988;111:229–236.
30. Francis RB Jr, Neely S. Effect of the lupus anticoagulant on endothelial fibrinolytic activity in vitro. Thromb Haemost 1989;61:314–317.
31. Tsakiris DA, Marbet GA, Makris PE, Settas L, Duckert F. Impaired fibrinolysis as an essential contribution to thrombosis in patients with lupus anticoagulant. Thromb Haemost 1989;61:175–177.
32. Violi F, Ferro D, Valesini G, et al. Tissue plasminogen activator inhibitor in patients with systemic lupus erythematosus and thrombosis. BMJ 1990;300:1099–1102.
33. Jurado M, Paramo JA, Gutierrez-Pimentel M, Rocha E. Fibrinolytic potential and antiphospholipid antibodies in systemic lupus erythematosus and other connective tissue disorders. Thromb Haemost 1992;68:516–520.
34. Ferro D, Pittoni V, Quintarelli C, et al. Coexistence of anti-phospholipid antibodies and endothelial perturbation in systemic lupus erythematosus patients with ongoing prothrombotic state. Circulation 1997;95:1425–1432.
35. Kohler HP, Grant PJ. Plasminogen-activator inhibitor type 1 and coronary artery disease. N Engl J Med 2000;342:1792–1801.
36. Cockwell P, Tse WY, Savage CO. Activation of endothelial cells in thrombosis and vasculitis. Scand J Rheumatol 1997;26:145–150.
37. Boyer-Neumann C, Brenot F, Wolf M, et al. Continuous infusion of prostacyclin decreases plasma levels of t-PA and PAI-1 in primary pulmonary hypertension. Thromb Haemost 1995;73:735–736.
38. Asherson RA, Cervera R. Antiphospholipid antibodies and the lung. J Rheumatol 1995;22:62–66.
39. Ames PR, Tommasino C, Iannaccone L, Brillante M, Cimino R, Brancaccio V. Coagulation activation and fibrinolytic imbalance in subjects with idiopathic antiphospholipid antibodies – a crucial role for acquired free protein S deficiency. Thromb Haemost 1996;76:190–194.
40. Gris JC, Ripart-Neveu S, Maugard C, et al. Respective evaluation of the prevalence of haemostasis abnormalities in unexplained primary early recurrent miscarriages. The Nimes Obstetricians and Haematologists (NOHA) Study. Thromb Haemost 1997;77:1096–1103.

41. Keeling DM, Campbell SJ, Mackie IJ, Machin SJ, Isenberg DA. The fibrinolytic response to venous occlusion and the natural anticoagulants in patients with antiphospholipid antibodies both with and without systemic lupus erythematosus. Br J Haematol 1991;77:354–359.

42. Patrassi GM, Sartori MT, Ruffatti A, et al. Fibrinolytic pattern in recurrent spontaneous abortions: no relationship between hypofibrinolysis and anti-phospholipid antibodies. Am J Hematol 1994;47:266–272.

43. Mackworth-Young CG, Andreotti F, Harmer I, et al. Endothelium-derived haemostatic factors and the antiphospholipid syndrome. Br J Rheumatol 1995;34:201–206.

44. McCrae KR, DeMichele A, Samuels P, et al. Detection of endothelial cell-reactive immunoglobulin in patients with anti-phospholipid antibodies. Br J Haematol 1991;79:595–605.

45. Hill MB, Phipps JL, Malia RG, Greaves M, Hughes P. Characterization and specificity of anti-endothelial cell membrane antibodies and their relationship to thrombosis in primary antiphospholipid syndrome (APS). Clin Exp Immunol 1995;102:368–372.

46. Lanir N, Zilberman M, Yron I, Tennenbaum G, Shechter Y, Brenner B. Reactivity patterns of antiphospholipid antibodies and endothelial cells: effect of antiendothelial antibodies on cell migration. J Lab Clin Med 1998;131:548–556.

47. Simantov R, LaSala JM, Lo SK, et al. Activation of cultured vascular endothelial cells by antiphospholipid antibodies. J Clin Invest 1995;96:2211–2219.

48. Pierangeli SS, Colden-Stanfield M, Liu X, Barker JH, Anderson GL, Harris EN. Antiphospholipid antibodies from antiphospholipid syndrome patients activate endothelial cells in vitro and in vivo. Circulation 1999;99:1997–2002.

49. Meroni PL, Raschi E, Testoni C, Borghi MO. Endothelial cell activation by antiphospholipid antibodies. Clin Immunol 2004;112:169–174.

50. Dignat-George F, Camoin-Jau L, Sabatier F, et al. Endothelial microparticles: a potential contribution to the thrombotic complications of the antiphospholipid syndrome. Thromb Haemost 2004;91:667–673.

51. Sheng Y, Sali A, Herzog H, Lahnstein J, Krilis SA. Site-directed mutagenesis of recombinant human beta 2-glycoprotein I identifies a cluster of lysine residues that are critical for phospholipid binding and anti-cardiolipin antibody activity. J Immunol 1996;157:3744–3751.

52. Bouma B, de Groot PG, van den Elsen, et al. Adhesion mechanism of human beta(2)-glycoprotein I to phospholipids based on its crystal structure. EMBO J 1999;18:5166–5174.

53. Guerin J, Sheng Y, Reddel S, Iverson GM, Chapman MG, Krilis SA. Heparin inhibits the binding of beta 2-glycoprotein I to phospholipids and promotes the plasmin-mediated inactivation of this blood protein. Elucidation of the consequences of the two biological events in patients with the antiphospholipid syndrome. J Biol Chem 2002;277:2644–2649.

54. Ma K, Simantov R, Zhang JC, Silverstein R, Hajjar KA, McCrae KR. High affinity binding of beta 2-glycoprotein I to human endothelial cells is mediated by annexin II. J Biol Chem 2000;275:15541–15548.

55. Shi T, Iverson GM, Qi JC, Cockerill KA, et al. Beta 2-Glycoprotein I binds factor XI and inhibits its activation by thrombin and factor XIIa: loss of inhibition by clipped beta 2-glycoprotein I. Proc Natl Acad Sci U S A 2004;101:3939–3944.

56. Hunt JE, Simpson RJ, Krilis SA. Identification of a region of beta 2-glycoprotein I critical for lipid binding and anti-cardiolipin antibody cofactor activity. Proc Natl Acad Sci U S A 1993;90:2141–2145.

57. Matsuura E, Inagaki J, Kasahara H, et al. Proteolytic cleavage of beta(2)-glycoprotein I: reduction of antigenicity and the structural relationship. Int Immunol 2000;12:1183–1192.

58. Ohkura N, Hagihara Y, Yoshimura T, Goto Y, Kato H. Plasmin can reduce the function of human beta2 glycoprotein I by cleaving domain V into a nicked form. Blood 1998;91:4173–4179.

59. Horbach DA, van Oort E, Lisman T, Meijers JC, Derksen RH, de Groot PG. Beta2-glycoprotein I is proteolytically cleaved in vivo upon activation of fibrinolysis. Thromb Haemost 1999;81:87–95.

60. Itoh Y, Inuzuka K, Kohno I, et al. Highly increased plasma concentrations of the nicked form of beta(2) glycoprotein I in patients with leukemia and with lupus anticoagulant: measurement with a monoclonal antibody specific for a nicked form of domain V. J Biochem (Tokyo) 2000;128:1017–1024.

61. Yasuda S, Atsumi T, Ieko M, et al. Nicked beta2-glycoprotein I: a marker of cerebral infarct and a novel role in the negative feedback pathway of extrinsic fibrinolysis. Blood 2004;103:3766–3772.

62. Rouy D, Koschinsky ML, Fleury V, Chapman J, Angles-Cano E. Apolipoprotein(a) and plasminogen interactions with fibrin: a study with recombinant apolipoprotein(a) and isolated plasminogen fragments. Biochemistry 1992;31:6333–6339.

63. Rantapaa-Dahlqvist S, Wallberg-Jonsson S, Dahlen G. Lipoprotein (a), lipids, and lipoproteins in patients with rheumatoid arthritis. Ann Rheum Dis 1991;50:366–368.

64. Lotz H, Salabe GB. Lipoprotein(a) increase associated with thyroid autoimmunity. Eur J Endocrinol 1997;136:87–91.
65. Seriolo B, Accardo S, Fasciolo D, Sulli A, Bertolini S, Cutolo M. Lipoprotein (a) and anticardiolipin antibodies as risk factors for vascular disease in rheumatoid arthritis. Thromb Haemost 1995;74:799–800.
66. Matsuda J, Gotoh M, Gohchi K, Saitoh N, Tsukamoto M. Serum lipoprotein(a) level is increased in patients with systemic lupus erythematosus irrespective of positivity of antiphospholipid antibodies. Thromb Res 1994;73:83–84.
67. Kawai S, Mizushima Y, Kaburaki J. Increased serum lipoprotein(a) levels in systemic lupus erythematosus with myocardial and cerebral infarctions. J Rheumatol 1995;22:1210–1211.
68. Yamazaki M, Asakura H, Jokaji H, et al. Plasma levels of lipoprotein(a) are elevated in patients with the antiphospholipid antibody syndrome. Thromb Haemost 1994;71:424–427.
69. Borba EF, Santos RD, Bonfa E, et al. Lipoprotein(a) levels in systemic lupus erythematosus. J Rheumatol 1994;21:220–223.
70. Levy PJ, Cooper CF, Gonzalez MF. Massive lower extremity arterial thrombosis and acute hepatic insufficiency in a young adult with premature atherosclerosis associated with hyperlipoprotein(a)emia and antiphospholipid syndrome. A case report. Angiology 1995;46:853–858.
71. Atsumi T, Khamashta MA, Andujar C, et al. Elevated plasma lipoprotein(a) level and its association with impaired fibrinolysis in patients with antiphospholipid syndrome. J Rheumatol 1998;25:69–73.
72. Okawa-Takatsuji M, Aotsuka S, Sumiya M, Ohta H, Kawakami M, Sakurabayashi I. Clinical significance of the serum lipoprotein(a) level in patients with systemic lupus erythematosus: its elevation during disease flare. Clin Exp Rheumatol 1996;14:531–536.
73. Kochl S, Fresser F, Lobentanz E, Baier G, Utermann G. Novel interaction of apolipoprotein(a) with beta-2 glycoprotein I mediated by the kringle IV domain. Blood 1997;90:1482–1489.
74. Balasubramanian K, Schroit AJ. Characterization of phosphatidylserine-dependent beta2-glycoprotein I macrophage interactions. Implications for apoptotic cell clearance by phagocytes. J Biol Chem 1998;273:29272–29277.
75. O'Mullane MJ, Baker MS. Loss of cell viability dramatically elevates cell surface plasminogen binding and activation. Exp Cell Res 1998;242:153–164.
76. Witztum JL, Horkko S. The role of oxidized LDL in atherogenesis: immunological response and antiphospholipid antibodies. Ann N Y Acad Sci 1997;811:88–96; discussion 96–99.
77. Bouma BN, von dem Borne PA, Meijers JC. Factor XI and protection of the fibrin clot against lysis – a role for the intrinsic pathway of coagulation in fibrinolysis. Thromb Haemost 1998;80:24–27.
78. Angles-Cano E, Balaton A, Le Bonniec B, Genot E, Elion J, Sultan Y. Production of monoclonal antibodies to the high fibrin-affinity, tissue-type plasminogen activator of human plasma. Demonstration of its endothelial origin by immunolocalization. Blood 1985;66:913–920.

38 Lessons from Sequence Analysis of Monoclonal Antiphospholipid Antibodies

Ian P. Giles, David A. Isenberg, and Anisur Rahman

Introduction

The identification of antiphospholipid antibodies (aPL) is central to the diagnosis of the antiphospholipid syndrome (APS) [1]. A great deal of evidence exists from both clinical and laboratory studies to support the idea that aPL are directly pathogenic and not merely an epiphenomenon. Not all aPL, however, are associated with pathogenicity. aPL can occur in healthy adults and in some patients with infectious, malignant, or drug-related disorders, but do not cause thrombosis or fetal loss in those people. These non-pathogenic aPL mostly bind both neutral and negative phospholipid (PL) with low affinity and lack co-factor dependence [2]. In contrast, aPL found in patients with APS, whether primary or secondary, are generally IgG in isotype [3, 4], target predominantly negative PL, and require the presence of serum co-factors in order to bind PL [5–8]. The reason for this co-factor dependence is that the majority of pathogenic aPL are in fact not directed against PL at all but target serum proteins that bind PL. These proteins include protein C [9], protein S [9], prothrombin [10], and β2-glycoprotein I (β_2-GPI) [5–7]. β_2-GPI is the most extensively studied of these proteins and appears to be the most relevant clinically [11–13].

A wealth of evidence implicating aPL in the pathogenesis of thrombosis and pregnancy morbidity and suggesting potential mechanisms of action has been generated from the study of monoclonal aPL. These antibodies (Ab) are ideal for investigating the relationship between the structural properties that are important in determining the ability of pathogenic aPL to bind PL and/or β_2-GPI and the properties that determine their pathogenicity. This chapter will review the origin, binding characteristics, molecular properties, and biological function of all human monoclonal aPL for which sequence analysis has been published and the lessons learned from this with regard to the relationship between aPL structure and function.

Monoclonal Antibodies

The usefulness of monoclonal antibodies (mAb) stems from 4 characteristics: their specificity of binding; their homogeneity; their ability to be produced in unlimited quantities; and the relative ease with which their antigen binding site may be manipulated. In 1975, a method was devised that allowed Ab secreting cells isolated from an immunized mouse to be fused with a myeloma cell [14]. These hybrid cells (called *hybridomas*) have the immortal growth properties of the myeloma cell and the Ab producing properties of the B cell. The resultant cell lines can be maintained in vitro indefinitely and will continue to secrete Ab with a defined specificity, known as monoclonal Ab. This method was later adapted to produce human mAb from splenic and peripheral blood lymphocytes (PBL) [15, 16].

Hybridoma cells contain large quantities of mRNA encoding the light and heavy chains of the secreted mAb, which can be used to make and amplify cDNA. Sequence analysis of this cDNA gives the nucleotide and amino acid sequence of the mAb. This analysis is a powerful tool to gain greater understanding of features at the molecular level which distinguish natural (non-pathogenic) autoantibodies found in healthy individuals from pathogenic autoantibodies found in patients with autoimmune disease. It has been suggested that the properties of IgG isotype, specificity for negatively charged PL, and ability to bind β_2-GPI may define a population of pathogenic aPL which are particularly likely to cause APS. To investigate the factors that determine these properties at the molecular level, it is important to study the sequences and molecular structures of pathogenic aPL, and thus identify features which are common to those antibodies but are less commonly found in non-pathogenic aPL.

Analysis of Antibody Sequences to Identify Genes of Origin

An antibody molecule is composed of 2 identical heavy chains and 2 identical light chains which can be either κ or λ. The carboxyl terminal domains of both the heavy and light chains are highly conserved and are called the constant (C) regions. The amino terminal domains are much more variable in sequence and are responsible for binding antigen. These domains are known as the heavy chain variable region (V_H) and light chain variable region (V_L).

Antigen binding sites usually comprise 3 polypeptide loops from the V_H domain and 3 polypeptide loops from the V_L domain [17]. These 6 polypeptide loops are regions of high variability (in both sequence and length) known as the complementary determining regions (CDRs). The CDRs are separated by more conserved regions which perform a structural role and are hence called the framework regions (FRs) [18]. In analyzing those sequence features of aPL which are responsible for their binding properties, therefore, it is only necessary to consider the variable regions. Within these regions, the CDRs are likely to be of particular interest.

In humans, functional immunoglobulin (Ig) heavy, κ, and λ genes are found upon separate chromosomes. Sequences encoding the variable regions are assembled during early B cell development by the site specific recombination of three segments, the V_H, D_H, and J_H genes, to form the V_H domain and 2 segments, V_L and J_L, which then encode the V_L domain [19]. The genes in these loci have been sequenced and mapped [20–23]. The availability of a relatively large number of potentially functional variable region genes for recombination contributes to the diversity of possible Ab sequences (and therefore possible antigen binding sites) that can be produced. Diversity is amplified by imprecision at the joining of V_L–J_L, V_H–D_H, and D_H–J_H segments with deletion or insertion of nucleotides [19].

It is important to recognize that each locus shows an intrinsic bias towards the rearrangement of certain genes. Thus, some V_H, V_κ, and V_λ genes are more likely to be used to encode antibodies than others, regardless of the specificities of the antibodies produced [24–26]. Measurement of the frequency of expression of different V_H/V_L pairs has demonstrated that preferential pairing of specific genes or families does not occur. The most likely finding in a single B cell is the expression of a commonly rearranged V_H gene together with a commonly rearranged V_L gene [27, 28]. The pattern of V_H/V_L gene usage and pairing in PBL is not significantly different in patients with systemic lupus erythematosus (SLE) compared to healthy people [29].

Analysis of Number and Distribution of Somatic Mutations

After rearrangement of V_H, D_H, and J_H genes to produce a functional heavy chain and of either V_κ and J_κ or V_λ and J_λ genes to produce a functional light chain, a B lymphocyte begins to secrete IgM antibody. By entering a germinal center and recruiting T cell help, the B cell may then alter the isotype of the antibody produced by class switching and alter the sequence of the V_H and V_L domains by somatic hypermutation [30, 31].

Each mutation may be either silent (S), leading to no change in amino acid sequence, or replacement (R), leading to a change in amino acid sequence. Those R somatic mutations that increase affinity of the antibody for antigen are crucial in the production of the secondary repertoire. B cells expressing higher affinity Ig on their surface will be selected by limited amounts of antigen and stimulated to divide faster leading to clonal expansion of these somatically mutated B cells [32]. The presence of antigen leads to a selective pressure favoring the accumulation of particular R mutations in the CDRs, the areas of the sequence where such mutations can exert the greatest positive effects on binding affinity [33].

By comparing the V_H and V_L sequences of an antibody with those of the germline genes from which they were derived, the positions and nature (R or S) of the somatic mutations can be identified. The distribution of R and silent S mutations can then be analyzed statistically by the cumulative multinomial method of Lossos et al [34], to calculate a P value representing the probability that the observed distribution of mutations could have occurred due to chance alone. If this probability is very low, antigen driven selection is very likely to have occurred.

In antibodies which seem likely to have been modified by antigen driven selection of mutations, it is possible to identify particular sequence features which result from these modifications and which may therefore enhance binding to the driving antigen. For example, in both human and murine antibodies to double stranded DNA, somatic mutations creating arginine (Arg), lysine (Lys), and asparagine (Asn) residues in the CDRs occur very commonly [35, 36]. All of these amino acids may promote binding to the negatively charged DNA double helix by charge interactions or hydrogen bond formation. It is possible to generate hypotheses about the potential interactions between such amino acids and antigen by using computer modeling programs. These programs allow prediction of the three-dimensional structures of antibodies from their amino acid sequences [35, 37, 38].

Analysis of the known crystal structures of 26 different antigen–antibody complexes allowed MacCallum et al [37] to show that certain residues within CDRs of the heavy and light chains are more likely than others to contact antigens. These authors suggested that analyses of CDR amino acid composition could be much more informative when the likelihood that an amino acid at a particular position will be involved in antigen contact is taken into account.

Sequence Analysis of Monoclonal aPL

Using the principles of antibody sequence analysis outlined in the previous sections, we may pose the following questions about monoclonal aPL:

- **Do aPL preferentially use certain genes of origin?** In analyzing the sequences of the V_H and V_L domains of a particular antibody, it is possible to deduce which of the available genes in the repertoire have been used to encode these domains and the extent to which somatic mutations and modification at the junctions has occurred. By repeating this analysis for a large number of different monoclonal aPL, it is possible to deduce whether particular genes are used in these antibodies more frequently than in other antibodies.
- **What is the extent of somatic hypermutation in aPL and is it likely to have been driven by antigen?** Having identified the positions of R and S mutations within the V_H and V_L sequences, the distribution of these mutations using the multinomial method may be analyzed [34].
- **Are particular sequence motifs found characteristically in aPL?** The sequences of the CDRs are of particular interest because recurring motifs there might point to possible common features that enhance binding to PL.
- **Do these sequence motifs correspond with sites of somatic hypermutation and with the predicted contact sites of the antibody?** Analysis of CDR amino acid composition can be much more informative when the likelihood that an amino acid at a particular position will be involved in antigen contact is taken into account using the model of MacCallum et al [37].

Sequence Analysis of Murine Monoclonal aPL

Thus far aPL have been produced from animal models which show consistent serological features of the syndrome, but which generally show either the obstetric or thrombotic clinical features, but not both [39]. Studies of aPL derived from MRL lpr/lpr mice [40] and NZW x BXSB F1 mice [41, 42] do not reveal convincing evidence of any particular gene preference, somatic mutations, or specific residues in CDRs which are important for binding. The most commonly expressed V_H genes in these murine aPL were members of the J558 murine V_H family, but almost 50% of all spontaneously activated B cells in MRL lpr/lpr mice express J558 genes regardless of antigen specificity [43]. Despite some evidence of clonal expansion in development of aPL and some clustering of replacement mutations in V_H, CDRs found in one study [42], the extent to which antigen driven somatic mutations and the presence of certain residues in CDRs are important in murine aPL remains uncertain [44].

Sequence Analysis of Human Monoclonal aPL

Sequences of 51 human mAb that bind PL have been reported. Human aPL produced thus far can be divided into 3 groups: polyreactive IgM, more specific IgM, and IgG. Early published sequences were of polyreactive IgM antibodies, often produced from healthy individuals, that were primarily targeted against other antigens (mainly DNA) and found to bind PL with low affinity on panel antigen testing [45–51]. Later groups sought to produce more specific aPL and initially it proved easier to produce IgM aPL, which again were often derived from healthy individuals [52–58]. It is only in the last 5 years that human monoclonal IgG aPL with all 3 major pathogenic features (IgG isotype, binding to β_2-GPI, and preference for negatively charged PL) have been produced, sequenced, and their pathogenic effects studied [59–61]. Thus, more sequence information relating to clinically relevant antibodies is now available and it is now clear that a large proportion of pathogenic antibodies in APS probably bind epitopes on β_2-GPI.

We have identified all published human monoclonal aPL and anti–β_2-GPI sequences from PubMed and obtained additional information from original authors where necessary (J. L. Pasquali, personal communication). The V region DNA sequences of these antibodies were obtained and sequence alignment, using DNAplot software [62], and statistical analyses using the multinomial method [34] were carried out.

Sequences of Human aPL

Fifty-one human monoclonal aPL were identified. In this analysis, these have been subdivided according to isotype and degree of relevance to pathogenesis of APS, as suggested by binding properties and/or activity in assays of pathogenicity.

Twenty-three of these aPL were of IgM isotype and were derived from lymphocytes immortalized by Epstein–Barr transformation or by fusion with immortal cells to form hybridomas. The genes of origin, homology values, and binding characteristics of these IgM antibodies are shown in Table 38.1. Homology values show the extent of shared sequence between the V_H or V_L sequence of an antibody and the germline genes of origin. Lower homology values indicate more somatic mutation.

These IgM antibodies can be divided into 2 groups, shown as groups A and B in Table 38.1. The first group (A) of 15 antibodies are polyreactive and were not selected for specific binding to PL or for relevance to APS [45–51]. Most of these mAb were actually selected for binding to DNA and were incidentally found to bind PL (often with low affinity) on panel Ag testing. Most of the antibodies in group A were derived from PBL of healthy individuals. Only four (18/2, 1/17, C119, and C471) of the 15 aPL identified in this group were derived from patients with SLE, none of whom had features of the APS. Binding to β_2-GPI was not reported for any of these Ab.

Although the antibodies in group A seem likely to have limited relevance to the pathogenesis of APS, they are included in this analysis to ensure a comprehensive analysis of all human aPL sequences. The group A antibodies are likely to be representative of non-pathogenic natural autoantibodies and thus their sequence charac-

Table 38.1. Sequence features of polyreactive IgM, group A, and more specific IgM, group B antiphospholipid antibodies.

mAb	Origin	Nucleotide Homology	VH gene	D_H	J_H	VL family	VL gene	Nucleotide Homology	J_L	Binding	Reference
Group A											
m18/2	SLE PBL	100	V3-23	NM	NM	NP	NP	NP	NP	ssDNA, poly-I, poly-dT, Plt	45
m1/17	SLE PBL	100	V3-23	NM	NM	NP	NP	NP	NP	ssDNA, Plt, Vimentin	45
C6B2	Sickle cell	97.5	V4-61	D3-10	J_H3b	NP	NP	NP	NP	Poly-G/I/U, ss/dsDNA	46
spleen										Poly-dAdT-PolydAdT PA, CL, PI, PG	
Kim4.6	Healthy tonsil	100	V3-30	D3-10	J_H6a	$V_\lambda1$	1b	100	NM	ss/dsDNA, poly-dAdT poly-dG-Poly-dC, RNA, CL	47, 48
A10	Healthy PBL	99	V6-01	NM	J_H6a	NP	NP	NP	NP	ss/dsDNA, CL, PdT, Hel	49
A431	Healthy PBL	98	V6-01	NM	J_H6a	NP	NP	NP	NP	ss/dsDNA, CL, PdT, Cyt c	49
L16	Fetal liver	100	V6-01	NM	J_H6a	NP	NP	NP	NP	ssDNA, CL, PdT	49
C119 *	SLE, PBL	95.5	V3-23	NM	NM	$V_\kappa3$	L6	100	$J_\kappa4$	ssDNA, Plt, CL, DOPE	50
B122	Healthy PBL	97	V1-18	NM	NM	$V_\kappa1$	L12a	98.3	NM	ssDNA, Plt, CL, DOPE	50
B6204	Healthy PBL	97	V3-23	NM	NM	$V_\kappa3$	A27	99.6	NM	ssDNA, Plt, CL, DOPE, RF	50
C471	SLE, PBL	99.6	V3-64	NM	NM	$V_\kappa3$	L2	100	$J_\kappa2$	ssDNA, Plt, DOPE	50
H3	Healthy PBL	97	V1-46	D6-13	J_H4	$V_\kappa3$	3l	97	$J_\lambda2/3a$	CL, PS, PE, DT, TT	51
H5	Healthy PBL	96	V4-30	DIRL	J_H4	NP	NP	NP	NP	CL, DT, TT	51
A5	Healthy PBL	100	V3-23	DHF16	J_H6	$V_\lambda3$	3p	97	$J_\lambda2/3a$	CL, DT, TT, ssDNA	51
Bou 53.6	Healthy tonsil	100	V3-23	D4	J_H6	$V_\kappa1$	L12	99	$J_\kappa2$	CL, polyreactive	51
Group B											
Kim 13.1	Healthy tonsil	100	1-e	NM	J_H5b	$V_\kappa3$	L6	100	$J_\kappa4$	CL, RF	52
REN †	CLL	100	V4-61	NM	J_H3b	$V_\lambda8$	8a	99.7	$J_\lambda3b$	CL, ssDNA	53
BH1 *†	PAPS PBL	100	V3-30	NM	NM	$V_\lambda3$	3r	97.5	$J_\lambda3b$	anionic PL	54
STO 103	Healthy tonsil	100	V4-61	D3-03	J_H4a	$V_\kappa IV$	B3	100	$J_\kappa2$	Plt, anionic PL	55
RSP 4	SLE PBL	96	V3-30	D4-23	J_H4b	$V_\lambda1$	le	98.3	$J_\lambda1$	CL	56
B9421 *	SLE/APS PBL	100	V3-72	D21-9	J_H3	$V_\lambda2$	2a2	99.3	$J_\lambda3b$	LA	57
B9427 *†	SLE/APS PBL	100	V3-15	D21-9	J_H4	$V_\kappa2$	A17	100	$J_\kappa3$	LA	57
HY-FRO*	LPL	97.9	V3-30	D3-22	J_H2	$V_\lambda2$	3l	97.6	$J_\lambda3b$	CL, PS	58

The symbols denote: * = lupus anticoagulant activity; † = binding to β_2-GPI; ‡ = pathogenicity in biological assay.

Abbreviations: NM = no match; NP = not published; SLE = systemic lupus erythematosus; PBL = peripheral blood lymphocyte; PD = phage display; CLL = chronic lymphocytic leukaemia; LPL = lymphoplasmacytic lymphoma; ss/ds DNA = single/double stranded DNA; Poly I = polyirosinic acid; Poly U = polyuracil; Poly G = polyguanolic acid; Poly dA-dT = polydeoxyadenylate-thymidylate sodium salt; Poly dG-Poly dC = polydeoxyguanylate-polydeoxycytidylate; Plt = platelet; CL = cardiolipin; Hel = hen egg lysozyme; Cyt c = cytochrome c; DOPE = dioleoylphosphatidylethanolamine; RF = rheumatoid factor; PT = prothrombin; OVA = chicken ovalbumin; BSA = bovine serum albumin.

teristics serve as a useful comparison with those of the more specific and probably more pathogenic IgM aPL in group B and of the IgG aPL.

Members of the second group (B) of 8 IgM antibodies are likely to be more relevant to the pathogenesis of APS [52–58]. Most of these antibodies showed specific binding to PL alone despite testing against a range of other antigens. REN, which also binds ssDNA, is an exception. Four antibodies in group B showed LA activity (BH1, B9421, B9427, and HY-FRO). B9427 bound β_2-GPI, REN showed β_2-GPI–dependent binding to PL, and BH1 showed serum dependent binding to PL (the effect of β_2-GPI was not tested formally). Three antibodies (BH1, B9427, and B9421) were produced from the lymphocytes of patients with APS and another one (RSP4) from a patient with SLE and serum aPL, who did not have clinical features of APS.

The other 28 aPL identified were IgG antibodies [61, 63–69]. The genes of origin, homology values, and binding characteristics of these antibodies are shown in Table 38.2. Seventeen of these IgG antibodies were derived from immortalized lymphocytes, 4 (P11, B22, B27, and B14) by repertoire cloning using the phage display method [65], and 6 (CIC01, CIC03, CIC11, CIC14, CIC15, and CIC19) by cloning of V_H and V_L genes originating from aPL specific B cells into a baculovirus expression system [61, 69]. The 4 antibodies produced by phage display were derived from lymphocytes of a patient who had circulating anti–β_2-GPI antibodies, but did not have APS. The cDNA was cloned into phage display vectors from which a library of phages were produced carrying surface Fab derived from heavy and light chain sequences expressed in that patient's lymphocytes. These V_H/V_L gene combinations, however, were artificial and not all may have been expressed in patient serum. Phages carrying anti–β_2-GPI Fab were selected by binding to plates carrying β_2-GPI. Thus, the heavy and light chain gene combinations of the aPL selected by phage display may not be representative of naturally occurring aPL. Such a discrepancy does not occur in monoclonal aPL that are derived from immortalized B cells or specifically selected B cells in which the V_H/V_L gene combination is definitely expressed by at least one B cell in the individual from which it was produced.

Of the other 24 IgG aPL, 11 were derived from patients with SLE (4 of whom had APS) and 12 were produced from patients with primary APS (PAPS). Most of the monoclonal IgG aPL showed specificity for PL or β_2-GPI (see Table 38.2). The functional activities of 13 IgG monoclonal aPL have been examined in various biological assays and 8 were shown to be pathogenic compared to control monoclonal Ab. Two aPL derived from patients with PAPS (516, CIC15) and 1 from a healthy subject (519) induced a significantly higher rate of fetal resorptions and a significant reduction in fetal and placental weight following intravenous injection into mated BALB/c mice [61, 66]. Five aPL derived from patients with PAPS (IS2, IS3, and IS4) and SLE/APS (CL15 and CL24) were found to be thrombogenic – inducing larger thrombi which persist for longer – in an in vivo model of thrombosis [60].

Which Were the Genes of Origin?

The frequency of use of V, D, and J genes to encode monoclonal aPL was compared with that which would be expected from the intrinsic bias of the Ig gene recombination process.

Table 38.2. Sequence features of IgG antiphospholipid antibodies.

mAb	Origin	VH gene	Nucleotide homology	D_H	J_H	VL family	VL gene	Nucleotide Homology	J_L	Binding to other Ag	Reference
R149	SLE PBL	V1-69	96.6	NM	J_H6a	$V_\kappa2$	A19	99.3	$J_\kappa2$	ssDNA	63
LJ-1	SLE PBL	NP	NP	NP	NP	$V_\lambda3$	3h	98.6	$J_\lambda2/J_\lambda3a$	histone	64
AH-2	SLE PBL	V5-51	94.9	D4-23	J_H6b	$V_\lambda1$	le	99	$J_\lambda3b$	no	64
DA-3	SLE PBL	V5-51	95.2	D3-09	J_H6a	$V_\lambda1$	le	98.3	$J_\lambda3b$	histone	64
UK-4	SLE PBL	V3-74	95	NM	J_H4b	$V_\kappa2$	2a2	94	$J_\lambda2/J_\lambda3a$	No	64
B3	SLE PBL	V3-23	94	NM	J_H4	$V_\kappa2$	2a2	93	$J_\lambda2/J_\lambda3$	dsDNA	64
516‡	PAPS PBL	V1-69	97.3	D3-10	J_H6b	$V_\kappa1$	L19	96.9	$J_\kappa4$	ssDNA, recombinant human insulin, tetanus toxoid, human thyroglobulin, BSA	68
519‡	Healthy PBL	V4-34	97.9	NM	J_H5a	$V_\kappa3$	L2	98.9	$J_\kappa4$	No	66
B9416 *	SLE/APS PBL	V3-23	98	NM	J_H4b	$V_\kappa1$	012/02	98.6	$J_\kappa1$	No	66
HL-5B *	PAPS PBL	V3-53	89	NM	NM	NP	NP	NP	NP	oxLDL	57
RR-7F	SLE PBL	V3-24	86.1	NM	NM	NP	NP	NP	NP	oxLDL	67
B14 †	Healthy PD	V3-23	91.9	D2-15	J_H4b	$V_\kappa1$	A20	97.6	$J_\kappa2$	No	65
B22 †	Healthy PD	V6-01	93.7	NM	J_H4b	$V_\kappa1$	A20	98.1	$J_\kappa3$	No	65
B27 †	Healthy PD	V6-01	93.7	NM	J_H4b	$V_\kappa1$	L15	95.8	$J_\kappa4$	No	65
P11 †	Healthy PD	V4-30	92.7	D3-03	J_H4b	$V_\kappa1$	L8	96	$J_\kappa3$	PT, OVA, ssDNA	65
IS1	PAPS PBL	V4-39	97	NM	J_H4	$V_\varrho1$	L12a	95	$J_\varrho4$	No	59
IS2‡	PAPS PBL	V4-39	97	NM	J_H4	$V_\varrho1$	L12a	97	$J_\varrho4$	No	59
IS3 †‡	PAPS PBL	V4-39	93	NM	J_H1	$V_\varrho2$	A3/A19	99	$J_\varrho2$	No	59
IS4 †‡	PAPS PBL	V1-03	93	NM	J_H4b	$V_\varrho2$	2a2	93	$J_\varrho3b$	No	59
CL1 †	SLE/APS PBL	V1-02	96	NM	J_H5	$V_\varrho3$	3j	93	$J_\varrho2/3$	No	59
CL15‡	SLE/APS PBL	V4-34	90	NM	J_H6	$V_\varrho1$	O12	96	$J_\varrho2$	No	59
CL24*†‡	SLE/APS PBL	V3-23	84	D6-19	J_H4b	$V_\varrho3$	A27	92	$J_\varrho2$	No	59
ClC01*	PAPS PBL	V5-51	85.1	D5-24	J_H5	$V_\varrho1$	L8	89.6	$J_\kappa1$	No	69
ClC03 †	PAPS PBL	V4-04	92.9	D1-01	J_H3	$V_\varrho1$	L12a	91.8	$J_\kappa1$	No	69
ClC11	PAPS PBL	V3-48	95.9	D2-21	J_H4	$V_\varrho1$	L8	97.8	$J_\kappa5$	PT	69
ClC14 †	PAPS PBL	V3-13	96.9	D3-10	J_H6	$V_\varrho1$	L8	98.1	$J_\kappa3$	PT	69
ClC15‡	PAPS PBL	V4-61	99.3	D3-03	J_H4d	$V_\varrho1$	L12a	97.9	$J_\kappa1$	Annexin A5	61
ClC19	PAPS PBL	V3-30	100	D3-16	J_H4	$V_\varrho3$	A27	99.7	$J_\kappa1$	PT	69

For key to abbreviations, see legend to Table 38.1. Only binding to antigens other than anionic PL is indicated.

Heavy Chain Genes

Twelve of the 15 polyreactive aPL in group A, all 8 of the more specific IgM aPL in group B, and 22 of 27 published IgG aPL used genes from the V_H 1,3, or 4 families. These are the largest and most commonly expressed V_H families in both normal donors and patients with SLE [29]. The other 3 polyreactive antibodies used the V_H 6 gene V6-01, but were derived from an experiment which set out specifically to produce monoclonal Ab encoded by that gene [49].

The most commonly used gene amongst polyreactive IgM aPL and IgG aPL is V3-23 which is the most commonly rearranged V_H gene in IgM secreting B cells regardless of Ag specificity [26]. A group of V_H genes that are particularly likely to be rearranged due to the intrinsic bias in the recombination process has been identified by single cell PCR in peripheral B cells [26, 29]. This group includes V3-23, V3-30, V3-07, V4-34, V4-39, V4-59, V1-18, V1-69, and V5-51. Members of this group of genes encode V_H sequences in 8 of the 15 polyreactive IgM antibodies, 15 of the 27 published IgG aPL, but only 3 of the 8 more specific IgM antibodies.

For a number of the antibodies studied, it was not possible to match the heavy chain CDR3 sequence to any known D_H gene because the DNAPLOT software used very stringent criteria for aligning Ab sequences to germline D segments [70]. Six of the 15 IgM sequences in group A, 5 of the 8 in group B, and 12 of the 27 IgG sequences could be matched to known D genes. The majority of the D segments matched were from the D2 and D3 families, which have previously been shown to dominate the expressed repertoire [26, 29, 70].

J_H genes of origin could be identified for 9 IgM antibodies in group A, 7 in group B, and 25 IgG antibodies. Where no match could be made, this was usually because the published sequence did not extend as far as the J region. The majority of the sequences matched the J_H3, J_H4, or J_H6 genes, which are the most commonly rearranged J_H genes in peripheral B cells [29].

Light Chain Genes

Of the light chain sequences of these aPL, all polyreactive IgM, all IgG, and 5 of 7 more specific IgM aPL used genes which are members of the 3 largest and most commonly expressed V_λ (I–III) or V_κ (1–3) families. Six of the 8 published V_L sequences of IgM in group A, 7 of 8 sequences in group B, and 22 of 26 published IgG aPL sequences utilized V_κ or V_λ genes which are known to be commonly rearranged and expressed [24, 71]. The most commonly rearranged V_κ genes include A3, A17, A20, 02/12, L8, L12, L6, A27, L2, and B3, while commonly rearranged V_λ genes include 1b, 1c, 1e, 2a2, 2b2, 2c, 3h, and 3r.

In the cases where assignment to a J_L gene could be made, it was found that λ encoded sequences always used $J_\lambda2$ or $J_\lambda3$ genes, whereas the κ encoded sequences were mostly $J_\kappa1$, $J_\kappa2$, $J_\kappa3$, or $J_\kappa4$. There was no difference between IgM and IgG antibodies. These results mirror the known usage of these genes in peripheral lymphocytes [29, 72].

In summary, therefore, the pattern of gene usage in these aPL antibodies is generally that which would be expected from the intrinsic bias of the recombination mechanism. Genes that are commonly rearranged by that mechanism are also commonly used to encode both IgM and IgG aPL. Interestingly, in the group of more specific IgM aPL, 5 of 8 antibodies use V_H genes which are not commonly rearranged in other antibodies (including V1-e, V3-72, and V3-15) and 4 of these antibodies use genes that are not used to encode either polyreactive IgM aPL or IgG aPL. Although each of these genes is used in its germline configuration there is no evidence to support the idea that these genes confer any common structural property (from sequence analysis or knowledge of three-dimensional structures) which promotes the formation of a PL binding site. It is therefore not possible to conclude that these results represent preferential use of these particular genes to encode a PL binding site in specific IgM aPL.

What is the Extent of Somatic Hypermutation?

Overall, IgG aPL carried more somatic mutations than IgM aPL, and this difference was most pronounced when considering the heavy chains. Twenty-five of 27 published IgG V_H sequences compared to 16 of 26 published IgG V_L sequences showed homology of 98% or less to the corresponding germline gene (see Table 38.2). The high degree of somatic mutation in IgG antibodies was expected, because class switching and somatic hypermutation are closely linked processes in the B lymphocyte [73].

Nevertheless, somatic hypermutation can take place in the absence of class switching, leading to the production of IgM antibodies carrying many mutations. A number of such antibodies were seen in group A, where 7 of 15 V_H sequences and 2 of 8 published V_L sequences had homology values less than or equal to 98%.

The more specific IgM aPL in group B, however, contained very few somatic mutations with 2 V_H chains having less than 98% nucleotide homology and the other 6 V_H chains having 100% homology. Five of the 8 V_L chains showed greater than 99% homology to germline genes with only 2 V_L chain having less than 98% (but greater than 97%) nucleotide homology.

Are the Somatic Mutations Antigen Driven?

Statistical analysis of the distribution of R and S mutations in the CDR and FR regions of the V_H and V_L sequences was performed using the multinomial (Pm) method [34]. A Pm value of less than 0.05 for either FRs or CDRs in the heavy or light chain is taken as representing strong evidence of antigen drive. Eighteen of the 26 IgG aPL analyzed fulfill this criterion.

Eight IgG aPL did not have Pm values of less than 0.05 in either chain: AH-2, DA-3, 519, RR-7F, P11, IS2, IS3, and CIC11. No conclusion can be made as to whether antigen drive plays a role in the development of RR-7F, because the sequence of RR-7FV_L is unpublished. There is good evidence that AH-2 and DA-3 are derived from a clone of B cells which has been subject to antigen driven expansion, despite the non-significant Pm values. AH-2 and DA-3 are distinct monoclonal Ab derived from descendants of the same B cell clone in a single patient, because they share exactly the same V_H and V_L sequences, except at a few sites of somatic mutation. The fact that the same clone has given rise to 2 distinct monoclonal Ab implies that it is a highly expanded clone, and the fact that the sequences contain multiple somatic mutations implies that this has been driven by antigen. Similarly, IS2 is clonally related to IS1 because both aPL share an identical heavy chain and their light chains differ by only 5 amino acid residues. Thus, in only 4 IgG antibodies was the evidence clearly against the influence of antigen drive.

It is therefore apparent that most of the IgG aPL have been subject to antigen driven expansion and accumulation of somatic mutations. Because, on testing for binding to a range of other antigens, these antibodies showed specificity for either PL or β_2-GPI, these seem likely to have been the driving antigens.

The results for the more specific IgM aPL in group B are completely different from those of the IgG aPL. Most have very few mutations, and even the 3 aPL with less than 98% nucleotide homology in 1 or both chains do not show any evidence of antigen drive on statistical analysis. Indeed, the majority of the more specific IgM aPL had very few somatic mutations. This suggests that these IgM attain specificity due to features inherent in their germline sequence or produced at the V_H–D_H, D_H–J_H, or V_L–J_L junctions. Antigen drive would then tend to select against somatic mutations because mutations would tend to alter the favorable germline sequence. Conversely, IgG aPL would attain specificity and high affinity for PL or β_2-GPI due to accumulation of somatic mutations.

Seven polyreactive IgM aPL had V_H or V_L sequences with less than 98% nucleotide homology but in 3 antibodies (H3, H5, and A5) nucleotide sequences were not published and therefore could not be analyzed [51]. Of the remaining 4 antibodies (C6B2, C119, B122, and B6204), statistical analysis gave Pm values of less than 0.05 in 3 cases. This shows that antigen driven accumulation of mutations in IgM antibodies is not always associated with the loss of polyreactivity. However, extensive somatic mutation was the exception rather than the rule in polyreactive IgM antibodies, in contrast to the IgG aPL discussed above.

Are Particular Residues Important in CDRs and Contact Regions?

Somatic mutations occur frequently in the contact H1 and H2 regions of the IgG antibodies, less commonly in L1, L2, and L3 of the IgG antibodies, and are very rare in the IgM antibodies. We were unable to analyze H3 because it is very difficult to be sure where somatic mutations occur, due to the contribution of junctional diversity and the large number of cases in which germline D genes of origin cannot be identified.

The hypothesis that somatic mutation to create Arg, Lys and Asn residues in the contact regions may play a major role in IgG aPL is examined in Tables 38.3 and 38.4. The proportion of somatic mutations in the contact regions which give rise to these amino acids is compared with the proportion of mutations in the same regions which give rise to aspartic acid (Asp) or glutamic acid (Glu). These residues were chosen for comparison because they are acidic and negatively charged as opposed to the basic, positively charged Arg and Lys.

Table 38.3 clearly shows an excess of mutation to Arg, Lys, and Asn in the contact sites of the IgG aPL in comparison to Asp and Glu. In Table 38.4, the total numbers of Arg, Asn, and Lys residues in the contact regions of both the IgG aPL and the more specific IgM aPL are compared with the numbers of Asp and Glu residues in those regions. This table includes both germline encoded residues and those

Table 38.3. Analysis of somatic mutations at contact residues.

V region	Number of antibodies	Number of somatically mutated contact residues that are Arg, Asn, or Lys/number of contact residues that are somatic mutations			Number of somatically mutated contact residues that are Asp or Glu/number of contact residues that are somatic mutations		
		Contact Region 1	Contact egion 2	Contact Region 3	Contact Region 1	Contact Region 2	Contact Region 3
IgG V$_H$	27	11/44	13/51	–	3/42	2/48	–
IgG V$_\kappa$	19	6/18	1/9	4/10	0/18	1/9	2/10
IgGV$_\lambda$	7	1/6	1/8	2/7	0/5	3/7	0/5

Table 38.4. Analysis of all amino acids present at sites of contact.

V region	Number of antibodies	Total Arg, Asn or Lys residues present at contact sites (in brackets; total not including somatically mutated residues)			Total Asp or Glu residues present at contact sites (in brackets; total not including somatically mutated residues)		
		Contact Region 1	Contact egion 2	Contact Region 3	Contact Region 1	Contact Region 2	Contact Region 3
IgG V$_H$	27	15 (4)	37 (24)	27 (–)	5 (2)	15 (12)	26 (–)
IgG V$_\kappa$	19	14 (8)	6 (5)	10 (6)	2 (1)	3 (3)	2 (0)
IgGV$_\lambda$	7	7 (6)	5 (4)	2 (0)	2 (2)	4 (2)	3 (2)
IgM V$_H$	8	2 (1)	14 (14)	15 (–)	3 (2)	6 (6)	9 (–)
IgM V$_\kappa$	3	5 (5)	4 (4)	2 (2)	1 (1)	3 (3)	0 (0)
IgM V$_\lambda$	5	3 (3)	7 (6)	3 (3)	2 (2)	2 (0)	3 (3)

derived by somatic mutation. This comparison is particularly important for the IgM antibodies, where somatic mutation plays no major role. In general, there is an excess of Arg, Lys, and Asn residues over Asp and Glu residues in the contact regions of the V$_H$ and V$_\kappa$, but not the V$_\lambda$ sequences. Interestingly, this does not hold true for the H3 regions of the IgG antibodies. Accumulation of basic residues (particularly Arg) in H3 has been noted to be a common feature of human and murine IgG anti-DNA antibodies [35, 36], but does not outweigh accumulation of acidic residues in the IgG aPL considered as a whole here. However, Arg residues in H3 may be a distinguishing feature of the subset of these antibodies which are pathogenic (see below).

Thus, whereas both the group B IgM aPL and the IgG aPL show some evidence of accumulation of Asn, Arg, and Lys at the contact sites, these are mostly encoded in the germline in IgM and derived from somatic mutation in IgG. The presence of CDRs and contact regions which are rich in Arg, Asn, and Lys residues in both the more specific IgM aPL and IgG aPL is relevant to the nature of the epitope bound by these antibodies. Pathogenic aPL have a predilection for negatively charged PL and β$_2$-GPI, which has a potential epitope rich in negatively charged residues within domain I [reviewed in 74]. Therefore, the presence of Arg, Asn, and Lys residues in the contact regions of aPL may increase the affinity of binding via electrostatic interactions and hydrogen bonds with negatively charged epitopes upon PL and domain I of β$_2$-GPI.

Are There Differences Between Antibodies Which Bind β_2-GPI and Those Which Do Not?

Thirteen antibodies were either known to bind β_2-GPI or there was strong evidence to suggest that β_2-GPI was required for them to bind phospholipids. Three of these antibodies (BH1, REN, and B9427) were IgM antibodies from group B while the other 10 (B14, B22, B27, P11, IS3, IS4, CL1, CL24, CIC03, and CIC14) were IgG antibodies. When these antibodies are considered as one group, the results are similar to those noted for the whole set of aPL. Thus, the 10 IgG antibodies which bound β_2-GPI all had many somatic mutations and Pm values suggested antigen drive in 8 cases (P11 and IS3 were the exceptions). The 3 IgM antibodies had few or no mutations with no evidence of antigen drive. All the IgG antibodies except P11 and CIC14 contained somatic mutations to Arg, Asn, or Lys in their contact regions whereas none of the IgM antibodies had mutations to those residues in their contact regions.

Are There Differences Between Pathogenic and Non-pathogenic Antibodies?

The 8 IgG aPL shown to be directly pathogenic compared to control monoclonal Ab in biological assays all used the most commonly expressed genes apart from IS4V_H, CIC15V_H, and 516V_L. In each of the 8 aPL, at least 1 of the heavy or light chains contained numerous somatic mutations and in 5 of these antibodies the Pm values suggested antigen drive (519, IS2, and IS3 were the exceptions). In comparison, the 5 aPL found to be non-pathogenic on testing use commonly expressed genes apart from CL1V_H, CIC03V_H, CIC11V_H, and CL1V_L. Four of the non-pathogenic antibodies contain numerous mutations and 3 had evidence of antigen drive. It is striking however that 7 of the 8 pathogenic aPL contain at least 1 Arg residue in V_HCDR3 with 6 of them containing at least 2. Of the 5 non-pathogenic aPL, 3 contained Arg residues in V_HCDR3 with 2 of them containing only a single Arg residue.

Computer Modeling of aPL

Computer models of the IgG aPL IS4 and CL24, shown in Figure 38.1, support the idea that Arg residues are important at the binding sites of these aPL. These Ab are likely to be representative of pathogenic aPL for a number of reasons. Both aPL were isolated from patients with APS, shown to be pathogenic in a murine model, show β_2-GPI–dependent binding to PL, and contain numerous somatic mutations in an antigen driven pattern. Overall the heavy chain CDRs of both IS4 and CL24 display an accumulation of predominantly Arg and Asn residues compared to acidic residues. This accumulation is greater than that seen in the light chains. IS4V_HCDR3 is long (15 amino acids) with a very high content of 5 Arg residues. It seems likely that the length and Arg content of this CDR3 arise from N addition and somatic mutation and that selection by antigen has acted to promote expansion of the clone containing these Arg residues. Models in Figure 38.1(C,D) support this hypothesis because 4 of the 5 Arg residues in IS4V_HCDR3 are surface exposed and

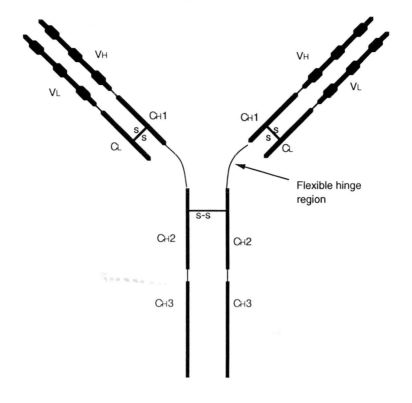

In each V region CDRs and FRs are distinguished as shown below.

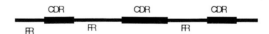

Figure 38.1. Modeling studies of CL24V$_L$, IS4VL, and IS4V$_H$. (A) Model of the light chain of CL24 is shown in *secondary structure mode*. (B) A model of the light chain of IS4 in *secondary structure mode*. (C) Spacefill model of the heavy chain of IS4. The labeled arginines (Arg) in the large CDR3 loop region of IS4V$_H$ are predicted to importantly contribute to CL binding specificity. (D) The heavy chain of IS4 in *secondary structure mode*. In all models Arg residues predicted to be exposed are shown in *dark blue* (*spacefill mode*); CDR1 in light and heavy chains is depicted in *yellow*, CDR2 in *orange*, and CDR3 in *red*.

could therefore be important in contributing to CL-binding specificity. The model of CL24V$_L$ in Figure 38.1(A) clearly shows that the 2 Arg residues created by somatic mutation in CDR1 (at position 28 and 31) are surface exposed. In contrast, IS4V$_L$ shown in Figure 38.1(B) has no somatic mutations to Arg at all but does contain a germline encoded Arg at position 54 which is also present in CL24V$_L$.

Once computer models such as these have been used to identify particular amino acids that potentially affect the aPL–β_2-GPI–PL interaction, further experiments may be performed to produce variant forms of monoclonal aPL in which these key residues are altered. The wild-type and altered antibodies can be compared to test the effect this has upon binding and/or pathogenic properties of the antibody. There are a number of different systems available for expressing antibody sequences as whole Ig molecules or antigen binding fragments.

Expression Systems for Monoclonal Antibodies

All expression systems involve cloning V_H and/or V_L sequences of a selected Ab into an expression vector containing the appropriate amount of C_H and/or C_L as well as the components required to enable the plasmid vector to express Ig once transfected into either a bacterial or eukaryotic cell. In this way, either part or the whole Ig molecule is expressed containing a functional binding site. A major disadvantage of bacterial expression of eukaryotic proteins is that post-translational modifications are absent and it is not possible to express a stable, functional whole Ig molecule in bacteria [75]. It has proved possible, however, to express smaller fragments of Ab which contain a functional binding site.

The simplest expression products are single chain fused variable region (scFv) molecules. In scFv expression plasmids, V_H and V_L sequences are cloned either side of a sequence encoding a short flexible linker fragment which when expressed from bacterial cells allows the V_H and V_L to interact with each other and produce an antigen binding site [76]. Fab fragments may also be expressed from bacteria. Expression vectors for these fragments contain V_H and V_L followed by a C_H1 sequence and a C_L sequence, respectively. Hence, the products of expression are the whole light chain and half the heavy chain which combine covalently to form Fab [77].

Fab and scFv molecules however, are both unsuitable for use in functional assays because they lack some or all C region domains. Therefore, despite the usefulness of these Ab fragments in determining the binding properties of the V region of an antibody they cannot be used to investigate how altering these binding properties may affect pathogenicity of these antibodies in vivo. Whole IgG molecules – expressed from eukaryotic cells – are required for this purpose.

The expression of whole Ig in mammalian cells may be achieved in a variety of ways which give rise to either transient expression of Ab or the selection of stably transfected cell lines. Transient expression allows rapid screening of large combinations of different Ab and does not require the selection of cells for drug resistance markers or long-term maintenance of cell lines but the total yield of Ab is generally low. In contrast, stable expression systems allow the production of much larger quantities of Ab than with transient expression but are more difficult and time consuming to produce.

The Use of Different Expression Systems in the Further Investigation of Links Between Sequence, Structure, and Function of aPL

There have been few studies of the relative importance of heavy and light chain sequence motifs in the binding of aPL to PL–β_2-GPI. Several groups have studied murine aPL expressed as scFv. One group found the heavy chain of a pathogenic aPL to be important in conferring β_2-GPI dependent binding to PL as well as LA activity [78]. Another group studied the murine anti-DNA antibody 3H9, which has dual specificity for DNA and PL [79]. They found that the introduction of Arg residues into the heavy chain of 3H9 variable region at positions known to mediate DNA binding enhanced binding to PS–β_2-GPI complexes. In contrast, the CL binding activity of different monoclonal antibodies A1.72 and A1.84 was found to be solely mediated by the light chain sequence [80]. The direct relevance of these studies to APS in humans is limited, however, by the use of murine antibodies in the form of scFv, which do not contain any constant region sequence, and are therefore not representative of antibodies found in patients with APS.

A murine monoclonal anti-phosphorylcholine (PC) antibody 6G6 was expressed as whole IgM molecules [81]. It was demonstrated that both the light chain and CDR3 of the heavy chain were necessary for binding to PC. A later study expressed a number of human antibodies in the form of Fab produced by *Escherichia coli* [82]. These experiments showed that the ability to bind CL was mainly dependent on the light chain of some human antibodies, but the heavy chain of others. In further experiments which optimized conditions to improve the quality and quantity of purified Fabs produced by *E. coli* significantly, the light chain of 2 human autoantibodies conferred the ability to bind DNA and CL [83] as well as β_2-GPI [84]. These studies, however, were primarily directed at investigating the origin and properties of anti-DNA Ab and did not study antibodies that were known to be relevant to APS on the basis of pathogenicity in mouse models. Indeed the first report of in vitro expression of whole human aPL antibodies with these pathogenic properties has stemmed from our group [85].

We used a transient expression system to test the binding properties of combinations of heavy and light chains derived from a range of human mAb. These included the mAb IS4 and CL24 described above. We found that the sequence of IS4V$_H$ was dominant in conferring the ability to bind CL whilst the identity of the V$_L$ paired with this heavy chain was important in determining the strength of CL binding [85]. Modeling studies showed that multiple surface exposed Arg residues were prominent features of the heavy and light chains that conferred the highest ability to bind CL, particularly IS4V$_H$CDR3 (shown in Fig. 38.1).

In a subsequent study, we examined the importance of specific Arg residues in IS4V$_H$ and paired V$_L$ in CL binding (Giles et al., manuscript submitted). The distribution of Arg residues in CDRs of V$_H$ and V$_L$ sequences was altered by site-directed mutagenesis or CDR exchange. Of 4 Arg residues in IS4V$_H$CDR3 substituted to serines (Ser), 2 at positions 100 and 100g had a major influence on the strength of CL binding whilst 2 at positions 96 and 97 had no effect. In CDR exchange studies, V$_L$ containing 2 somatically mutated Arg residues in CDR1 were associated with elevated CL binding which was reduced significantly by substitution of one of these Arg residues with Ser. In contrast, Arg residues in V$_L$ CDR2 or CDR3 did not enhance CL binding, and in one case may have contributed to inhibition of this binding. In conclusion we found that subsets of Arg residues at specific locations in the CDRs of heavy and light chains of pathogenic aPL are important in determining their ability to bind CL as had been predicted previously by both sequence analysis and computer modeling.

There have been very few studies examining the relationship between sequence, structure, and pathogenicity of aPL. Sequence analysis of a range of aPL tested in the in vivo models of microcirculation by Pierangeli et al [60] revealed that there is no simple relationship between pathogenicity and strength of binding to CL. Two of the antibodies tested, IS1 and IS2 as previously mentioned, contained identical V_H and their light chains differed from each other by only 5 amino acids [59]. $IS1V_L$ contained slightly more mutations than $IS2V_L$ which improved its reactivity for antigen but abrogated its thrombogenic activity [60, 86].

Recently, Lieby et al [61] studied the effects of 5 randomly selected monoclonal aPL from a single patient with PAPS upon pregnant BALB/c mice and found that only 1 aPL (CIC15) induced fetal losses. The PL binding of this aPL was dependent upon annexin A5 but not β_2-GPI. $CIC15V_H$ contains only 2 R mutations in FR1 whilst $CIC15V_L$ has 3 R mutations – all Ser to Asn – in CDR1 2 of which are at sites of antigen contact. To clarify the role of these light chain mutations in pathogenicity of the Ab they were reverted to the germline configuration and expressed with the native $CIC15V_H$ sequence. The resulting almost germline Ab reacted with multiple self antigens, only partially lost its reactivity against PL, but was no longer dependent on annexin A5 and more importantly no longer induced fetal loss in BALB/c mice.

Therapeutic Implications

Currently, therapeutic recommendations in patients with APS consist of aspirin +/- anticoagulation with warfarin or heparin, depending upon whether the patient has previously experienced a vascular thrombotic event or pregnancy morbidity. Recurrence rates of up to 29% for thrombosis and mortality of up to 10% over a follow-up period of 10 years have been reported, despite the currently best available treatment of life long anticoagulation [87, 88]. Thus, it is important to develop new treatments for APS which are both more effective and more accurately targeted to the disease process. In particular, it may be advantageous to block or manipulate interactions between aPL and their major epitopes.

Sequence analysis of monoclonal aPL allows a greater understanding of how pathogenic aPL interact with their target antigen. Several groups have shown that the pathogenic effects of monoclonal anti– β_2-GPI antibodies in mice could be neutralized with synthetic peptides that bound to DI-II, DIII, and DIV [89, 90]. To be therapeutically useful, however, this approach requires the ability to identify a broadly cross-reactive peptide capable of binding with aPL in the majority of APS patients. Not all of these peptides meet these criteria [89].

An alternative approach would be to develop a drug containing the epitope for aPL that was able to tolerize aPL specific B cells leading to their anergy or deletion. Various studies using monoclonal aPL have identified possible epitopes on β_2-GPI, and the results from a number of studies are consistent with the location of dominant epitopes on domain I [reviewed in 74]. These findings have led to the development of a β_2-GPI–domain I-specific B cell tolerogen, LJP 1082, which has recently been evaluated in a phase I/II clinical trial [91]. The drug was well tolerated and led to a reduction in anti–β_2-GPI Ab titers in patients with APS. Further clinical trials are required to evaluate whether this reduction in anti–β_2-GPI Ab titers will lead to a reduction in manifestations of the APS.

Conclusion

From the published sequences of monoclonal aPL there is no evidence that particular human Ig V region genes are used preferentially to encode aPL. Somatic mutations which are antigen driven confer high specificity binding in IgG aPL but do not play a role in the formation of similar binding characteristics in the more specific IgM aPL. We have identified a common factor between these 2 groups of aPL, which is the presence of Arg, Asn, and Lys residues in CDRs and contact sites. These are germline encoded in the more specific IgM aPL but often arise due to somatic mutations in the IgG aPL. Our hypothesis is that the Arg, Asn, and Lys residues increase the affinity of binding via electrostatic interactions and hydrogen bonds with negatively charged epitopes upon PL and domain I of β_2-GPI. We have demonstrated the relative importance of certain surface exposed Arg residues at critical positions within the light chain CDR1 and heavy chain CDR3 of different human monoclonal aPL in conferring the ability to bind CL. It is now important to test the effects of sequence changes involving these amino acids on pathogenic functions of these aPL. Such tests may help to define the nature of interactions between aPL, PL, and β_2-GPI. This may eventually help in the development of drugs to interfere with those interactions, and thereby improve the treatment of APS.

References

1. Wilson WA, Gharavi AE, Koike T, et al. International consensus statement on preliminary classification criteria for definite antiphospholipid syndrome: report of an international workshop. Arthritis Rheum 1999;42:1309–1311.
2. Loizou S, Mackworth-Young CG, Cofiner C, et al. Heterogeneity of binding reactivity to different phospholipids of antibodies from patients with systemic lupus erythematosus (SLE) and with syphilis. Clin Exp Immunol 1990;80:171–176.
3. Alarcon-Segovia D, Deleze M, Oria CV, et al. Antiphospholipid antibodies and the antiphospholipid syndrome in systemic lupus erythematosus. A prospective analysis of 500 consecutive patients. Medicine (Baltimore) 1989;68:353–365.
4. Lynch A, Marlar R, Murphy J, et al. Antiphospholipid antibodies in predicting adverse pregnancy outcome. A prospective study. Ann Intern Med 1994;120:470–475.
5. Galli M, Comfurius P, Maassen C, et al. Anticardiolipin antibodies (ACA) directed not to cardiolipin but to a plasma protein cofactor. Lancet 1990;335:1544–1547.
6. McNeil HP, Simpson RJ, Chesterman CN, et al. Anti-phospholipid antibodies are directed against a complex antigen that includes a lipid-binding inhibitor of coagulation: beta 2- glycoprotein I (apolipoprotein H). Proc Natl Acad Sci U S A 1990;87:4120–4124.
7. Matsuura E, Igarashi Y, Fujimoto M, et al. Anticardiolipin cofactor(s) and differential diagnosis of autoimmune disease. Lancet 1990;336:177–178.
8. Ordi J, Selva A, Monegal F, et al. Anticardiolipin antibodies and dependence of a serum cofactor. A mechanism of thrombosis. J Rheumatol 1993;20:1321–1324.
9. Oosting JD, Derksen RH, Bobbink IW, et al. Antiphospholipid antibodies directed against a combination of phospholipids with prothrombin, protein C, or protein S: an explanation for their pathogenic mechanism? Blood 1993;81:2618–2625.
10. Bevers EM, Galli M, Barbui T, et al. Lupus anticoagulant IgG's (LA) are not directed to phospholipids only, but to a complex of lipid-bound human prothrombin. Thromb Haemost 1991;66:629–632.
11. Tsutsumi A, Matsuura E, Ichikawa K, et al. Antibodies to beta 2-glycoprotein I and clinical manifestations in patients with systemic lupus erythematosus. Arthritis Rheum 1996;39:1466–1474.
12. McNally T, Mackie IJ, Machin SJ, et al. Increased levels of beta 2 glycoprotein-I antigen and beta 2 glycoprotein-I binding antibodies are associated with a history of thromboembolic complications in patients with SLE and primary antiphospholipid syndrome. Br J Rheumatol 1995;34:1031–1036.

13. Kandiah DA, Sali A, Sheng Y, et al. Current insights into the "antiphospholipid" syndrome: clinical, immunological, and molecular aspects. Adv Immunol 1998;70:507–563.
14. Kohler G, Milstein C. Continuous cultures of fused cells secreting antibody of predefined specificity. Nature 1975;256:495–497.
15. Olsson L, Kaplan HS. Human-human hybridomas producing monoclonal antibodies of predefined antigenic specificity. Proc Natl Acad Sci U S A 1980;77:5429–5431.
16. Teng NN, Lam KS, Calvo Riera F, et al. Construction and testing of mouse–human heteromyelomas for human monoclonal antibody production. Proc Natl Acad Sci U S A 1983;80:7308–7312.
17. Chothia C, Lesk AM, Tramontano A, et al. Conformations of immunoglobulin hypervariable regions. Nature 1989;342:877–883.
18. Wu TT, Kabat EA. An analysis of the sequences of the variable regions of Bence Jones proteins and myeloma light chains and their implications for antibody complementarity. J Exp Med 1970;132:211–250.
19. Tonegawa S. Somatic generation of antibody diversity. Nature 1983;302:575–581.
20. Matsuda F, Shin EK, Nagaoka H, et al. Structure and physical map of 64 variable segments in the 3'0.8- megabase region of the human immunoglobulin heavy-chain locus. Nat Genet 1993;3:88–94.
21. Cook GP, Tomlinson IM, Walter G, et al. A map of the human immunoglobulin VH locus completed by analysis of the telomeric region of chromosome 14q. Nat Genet 1994;7:162–168.
22. Schable KF, Zachau HG. The variable genes of the human immunoglobulin kappa locus. Biol Chem Hoppe Seyler 1993;374:1001–1022.
23. Williams SC, Frippiat JP, Tomlinson IM, et al. Sequence and evolution of the human germline V lambda repertoire. J Mol Biol 1996;264:220–232.
24. Ignatovich O, Tomlinson IM, Jones PT, et al. The creation of diversity in the human immunoglobulin V(lambda) repertoire. J Mol Biol 1997;268:69–77.
25. Ignatovich O, Tomlinson IM, Popov AV, et al. Dominance of intrinsic genetic factors in shaping the human immunoglobulin Vlambda repertoire. J Mol Biol 1999;294:457–465.
26. Brezinschek HP, Foster SJ, Brezinschek RI, et al. Analysis of the human VH gene repertoire. Differential effects of selection and somatic hypermutation on human peripheral CD5(+)/IgM+ and CD5(-)/IgM+ B cells. J Clin Invest 1997;99:2488–2501.
27. Brezinschek HP, Foster SJ, Dorner T, et al. Pairing of variable heavy and variable kappa chains in individual naive and memory B cells. J Immunol 1998;160:4762–4767.
28. de Wildt RM, Hoet RM, van Venrooij WJ, et al. Analysis of heavy and light chain pairings indicates that receptor editing shapes the human antibody repertoire. J Mol Biol 1999;285:895–901.
29. de Wildt RM, Tomlinson IM, van Venrooij WJ, et al. Comparable heavy and light chain pairings in normal and systemic lupus erythematosus IgG(+) B cells. Eur J Immunol 2000;30:254–261.
30. Storb U. The molecular basis of somatic hypermutation of immunoglobulin genes. Curr Opin Immunol 1996;8:206–214.
31. Berek C, Milstein C. The dynamic nature of the antibody repertoire. Immunol Rev 1988;105:5–26.
32. Wagner SD, Neuberger MS. Somatic hypermutation of immunoglobulin genes. Annu Rev Immunol 1996;14:441–457.
33. Shlomchik MJ, Marshak-Rothstein A, Wolfowicz CB, et al. The role of clonal selection and somatic mutation in autoimmunity. Nature 1987;328:805–811.
34. Lossos IS, Tibshirani R, Narasimhan B, et al. The inference of antigen selection on Ig genes. J Immunol 2000;165:5122–5126.
35. Radic MZ, Weigert M. Genetic and structural evidence for antigen selection of anti-DNA antibodies. Annu Rev Immunol 1994;12:487–520.
36. Rahman A, Latchman DS, Isenberg DA. Immunoglobulin variable region sequences of human monoclonal anti-DNA antibodies. Semin Arthritis Rheum 1998;28:141–154.
37. MacCallum RM, Martin AC, Thornton JM. Antibody-antigen interactions: contact analysis and binding site topography. J Mol Biol 1996;262:732–745.
38. Chothia C, Gelfand I, Kister A. Structural determinants in the sequences of immunoglobulin variable domain. J Mol Biol 1998;278:457–479.
39. Radway-Bright EL, Inanc M, Isenberg DA. Animal models of the antiphospholipid syndrome. Rheumatology (Oxford) 1999;38:591–601.
40. Kita Y, Sumida T, Ichikawa K, et al. V gene analysis of anticardiolipin antibodies from MRL-lpr/lpr mice. J Immunol 1993;151:849–856.
41. Kita Y, Sumida T, Iwamoto I,, et al. V gene analysis of anti-cardiolipin antibodies from (NZW x BXSB) F1 mice. Immunology 1994;82:494–501.
42. Monestier M, et al. Monoclonal antibodies from NZW x BXSB F1 mice to beta2 glycoprotein I and cardiolipin. Species specificity and charge-dependent binding. J Immunol 1996;156:2631–2641.

43. Foster MH, MacDonald M, Barrett KJ, et al. VH gene analysis of spontaneously activated B cells in adult MRL- lpr/lpr mice. J558 bias is not limited to classic lupus autoantibodies. J Immunol 1991;147:1504–1511.

44. Rahman A, Menon S, Latchman DS, et al. Sequences of monoclonal antiphospholipid antibodies: variations on an anti-DNA antibody theme. Semin Arthritis Rheum 1996;26:515–525.

45. Dersimonian H, Schwartz RS, Barrett KJ, et al. Relationship of human variable region heavy chain germ-line genes to genes encoding anti-DNA autoantibodies. J Immunol 1987;139:2496–2501.

46. Hoch S, Schwaber J. Identification and sequence of the VH gene elements encoding a human anti-DNA antibody. J Immunol 1987;139:1689–1693.

47. Siminovitch KA, Misener V, Kwong PC, et al. A natural autoantibody is encoded by germline heavy and lambda light chain variable region genes without somatic mutation. J Clin Invest 1989;84:1675–1678.

48. Cairns E, Kwong PC, Misener V, et al. Analysis of variable region genes encoding a human anti-DNA antibody of normal origin. Implications for the molecular basis of human autoimmune responses. J Immunol 1989;143:685–691.

49. Logtenberg T, Young FM, Van Es JH, et al. Autoantibodies encoded by the most Jh-proximal human immunoglobulin heavy chain variable region gene. J Exp Med 1989;170:1347–1355.

50. Rioux JD, Zdarsky E, Newkirk MM, et al. Anti-DNA and anti-platelet specificities of SLE-derived autoantibodies: evidence for CDR2H mutations and CDR3H motifs. Mol Immunol 1995;32:683–696.

51. Hohmann A, Cairns E, Brisco M, et al. Immunoglobulin gene sequence analysis of anti-cardiolipin and anti- cardiolipin idiotype (H3) human monoclonal antibodies. Autoimmunity 1995;22:49–58.

52. Siminovitch KA, Misener V, Kwong PC, et al. A human anti-cardiolipin autoantibody is encoded by developementally restricted heavy and light chain variable region genes. Autoimmunity 1990;8:97–105.

53. Mariette X, Levy Y, Dubreuil ML, et al. Characterization of a human monoclonal autoantibody directed to cardiolipin/beta 2 glycoprotein I produced by chronic lymphocytic leukaemia B cells. Clin Exp Immunol 1993;94:385–390.

54. Harmer IJ, Loizou S, Thompson KM, et al. A human monoclonal antiphospholipid antibody that is representative of serum antibodies and is germline encoded. Arthritis Rheum 1995;38:1068–1076.

55. Denomme GA, Mahmoudi M, Cairns E, et al. Immunoglobulin V region sequences of two human antiplatelet monoclonal autoantibodies derived from B cells of normal origin. J Autoimmun 1994;7:521–535.

56. Demaison C, Ravirajan CT, Isenberg DA, et al. Analysis of variable region genes encoding anti-Sm and anti-cardiolipin antibodies from a systemic lupus erythematosus patient. Immunology 1995;86:487–494.

57. Lai CJ, Rauch J, Cho CS, et al. Immunological and molecular analysis of three monoclonal lupus anticoagulant antibodies from a patient with systemic lupus erythematosus. J Autoimmun 1998;11:39–51.

58. Gallart T, Benito C, Reverter JC, et al. True anti-anionic phospholipid immunoglobulin M antibodies can exert lupus anticoagulant activity. Br J Haematol 2002;116:875–886.

59. Chukwuocha RU, Zhu M, Cho CS, et al. Molecular and genetic characterizations of five pathogenic and two non- pathogenic monoclonal antiphospholipid antibodies. Mol Immunol 2002;39:299–311.

60. Pierangeli SS, Liu X, Espinola R, et al. Functional analyses of patient-derived IgG monoclonal anti-cardiolipin antibodies using in vivo thrombosis and in vivo microcirculation models. Thromb Haemost 2000;84:388–395.

61. Lieby P, Poindron V, Roussi S, et al. Pathogenic antiphospholipid antibody: an antigen selected needle in a haystack. Blood 2004. Epub ahead of print.

62. Tomlinson IM, et al. VBASE: A database of human immunoglobulin variable region genes. Cambridge, UK: MRC Centre for Protein Engineering: 1998.

63. Van Es JH, Aanstoot H, Gmelig-Meyling FH, et al. A human systemic lupus erythematosus-related anti-cardiolipin/single- stranded DNA autoantibody is encoded by a somatically mutated variant of the developmentally restricted 51P1 VH gene. J Immunol 1992;149:2234–2240.

64. Menon S, Rahman MA, Ravirajan CT, et al. The production, binding characteristics and sequence analysis of four human IgG monoclonal antiphospholipid antibodies. J Autoimmun 1997;10:43–57.

65. Chukwuocha RU, Hsiao ET, Shaw P, et al. Isolation, characterization and sequence analysis of five IgG monoclonal anti-beta 2-glycoprotein-1 and anti-prothrombin antigen- binding fragments generated by phage display. J Immunol 1999;163:4604–4611.

66. Ikematsu W, Luan FL, La Rosa L, et al. Human anticardiolipin monoclonal autoantibodies cause placental necrosis and fetal loss in BALB/c mice. Arthritis Rheum 1998;41:1026–1039.

67. von Landenberg C, Lackner KJ, von Landenberg P, et al. Isolation and characterization of two human monoclonal anti- phospholipid IgG from patients with autoimmune disease. J Autoimmun 1999;13:215–223.
68. Ehrenstein MR, Longhurst CM, Latchman DS, et al. Serological and genetic characterization of a human monoclonal immunoglobulin G anti-DNA idiotype. J Clin Invest 1994;93:1787–1797.
69. Lieby P, Soley A, Levallois H, et al. The clonal analysis of anticardiolipin antibodies in a single patient with primary antiphospholipid syndrome reveals an extreme antibody heterogeneity. Blood 2001;97:3820–3828.
70. Corbett SJ, Tomlinson IM, Sonnhammer EL, et al. Sequence of the human immunoglobulin diversity (D) segment locus: a systematic analysis provides no evidence for the use of DIR segments, inverted D segments, "minor" D segments or D-D recombination. J Mol Biol 1997;270:587–597.
71. Cox JP, Tomlinson IM, Winter G. A directory of human germ-line V kappa segments reveals a strong bias in their usage. Eur J Immunol 1994;24:827–836.
72. Dorner T, Farner NL, Lipsky PE. Ig lambda and heavy chain gene usage in early untreated systemic lupus erythematosus suggests intensive B cell stimulation. J Immunol 1999;163:1027–1036.
73. Muramatsu M, Kinoshita K, Fagarasan S, et al. Class switch recombination and hypermutation require activation-induced cytidine deaminase (AID), a potential RNA editing enzyme. Cell 2000;102:553–563.
74. Giles IP, Isenberg DA, Latchman DS, et al. How do antiphospholipid antibodies bind beta2-glyco-protein I? Arthritis Rheum 2003;48:2111–2121.
75. Rahman A, Haley J, Latchman DS. Molecular expression systems for anti-DNA antibodies–1. Lupus 2002;11:824–832.
76. Bird RE, Hardman KD, Jacobson JW, et al. Single-chain antigen-binding proteins. Science 1988;242:423–426.
77. Better M, Chang CP, Robinson RR, et al. Escherichia coli secretion of an active chimeric antibody fragment. Science 1988;240:1041–1043.
78. Blank M, Waisman A, Mozes E, et al. Characteristics and pathogenic role of anti-beta2-glycoprotein I single- chain Fv domains: induction of experimental antiphospholipid syndrome. Int Immunol 1999;11:1917–1926.
79. Cocca BA, Seal SN, D'Agnillo P, et al. Structural basis for autoantibody recognition of phos-phatidylserine- beta 2 glycoprotein I and apoptotic cells. Proc Natl Acad Sci U S A 2001;98:13826–13831.
80. Pereira B, Benedict CR, Le A, et al. Cardiolipin binding a light chain from lupus-prone mice. Biochemistry 1998;37:1430–1437.
81. Pewzner-Jung Y, Simon T, Eilat D. Structural elements controlling anti-DNA antibody affinity and their relationship to anti-phosphorylcholine activity. J Immunol 1996;156:3065–3073.
82. Kumar S, Kalsi J, Ravirajan CT, et al. Molecular cloning and expression of the Fabs of human autoantibodies in Escherichia coli. Determination of the heavy or light chain contribution to the anti-DNA/-cardiolipin activity of the Fab. J Biol Chem 2000;275:35129–35136.
83. Kumar S, Kalsi J, Latchman DS, et al. Expression of the Fabs of human auto-antibodies in Escherichia coli: optimization and determination of their fine binding characteristics and cross-reac-tivity. J Mol Biol 2001;308:527–539.
84. Kumar S, Nagl S, Kalsi JK, et al. Anti-cardiolipin/beta-2 glycoprotein activities co-exist on human anti-DNA antibody light chains. Mol Immunol 2003;40:517–530.
85. Giles IP, Haley J, Nagl S, et al. Relative importance of different human aPL derived heavy and light chains in the binding of aPL to cardiolipin. Mol Immunol 2003;40:49–60.
86. Zhu M, Olee T, Le DT, et al. Characterization of IgG monoclonal anti-cardiolipin/anti-beta2GP1 anti-bodies from two patients with antiphospholipid syndrome reveals three species of antibodies. Br J Haematol 1999;105:102–109.
87. Shah NM, Khamashta MA, Atsumi T, et al. Outcome of patients with anticardiolipin antibodies: a 10 year follow- up of 52 patients. Lupus 1998;7:3–6.
88. Schulman S, Svenungsson E, Granqvist S. Anticardiolipin antibodies predict early recurrence of thromboembolism and death among patients with venous thromboembolism following anticoagu-lant therapy. Duration of Anticoagulation Study Group. Am J Med 1998;104:332–338.
89. Blank M, Shoenfeld Y, Cabilly S, et al. Prevention of experimental antiphospholipid syndrome and endothelial cell activation by synthetic peptides. Proc Natl Acad Sci U S A 1999;96:5164–5168.
90. Pierangeli SS, Blank M, Liu X, et al. A peptide that shares similarity with bacterial antigens reverses thrombogenic properties of antiphospholipid antibodies in vivo. J Autoimmun 2004;22:217–225.
91. Horizon A, et al. Results of a randomised, placebo controlled, double blind phase 1/2 clinical trial (RCT) to assess the safety and tolerability of LJP 1082 in patients with antiphospholipid syndrome. Arthritis Rheum 2003;48:S364.

92. Radic MZ, Mackle J, Erikson J, et al. Residues that mediate DNA binding of autoimmune antibodies. J Immunol 1993;150:4966–4977.
93. Rahman A, Haley J, Radway-Bright E, et al. The Importance of somatic mutations in the V(lambda) gene 2a2 in human monoclonal anti-DNA antibodies. J Mol Biol 2001;307:149–160.
94. Katz JB, Limpanasithikul W, Diamond B. Mutational analysis of an autoantibody: differential binding and pathogenicity. J Exp Med 1994;180:925–932.
95. Giles IP, Haley JD, Nagl S, et al. A systematic analysis of sequences of human antiphospholipid and anti- beta2-glycoprotein I antibodies: the importance of somatic mutations and certain sequence motifs. Semin Arthritis Rheum 2003;32:246–265.

39   Apoptosis and Antiphospholipid Antibodies

Keith B. Elkon, Neelufar Mozaffarian, and Natalia Tishkevich

Introduction

In the early 1980s, a motley crew of itinerants strove to discover the cause of systemic lupus erythematosus (SLE) in Graham Hughes' laboratory at the Hammersmith Hospital, London. The crew included myself (KBE), Azzudin Gharavi, Bernie Colaco, and others. Having presented a stimulating paper by Robert Schwartz at a journal club demonstrating that some murine anti-DNA monoclonal antibodies cross react with phospholipids [1], Aziz, Bernie, and I decided to test the same idea in human SLE, and Graham decided to re-explore the clinical associations of anticardiolipin (aCL) autoantibodies. The resulting publications [2, 3] were a start and led to the subsequent collaboration between Aziz and Nigel Harris, and the development of the quantitative solid-phase immunoassay for antiphospholipid antibodies (aPL) that transformed the field.

In this brief review, we will provide an outline of apoptosis and discuss its relevance to aPL and the development of systemic autoimmunity.

Why Is Apoptosis Clinically Relevant to aPL and Systemic Autoimmunity?

A number of clinical observations have focused attention on the products of apoptotic cells as antigens or immunogens in SLE:

1. An increase in apoptosis of SLE peripheral blood mononuclear cells (PBMC) in vitro has been observed [4] and has been correlated with lymphopenia in the patient [5]. Freshly isolated lymphocytes from patients show high annexin V binding [6] and elevated caspase 3 functional activity [7], suggesting that accelerated apoptosis occurs in vivo.
2. SLE macrophages *may* have a reduced uptake of apoptotic cells in vitro [8].
3. Nucleosomes (histones complexed to DNA), a product of apoptotic cells (see below) are detected in the circulation of SLE patients with active disease [9].
4. Nucleosomes are more strongly antigenic than DNA or histones alone, and antibodies to nucleosomes precede those to DNA and histones [10, 11].

5. Nucleosomes, but not isolated DNA or histones, deposit in the glomeruli, suggesting that it is in situ fixation of nucleosomes, rather than DNA/anti-DNA immune complexes that causes lupus nephritis [12, 13].
6. SLE antigens are redistributed to apoptotic blebs when cells such as keratinocytes undergo programmed cell death [14]. Some, but not all of these antigens undergo modification, including cleavage and phosphorylation. It is possible that this makes them more antigenic.
7. Phosphatidylserine (PS), the negatively charged phospholipids that flips from the inside to outside of the dying cell (see below), may serve as an antigen for aCL [15] and PS (either on activated platelets or apoptotic cells) provides a scaffold for the coagulation cascade [16, 17].

In addition to SLE, aPL have been detected in other autoimmune diseases where apoptosis is abnormal. For example, impaired Fas mediated apoptosis results in massive lymphadenopathy and systemic autoimmunity in humans [18, 19]. It appears that aPL directed at phospholipids and at related proteins such as β_2-glycoprotein I (β_2-GPI), prothrombin, and annexin V are a common feature in these patients [20].

aPL Bind to Many Different Antigens Derived from Apoptotic Cells

The aPL traditionally refer to both aCL and lupus anticoagulant antibodies (LA), identified by in vitro assays that quantify aCL binding or prolongation of coagulation, respectively. Although prototypic aPL bind to negatively charged phospholipids, aPL react with a broad array of cell membrane derived phospholipids and their associated proteins that include not only cardiolipin (CL), but also phosphatidylserine (PS), phosphatidycholine (PC), phosphatidyethanolamine (PE), β_2-GPI, prothrombin, protein C, protein S, kininogen, and annexin V (see other chapters in this volume).

The polyclonal autoantibodies that occur in patients are heterogeneous with respect to their fine binding specificities, affinities, effects on coagulation, and their role in the antiphospholipid syndrome (APS). Although these antibodies could be generated by polyclonal B cell activation or cross-reactivity in an immune response to foreign antigen (for a review of aPL generated via infectious disease-related molecular mimicry see [21]), in this chapter we will provide evidence to support the argument that aPL are generated in response to dead and dying cells. This evidence includes the localization of CL in mitochondrial membranes (a critical site involved in the regulation of apoptosis as discussed below); the translocation of another negatively charged phospholipid, PS, which is normally located on the inner cytoplasmic leaflet of the lipid bilayer to the outer cell surface during apoptosis; and, finally, we review studies showing that aPL can be generated by immunization of animals with dying cells.

What Is Apoptosis?

The term *apoptosis* was coined by Kerr, Wyllie, and Currie in 1972 to describe the form of cell death characterized by shrinkage, nuclear condensation, and cell blebbing [22]. Notably, the process of apoptosis is ATP dependent, and the observable changes in the nucleus and cell membrane are preceded by active bi-directional redistribution of phospholipids in the cytosolic membrane via the activity of scramblase, a non-specific lipid translocator [23]. Following re-distribution of these molecules, the orderly death program of apoptosis results in the formation of smaller blebs or "apoptotic bodies," membrane bound packages of cytosolic contents which elicit phagocytosis and an anti-inflammatory response (characterized by the production of transforming growth factor-beta and prostaglandin E2) [24]. The apoptosis-induced activation of scramblase is integral to this process, as the appropriate recognition of and response to apoptotic bodies by phagocytes depends upon the surface presentation of typically sequestered and less accessible phospholipids and associated intracellular proteins. Because patients with Scott's syndrome, an inherited defect in calcium-induced scramblase activity, still flip PS to the outside of the membrane of apoptotic cells, it is suggested that ABC1 may be the key lipid transporter in apoptotic cells [25].

Cellular necrosis differs from apoptosis in that it is typified by disorderly fragmentation of chromatin as well as severe damage to the mitochondria, resulting in uncontrolled release of cell products and a reactive pro-inflammatory response with the production of cytokines such as tumor necrosis factor-alpha, interleukin (IL)-1, and IL-6 [24]. However, it should be noted that the distinction between apoptosis and necrosis is not absolute. The same inducers (e.g., ischemia, hydrogen peroxide) may produce either apoptosis or necrosis depending on the dose and, consequently, the severity of the injury. The cell fate decision is determined, in part, by cellular energy reserves such as ATP [26]. Some types of injury may initially cause apoptosis followed by necrosis ("post-apoptotic necrosis"), especially if there is a delay in removal of the apoptotic cells. This overlap is important, as leakage of cellular material (heat shock proteins, HMGB-1, or nucleic acids themselves) promote activation of the innate immune system and may be necessary for immune responses to self.

How Does Apoptosis Occur?

A simplified schematic diagram of an apoptotic cell and the key pathways that regulate apoptosis are shown in Figure 39.1. For a much more detailed discussion of the biochemistry of apoptosis, the reader is referred to a series of reviews in *Oncogene* (Nov. 24 and 27, 2003). Death of a cell may forced upon the cell by a receptor mediated pathway such as Fas/ APO-1/ CD95 [Fig. 39.1(A)] or be the result of an intrinsic program that works through the mitochondria [Fig. 39.1(B) or endoplasmic reticulum [Fig. 39.1(C)]. Regardless of the initiating event, cysteine rich proteases (caspases) that have specificity for aspartic acid residues become activated (caspase 8 or 10 in the case of Fas) or caspase 9 in the case of mitochondrial pathways. These initiator caspases induce a cascade that activates the effector caspases such as caspase 3, 6, and 7. The caspase cascade results in the cleavage of a number of substrates that include certain autoantigens (e.g., chromatin through the cleavage of ICAD releasing CAD [27],U1- RNP, DNA-protein kinase [28]) as well as structural proteins within the cytosol, nuclear, and plasma membranes. Of particular interest to autoimmunity is the cleavage of chromatin into nucleosome fragments and the translocation of negatively charged phospholipids from the inside to the outside of the cell membrane as mentioned above (Fig. 39.1). Also, in the context of the association between aCL and clotting disorders discussed extensively in this volume, the

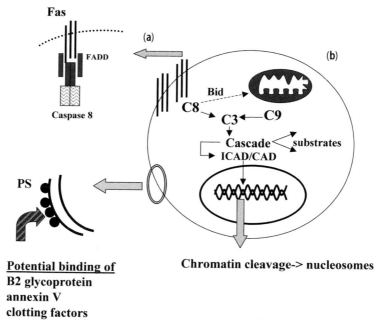

Figure 39.1. The fundamental pathways of apoptosis. Cell death can be initiated by multiple pathways, including an extrinsic ligand induced pathway (left panel), an intrinsic pathway mediated by the mitochondria (middle panel), and an intrinsic pathway mediated through the endoplasmic reticulum (ER) (right panel). Death receptors may activate the intrinsic pathway in that caspase 8 cleaves a pro-apoptotic molecule, Bid, which causes release of cytochrome c from mitochondria and amplification of the caspase cascade. Examples of stimuli that can induce each of these pathways are shown. Note that these pathways differ in the upstream caspases activated, but converge to cleave the effector caspases such as caspase 3 during execution of apoptosis. During ER stress, unfolded proteins release the ER chaperone protein, Bip, from the stress sensor proteins, IRE and PERK. The alterations that occur during dissolution of the cell are too numerous to mention but a few are highlighted in view of their potential relevance to aPL and autoimmunity. Exposure of phosphatidylserine (PS) on the cell surface (lower left) provides a simple means for detection of apoptotic cells through binding to annexin V and may be relevant to the generation of aPL autoantibodies and coagulation disorders in vivo. Cleavage products of chromatin (lower middle) as well as proteins, such as lamins and DNA-PK, may be antigenic in lupus. Abbreviations: Cyt C = cytochrome c; PS = phosphatidylserine; LPC = lysophosphatidylcholine.

exposure of membrane PS potentiates the coagulation cascade by acting as a scaffold for the tenase and prothrombinase complexes [25].

What Happens to Apoptotic Cells In Vivo?

Within the immune system alone, more than 10^8 apoptotic cells are removed from the body each day. These apoptotic cells are generated in vast numbers in the central lymphoid organs such as the thymus and bone marrow by out-of-frame rearrangements of antigen receptors, negative selection, or simple "neglect." In addition, a significant load of apoptotic cells is also produced in the peripheral immune system due to the relatively short life span of lymphocytes and myeloid cells as well as specialized sites of secondary selection of high-affinity B cells in germinal centers. The specialized sites of selection (thymus, bone marrow, and lymphoid follicles) have remarkably efficient phagocytes that remove the dying cells rapidly. Apoptotic cells not only induce immunosuppressive cytokines by macrophages, but also inhibit pro-inflammatory responses by dendritic cells. Both of these phenomena likely result in tolerization of T cells to self antigens [29].

Key alterations occur in the cell membrane of the dying cell that alert macrophages to phagocytose the cell and degrade it in a non-inflammatory fashion. Although a large number of receptors and ligands have been implicated in a two-step tether-and-tickle process of phagocytosis [30], here we will focus on the 2 categories of receptors that involve the phospholipids, PS and PC. The negatively charged phospholipid, PS is recognized by a specific PS receptor (PSR) on macrophages and promotes phagocytosis [31]. In view of the proposed cross-reactivity of aPL between PS and CL [15], it is of considerable interest that aCL antibodies appear to preferentially bind to oxidized CL and that PS on the surface of apoptotic cells is also frequently oxidized [32]. PS is also known to bind to a number of proteins including β_2-GPI), Gas6, milk fat globule epidermal growth factor 8 (MFGE-8), and annexins I and V, thereby allowing the protein bridges to interact with different receptors (Fig. 39.2). Significantly, deletion of at least 2 of these pathways in mice results in defective clearance of apoptotic cells and lupus-like autoimmunity [34, 35]. It remains to be determined what role, if any, anti-CL antibodies have in altering the clearance of dying cells (see Fig. 39.3).

A second mechanism involving aPL and the clearance of apoptotic cells relates to complement deposition on the cell surface [38]. It is well known that deficiencies of early complement components leads to lupus, but only recently has it been reported that deficiency of early complement components lead to defective phagocytosis of apoptotic cells [39]. Because IgM deficiency also predisposes to lupus, at least in mice [40, 41], we recently related these observations by showing that polyclonal

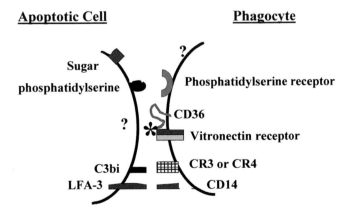

Figure 39.2. The role of phospholipids as ligands for the phagocytosis of apoptotic cells. There are numerous receptors and ligands implicated in the clearance of apoptotic cells [33]. At least 2 phospholipids, LPC and PS, serve as antigens, scaffolds, or activators of cascades as shown. Abbreviations: $av\beta_{3/5}$ = the vitronectin receptor; β_2-GPI = β_2-glycoprotein I; C = complement; MFGE-8 = milk fat globule epidermal growth factor 8; PSR = phosphatidylserine receptor.

Apoptotic Cell   B cell

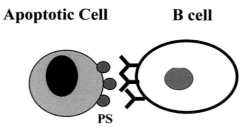

PS

Figure 39.3. Possible immunological consequences of apoptosis in relation to aPL and autoimmunity. Antibodies to the different (modified) phospholipids on the cell surface may have different consequences for immune activation or tolerance. As shown on the left, IgM anti-LPC antibody activation of complement promotes clearance, which is associated with immunosuppressive cytokines [36]. Similarly, bridging proteins (see Fig. 39.2) presumably also facilitate silent clearance of apoptotic cells [24]. However, excess coating with certain bridging proteins can, under certain circumstances, reduce phagocytosis and lead to immunization [37]. Another way in which aCL may activate phagocytes is through engagement of FcgR. Finally, it is possible that PS exposure may act as a polyvalent, T independent antigen capable of cross-linking surface immunoglobulin on the surface of B lymphocytes.

natural IgM antibodies bind to lyso-phosphatidylcholine (LPC) and activate complement [42] (Fig. 39.2). The potential role of IgM and complement in the clearance of apoptotic cells and tolerization of T cells is illustrated in Figure 39.3. This topic is dealt with in greater depth elsewhere [43]. It should be emphasized that the beneficial functions of the early complement components should be contrasted with the damaging effects of the later complement components (C5-9) that are implicated in nephritis and fetal loss (the latter associated with aCL).

Can Dying Cells Induce aPL In Vivo?

The fact that autoantibodies target many of the products of apoptotic cells does not necessarily mean that the apoptotic cells *induced* the immune response. It is, however, particularly intriguing that aCL have been shown to bind with greater affinity to oxidized CL [44] and there is good evidence that PS that has translocated to the outside of the cell is also oxidized [32]. To address whether apoptotic cells can be immunogenic, apoptotic thymocytes were injected in the absence of adjuvant into normal syngeneic mice and autoantibody production was monitored. The results of these studies showed that low levels of autoantibodies against ssDNA and negatively charged phospholipids can be generated following immunization with apoptotic cells, but that autoantibodies against protein antigens were not [45]. Although it is possible that the dose, duration, or mode of administration may not accurately mimic exposure that occurs in spontaneous disease, it appears that a large load of dying cells can initiate humoral autoimmunity, but does not lead to clinical expression of disease. In a recent study, it was shown that immunization of apoptotic cells with a mutant form of MFGE-8 that binds to PS on apoptotic cells but is not efficiently phagocytosed, also stimulates the production of aCL autoantibodies [46].

The generation of aPL in these studies is intriguing. It is possible that exposure of a multivalent antigen like PS on the cell surface may be sufficient to break B, but not T, cell tolerance, accounting for the transient nature of the immune response [45] (see Fig. 39.3). An important question for the future is what are the *additional* requirements for protracted autoimmunity? Could exposure to larger numbers of apoptotic cells, defective uptake of apoptotic cells, alteration of macrophage or dendritic cell responses (cytokine production, antigen processing), or T cell defects generate clinical expression of disease?

Conclusions and Future Directions

In an editorial on apoptosis published more than a decade ago, we asked whether there was "too little or too much apoptosis" in SLE [47]. It is now apparent that only rare SLE patients have reduced apoptosis signaling through Fas or Fas ligand [48, 49]. As discussed above, there is some evidence of enhanced apoptosis in SLE and this is also suggested by lymphopenia, an ACR criterion for the disease. More information is required on cell turnover in patients in vivo. In contrast to these quantitative aspects, increasing emphasis has recently been placed on qualitative aspects of apoptosis (how cells die) and how the corpses are dealt with (Fig. 39.3). As mentioned, the complement deficiencies in humans and the knockout experiments in mice argue strongly that deficient opsonization or aberrant handling of the dying cells lead to immune responses to self. This insight needs to be translated to the human situation and, once well understood, to be corrected.

While it is reasonable to propose that aCL are generated in response to PS or CL in apoptotic cells, and there is experimental evidence to support the induction of aCL by dying cells, it must be acknowledged that the stimulus for aPL generation in human disease remains uncertain. It would be useful to gain at least correlative data linking apoptosis and aPL. Finally, the discovery that a different category of aPL, IgM natural antibodies to LPC, provide a protective function by promoting complement fixation and clearance of apoptotic cells [42, Kowalewski, submitted], provides a new window for exploration of the mechanisms of autoantibody production and the clinical expression of disease.

References

1. Lafer E, Rauch J, Andrzejewski C, et al. Polyspecific monoclonal lupus autoantibodies reactive with both polynucleotides and phospholipids. J Exp Med 1981;153:897–904.
2. Boey ML, Gharavi AE, Elkon KB, Loizou S, Hughes GRV. Thrombosis in SLE, striking association with the presence of circulating "lupus anticoagulant". Br Med J 1983;287:1021–1023.
3. Colaco CB, Elkon KB. The lupus anticoagulant, a disease marker in ANA negative lupus, yet cross reactive with autoantibodies to ds DNA. Arthritis Rheum 1985;28:67–74.
4. Emlen W, Niebur J-A, Kadera R. Accelerated in vitro apoptosis of lymphocytes from patients with systemic lupus erythematosus. J Immunol 1994;152:3685–3692.
5. Georgescu L, Vakkalanka RK, Elkon KB, Crow MK. Interleukin-10 promotes activation-induced cell death of SLE lymphocytes mediated by Fas ligand. J Clin Invest 1997;100:2622–2633.
6. Perniok A, Wedekind F, Herrmann M, Specker C, Schneider M. High levels of circulating early apoptotic peripheral blood mononuclear cells in systemic lupus erythematosus. Lupus 1998;7:113–118.
7. Ohsako S, Elkon KB. Increased caspase-like activity in freshly isolated lymphocytes from SLE patients. Arthritis Rheum 1998;41:S70.
8. Herrmann M, Voll RE, Zoller OM, Hagenhofer M, Ponner BB, Kalden JR. Impaired phagocytosis of apoptotic cell material by monocyte-derived macrophages from patients with systemic lupus erythematosus. Arthritis Rheum 1998;41:1241–1250.

9. Rumore PM, Steinman CR. Endogenous circulating DNA in systemic lupus erythematosus, occurrence as multimeric complexes bound to histone. J Clin Invest 1990;86:69–74.
10. Burlingame RW, Rubin RL, Balderas RS, Theofilopoulos AN. Genesis and evolution of anti-chromatin autoantibodies in murine lupus implicates T-dependent immunization and self antigen. J Clin Invest 1993;91:1687–1696.
11. Amoura Z, Chabre H, Koutouzov S, et al. Nucleosome restricted antibodies are detected before anti-ds DNA and/ or anti-histone antibodies in serum of MRL-Mp lpr/lpr and +/+ mice, and are present in kidney eluates of lupus mice with proteinuria. Arthritis Rheum 1994;37:1684–1688.
12. Termaat RM, Assmann KJ, Dijkman HB, van Gompel F, Smeenk RJ, Berden JH. Anti-DNA antibodies can bind to the glomerulus via two distinct mechanisms. Kidney Int 1992;42:1363–1371.
13. Kramers C, Hylkema MN, van Bruggen MCJ, et al. Anti-nucleosome antibodies complexed to nucleosomal antigens show anti-DNA reactivity and bind to rat glomerular basement membrane in vivo. J Clin Invest 1994;94:568–577.
14. Casciola-Rosen LA, Anhalt G, Rosen A. Autoantigens targeted in systemic lupus erythematosus are clustered in two populations of surface structures on apoptotic keratinocytes. J Exp Med 1994;179:1317–1330.
15. Price BE, Rauch J, Shia MA, et al. Antiphospholipid autoantibodies bind to apoptotic, but not viable, thymocytes in a beta2-glycoprotein I-dependent manner. J Immunol 1996;157:2201–2208.
16. Bach R, Gentry R, Nemerson Y. Factor VII binding to tissue factor in reconstituted phospholipid vesicles: induction of cooperativity by phosphatidylserine. Biochemistry 1986;25:4007–4020.
17. Rosing J, van Rijn JL, Bevers EM, van Dieijen G, Comfurius P, Zwaal RF. The role of activated human platelets in prothrombin and factor X activation. Blood 1985;65:319–332.
18. Vaishnaw AK, Orlinick JR, Chu JL, Krammer PH, Chao MV, Elkon KB. Molecular basis for the apoptotic defects in patients with CD95 (Fas/Apo-1) mutations. J Clin Invest 1999;103:355–363.
19. Martin DA, Zheng L, Siegel RM, et al. Defective CD95/APO-1/Fas signal complex formation in the human autoimmune lymphoproliferative syndrome, type Ia [in process citation]. Proc Natl Acad Sci U S A 1999;96:4552–4557.
20. Pittoni V, Sorice M, Circella A, et al. Specificity of antinuclear and antiphospholipid antibodies in sera of patients with autoimmune lymphoproliferative disease (ALD). Clin Exp Rheumatol 2003;21:377–385.
21. Gharavi AE, Pierangeli SS, Harris EN. Viral origin of antiphospholipid antibodies: endothelial cell activation and thrombus enhancement by CMV peptide-induced APL antibodies. Immunobiology 2003;207:37–42.
22. Kerr JFR, Wyllie AH, Currie AR. Apoptosis: a basic biological phenomenon with wide-ranging implications in tissue kinetics. Br J Cancer 1972;26:239–257.
23. Zwaal RF, Schroit AJ. Pathophysiologic implications of membrane phospholipid asymmetry in blood cells. Blood 1997;89:1121–1132.
24. Fadok VA, Bratton DL, Konowal A, Freed PW, Westcott JY, Henson PM. Macrophages that have ingested apoptotic cells in vitro inhibit proinflammatory cytokine production through autocrine/paracrine mechanisms involving TGF-beta, PGE2, and PAF. J Clin Invest 1998;101:890–898.
25. Zwaal RF, Comfurius P, Bevers EM. Scott syndrome, a bleeding disorder caused by defective scrambling of membrane phospholipids. Biochim Biophys Acta 2004;1636:119–128.
26. Leist M, Single B, Castoldi AF, Kuhnle S, Nicotera P. Intracellular adenosine triphosphate (ATP) concentration: a switch in the decision between apoptosis and necrosis. J Exp Med 1997;185:1481–1486.
27. Enari M, Sakahira H, Yokoyama H, Okawa K, Iwamatsu A, Nagata S. A caspase-activated DNase that degrades DNA during apoptosis, and its inhibitor ICAD. Nature 1998;391:43–50.
28. Casciola-Rosen LA, Anhalt GJ, Rosen A. DNA-dependent protein kinase is one of a subset of autoantigens specifically cleaved early during apoptosis. J Exp Med 1995;182:1625–1634.
29. Hawiger D, Inaba K, Dorsett Y, et al. Dendritic cells induce peripheral T cell unresponsiveness under steady state conditions in vivo. J Exp Med 2001;194:769–779.
30. Somersan S, Bhardwaj N. Tethering and tickling: a new role for the phosphatidylserine receptor. J Cell Biol 2001;155:501–504.
31. Fadok VA, Voelker DR, Campbell PA, Cohen JJ, Bratton DL, Henson PM. Exposure of phosphatidyl serine on the surface of apoptotic lymphocytes triggers specific recognition and removal by macrophages. J Immunol 1992;148:2207–2216.
32. Kagan VE, Gleiss B, Tyurina YY, et al. A role for oxidative stress in apoptosis: oxidation and externalization of phosphatidylserine is required for macrophage clearance of cells undergoing Fas-mediated apoptosis. J Immunol 2002;169:487–499.

33. Savill J, Dransfield I, Gregory C, Haslett C. A blast from the past: clearance of apoptotic cells regulates immune responses. Nat Rev Immunol 2002;2:965–975.
34. Scott RS, McMahon EJ, Pop SM, et al. Phagocytosis and clearance of apoptotic cells is mediated by MER. Nature 2001;411:207–211.
35. Hanayama R, Tanaka M, Miyasaka K, et al. Autoimmune disease and impaired uptake of apoptotic cells in MFG-E8-deficient mice. Science 2004;304:1147–1150.
36. Gershov D, Kim S, Brot N, Elkon KB. C-reactive protein binds to apoptotic cells, protects the cells from assembly of the terminal complement components, and sustains an antiinflammatory innate immune response. Implications for systemic autoimmunity. J Exp Med 2000;192:1353–1364.
37. Stach CM, Turnay X, Voll RE, et al. Treatment with annexin V increases immunogenicity of apoptotic human T-cells in Balb/c mice. Cell Death Differ 2000;7:911–915.
38. Mevorach D, Mascarenhas J, Gershov DA, Elkon KB. Complement-dependent clearance of apoptotic cells by human macrophages. J Exp Med 1998;188:2313–2320.
39. Botto M, Dell'Agnola C, Bygrave AE, et al. Homozygous C1q deficiency causes glomerulonephritis associated with multiple apoptotic bodies. Nat Genet 1998;19:56–59.
40. Boes M, Schmidt T, Linkemann K, Beaudette BC, Marshak-Rothstein A, Chen J. Accelerated development of IgG autoantibodies and autoimmune disease in the absence of secreted IgM. Proc Natl Acad Sci U S A 2000;97:1184–1189.
41. Ehrenstein MR, Cook HT, Neuberger MS. Deficiency in serum immunoglobulin (Ig)M predisposes to development of IgG autoantibodies. J Exp Med 2000;191:1253–1258.
42. Kim SJ, Gershov D, Ma X, Brot N, Elkon KB. I-PLA(2) activation during apoptosis promotes the exposure of membrane lysophosphatidylcholine leading to binding by natural immunoglobulin M antibodies and complement activation. J Exp Med 2002;196:655–665.
43. Kim SJ, Gershov D, Ma X, Brot N, Elkon KB. Opsonization of apoptotic cells and its effect on macrophage and T cell immune responses. Ann N Y Acad Sci 2003;987:68–78.
44. Matsuura E, Igarashi Y, Yasuda T, Triplett DA, Koike T. Anticardiolipin antibodies recognize beta 2-glycoprotein I structure altered by interacting with an oxygen modified solid phase surface. J Exp Med 1994;179:457–462.
45. Mevorach D, Zhou J-L, Song X, Elkon KB. Systemic exposure to irradiated apoptotic cells induces autoantibody production. J Exp Med 1998;188:387–392.
46. Asano K, Miwa M, Miwa K, et al. Masking of phosphatidylserine inhibits apoptotic cell engulfment and induces autoantibody production in mice. J Exp Med 2004;200:459–67.
47. Elkon KB. Apoptosis in SLE – too little or too much? Clin Exp Rheum 1994;12:553–559.
48. Wu J, Wilson J, He J, Xiang L, Schur PH, Mountz JD. Fas ligand mutation in a patient with systemic lupus erythematosus and lymphoproliferative disease. J Clin Invest 1996;98:1107–1113.
49. Vaishnaw AK, Toubi E, Ohsako S, et al. Both quantitative and qualitative apoptotic defects are associated with the clinical spectrum of disease, including systemic lupus erythematosus in humans with Fas (APO-1/CD95) mutations. Arthritis Rheum 1999;42:1833–1842.

40 Accelerated Atherogenesis and Antiphospholipid Antibodies

Eiji Matsuura, Kazuko Kobayashi, and Luis R. Lopez

Introduction

Atherosclerosis is a major health concern of worldwide importance. The causal relationship between atherosclerosis and cholesterol metabolism is well established. However, newer inflammatory and immunologic mechanisms are emerging as relevant factors for the initiation and progression of atherosclerotic lesions. In particular, the oxidation of low-density lipoprotein (LDL) has been identified as an early pro-atherogenic event that promotes the formation of macrophage derived foam cells [1–4].

The increased cardiovascular morbidity and mortality recently reported in patients with systemic autoimmune diseases is a likely consequence of the accelerated (or premature) development of atherosclerosis. These findings have suggested a contributing role of autoimmunity in the development of atherosclerosis. Antiphospholipid syndrome (APS) is characterized by venous and arterial thromboembolic complications associated with high serum levels of antiphospholipid antibodies. APS is frequently diagnosed in the context of an autoimmune disease [5, 6]. The exact mechanism(s) by which anticardiolipin (aCL), lupus anticoagulants (LA), and/or other antiphospholipid antibodies promote thrombosis is not completely understood. It is now widely agreed that β_2-glycoprotein I (β_2-GPI) plays a central role in APS, and more importantly, represents a major antigenic target for antiphospholipid antibodies [7–11].

Oxidized LDL (oxLDL) is the principal lipoprotein found in atherosclerotic lesions, and it co-localizes with β_2-GPI and immunoreactive lymphocytes [12]. It was also reported that aCL antibodies from patients with systemic lupus erythematosus (SLE) cross-reacted with malondialdehyde (MDA) modified LDL [13], and that anti–β_2-GPI antibodies were associated with arterial thrombosis [14, 15]. These findings further indicated the participation of antiphospholipid antibodies in atherogenesis. More recently, we have demonstrated that oxLDL binds to β_2-GPI, and that these complexes (oxLDL/β_2-GPI) can be found in the blood stream of patients with various autoimmune and chronic inflammatory diseases, such as SLE, APS, chronic renal disease, diabetes mellitus, as well as in some patients with "acute" myocardial infarction [16].

IgG antibodies to oxLDL/β_2-GPI were detected only in SLE and APS patients and were strongly associated with arterial thrombosis. Further, immune complexes containing oxLDL, β_2-GPI, and IgG anti–β_2-GPI antibodies have also been detected in SLE and APS patients [16]. Our recent in vitro experiments showed that oxLDL/β_2-GPI complexes were internalized by macrophages via an anti–β_2-GPI antibody mediated phagocytosis [17–19]. Thus, circulating IgG immune complexes containing oxLDL and β_2-GPI may be atherogenic. In contrast, recent reports indicated that natural antibodies (mainly of the IgM class) derived from hyperlipidemic mice reduced the incidence of atherosclerosis in experimental models [20–23].

Atherogenic Mechanisms

Atherosclerosis is a pathological condition in which arteries undergo thickening of the intima causing a decrease in their elasticity. The aorta, coronary, and cerebral arteries are blood vessels most commonly affected by atherosclerosis. The appearance of lipid laden foam cells is a characteristic hystologic finding in early atherosclerotic lesions. Figure 40.1(A) depicts a current consensus of different events leading to the initial stages of atherosclerosis. Hypercholesterolemia is commonly associated with an elevation of LDL, which is the lipoprotein that accumulates in foam cells. Increasing LDL blood levels together with arterial shear stress may produce a vascular inflammatory response, with the adherence of circulating monocytes to endothelial cells and the migration of these elements (LDL, oxLDL, and monocytes) into the intima. The oxidative modification of LDL may be further catalyzed by inflammatory cells at the site of the arterial lesion, resulting in foam cell formation (oxLDL loaded macrophages). Numerous pro-inflammatory molecules and/or adhesion molecules also participate in the development of atherosclerosis. These molecules participate under complicated interrelated conditions and include: monocyte chemo-attractant protein-1 (MCP-1), macrophage colony-stimulating factor (M-CSF), interferon-γ (IFN-γ), tumor necrosis factor-α (TNF-α), interleukine-4 (IL-4), platelet-derived growth factor (PDGF), heparin-binding EGF-like growth factor (HB-EGF), intercellular adhesion molecules (ICAMs), vascular cell adhesion molecules (VCAM-1), endothelial selectin (E-selectin), and so on [24–27]. In addition, macrophage scavenger receptors and various cell–cell interactions, possibly via CD40 and CD40 ligands, have been reported to be involved in the development of atheroma [28].

When the endothelial surface of the atherosclerotic lesion becomes damaged and unstable, it may rupture. This event is followed by the activation of blood coagulation mechanisms such as platelet aggregation and thrombi formation, which can result in a complete occlusion of the blood vessel and tissue or organ necrosis, as seen in acute myocardial and cerebral infarction.

Macrophages and Scavenger Receptors

Macrophages receptors for the specific uptake of LDL were first described by Goldstein and Brown [29, 30]. Theses receptors are downregulated to prevent lipid overloading. Another type of macrophage receptor was later described for chemically modified LDLs and named scavenger receptors [29, 31]. These scavenger receptors are not downregulated, and may lead to the accumulation of massive amounts of intracellular lipids in macrophages, resulting in the formation of macrophage derived foam cells. Initially, acetylated LDL was used as a ligand to study scavenger receptors, but this acetylation was not seen under physiological conditions. In contrast, oxLDL was described as a physiological ligand for scavenger receptors, and it was generated by peroxidation of LDL when co-cultured with endothelial cells or when incubated with a metal ion such as Cu^{2+} or Fe^{2+}.

Scavenger receptors (i.e., SR-A) were first cloned by Kodama and his colleagues [32, 33], and shown to be specific for both acetylated LDL and Cu^{2+}–oxLDL. This was followed by the description of several different types of scavenger receptors, that is, MARCO (a novel macrophage receptor with collagenous structure), SR-B1, CD36, Macrosialin, CD68, LOX-1, SREC, SRPSOX, etc. [34–41].

LDL Oxidation

The LDL particle contains phospholipids, free cholesterols, cholesteryl esters, triglycerides, and apolipoprotein B (apoB). Both the lipids and apoB are subjected to oxidation, and apoB breaks down into fragments of different sizes (from 14 kDa to over 550 kDa) by oxidative attack [42]. A key feature of LDL's oxidation is the breakdown of the polyunsaturated fatty acids to yield a broad array of smaller fragments including aldehydes and ketones that can become conjugated to amino lipids or to apoB [43]. The polyunsaturated fatty acids in cholesterol esters, phospholipids, and triglycerides are subject to free radical–initiated oxidation and can participate in chain reactions that amplify the damage. Recently, 2 oxidized fatty acid components have been described, 9- or 13-hydroxyoctadecadienoic acid (9-HODE and 13-HODE). These activate peroxisome proliferator–activator receptor γ (PPARγ), a transcriptional regulator of genes linked to lipid metabolism that upregulate the CD36 scavenger receptor [44]. Thus, lipid components of oxLDL generated by PPARγ activation can promote foam cell formation.

Linoleic acid is a predominant polyunsaturated fatty acid in LDL present mainly as a cholesterol ester [45]. In mildly oxidized LDL, cholesteryl hydroperoxyoctadecadienoic acid (Chol-HPODE) and cholesteryl hydroxyoctadecadienoic acid (Chol-HODE) are the main products of oxidation [46]. It has been reported that Cho-HPODE inactivate PDGF [47]. The oxidative breakdown of either free polyunsaturated fatty acids or those esterified at the sn-2 position of phospholipids result in fatty acid hydroperoxides which form highly reactive products containing aldehyde and ketone functions. Such active functions can form Schiff base adducts with lysine residues of the apoB moiety of LDL or other proteins, and with primary amine containing phospholipids such as phosphatidylserine and phosphatidylethanolamine.

Cholesterol is also converted to oxysterols, and it is especially oxidized at the 7-position. 7-Hydroxycholesterol (both free and esterified) is the major oxysterol formed during early events in LDL oxidation, with 7-ketocholesterol dominating at later stages [48]. Recent studies indicated that elevated plasma level of 7β-hydroxycholesterol is associated with an increased risk of atherosclerosis [49]. At a later stage of LDL oxidation, cholesterol or 7-ketocholesteryl esters of 9-oxononanoate derived from cholesteryl linoleate, are detected as the most abundant fraction of oxidized cholesteryl linoleate [50–52]. As a result of oxidation, a large number of oxidative structures are literally generated.

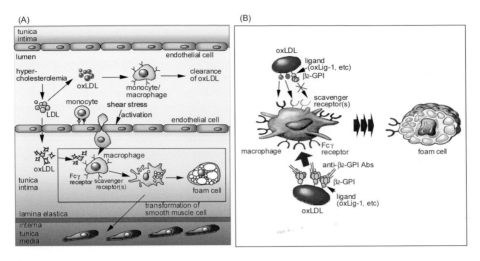

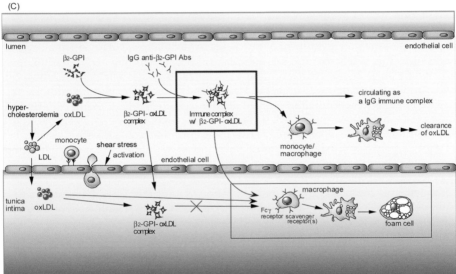

Figure 40.1. Mechanisms of development of atherosclerosis. (A) General consensus of atherogenesis. (B) Possible mechanism of anti–β_2-GPI autoantibody mediated oxLDL uptake by macrophages in APS. (C) Proposed mechanism of development of thrombosis in APS.

Chemically modified LDLs, such as MDA modified LDL, acetylated LDL, and Cu^{2+} mediated oxLDL, were extensively examined as experimental models of denatured LDL to study atherogenic mechanisms. Among these models, trace amounts of Cu^{2+} can induce LDL oxidation, resulting in highly reproducible LDL damage [53]. This process leads to an oxidized LDL structure that shares many functional properties with the LDL oxidized by cells or to oxLDL extracted from arterial atherosclerotic plaques. Incubation of LDL with several different types of cells, or with Cu^{2+} even in the absence of cells, results in an oxLDL structure with similar properties [54]. There is general consensus that Cu^{2+} oxidized LDL is a relevant autoantigen because the oxLDL found in atheromatous lesions and the oxLDL extracted from atherosclerotic lesions exhibited similar physicochemical and immunological properties to the Cu^{2+} oxLDL [55]. Thus, Cu^{2+} mediated oxLDL seems to be a more suitable model for physiological LDL rather than other chemically modified LDL, such as MDA-LDL. In vivo, LDL might be alternatively oxidized by released Cu^{2+} from ceruloplasmin, the major copper-containing component of mammalian plasma [56, 57].

OxLDL/β_2-GPI Complexes

β_2-GPI is a 50 kDa single chain polypeptide composed of 326 amino acid residues, arranged in 5 homologous repeats known as complement control protein domains. β_2-GPI's fifth domain contains a patch of positively charged amino acids that likely represents the binding region for phospholipids [58, 59]. β_2-GPI binds strongly to negatively charged molecules, such as phospholipids, heparin, and certain lipoproteins, as well as to activated platelets and apoptotic cell membranes. This binding may aid the clearance of apoptotic cells from circulation [60]. Further, β_2-GPI may have anticoagulant properties, as it has been shown to inhibit the intrinsic coagulation pathway, prothrombinase activity, and ADP dependent platelet aggregation [61]. It has also been reported to interact with several components of the protein C, protein S anticoagulant system [62].

   We recently demonstrated [16–19] the specific interaction between Cu^{2+}-oxLDL and β_2-GPI by ELISA, optical biosensor (Fig. 40.2) and ligand blot analysis on a silica gel plate for thin layer chromatography (TLC) (Fig. 40.3). Thus, oxLDL but not native LDL, binds β_2-GPI and anti-β_2-GPI autoantibodies. Two chloroform extractable lipids (oxLig-1 and oxLig-2) were identified as the ligands for the specific interaction between oxLDL and β_2-GPI. These oxLDL-derived β_2-GPI specific ligands were further purified by reverse-phase HPLC and their structures

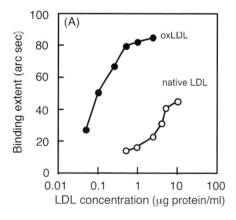 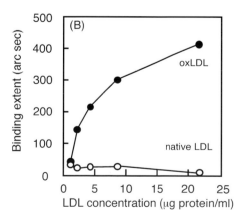

Figure 40.2. Molecular interactions among LDL, β_2-GPI, and anti–β_2-GPI autoantibodies detected by optical biosensor (IAsys). (A) Native LDL or oxLDL binding to solid phase β_2-GPI. (B) Native LDL or oxLDL binding to solid phase WB-CAL-1 antibody (anti–β_2-GPI autoantibody) in the presence of β_2-GPI.

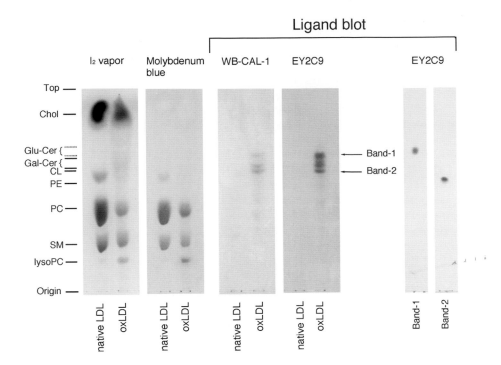

Figure 40.3. Thin layer chromatography (TLC) and ligand blot of lipid extracts from LDL. Lipids were spotted on a TLC plate, developed in chloroform/methanol/30% ammonia/water (120:80:10:5, v/v/v/v). Plates were stained with I2 vapor, molybdenum blue. Ligand blot was performed with β_2-GPI and anti–β_2-GPI antibody (WB-CAL-1 and EY2C9). WB-CAL-1 and EY2C9 are monoclonal anti–β_2-GPI autoantibodies derived from NZW x BXSB F1 mouse (an animal model of APS) and APS patient, respectively.

were identified as 7-ketocholesteryl-9-carboxynonanoate [9-oxo-9-(7-ketocholest-5-en-3β-yloxy) nonanoic acid (IUPAC)] and 7-ketocholesteryl-12-carboxy (keto) dodecanoate, respectively (Fig. 40.4). Cholesteryl linoleate present in LDL is a major core lipid and represents the most probable candidate for a precursor of these ligands.

The initial in vitro interaction of Cu^{2+}-oxLDL with β_2-GPI is due to electrostatic interactions between ω-carboxyl functions and lysine residues of β_2-GPI and is reversible by Mg^{2+} treatment. This interaction later progresses to a much more stable bond such as Schiff base formation with an ω-aldehyde (Fig. 40.5). Interestingly, the negative charges generated by Cu^{2+}-oxLDL were neutralized by the interaction with β_2-GPI (Fig. 40.6). These complexes are occasionally present in APS and SLE patients as IgG immune complexes with anti–β_2-GPI antibodies [16]. The strength of the bond formed and the neutralization of the charges by the complexes may contribute to their stability in the blood stream.

Role of Macrophage Fcγ Receptors

We first demonstrated in 1997 that the in vitro macrophage uptake of ^{125}I-Cu^{2+}-oxLDL was significantly enhanced in the presence of β_2-GPI and IgG anti–β_2-GPI

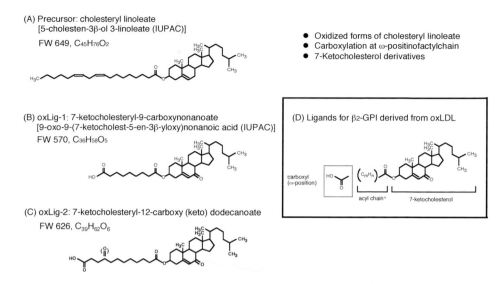

Figure 40.4. Structures of oxLDL derived ligands, specific for β_2-GPI. (A) Cholesteryl linoleate (as a precursor). (B, C) Major ligands for β_2-GPI (oxLig-1 and oxLig-2, respectively). (C) A common structure of the β_2-GPI ligands. oxLig-1: ^{1}H-NMR (300.1 MHz, CDCl$_3$): = 5.71 (s, 1 H, H-6), 4.78-4.69 (m, 1 H, H-3); ^{13}C-NMR (75.5 MHz, CDCl$_3$): = 202.5, 179.7, 173.4, 164.5, 127.1, 72.4, 55.2, 50.4, 50.2, 45.8, 43.5, 39.9, 38.7, 36.6, 36.1, 29.2, 28.9, 28.4, 25.3, 25.0, 24.2, 23.2, 23.0, 19.3, 17.7, 12.4; m/z (FD-MS): 571 [(M+H)$^+$, C$_{36}$H$_{59}$O$_5$ requires 571].

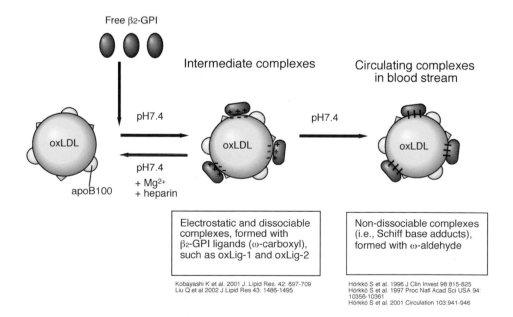

Figure 40.5. Mechanism of complex formation between oxLDL and β_2-GPI.

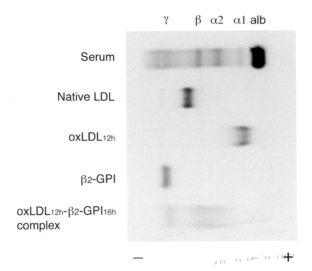

Figure 40.6. Agarose electrophoresis of oxLDL/?$_2$-GPI complexes. oxLDL12h: LDL was oxidized by incubating with Cu2+ ion for 12 hours. oxLDL12h–?$_2$-GPI16h: complexes prepared by incubating oxLDL12 and ?$_2$-GPI for 16 hours at 37°C.

autoantibodies [17]. Further, the macrophage uptake of liposomes containing β$_2$-GPI ligands (oxLig-1 and oxLig-2) was also enhanced confirming the previous results [16, 18, 19]. These findings indicate that IgG anti–β$_2$-GPI autoantibodies may be pro-atherogenic. The in vivo oxLDL uptake is likely mediated by Fcγ receptors rather than by scavenger receptors [Fig. 40.1(B)]. In contrast, Fcμ receptors have poor phagocytic properties, possibly making IgM class of autoantibodies and/or natural antibodies anti-atherogenic (or protective).

Both a ketone function at the 7 position (not at the 22 position) on the sterol backbone and the ω-carboxyl function on the acyl chain of the ligands are responsible either for the interaction between oxLDL and β$_2$-GPI or the β$_2$-GPI/anti–β$_2$-GPI mediated uptake of oxLDL by macrophages [16].

oxLDL/β$_2$-GPI and anti–oxLDL/β$_2$-GPI Complex ELISA

We established a novel ELISA system for oxLDL/β$_2$-GPI complexes utilizing an anti–β$_2$-GPI monoclonal antibody, WB-CAL-1, derived from a NZW x BXSB F1 mouse [63] (Fig. 40.7). Microwells were coated with WB-CAL-1, diluted serum samples applied, and bound oxLDL/β2GPI complexes determined with an enzyme-labeled anti-apoB antibody. WB-CAL-1 antibody only captured β$_2$-GPI when complexed with oxLDL, it did not react with free β$_2$-GPI in solution. ELISA for anti–oxLDL/β$_2$-GPI antibodies used oxLDL/B$_2$-GPI complexes as the antigenic substrate. OxLDL/B$_2$-GPI coated microwells were reacted with diluted samples and bound antibodies determined with an enzyme-labeled anti-human antibody [16, 18, 19].

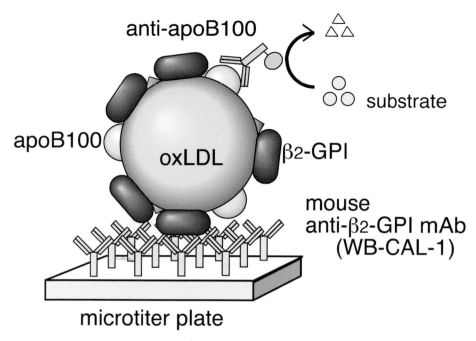

Figure 40.7. Detection system (ELISA) for oxLDL/β_2-GPI complexes. OxLDL/β_2-GPI complexes in serum samples are detected in a sandwich ELISA using WB-CAL-1 (anti–β_2-GPI monoclonal antibody) coated plate and labeled anti-apoB100 as probe antibody.

Oxidation of LDL and Atherogenesis

Traditional risk factors for atherosclerosis include high blood cholesterol levels from either dietary or familial (hereditary) sources, high blood pressure, diabetes mellitus, obesity, smoking, and inactive lifestyles. These risk factors may contribute to both the initiation and the progression of atherosclerotic lesions, and thought to disrupt a number of regulatory and inflammatory mechanisms within the arterial wall. The causal relationship between atherosclerosis and blood cholesterol has been established. The cholesterol that accumulates in macrophage-derived foam cells is derived from circulating lipoproteins, mainly from the pro-atherogenic LDL [2–4]. However, LDL must be modified before is taken up by macrophages via scavenger receptors, and oxidation of LDL represent one such mechanism [64]. Native (unmodified) LDL and perhaps, minimally modified LDL are removed from circulation by LDL receptors located on endothelial and monocyte–macrophage cells. These LDL receptors are downregulated to prevent excessive intracellular lipid accumulation. In contrast, LDL modified by lipid peroxidation is removed at a higher rate by macrophage scavenger receptors. Scavenger receptors are not downregulated, making possible an excessive intracellular accumulation of oxLDL that leads to foam cell formation.

Several studies have demonstrated an inflammatory component in atherosclerosis which involves the dysregulation of cholesterol homeostasis by aberrant interactions between lipid modulating elements and mediators of inflammation [65]. Although the initiating inflammatory factor(s) remain to be identified, likely candidates include immunological injury, homocysteine or other biochemical/metabolic factors and possibly certain infectious agents. More recently, it has been proposed an active participation of antibodies in atherogenesis [66]. These inflammatory and immunologic mechanisms contrast with the purely degenerative or metabolic origin of atherosclerosis as previously thought.

oxLDL plays an important pathogenic role in early events leading to atherosclerosis [3, 67], acting as a pro-inflammatory chemotactic agent for macrophages and T lymphocytes [68], being cytotoxic for endothelial cells, and stimulating the release of soluble inflammatory molecules. In addition, oxLDL has been found in both human and rabbit atherosclerotic lesions [55]. Oxidation of LDL may generate immunogenic epitopes capable of producing autoantibodies. These autoantibodies have been demonstrated in patients with autoimmune disorders, such as SLE and APS [13, 69, 70]. Further, β_2-GPI has also been localized with oxLDL in human atherosclerotic lesions by immunohistochemical staining [12], finding that suggested a role of β_2-GPI (and antiphospholipid antibodies, i.e., anti–β_2-GPI antibodies) in atherosclerosis.

Regulation of Lipid (LDL) Oxidation

Increased lipid peroxidation (oxidative stress) has been demonstrated in patients with rheumatic diseases and vascular involvement [71], including patients with APS [72]. The high-density lipoprotein (HDL) associated enzyme paraoxonase 1 (PON) has antioxidant activity that protects LDL from oxidation [73]. Decreased PON activity has been shown in patients with high serum levels of aCL antibodies [74]. Furthermore, IgG anti–β_2-GPI antibodies have been associated with reduced PON activity in patients with SLE and primary APS [75]. PON activity is also known to increase with lipid lowering drugs [76], and in one study, cholesterol lowering statins prevented the in vitro endothelial cell activation induced by anti–β_2-GPI antibodies [77]. Antioxidant treatment for 4 to 6 weeks has been observed to decrease the titer of circulating aCL antibodies in patients with SLE and APS [78]. Vascular (endothelial) injury as seen in autoimmune patients may affect PON activity or any other antioxidant mechanism, triggering the oxidation of LDL.

In addition to PON, other lipid oxidation mechanisms operating in autoimmune diseases have been investigated. Increased activity of vasoactive isoprostanes (F2α-III and F2α-VI) has been reported in these patients indicating in vivo oxidative stress, likely resulting in oxLDL formation [79]. Also, increased hydrolytic activity of phospholipase A2 and PAF-AH (Lp-PLA2) damaging LDL phospholipids may be responsible for the generation of pro-inflammatory molecules, possibly perpetuating a cycle of inflammation and oxidation of LDL [80].

Autoimmunity and Atherogenesis

The premature (or accelerated) development of atherosclerosis has been recently recognized in patients with systemic autoimmune diseases [81–83]. The traditional risk factors for atherosclerosis and treatment for autoimmune disorders (i.e., steroids) failed to account for the atherosclerotic changes [84]. Today's SLE survival rate (> 80% over a 10-year follow up) may have uncovered hidden causes of mortality and morbidity. SLE mortality rates due to cardiovascular disease have surpassed that from SLE disease itself or from complications such as infections in most studies [85]. In addition, abnormal myocardial perfusion results by Tc99m emission tomography have been reported in about 43% of asymptomatic SLE patients, and increased carotid intima medial thickness (IMT) with atherosclerotic plaques have also been demonstrated by B-mode ultrasound in over 33% of these patients.

Venous thromboembolic complications are the most common clinical finding in APS patients [86, 87]. However, about 25% of the APS patients enrolled into a European cohort of 1000 patients presented an arterial thrombotic event (myocardial infarction, cerebrovascular accident, angina, etc.) as the initial clinical manifestation. If all the initial and late arterial thrombotic events were considered, up to 31% of the patients presented these complications [88]. These observations not only support the hypothesis of autoimmune mechanism(s) but also suggest a role for antiphospholipid antibodies in atherosclerosis. Systemic autoimmune diseases may cause generalized vascular inflammation, decreased antioxidant activity and/or direct oxidation of LDL, the interaction of oxLDL with β_2-GPI, all favoring autoantibody production.

APS and Atherosclerosis

Antiphospholipid antibodies (aCL or LA) are a heterogeneous group of autoantibodies characterized by their reactivity to negatively charged phospholipids, phospholipid/protein complexes, and certain proteins presented on suitable surfaces (i.e., activated cell membranes, oxygenated polystyrene) [11, 89]. Several plasma proteins that participate in coagulation and interact with phospholipids have been described as antiphospholipid cofactors, that is, β_2-GPI, prothrombin, and annexin V, etc. β_2-GPI has been shown to be a relevant antigenic target for antiphospholipid antibodies [7, 9–11]. Antiphospholipid antibodies, β_2-GPI dependent aCL and antiprothrombin, have been associated with several forms of cardiovascular diseases such as myocardial infarction, stroke, carotid stenosis, etc. [90, 91]. Anti–β_2-GPI antibodies have been reported as more specific for thrombosis and APS than aCL antibodies [92], and recent prospective studies have shown that aCL antibodies, particularly β_2-GPI dependent, or anti–β_2-GPI antibodies are important predictors for arterial thrombosis (myocardial infarction and stroke) in men [90, 91, 93].

APS is the most common cause of acquired hypercoagulability in the general population [94, 95]. Elevated serum levels of antiphospholipid antibodies along with thrombotic events of both the venous and arterial vasculature, or with pregnancy morbidity (miscarriages and fetal loss) represent the major features of the APS. APS may be present in the context of a systemic autoimmune disorder, for example, SLE, and referred to as secondary APS, or in the absence of an obvious underlying disease (primary APS) [5]. Antiphospholipid antibodies increase the risk of thrombosis by at least 2-fold when present in the context of an autoimmune disease [96]. In both primary and secondary APS, recurrence rates of up to 30% for thrombosis with a mortality of up to 10% over a 10-year follow-up period have been reported [97, 98]. Some aCL obtained from patients with APS cross-reacted with oxLDL [13], providing initial clues that antiphospholipid antibodies promote atherosclerosis. β_2-GPI found in atherosclerotic lesions co-localizes with immunoreactive CD4 lymphocytes [12]. These findings provide additional support to the hypothesis that β_2-GPI and anti–β_2-GPI antibodies play a pathogenic role in the development of thrombosis, particularly arterial thrombosis (atherosclerosis) in SLE and APS patients.

OxLDL/β_2-GPI Complexes in Autoimmune Diseases

Lipid peroxidation resulting in oxLDL is a common occurrence in patients with some systemic autoimmune diseases [71]. OxLDL, not native LDL, binds β_2-GPI in vitro initially forming dissociable electrostatic complexes followed by more stable complexes bound by covalent interactions. Circulating oxLDL/β_2-GPI complexes have been detected in patients with autoimmune diseases [Fig. 40.1(C)] [16]. High serum levels of stable oxLDL/β_2-GPI complexes were detected by ELISA in 75% to 80% of patients with SLE and systemic sclerosis (SSc). OxLDL/β_2-GPI complex levels of patients with rheumatoid arthritis (RA) were slightly elevated compared to healthy controls but this difference did not reach statistical significance [Fig. 40.8(A)]. Unlike RA, both SLE and SSc are characterized by widespread vascular abnormalities. Serum levels of oxLDL/β_2-GPI complexes were also significantly elevated in patients with secondary APS and in SLE patients without APS compared to healthy controls [Fig. 40.8(B)]. However, these complexes were not associated with SLE disease activity or any major clinical manifestation of APS [99]. Although it can be hypothesized that this interaction might be related to chronic inflammation of the vasculature that occurs in autoimmune patients, the exact mechanism(s) for the increased oxidation of LDL and oxLDL/β_2-GPI complex formation are not fully understood. It is possible that the interaction between oxLDL and β_2-GPI may promote the clearance of oxLDL from circulation to prevent thrombus formation. Serum levels of oxLDL/β_2-GPI complexes fluctuated widely when measured in samples obtained at different time intervals over a 12-month follow up from 6 SLE patients. This suggests that oxidation and formation of complexes are very active processes under unknown regulatory mechanism(s). Stable oxLDL/β_2-GPI complexes may be clinically relevant as they have been implicated as atherogenic autoantigens, and their presence may represent a risk factor or an indirect but significant contributor for thrombosis and atherosclerosis in patients with an autoimmune background [16].

Anti–oxLDL/β_2-GPI Antibodies in Autoimmune Diseases

Serum levels of IgG anti–oxLDL/β_2-GPI antibodies were measured in the same group of SLE, SSc, and RA patients. SLE and SSc patients had significantly higher levels of anti–oxLDL/β_2-GPI antibodies compared to the controls [Fig. 40.9(A)]. RA patients showed higher antibody levels than the controls but this difference was not statistically significant. When IgG anti–oxLDL/β_2-GPI antibodies were evaluated for

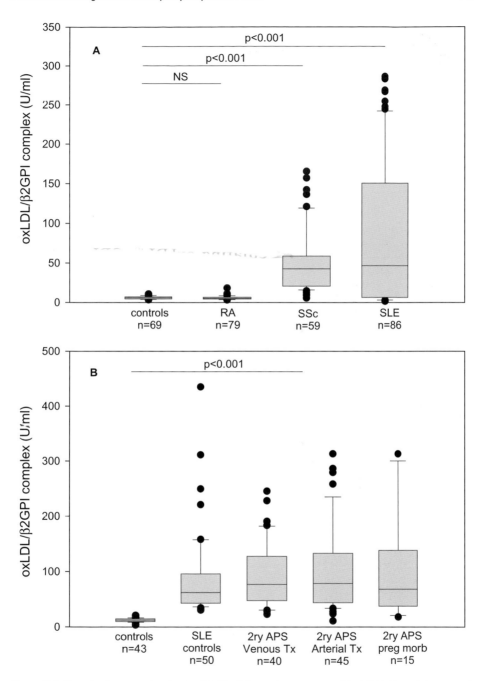

Figure 40.8. Box plot for serum levels of oxLDL/β_2-GPI complexes measured by ELISA (A, top) in systemic autoimmune diseases (RA = rheumatoid arthritis; SSc = systemic sclerosis; SLE = systemic lupus erythematosus) and healthy controls; and (B, bottom) in secondary antiphospholipid syndrome (APS) patients classified into venous thrombosis (venous Tx), arterial thrombosis (arterial Tx), or pregnancy morbidity (preg morb) subgroups. SLE without APS and healthy individuals served as controls. OxLDL/β2GPI complex levels were expressed in arbitrary units (U/mL). Boxes represent 75/25 percentiles and horizontal line the median for the group. Dots are samples reacting outside the 90/10 percentile bars. *P* values of 0.05 or less were considered as significant (Mann–Whitney Rank Sum test).

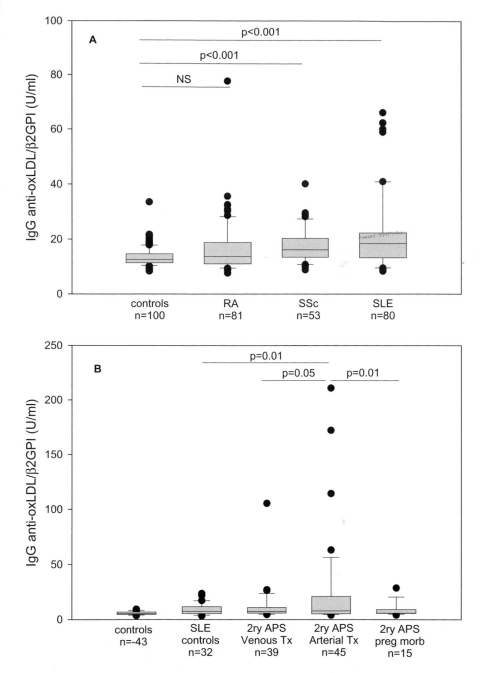

Figure 40.9. Box plot for serum levels of IgG anti–oxLDL/β_2-GPI antibodies measured by ELISA (A, top) in sys-temic autoimmune diseases (RA = rheumatoid arthritis; SSc = systemic sclerosis; SLE = systemic lupus erythe-matosus) and healthy controls; and (B, bottom) in secondary antiphospholipid syndrome (APS) patients classified into venous thrombosis (venous Tx), arterial thrombosis (arterial Tx), or pregnancy morbidity (preg morb) subgroups. SLE without APS and healthy individuals served as controls. IgG anti–oxLDL/β_2-GPI antibody levels were expressed in arbitrary units (U/mL). Boxes represent 75/25 percentiles and horizontal line the median for the group. Dots are samples reacting outside the 90/10 percentile bars. *P* values of 0.05 or less were considered as significant (Mann–Whitney Rank Sum test).

Table 40.1. Association of IgG anti–oxLDL/β_2-GPI antibodies with clinical manifestations of the antiphospholipid syndrome.

APS manifestation (n)	Sensitivity (%)	Positive predictive value (%)	Chi-square (P)
Total thrombosis (79)	29.1	92.1	0.018
Arterial thrombosis (42)	38.1	88.9	0.004
Venous thrombosis (37)	18.9	77.7	ns
Pregnancy morbidity (14)	0	0	Ns

ns = not statistically significant.

their association with the major clinical manifestations of APS [16, 100], a stronger correlation with arterial thrombosis compared to venous thrombosis and pregnancy morbidity was observed [Fig. 40.9(B)]. Further, the positive predictive value of IgG anti–oxLDL/β_2-GPI antibodies for total thrombosis (arterial and venous) in patients with secondary APS was 92% and for arterial thrombosis was 88.9%. In contrast, the positive predictive value for venous thrombosis was not statistically significant at 77.7% (Table 40.1). In addition, anti–oxLDL/β_2-GPI antibodies were present in 3 of 4 SLE patients with active disease followed over a 12-month period, while 2 patients with inactive disease and oxLDL/β_2-GPI complexes did not have these antibodies [99].

The co-existence of oxLDL-1/β_2-GPI autoantibodies with oxLDL/β_2-GPI complexes, suggest that these 2 elements interact perhaps forming circulating immune complexes (oxLDL/β_2-GPI/antibody). Such immune complexes have been recently detected in patients with SLE and/or APS [16]. These observations along with the increased in vitro uptake of oxLDL/β_2-GPI complexes by macrophage in the presence of anti–oxLDL/β_2-GPI antibodies [14, 17–19] provide an explanation for the accelerated (premature) development of atherosclerosis in autoimmune patients. Although preliminary, IgG anti–oxLDL/β_2-GPI antibodies represent a distinct subset of antiphospholipid antibodies (i.e., anti–β_2-GPI) that co-exist with other antiphospholipid antibodies. Thus, IgG anti–oxLDL/β_2-GPI antibodies appear to be useful serologic markers for atherosclerotic risk in autoimmune patients with high specificity for APS.

Summary and Clinical Relevance

The interaction between oxLDL and β_2-GPI to form circulating complexes strongly suggests that this complex is an atheroantigen. This interaction has been further characterized and the oxLDL derived ligand (oxLig-1) specific for β_2-GPI has been identified and synthesized. APS patients may produce antibodies to this complex and the resulting circulating immune complexes trigger atherosclerotic changes. The physiologic relevance of this finding has been demonstrated in vitro by the enhanced macrophage uptake of oxLDL/β_2-GPI/antibody complexes. The participation of macrophage Fcγ receptors in the uptake of oxLDL containing complexes seems to be particularly important in the development of foam cells and atherosclerotic plaques.

Are there other molecules, antigens, antibodies, or other interactions playing a role in the development of atherosclerosis? It has been reported that β_2-GPI may interact with various negatively charged molecules. Inflammatory reactions may modify certain molecules, making them reactive with β_2-GPI. The resulting complexes may exert unwanted effects and even trigger immune responses. For example, C-reactive protein (CRP), fibrinogen, tumor necrosis factor-α (TNF-α), heat-shock protein (HSP), homocysteine, etc. are being use to assess the risk for cardiovascular disease. However, the exact mode of action(s) of these molecules is not complete understood. It is possible that β_2-GPI may participate in additional, yet unknown, molecular interactions. The product of these interactions may cause vascular inflammation and/or trigger the production of autoantibodies, including immune complexes that promote atherosclerosis.

The development of ELISA systems to measure oxLDL/β_2-GPI complexes and anti-oxLDL/β_2-GPI antibodies had provided additional tools to further study the role of the humoral immune response in the atherosclerotic process. Stable and likely pathogenic oxLDL/β_2-GPI complexes were demonstrated in the serum of SLE, SSc, and APS patients. Anti–oxLDL/β_2-GPI antibodies were detected in SLE and SSc patients, both diseases characterized by generalized vascular complications. Further, the association of these antibodies with arterial thrombosis was stronger than venous thrombosis in APS patients. The role of oxLDL/β_2-GPI complexes and autoantibodies to these complexes in the vascular complications of SSc remain to be further studied. At this point, these results should be interpreted in the context of an autoimmune disease. However, oxLDL/β_2-GPI complexes have been demonstrated in patients with syphilis, infectious endocarditis, diabetes mellitus, and chronic nephritis, indicating that oxidation of LDL and the formation of complexes with β_2-GPI is not restricted to SLE. In contrast, none of these patients developed significant levels of anti–oxLDL/β_2-GPI antibodies. These antibodies seem to be restricted to patients with SLE and APS. Thus, it can be hypothesized that these antibodies accelerate the development of atherosclerosis in autoimmune patients.

References

1. Steinbrecher UP, Parthasarathy S, Leake DS, Witztum JL, Steinberg D. Modification of low-density lipoprotein by endothelial cells involves lipid peroxidation and degradation of low-density lipoprotein phospholipids. Proc Natl Acad Sci U S A 1984;81:3883–3887.
2. Steinberg D, Parthasarathy S, Carew TE, Khoo JC, Witztum JL. Beyond cholesterol. Modifications of low-density lipoprotein that increase its atherogenicity. N Engl J Med 1989;320:915–924.
3. Steinberg D. Low-density lipoprotein oxidation and its pathobiological significance. J Biol Chem 1997;272:20963–20966.
4. Heinecke JW. Mechanisms of oxidative damage of low-density lipoprotein in human atherosclerosis. Curr Opin Lipid 1997;8:268–274.
5. Hughes GRV, Harris EN, Gharavi AE. The anticardiolipin syndrome. J Rheumatol 1986;13:486–489.
6. Harris EN, Gharavi AE, Boey ML, et al. Anticardiolipin antibodies: detection by radioimmunoassay and association with thrombosis in systemic lupus erythematosus. Lancet 1983;2:1211–1214.
7. McNeil HP, Simpson RJ, Chesterman CN, Krilis SA. Anti-phospholipid antibodies are directed against a complex antigen that includes a lipid-binding inhibitor of coagulation: β2-glycoprotein I (apolipoprotein H). Proc Natl Acad Sci U S A 1990;87:4120–4124.
8. Galli M, Comfurius P, Maassen C, et al. Anticardiolipin antibodies (ACA) directed not to cardiolipin but to a plasma protein cofactor. Lancet 1990;335:1544–1547.
9. Matsuura E, Igarashi Y, Fujimoto M, Ichikawa K, Koike T. Anticardiolipin cofactor(s) and differential diagnosis of autoimmune disease. Lancet 1990;336:177–178.
10. Matsuura E, Igarashi Y, Fujimoto M, et al. Heterogeneity of anticardiolipin antibodies defined by the anticardiolipin cofactor. J Immunol 1992;148:3885–3891.

11. Matsuura E, Igarashi Y, Yasuda T, Triplett DA, Koike T. Anticardiolipin antibodies recognize β2-glycoprotein I structure altered by interacting with an oxygen modified solid phase surface. J Exp Med 1994;179:457–462.

12. George J, Harats D, Gilburd B, et al. Immunolocalization of β2-glycoprotein I (apolipoprotein H) to human atherosclerotic plaques: potential implications for lesion progression. Circulation 1999;99:2227–2230.

13. Vaarala O, Alfthan G, Jauhiainen M, Leirisalo-Repo M, Aho K, Palosuo T. Crossreaction between antibodies to oxidised low-density lipoprotein and to cardiolipin in systemic lupus erythematosus. Lancet 1993;341:923–925.

14. Tinahones FJ, Cuadrado MJ, Khamashta MA, et al. Lack of cross reaction between antibodies to β2-glycoprotein-I and oxidized low-density lipoprotein in patients with antiphospholipid syndrome. Br J Rheumatol 1998;37:746–749.

15. Romero FI, Amengual O, Atsumi T, Khamashta MA, Tinahones FJ, Hughes GRV. Arterial disease in lupus and secondary antiphospholipid syndrome: Association with anti-β2-glycoprotein I antibodies but not with antibodies against oxidized low-density lipoprotein. Br J Rheumatol 1998;37:883–888.

16. Kobayashi K, Kishi M, Atsumi T, et al. Circulating oxidized LDL forms complexes with β2-glycoprotein I: implication as an atherogenic autoantigen. J Lipid Res 2003;44:716–726.

17. Hasunuma Y, Matsuura E, Makita Z, Katahira T, Nishi S, Koike T. Involvement of β2-glycoprotein I and anticardiolipin antibodies in oxidatively modified low-density lipoprotein uptake by macrophages. Clin Exp Immunol 1997;107:569–573.

18. Kobayashi K, Matsuura E, Liu Q, et al. A specific ligand for β2-glycoprotein I mediates autoantibody-dependent uptake of oxidized low density lipoprotein by macrophages. J Lipid Res 2001;42:697–709.

19. Liu Q, Kobayashi K, Inagaki J, et al. ω-carboxyl variants of 7-ketocholesteryl esters are ligands for β2-glycoprotein I and mediate antibody-dependent uptake of oxidized LDL by macrophages. J Lipid Res 2002;43:1486–1495.

20. Chang MK, Bergmark C, Laurila A, et al. Monoclonal antibodies against oxidized low-density lipoprotein bind to apoptotic cells and inhibit their phagocytosis by elicited macrophages: evidence that oxidation-specific epitopes mediate macrophage recognition. Proc Natl Acad Sci U S A 1999;96:6353–6358.

21. Horkko S, Bird DA, Miller E, et al. Monoclonal autoantibodies specific for oxidized phospholipids or oxidized phospholipid-protein adducts inhibit macrophage uptake of oxidized low-density lipoproteins. J Clin Invest 1999;103:117–128.

22. Binder CJ, Horkko S, Dewan A, et al. Pneumococcal vaccination decreases atherosclerotic lesion formation: molecular mimicry between Streptococcus pneumoniae and oxidized LDL. Nat Med 2003;9:736–743.

23. Rose N, Afanasyeva M. Autoimmunity: busting the atheorsclerotic plaque. Nat Med 2003;9:641–642.

24. Cushing SD, Berliner JA, Valente AJ, et al. Minimally modified low-density lipoprotein induces monocyte chemotactic protein 1 in human endothelial cells and smooth muscle cells. Proc Natl Acad Sci U S A 1990;87:5134–5138.

25. Rajavashisth TB, Andalibi A, Territo MC, et al. Induction of endothelial cell expression of granulocyte and macrophage colony-stimulating factors by modified low-density lipoproteins. Nature 1990;344:254–257.

26. Nakata A, Miyagawa J, Yamashita S, et al. Localization of heparin-binding epidermal growth factor-like growth factor in human coronary arteries. Possible roles of HB-EGF in the formation of coronary atherosclerosis. Circulation 1996;94:2778–2786.

27. Frostegard J, Wu R, Haegerstrand A, Patarroyo M, Lefvert AK, Nilsson J. Mononuclear leukocytes exposed to oxidized low density lipoprotein secrete a factor that stimulates endothelial cells to express adhesion molecules. Atherosclerosis 1993;103:213–219.

28. Mach F, Schonbeck U, Sukhova GK, Atkinson E, Libby P. Reduction of atherosclerosis in mice by inhibition of CD40 signalling. Nature 1998;394:200–203.

29. Goldstein JL, Ho YK, Basu SK, Brown MS. Binding site on macrophages that mediates uptake and degradation of acetylated low-density lipoprotein, producing massive cholesterol deposition. Proc Natl Acad Sci U S A 1979;76:333–337.

30. Yamamoto T, Davis CG, Brown MS, et al. The human LDL receptor: a cysteine-rich protein with multiple Alu sequences in its mRNA. Cell 1984;39:27–38.

31. Brown MS, Goldstein JL. Scavenger cell receptor shared. Nature 1985;316:680–681.

32. Kodama T, Reddy P, Kishimoto C, Krieger M. Purification and characterization of a bovine acetyl low-density lipoprotein receptor. Proc Natl Acad Sci U S A 1998;85:9238–9242.

33. Kodama T, Freeman M, Rohrer L, Zabrecky J, Matsudaira P, Krieger M. Type I macrophage scavenger receptor contains alpha-helical and collagen-like coiled coils. Nature 1990;343:531–535.
34. Elomaa O, Kangas M, Sahlberg C, et al. Cloning of a novel bacteria-binding receptor structurally related to scavenger receptors and expressed in a subset of macrophages. Cell 1995;80:603–609.
35. Elomaa O, Sankala M, Pikkarainen T, et al. Structure of the human macrophage MARCO receptor and characterization of its bacteria-binding region. J Biol Chem 1998;273:4530–4538.
36. Ramprasad MP, Fischer W, Witztum JL, Sambrano GR, Quehenberger O, Steinberg D. The 94- to 97-kDa mouse macrophage membrane protein that recognizes oxidized low density lipoprotein and phosphatidylserine-rich liposomes is identical to macrosialin, the mouse homologue of human CD68. Proc Natl Acad Sci U S A 1995;92:9580–9584.
37. Sambrano GR, Steinberg D. Recognition of oxidatively damaged and apoptotic cells by an oxidized low density lipoprotein receptor on mouse peritoneal macrophages: role of membrane phosphatidylserine. Proc Natl Acad Sci U S A 1995;92:1396–1400.
38. Rigotti A, Acton SL, Krieger M. The class B scavenger receptors SR-BI and CD36 are receptors for anionic phospholipids J Biol Chem 1995;270:16221–16224.
39. Sawamura T, Kume N, Aoyama T, et al. An endothelial receptor for oxidized low-density lipoprotein. Nature 1997;386:73–77.
40. Minami M, Kume N, Shimaoka T, et al. Expression of SR-PSOX, a novel cell-surface scavenger receptor for phosphatidylserine and oxidized LDL in human atherosclerotic lesions. Arterioscler Thromb Vasc Biol 2001;21:1796–1800.
41. Shimaoka T, Kume N, Minami M, et al. Molecular cloning of a novel scavenger receptor for oxidized low-density lipoprotein, SR-PSOX, on macrophages. J Biol Chem 2000;275:40663–40666.
42. Fong LG, Parthasarathy S, Witztum JL, Steinberg D. Nonenzymatic oxidative cleavage of peptide bonds in apoprotein B-100. J Lipid Res 1997;28:1466–1477.
43. Esterbauer H, Jurgens G, Quehenberger O, Koller E. Autoxidation of human low density lipoprotein: loss of polyunsaturated fatty acids and vitamin E and generation of aldehydes. J Lipid Res 1987;28:495–509.
44. Nagy L, Tontonoz P, Alvarez JG, Chen H, Evans RM. Oxidized LDL regulates macrophage gene expression through ligand activation of PPAR. Cell 1998;93:229–240.
45. Weidtmann A, Scheithe R, Hrboticky N, Pietsch A, Lorenz R, Siess W. Mildly oxidized LDL induces platelet aggregation through activation of phsopholipase A2. Arterioscler Thromb Vasc Biol 1995;15:1131–1138.
46. Kritharides L, Jessup W, Gifford J, Dean RT. A method for defining the stages of low density lipoprotein oxidation by the separation of cholesterol and cholesteryl ester-oxidation products using HPLC. Anal Biochem 1993;213:79–89.
47. van Heek M, Schmitt D, Toren P, Cathcart MK, DiCorleto PE. Cholesteryl hydroperoxyoctadecadienoate from oxidized low-density lipoprotein inactivated platelet-derived growth factor. J Biol Chem 1998;273:19405–19410.
48. Brown AJ, Leong SL, Dean RT, Jessup W. 7-Hydroperoxycholesterol and its products in oxidized low-density lipoprotein and human atherosclerotic plaque. J Lipid Res 1997;38:1730–1745.
49. Brown AJ, Jessup W. Oxysterols and atherosclerosis. Atherosclerosis 1999;142:1–28.
50. Kamido H, Kuksis A, Marai L, Myher JJ. Identification of cholesterol-bound aldehydes in copper-oxidized low-density lipoprotein. FEBS Lett 1992;304:269–272.
51. Kamido H, Kuksis A, Marai L, Myher JJ. Lipid ester-bound aldehydes among copper-catalyzed peroxidation products of human plasma lipoproteins. J Lipid Res 1995;36:1876–1886.
52. Hoppe G, Ravandi A, Herrera D, Kuksis A, Hoff HF. Oxidation products of cholesteryl linoleate are resistant to hydrolysis in macrophages, form complexes with proteins, and are present in human atherosclerotic lesions. J Lipid Res 1997;38:1347–1360.
53. Kleinveld HA, Hak-Lemmers HLM, Stalenhoef AFH, Demacker PNM. Improved measurement of low-density-lipoprotein susceptibility to copper-induced oxidation: application of a short procedure for isolating low-density lipoprotein. Clin Chem 1992;38:2066–2072.
54. Parthasarathy S, Fong LG, Quinn MT, Steinberg D. Oxidative modification of LDL: comparison between cell-mediated and copper-mediated modification. Eur Heart J 1990;11(suppl E):83–87.
55. Yla-Herttuala S, Palinski W, Rosenfeld ME, et al. Evidence for presence of oxidatively modified low-density lipoprotein in atherosclerotic lesions of rabbit and man. J Clin Invest 1989;85:1086–1095.
56. Ehrenwald E, Chisolm GM, Fox PL. Intact ceruloplasmin oxidatively modifies low-density lipoprotein. J Clin Invest 1994;93:1493–1501.
57. Lamb D, Leake DS. Acidic pH enables caeruloplasmin to catalyse the modification of low-density lipoprotein. FEBS Lett 1994;338:122–126.

58. Bouma B, de Groot PG, van den Elsen JM, et al. Adhesion mechanism of human β2-glycoprotein I to phospholipids based on its crystal structure. EMBO J 1999;18:5166–5174.

59. Hoshino M, Hagihara Y, Nishii I, Yamazaki T, Kato H, Goto Y. Identification of the phospholipid-binding site of human β2-glycoprotein I domain V by heteronuclear magnetic resonance. J Mol Biol 2000;304:927–939.

60. Inanc M, Radway-Bright EL, Isenberg DA. β2-glycoprotein I and anti-β2-glycoprotein I antibodies: where are we now? Br J Rheumatol 1997;36:1247–1257.

61. Sheng Y, Kandiah DA, Krilis SA. β2-glycoprotein I: Target antigen for 'antiphospholipid' antibodies. Immunological and molecular aspects. Lupus 1998;7:S5–S9.

62. Merrill JT, Zhang HW, Shen C, et al. Enhancement of protein S anticoagulant function by β2-glycoprotein I, a major target antigen of antiphospholipid antibodies: β2-glycoprotein I interferes with binding of protein S to its plasma inhibitor, C4b-binding protein. Thromb Haemost 1999;81:748–757.

63. Hashimoto Y, Kawamura M, Ichikawa K, et al. Anticardiolipin antibodies in NZW x BXSB F1 mice. A model of antiphospholipid syndrome. J Immunol 1992;149:1063–1068.

64. Ross R. Atherosclerosis: an inflammatory disease. N Engl J Med 1999;340:115–126.

65. Steinberg D. Atherogenesis in perspective: hypercholesterolemia and inflammation as partners in crime. Nat Med 2002;8:1211–1217.

66. Virella G, Atchley DH, Koskinen S, Zheng D, Lopes-Virella M. Pro-atherogenic and pro-inflammatory properties of immune complexes prepared with purified human oxLDL antibodies and human oxLDL. Clin Immunol 2002;105:81–92.

67. Berliner JA, Heinecke JW. The role of oxidized lipoproteins in atherogenesis. Free Radic Biol Med 1996;20:707–727.

68. McMurray HF, Parthasarathy S, Steinberg D. Oxidatively modified low-density lipoprotein is a chemoattractant for human T lymphocytes. J Clin Invest 1993;92:1004–1008.

69. Salonen JT, Yla-Herttuala S, Yamamoto R, et al. Autoantibodies against oxidized LDL and progression of carotid atherosclerosis. Lancet 1992;339:883–887.

70. Vaarala O. Antiphospholipid antibodies and atherosclerosis. Lupus 1996;5:442–447.

71. Ames PRJ, Alves J, Murat I, Isenberg DA, Nourooz-Zadeh J. Oxidative stress in systemic lupus erythematosus and allied conditions with vascular involvement. Rheumatology 1999;38:529–534.

72. Ames PRJ, Tommasino C, Alves J, et al. Antioxidant susceptibility of pathogenic pathways in subjects with antiphospholipid antibodies: a pilot study. Lupus 2000;9:688–695.

73. Durrington PN, Mackness B, Mackness MI. Paraoxonase and atherosclerosis. Arterioscler Thromb Vasc Biol 2001;21:473–480.

74. Lambert M, Boullier A, Hachulla E, et al. Paraoxonase activity is dramatically decreased in patients positive for anticardiolipin antibodies. Lupus 2000;9:299–300.

75. Delgado Alves J, Ames PR, Donohue S, et al. Antibodies to high-density lipoprotein and β2-glycoprotein I are inversely correlated with paraoxonase activity in systemic lupus erythematosus and primary antiphospholipid syndrome. Arthritis Rheum 2002;46:2686–2694.

76. Belogh Z, Seres I, Harangi M, Kovacs P, Kakuk G, Paragh G. Gemfibrozil increases paraoxonase activity in type 2 diabetic patients: a new hypothesis of the beneficial action of fibrates? Diabetes Metab 2001;27:604–610.

77. Meroni PL, Raschi E, Testoni C, et al. Statins prevent endothelial cell activation induced by antiphospholipid (anti-β2-glycoprotein I) antibodies. Effect on the proadhesive and proinflammatory phenotype. Arthritis Rheum 2001;44:2870–2878.

78. Ferro D, Iuliano L, Violi F, Valesini G, Conti F. Antioxidant treatment decreases the titer of circulating anticardiolipin antibodies. Arthritis Rheum 2002;46:3110–3112.

79. Pratico D, Ferro D, Rokach J, et al. Ongoing prothrombotic state in patients with antiphospholipid antibodies: a role for increased lipid peroxidation. Blood 1999;93:3401–3407.

80. Hurt-Camejo E, Paredes S, Masana L, et al. Elevated levels of small, low-density lipoprotein with high affinity for arterial matrix components in patients with rheumatoid arthritis. Possible contribution of phospholipase A2 to this atherogenic profile. Arthritis Rheum 2001;44:2761–2767.

81. Van Doornum S, McColl G, Wicks IP. Accelerated atherosclerosis. An extraarticular feature of rheumatoid arthritis? Arthritis Rheum 2002;46:862–873.

82. Ward MM. Premature morbidity from cardiovascular and cerebrovascular diseases in women with systemic lupus erythematosus. Arthritis Rheum 1999;42:338–346.

83. Aranow C, Ginzler EM. Epidemiology of cardiovascular disease in systemic lupus erythematosus. Lupus 2000;9:166–169.

84. Esdaile JM, Abrahamowicz M, Grodzicky T, et al. Traditional Framingham risk factors fail to fully account for accelerated atherosclerosis in systemic lupus erythematosus. Arthritis Rheum 2001;44:2331–2337.

85. Schattner A, Liang MH. The cardiovascular burden of lupus; a complex challenge. Arch Intern Med 2003;163:1507–1510.

86. Harris EN, Chan JKH, Asherson RA, Hughes GRV. Thrombosis, recurrent fetal loss and thrombocytopenia – predictive value of the anticardiolipin antibody test. Arch Intern Med 1986;146:2153–2156.

87. Ginsburg KS, Liang MH, Newcomer L, et al. Anticardiolipin antibodies and the risk for ischemic stroke and venous thrombosis. Ann Intern Med 1992;117:997–1002.

88. Cervera R, Piette JC, Font J, et al, Euro-Phospholipid Project Group. Antiphospholipid syndrome. Clinical and immunologic manifestations and patterns of disease expression in a cohort of 1,000 patients. Arthritis Rheum 2002;46:1019–1027.

89. Roubey RA. Autoantibodies to phospholipid-binding plasma proteins: a new view of lupus anticoagulants and other "antiphospholipid" autoantibodies. Blood 1994;84:2854–2867.

90. Vaarala O. Antiphospholipid antibodies in myocardial infarction. Lupus 1998;7:S132–S134.

91. Brey RL, Abbott RD, Curb JD, et al. β2-glycoprotein I dependent anticardiolipin antibodies and the risk of ischemic stroke and myocardial infarction. Stroke 2001;32:1701–1706.

92. Tsutsumi A, Matsuura E, Ichikawa K, et al. Antibodies to β2-glycoprotein I and clinical manifestations in patients with systemic lupus erythematosus. Arthritis Rheum 1996;39:1466–1474.

93. Lopez LR, Dier, KJ, Lopez D, Merrill JT, Fink CA. Anti-β2-glycoprotein I and antiphosphatidylserine antibodies are predictors of arterial thrombosis in patients with antiphospholipid syndrome. Am J Clin Pathol 2004;121:142–149.

94. Petri M. Autoimmune thrombosis. In: Asherson RA, Cervera R, Piette J, Schoenfeld Y, eds. The antiphospholipid syndrome. Amsterdam: Elsevier Science; 2002:11–20.

95. Thomas RH. Hypercoagulability syndromes. Arch Intern Med 2001;161:2433–2439.

96. Wahl DG, Guillemin F, de Maistre E, Perret C, Lecompte T, Thibaut G. Risk for venous thrombosis related to antiphospholipid antibodies in systemic lupus erythematosus: a meta analysis. Lupus 1997;6:467–473.

97. Shah NM, Khamashta MA, Atsumi T, Hughes GRV. Outcome of patients with anticardiolipin antibodies: a 10 year follow-up of 52 patients. Lupus 1998;7:3–6.

98. Khamashta MA, Cuadrado MJ, Mujic F, Taub NA, Hunt BJ, Hughes GRV. The management of thrombosis in the antiphospholipid-antibody syndrome. N Engl J Med 1995;332:993–997.

99. Lopez D, Garcia-Valladares I, Palafox-Sanchez C, et al. Oxidized low-density lipoprotein/β2-glycoprotein I complexes and autoantibodies to oxLig-1/β2-glycoprotein I in patients with systemic lupus erythematosus and antiphospholipid syndrome. Am J Clin Pathol 2004;121:426–436.

100. Lopez D, Kobayashi K, Merrill JT, Matsuura E, Lopez LR. IgG Autoantibodies against β2-glycoprotein I complexed with a lipid ligand derived from oxidized low-density lipoprotein are associated with arterial thrombosis in antiphospholipid syndrome. Clin Dev Immunol 2003;10:203–211.

41 Genetics of Antiphospholipid Syndrome

Tatsuya Atsumi and Olga Amengual

Introduction

The phenotypes of autoimmune diseases are related with both genetic and environmental factors. The antigen specificity of antiphospholipid antibodies (aPL) and the pathophysiology of thrombosis in antiphospholipid syndrome (APS) are highly heterogeneous and multifactorial, thus a single scenario cannot explain the mechanisms of thrombophilia or pregnancy morbidity present in affected patients.

A genetic predisposition for developing diseases is supported by various facts, such as concordance of disease in identical twins and in patients' relatives, increased frequency in certain ethnic groups, and elevated frequency of some genetic polymorphisms including the major histocompatibility complex (MHC) region. Since the early 1980s, familial occurrence of aPL with or without clinical manifestations of APS has been reported, and many researchers have investigated the immunogenetic predisposition to aPL or APS, including the role of HLA region which is involved in the control of immune recognition and the following response.

It is now widely recognized that the most common autoantigens for aPL are β_2-glycoprotein I (β_2-GPI) and prothrombin. In particular, the molecular structure and properties of β_2-GPI have been intensively studied. A number of polymorphisms of β_2-GPI gene have been described, and the biological significance and its relation to anti–β_2-GPI antibodies have been discussed.

Further, thrombotic genetic factors, as additional risks for the onset of thrombotic events, have been examined in patients with aPL.

In this chapter, we summarize family studies on APS and describe several disease-susceptible genetic factors that have been evaluated in patients with APS, including HLA haplotypes, β_2-GPI gene, and other genetic variants on disease development.

Family Studies

The first description regarding familial occurrence of aPL, reported by Exner et al [1], showed 2 pairs of siblings with lupus anticoagulant (LA). Subsequently, Matthey et al [2] described primary APS in 4 members of 1 family and Cevallos et al [3] reported the development of primary APS in 1 woman whose identical twin sister was an asymptomatic carrier of aPL.

The first degree relatives of patients with systemic lupus erythematosus (SLE) or primary APS had a higher incidence of anticardiolipin antibodies (aCL) [4, 5], suggesting that a genetic predisposition may influence the appearance of aPL. Evidence of familial form of APS could be obtained by the identification of several kindreds with an increased frequency of aPL and/or clinical manifestations of APS. In 1987, Mackie et al [6] reported 3 families having more than 1 member with LA and called familial lupus anticoagulants [6]. Later on, Ford et al reported a large kindred in which 9 out of 23 members of 4 generations (4 had neurologic symptoms and 5 asymptomatic) were positive for LA [7]. Primary APS, in the absence of SLE, was also reported to cluster in families and has been described as familial primary antiphospholipid antibody syndrome [8, 9]. Goel et al [10] studied clinical and laboratory abnormalities in 7 families with more than 1 affected members with segregation analysis. They proposed a set of criteria for a familial form of APS and suggested that a susceptibility gene is inherited in an autosomal dominant pattern.

Many family studies have explored familial aPL or APS with a documented HLA linkage [6, 11–17], suggesting that haplotypes containing either DR4, DR6, or DR7 related phenotype/genotype have some sort of link to aPL production. However, some affected family members were clinically and serologically normal despite of sharing the HLA haplotype with aPL positive siblings [13, 14], postulating that HLA contributions are not the only determinant of aPL production or development of APS.

HLA Haplotype and aPL

HLA class II (DP, DQ, and DR) loci is located on chromosome 6, being the main function of this locus to mediate specific T lymphocyte dependent immune responses. HLA associations with SLE and autoantibodies in SLE have been extensively studied in various ethnic groups.

The HLA associations with aPL are the center of interest due to the clinically relevant prothrombotic effects of these autoantibodies. Asherson et al [18] reported the increased frequency of DR4 in 13 patients with primary APS in a British population, data confirmed by Camps et al [19] in a population from the south of Spain and by Goldstein et al [20] in Canadian patients. HLA DR4 is typically in linkage disequilibrium with HLA-DQB1*0302 (DQ8) or DQB1*0301 (DQ7) [21]. Vargas-Alarcon et al [22] found that HLA DR5 was increased in 17 Mexican patients with primary APS. However, considering the antigen heterogeneity of aPL, specific autoantibody subgroup analysis needs to be done.

Studies of HLA alleles in patients with conventional aCL showed increased frequencies of HLA DR4 [23–25] or DR7 [19, 26] in SLE population. DR7 was also increased in Mexican patients with aCL [27]. After a specific β_2-GPI-based ELISA assay became available, positive correlations were found between anti-β_2-GPI antibodies and DQB1*0604/5-DRB1*1302 in African Americans, DR4-DQB1*0302 in white/Mexican Americans [28], and DRB1*0901 in Japanese [29]. Galeazzi et al [30] showed increased frequency of DRB1*0402/3 and DQB1*0302 in a large series of European lupus patients with anti-β_2-GPI antibodies. These studies were done in SLE or mixture population. In patients with primary APS, we [31] showed in a detailed haplotype analysis that HLA DQB1*0604/5/6/7/9-DQA1*0102-DRB1*1302 and DQB1*0303-DQA1*0201-DRB1*0701 haplotypes and their components may be responsible for anti–β_2-GPI antibody production in the British Caucasoid population.

LA activity is due to a highly heterogeneous population of antibodies and it may be difficult to confirm HLA linkage to LA. Arnett et al [32] suggested that the risk factor for aPL was an HLA DQB1 sequence comprising a specific amino acid sequence ([71]TRAELDT[77]) in the third hypervariable region in the DQB1 outer domain. As this region in the domain is involved in presentation of the antigens to the T lymphocyte receptor, it may influence the resulting immune response. HLA DQB1*0301, DQB1*0302, DQB1*0303, and DQB1*06 alleles share the same sequence in the 71–77 region, as described above, and may be genetic determinants of LA. LA may include autoantibodies to at least 2 phospholipid bound plasma proteins, β_2-GPI and prothrombin [33]. In their study, Arnett et al [32], however, did not discriminate between β_2-GPI dependent LA and prothrombin dependent LA. DQB1*0301/4 was found to be increased in patients with phosphatidylserine dependent antiprothrombin antibodies (aPS/PT) [34]. The increased frequency of HLA DQB1*0301/4-DQA1*0301/2-DRB1*04 haplotype in aPS/PT-positive patients makes this haplotype and its components to be a possible marker for antiprothrombin antibodies production in APS. We demonstrated that the presence of aPS/PT is more closely associated with LA than antiprothrombin antibodies detected using the irradiated plate system [35, 36], and at least the linkage between HLA DQB1*0301/4-DQA1*0301/2-DRB1*04 haplotype and aPS/PT partly explains the correlation between LA and DQB1*03 (Fig. 41.1).

Extended Haplotype and aPL

HLA class II gene polymorphisms may correlate with the immune response against thrombosis related autoantigens. It is also possible that yet to be defined polymor-

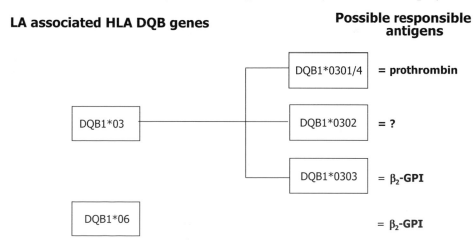

LA associated HLA DQB genes

Possible responsible antigens

DQB1*03

DQB1*0301/4 = prothrombin

DQB1*0302 = ?

DQB1*0303 = β_2-GPI

DQB1*06 = β_2-GPI

Figure 41.1. Lupus anticoagulant (LA) associated HLA-DQB genes and possible responsible antibodies. β_2-GPI = β_2-glycoprotein I.

phisms in linkage disequilibrium with HLA region are responsible for the induction of autoimmune aPL.

HLA-DP, HLA-DM, C4, and tumor necrosis factor α (TNF-α) regions have linkage disequilibrium with HLA-DR/DQ haplotype, and their link to aPL/APS have been investigated. Two studies reported a positive correlation between DPB1* genotypes and aCL [37, 38]. Recently Sanchez et al [39] presented that DMA*0102 variation is 1 of the genetic risks for aPL production. The biological significance of those genotypes is not known, presumably reflecting the linkage disequilibrium with aPL associated DQ-DR haplotype; that is, DQB1*0303-DRB1*0701 for DMA*0102.

Wilson et al [40] described the association between aCL and C4Q0 allele in African-American populations, and some years later reported familial aCL with the C4 deficiency genotype [15]. Genetic C4 deficiency was associated with the development of autoantibodies and immune complex diseases because the classical pathway of complement activation plays a major role for removal of circulating immune complex. However, serum C4 levels do not relate with C4 null allele, and a further study did not confirm the correlation of C4a allele to aCL [41].

We focused on the TNF-α loci in MHC class III region [42]. TNF-α is a proinflammatory cytokine and may play a role to develop thrombosis by stimulating procoagulant cells. Plasma levels of TNF-α were higher in patients with APS compared with non-APS subjects. TNFA-238*A polymorphism in TNF-α promoter region was correlated with APS, but we failed to demonstrate an association of this genotype and plasma TNF-α level, suggesting that the polymorphism is not responsible for the level of TNF-α production. The TNFA-238*A has, again, linkage to DQB1*0303-DRB1*0701.

Genetics of β_2-GPI

Single Nucleotide Polymorphisms (SNPs) of β_2-GPI Gene

Amongst aPL, β_2-GPI, which bears the epitope(s) for aCL binding, has been widely studied. These epitopes are exposed when β_2-GPI binds to negatively charged phospholipids such as cardiolipin, or oxidized plastic plates [33], behaving thus as a cofactor for aCL binding. Several studies have highlighted the significance of anti–β_2-GPI antibodies as an alternative ELISA with higher specificity than the conventional aCL ELISA [43].

β_2-GPI, which binds to negatively charged phospholipids, interacts with phospholipid associated coagulation reactions. The human β_2-GPI gene is localized on chromosome 17q23-qter [44], and the genetic construction of β_2-GPI was reported [45]. When the molecular basis of β_2-GPI polymorphisms was defined, 4 major polymorphisms (Ser/Asn^{88}, Leu/Val^{247}, Cys/Gly^{306}, and Trp/Ser^{316}) became evident [46–48].

The significance of antigen polymorphisms in the production of autoantibodies or in the development of autoimmune diseases is being discussed. Amino acid differences can lead to differences in antigenic epitopes of a given protein. In particular, β_2-GPI undergoes conformational alteration upon interaction with phospholipids [49]. Amino acid differences of β_2-GPI can affect the nature of conformational alterations induced by interaction with phospholipids. Therefore, polymorphism on or near the phospholipid binding site of the antigenic site can affect aCL (anti–β_2-GPI antibodies) production and the development of APS. β_2-GPI Ser/Asn[88], Leu/Val[247], Cys/Gly[306], and Trp/Ser[316] polymorphisms correspond to sites on Exon 3, 7, 7, and 8 of the β_2-GPI gene, respectively. Cys/Gly[306] and Trp/Ser[316] polymorphisms may affect the structure of phospholipid binding site of domain 5 of β_2-GPI, thus Gly[306] or Ser[316] β_2-GPI has low phospholipid binding ability compared with wild-type β_2-GPI [50].

Among these polymorphisms, β_2-GPI Leu/Val[247] polymorphism locates in domain 5 of β2-GPI, between the phospholipid binding sites [51] and the potential site of the epitopes for anti–β_2-GPI antibodies [52, 53]. Therefore, the position 247 polymorphism, or polymorphisms in linkage equilibrium, can affect the conformational change of β_2-GPI and the exposure of the epitopes for aCL (anti–β_2-GPI antibodies).

Our team analyzed the genetic polymorphism of β_2-GPI in a British cohort of well-defined APS patients (88 Caucasoid patients with APS; 57 with primary APS and 31 with APS secondary to SLE) and reported that the allele containing Val[247] was significantly more frequent in primary APS patients with anti–β_2-GPI antibodies than in healthy controls or in primary APS patients without anti–β_2-GPI antibodies [54]. Val[247] of β_2-GPI may be important for β_2-GPI antigenicity. Hirose et al [55] also reported the predominance of Val[247] in patients with APS (including lupus patients) in Asian populations. Leucin was dominant in the Japanese or African-American normal populations in contrast with predominance of valine in Caucasians. Despite the lacking of epidemiological evidence, the prevalence of APS between races is varied, that is, APS is more common in Caucasians than in African Americans or in Asians. Considering the association between Val[247] and anti–β_2-GPI antibody production, the high frequency of Val[247] in Caucasians may explain the higher prevalence of APS in this population. Positive correlation between Val[247] allele and presence of anti–β_2-GPI antibodies was also reported in Mexican patients [56] and in Japanese population [57]. However, this correlation was not found in other American populations [55] or in patients with thrombosis or pregnancy complications in United Kingdom [58]. This discrepancy may be the result of the difference of the Val[247] allele frequency among races, or the difference in the background of investigated patients.

Recently we found that autoimmune anti–β_2-GPI antibodies showed stronger binding to Val[247]–β_2-GPI than that to Leu[247]–β_2-GPI [57]. Conformational optimization displayed that the replacement of Leu[247] to Val[247] lead to a significant alteration in the tertial structure of domain V and/or domain IV–V interaction.

No correlations were reported between other polymorphisms of β_2-GPI and aPL/APS [48, 54].

Genetics of β_2-GPI Deficiency

In European populations, the prevalence of low plasma β_2-GPI levels was reported to be 6.8% to 12.5% [59], but a correlation between low β_2-GPI plasma levels and thrombophilia was not found.

We examined serum β_2-GPI levels in disease-free Japanese populations [60]. We found a wide range in β_2-GPI concentration and identified 2 siblings with a complete β_2-GPI deficiency, 1 apparently healthy 36-year-old woman, and her brother. Analysis of their β_2-GPI genes revealed that a thymine corresponding to position

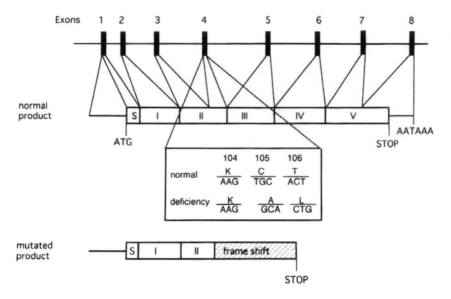

Figure 41.2. Construction of the β_2-glycoprotein I gene and protein in the β_2-glycoprotein I deficiency.

379 of the β_2-GPI cDNA was deleted (β_2-GPI Sapporo), hence, a frame shift would occur thus making the gene code for an amino acid sequence unrelated to β_2-GPI beyond this position (Fig. 41.2).

The siblings of homozygous β_2-GPI Sapporo subjects had no thrombotic episodes. In those individuals, elevated thrombin generation, enhancement of activated protein C response, or the fibrinolytic system were nil [61]. Thus, congenital β_2-GPI deficiency may not be a clinical risk for thrombosis, and apparently is not associated with increased/decreased thrombin formation (i.e., "subclinical" thrombotic/bleeding tendency) both in vivo and in vitro. Therefore, congenital β_2-GPI deficiency is not a risk factor for thrombosis or for bleeding tendencies.

In contrast, there was a case report of both Gly[306] and Ser[316] β_2-GPI mutation carrier, low phospholipid binding variant of β_2-GPI as described above, who had recurrence of deep vein thrombosis and stroke until the age of 35 [62]. β_2-GPI knockout mice showed decreased in vitro ability for thrombin generation [63]. Furthermore, although mice lacking β_2-GPI are fertile, the success of early pregnancy is moderately compromised, suggesting that β_2-GPI is necessary for optimal implantation and placental morphogenesis.

Genetics of β_2-GPI are summarized in Table 41.1.

Other Genetic Risk Factors for APS

Some patients with APS have artery related disorders, while others venous thrombosis only. Even some individuals with aPL do not have symptoms of APS. Such clinical heterogeneity of APS means that there are some additional risks to developing clinical manifestations of APS.

Table 41.1. Genetics of β_2-glycoprotein I.

Gene	Domain	Biological significance	Consequence	Reference
Ser/Asn[88]	II	Unknown	Unknown	46, 47
Leu/Val[247]	V	Alteration in the tertial structure domain V and/or domain IV–V interaction	(1) Correlation with high prevalence of anti–β_2-GPI antibodies (2) Anti–β_2-GPI autoantibody high binding	46, 47 54–58
Cys/Gly[306]	V	Gly[306]: low phospholipid binding	Gly[306]: low β_2-GPI property ?	47, 48
Trp/Ser[316]	V	Ser[316]: low phospholipid binding	Ser[316]: low β_2-GPI property ?	47, 48
Thymine(379) deletion	II	Cys[105] frame shift ?	β_2-GPI deficiency	60, 61

A number of genetic variants have been analyzed as risk factors for the development of APS. In particular, polymorphisms in genes involved in thrombus formation have been explored. Factor V Leiden is the most common thrombophilia in Caucasoid populations. However, the presence of factor V Leiden did not alter the clinical features of APS [64–68]. Prothrombin promotor G20210A, another common genetic risk for venous thrombosis, was found to be rare in patients with APS, implying that this genetic variant did not affect venous thrombosis in patients with aPL [68–71].

Impaired fibrinolytical outcomes may be 1 of the pathogenic factors for thrombotic events in patients with aPL. We studied the consequences of the well-known gene polymorphisms of tissue plasminogen activator (tPA) and plasminogen activator inhibitor-1 (PAI-1) in patients positive for aPL [72]. Alu-repeat insertion (I)/deletion (D) polymorphism of the tPA gene and 4G/5G polymorphism in the PAI-1 promoter gene were examined but there was no significant correlation between these gene polymorphisms and clinical symptoms of APS in patients with aPL. However, the presence of the 4G allele of the 4G/5G polymorphism of the PAI-1 gene was reported to be an additional risk factor for the development of arterial thrombosis in APS in a Spanish population [73]. An angiotensin converting enzyme gene polymorphism [74] or factor XIII Val34Leu polymorphism [75] were also explored in APS but those genotypes did not seem to have a role in APS.

The polymorphism of Fcγ receptor, FcγRIIA H/R131, is associated with the binding affinity for human IgG2 (i.e., FcgRIIA-H131 isoform has a higher affinity than FcgRIIA-R131). Because anti–β_2-GPI antibodies show IgG2 dominant distribution [76], we studied the prevalence of receptor isoforms in patients with aPL. We could not demonstrate a significant correlation between this polymorphism and any feature of APS [77], but meta-analysis suggested a possible link of R/R genotype to APS, mainly driven by secondary APS [78]. Despite the numerous studies on the immunogenetic predispostion on APS or aPL, the available data suggested that there are not apparent genetic risk factors for developing thrombosis in patients with aPL.

Conclusion

Genetic factors related to aPL and APS have been widely investigated. Many candidate genes, including HLA class II haplotype, have been presented to predispose aPL or APS. However, it is difficult to determine genetic risk factors related to aPL development and clinical manifestations of APS in these patients as there is a high heterogeneity in antigen specificity and in the pathophysiology of thrombosis.

References

1. Exner T, Barber S, Kronenberg H, Rickard KA. Familial association of the lupus anticoagulant. Br J Haematol 1980;45:89–96.
2. Matthey F, Walshe K, Mackie IJ, Machin SJ. Familial occurrence of the antiphospholipid syndrome. J Clin Pathol 1989;42:495–497.
3. Cevallos R, Darnige L, Arvieux J, Veyssier P, Gruel Y. Antiphospholipid and anti-beta 2 glycoprotein I antibodies in monozygotic twin sisters. J Rheumatol 1994;21:1970–1971.
4. Mackworth-Young C, Chan J, et al. High incidence of anticardiolipin antibodies in relatives of patients with systemic lupus erythematosus. J Rheumatol 1987;14:723–726.
5. Goldberg SN, Conti-Kelly AM, Greco TP. A family study of anticardiolipin antibodies and associated clinical conditions. Am J Med 1995;99:473–479.
6. Mackie IJ, Colaco CB, Machin SJ. Familial lupus anticoagulants. Br J Haematol 1987;67:359–363.
7. Ford PM, Brunet D, Lillicrap DP, Ford S. Premature stroke in a family with lupus anticoagulant and antiphospholipid antibodies. Stroke 1990;21:66–71.
8. Bansal AS, Hogan PG, Gibbs H, Frazer IH. Familial primary antiphospholipid antibody syndrome. Arthritis Rheum 1996;39:705–706.
9. Cantalapiedra A, Avello AG, Navarro JL, Cesar JM. Familial occurrence of primary antiphospholipid syndrome. Thromb Res 1999;95:127–129.
10. Goel N, Ortel TL, Bali D, et al. Familial antiphospholipid antibody syndrome: criteria for disease and evidence for autosomal dominant inheritance. Arthritis Rheum 1999;42:318–327.
11. Rouget JP, Goudemand J, Montreuil G, Cosson A, Jaillard J. Lupus anticoagulant: a familial observation. Lancet 1982;2:105.
12. Bussel J, Miller S, Hilgartner M, et al. Transient appearance of the lupus anticoagulant in three family members sharing the A11B35DR4 haplotype. Am J Pediatr Hematol Oncol 1983;5:275–278.
13. Dagenais P, Urowitz MB, Gladman DD, Norman CS. A family study of the antiphospholipid syndrome associated with other autoimmune diseases. J Rheumatol 1992;19:1393–1396.
14. May KP, West SG, Moulds J, Kotzin BL. Different manifestations of the antiphospholipid antibody syndrome in a family with systemic lupus erythematosus. Arthritis Rheum 1993;36:528–533.
15. Wilson WA, Scopelitis E, Michalski JP, et al. Familial anticardiolipin antibodies and C4 deficiency genotypes that coexist with MHC DQB1 risk factors. J Rheumatol 1995;22:227–235.
16. Hudson N, Busque L, Rauch J, Kassis J, Fortin PR. Familial antiphospholipid syndrome and HLA-DRB gene associations. Arthritis Rheum 1997;40:1907–1908.
17. Bhattacharya S, Kendra J, Schiach C. A case study of familial anti-phospholipid syndrome. Clin Lab Haematol 2002;24:313–316.
18. Asherson RA, Doherty DG, Vergani D, Khamashta MA, Hughes GR. Major histocompatibility complex associations with primary antiphospholipid syndrome. Arthritis Rheum 1992;35:124–125.
19. Camps MT, Cuadrado MJ, Ocon P, et al. Association between HLA class II antigens and primary antiphospholipid syndrome from the south of Spain. Lupus 1995;4:51–55.
20. Goldstein R, Moulds JM, Smith CD, Sengar DP. MHC studies of the primary antiphospholipid antibody syndrome and of antiphospholipid antibodies in systemic lupus erythematosus. J Rheumatol 1996;23:1173–1179.
21. Doherty DG, Vaughan RW, Donaldson PT, Mowat AP. HLA DQA, DQB, and DRB genotyping by oligonucleotide analysis: distribution of alleles and haplotypes in British caucasoids. Hum Immunol 1992;34:53–63.
22. Vargas-Alarcon G, Granados J, Bekker C, Alcocer-Varela J, Alarcon-Segovia D. Association of HLA-DR5 (possibly DRB1*1201) with the primary antiphospholipid syndrome in Mexican patients. Arthritis Rheum 1995;38:1340–1341.

23. McHugh NJ, Maddison PJ. HLA-DR antigens and anticardiolipin antibodies in patients with systemic lupus erythematosus. Arthritis Rheum 1989;32:1623–1624.
24. McNeil HP, Gavaghan T, Krilis SA, Geczy AF, Chesterman CN. HLA-DR antigens and anticardiolipin antibodies. Clin Exp Rheumatol 1990;8:425–426.
25. Hartung K, Coldewey R, Corvetta A, et al. MHC gene products and anticardiolipin antibodies in systemic lupus erythematosus results of a multicenter study. SLE Study Group. Autoimmunity 1992;13:95–99.
26. Savi M, Ferraccioli GF, Neri TM, et al. HLA-DR antigens and anticardiolipin antibodies in northern Italian systemic lupus erythematosus patients. Arthritis Rheum 1988;31:1568–1570.
27. Granados J, Vargas-Alarcon G, Andrade F, et al. The role of HLA-DR alleles and complotypes through the ethnic barrier in systemic lupus erythematosus in Mexicans. Lupus 1996;5:184–189.
28. Arnett FC, Thiagarajan P, Ahn C, Reveille JD. Associations of anti-beta2-glycoprotein I autoantibodies with HLA class II alleles in three ethnic groups. Arthritis Rheum 1999;42:268–274.
29. Hashimoto H, Yamanaka K, Tokano Y, et al. HLA-DRB1 alleles and beta 2 glycoprotein I-dependent anticardiolipin antibodies in Japanese patients with systemic lupus erythematosus. Clin Exp Rheumatol 1998;16:423–427.
30. Galeazzi M, Sebastiani GD, Tincani A, et al. HLA class II alleles associations of anticardiolipin and anti-beta2GPI antibodies in a large series of European patients with systemic lupus erythematosus. Lupus 2000;9:47–55.
31. Caliz T, Atsumi T, Kondeatis E, Amengual O, et al. HLA class II gene polymorphisms in antiphospholipid syndrome: haplotype analysis in 83 caucasoid patients. Rheumatology 2001;40:31–36.
32. Arnett FC, Olsen ML, Anderson KL, Reveille JD. Molecular analysis of major histocompatibility complex alleles associated with the lupus anticoagulant. J Clin Invest 1991;87:1490–1495.
33. Atsumi T, Matsuura E, Koike T. Immunology of antiphospholipid antibodies and co-factors. In: Lahita RG, ed. Systemic lupus erythematosus. San Diego: Academic Press; 2004:1081–1105.
34. Bertolaccini ML, Atsumi T, Caliz AR, et al. Association of antiphosphatidylserine/prothrombin autoantibodies with HLA class II genes. Arthritis Rheum 2000;43:683–688.
35. Atsumi T, Ieko M, Bertolaccini ML, Ichikawa K, et al. Association of autoantibodies against the phosphatidylserine-prothrombin complex with manifestations of the antiphospholipid syndrome and with the presence of lupus anticoagulant. Arthritis Rheum 2000;43:1982–1993.
36. Amengual O, Atsumi T, Koike T. Specificities, properties, and clinical significance of antiprothrombin antibodies. Arthritis Rheum 2003;48:886–895.
37. Galeazzi M, Sebastiani GD, Passiu G, et al. HLA-DP genotyping in patients with systemic lupus erythematosus: correlations with autoantibody subsets. J Rheumatol 1992;19:42–46.
38. Sebastiani GD, Galeazzi M, Tincani A, et al. HLA-DPB1 alleles association of anticardiolipin and anti-beta2GPI antibodies in a large series of European patients with systemic lupus erythematosus. Lupus 2003;12:560–563.
39. Sanchez ML, Katsumata K, Atsumi T, et al. Association of HLA-DM polymorphism with the production of antiphospholipid antibodies. Ann Rheum Dis 2004;63:1645–1648.
40. Wilson WA, Perez MC, Michalski JP, Armatis PE. Cardiolipin antibodies and null alleles of C4 in black Americans with systemic lupus erythematosus. J Rheumatol 1988;5:1768–1772.
41. Petri M, Watson R, Winkelstein JA, McLean RH. Clinical expression of systemic lupus erythematosus in patients with C4A deficiency. Medicine (Baltimore) 1993;72:236–244.
42. Bertolaccini ML, Atsumi T, Lanchbury JS, et al. Plasma tumor necrosis factor alpha levels and the -238*A promoter polymorphism in patients with antiphospholipid syndrome. Thromb Haemost 2001;85:198–203.
43. Amengual O, Atsumi T, Khamashta M, Koike T, Hughes GRV. Specificity of ELISA for antibody to β2-glycoprotein I in patients with antiphospholipid syndrome. Br J Rheumatol 1996;35:1239–1243.
44. Steinkasserer A, Estaller C, Weiss EH, Sim RB, Day AJ. Complete nucleotide and deduced amino acid sequence of human beta 2-glycoprotein I. Biochem J 1991;277:387–391.
45. Matsuura E, Igarashi M, Igarashi Y, et al. Molecular definition of human β2-glycoprotein I (β2-GPI) by cDNA cloning and inter species differences of β2-GPI in alternation anticardiolipin binding. Int Immunol 1991;3:1217–1221.
46. Steinkasserer A, Dorner C, Wurzner R, Sim RB. Human β2-glycoprotein I: molecular analysis of DNA and amino acid polymorphism. Hum Genet 1993;91:401–402.
47. Sanghera DK, Kristensen T, Hamman RF, Kamboh MI. Molecular basis of the apolipoprotein H (β2-glycoprotein I) protein polymorphism. Hum Genet 1997;100:57–62.
48. Gushiken FC, Arnett FC, Ahn C, Thiagarajan P. Polymorphism of beta2-glycoprotein I at codons 306 and 316 in patients with systemic lupus erythematosus and antiphospholipid syndrome. Arthritis Rheum 1999;42:1189–1193.

49. Matsuura E, Igarashi M, Igarashi Y, et al. Molecular studies on phospholipid-binding sites and cryptic epitopes appering on β2-glycoprotein I structure recognized by anticardiolipin antibodies. Lupus 1995;4(suppl1):S13–S17.
50. Kamboh MI, Mehdi H. Genetics of apolipoprotein H (beta2-glycoprotein I) and anionic phospholipid binding. Lupus 1998;7:S10–S13.
51. Hunt J, Krilis S. The fifth domain of β2-glycoprotein I contains a phospholipid binding site (Cys281-Cys288) and a region recognized by anticardiolipin antibodies. J Immunol 1994;152:653–659.
52. Ichikawa K, Khamashta M, Koike T, Matsuura E, Hughes GRV. Reactivity of monoclonal anticardiolipin antibodies from patients with the antiphospholipid syndrome to β2-glycoprotein I. Arthritis Rheum 1994;37:1453–1461.
53. Igarashi M, Matsuura E, Igarashi Y, et al. Human β2-glycoprotein I as an anticardiolipin cofactor determined using deleted mutants expressed by a Baculovirus system. Blood 1996;87:3262–3270.
54. Atsumi T, Tsutsumi A, Amengual O, et al. Correlation between beta2-glycoprotein I valine/leucine247 polymorphism and anti-beta2-glycoprotein I antibodies in patients with primary antiphospholipid syndrome. Rheumatology 1999;38:721–723.
55. Hirose N, Williams R, Alberts AR, et al. A role for the polymorphism at position 247 of the beta2-glycoprotein I gene in the generation of anti-beta2-glycoprotein I antibodies in the antiphospholipid syndrome. Arthritis Rheum 1999;42:1655–1661.
56. Prieto GA, Cabral AR, Zapata-Zuniga M, et al. Valine/valine genotype at position 247 of the beta2-glycoprotein I gene in Mexican patients with primary antiphospholipid syndrome: association with anti-beta2-glycoprotein I antibodies. Arthritis Rheum 2003;48:471–474.
57. Yasuda S, Atsumi T, Matsuura E, et al. Significance of valine/leucine247 polymorphism of β2-glycoprotein I in antiphospholipid syndrome: increased reactivity of anti-β2-glycoprotein I autoantibodies to the valine247 β2-glycoprotein I variant. Arthritis Rheum 2004;52:212–218.
58. Camilleri RS, Mackie IJ, Humphries SE, Machin SJ, Cohen H. Lack of association of beta2-glycoprotein I polymorphisms Val247Leu and Trp316Ser with antiphospholipid antibodies in patients with thrombosis and pregnancy complications. Br J Haematol 2003;120:1066–1072.
59. Bancsi LF, van der Linden IK, Bertina RM. β2-glycoprotein I deficiency and the risk of thrombosis. Thromb Haemost 1992;67:649–653.
60. Yasuda S, Tsutsumi A, Chiba H, et al. beta(2)-glycoprotein I deficiency: prevalence, genetic background and effects on plasma lipoprotein metabolism and hemostasis. Atherosclerosis 2000;152:337–346.
61. Takeuchi R, Atsumi T, Ieko M, et al. Coagulation and fibrinolytic activities in 2 siblings with beta(2)-glycoprotein I deficiency. Blood 2000;96:1594–1595.
62. Gushiken FC, Arnett FC, Thiagarajan P. Primary antiphospholipid antibody syndrome with mutations in the phospholipid binding domain of beta(2)-glycoprotein I. Am J Hematol 2000;65:160–165.
63. Sheng Y, Reddel SW, Herzog H, et al. Impaired thrombin generation in β2-glycoprotein I null mice. J Biol Chem 2001;276:13817–13821.
64. Montaruli B, Borchiellini A, Tamponi G, et al. Factor V Arg506 ? Gln mutation in patients with antiphospholipid antibodies. Lupus 1996;5:303–306.
65. Simantov R, Lo SK, Salmon JE, Sammaritano LR, Silverstein RL. Factor V Leiden increases the risk of thrombosis in patients with antiphospholipid antibodies. Thromb Res 1996;84:361–365.
66. Pablos JL, Caliz RA, Carreira PE, et al. Risk of thrombosis in patients with antiphospholipid antibodies and factor V Leiden mutation. J Rheumatol 1999;26:588–590.
67. Ames PR, Tommasino C, D'Andrea G, Iannaccone L, Brancaccio V, Margaglione M. Thrombophilic genotypes in subjects with idiopathic antiphospholipid antibodies–prevalence and significance. Thromb Haemost 1998;79:46–49.
68. Chopra N, Koren S, Greer W, et al. Factor V Leiden, prothrombin gene mutation, and thrombosis risk in patients with antiphospholipid antibodies. J Rheumatol 2002;29:1683–1688.
69. Bertolaccini ML, Atsumi T, Hunt BJ, Amengual O, Khamashta MA, Hughes GRV. Prothrombin mutation is not associated with thrombosis in patients with antiphospholipid syndrome. Thromb Haemost 1998;80:202–203.
70. Bentolila S, Ripoll L, Drouet L, Crassard I, Tournier-Lasserve E, Piette JC. Lack of association between thrombosis in primary antiphospholipid syndrome and the recently described thrombophilic 3'-untranslated prothrombin gene polymorphism. Thromb Haemost 1997;78:1415.
71. Ruiz-Arguelles GJ, Garces-Eisele J, Ruiz-Delgado GJ, Alarcon-Segovia D. The G20210A polymorphism in the 3'-untranslated region of the prothrombin gene in Mexican mestizo patients with primary antiphospholipid syndrome. Clin Appl Thromb Hemost 1999;5:158–160.
72. Yasuda S, Tsutsumi A, Atsumi T, et al. Gene polymorphisms of tissue plasminogen activator and plasminogen activator inhibitor-1 in patients with antiphospholipid antibodies. J Rheumatol 2002;29:1192–1197.

73. Tassies D, Espinosa G, Munoz-Rodriguez FJ, et al. The 4G/5G polymorphism of the type 1 plasminogen activator inhibitor gene and thrombosis in patients with antiphospholipid syndrome. Arthritis Rheum 2000;43:2349–2358.
74. Lewis NM, Katsumata K, Atsumi T, et al. An evaluation of an angiotensin-converting enzyme gene polymorphism and the risk of arterial thrombosis in patients with the antiphospholipid syndrome. Arthritis Rheum 2000;43:1655–1656.
75. Diz-Kucukkaya R, Hancer VS, Inanc M, Nalcaci M, Pekcelen Y. Factor XIII Val34Leu polymorphism does not contribute to the prevention of thrombotic complications in patients with antiphospholipid syndrome. Lupus 2004;13:32–35.
76. Amengual O, Atsumi T, Khamashta MA, Bertolaccini ML, Hughes GRV. IgG2 restriction of anti-beta2-glycoprotein I as the basis for the association between IgG2 anticardiolipin antibodies and thrombosis in the antiphospholipid syndrome: comment on the article by Sammaritano et al. Arthritis Rheum 1998;41:1513–1515.
77. Atsumi T, Caliz R, Amengual O, Khamashta MA, Hughes GRV. Fcgamma receptor IIA H/R131 polymorphism in patients with antiphospholipid antibodies. Thromb Haemost 1998;79:924–927.
78. Karassa FB, Bijl M, Davies KA, et al. Role of the Fcgamma receptor IIA polymorphism in the antiphospholipid syndrome: an international meta-analysis. Arthritis Rheum 2003;48:1930–1938.

42   Infection and Drug-Induced Antiphospholipid Antibodies

Silvia S. Pierangeli and Azzudin E. Gharavi[†]

Introduction

Antiphospholipid antibodies (aPL) have been subject of great interest for the past 90 years, first because they were found to be serological markers for syphilis, and later because of their association with clinical complications. A major sub-set of aPL are associated with infections. especially syphilis [1], and another sub-set of aPL are associated with an autoimmune disorder characterized by recurrent thrombosis, fetal death, and thrombocytopenia, called antiphospholipid syndrome (APS) [2, 3]. Neither the relationship between these 2 sub-groups, nor the cause and mechanism of production of aPL in these conditions are clearly understood.

Historical Background

Serological Test for Syphilis (STS)

aPL were detected for the first time in sera from patients with syphilis. Wassermann et al [1] in 1906 used saline extract of liver and spleen of fetus with congenital syphilis as an antigen in a complement fixation test and demonstrated positive reaction with syphilitic sera. The antibody was called Wassermann reagin and the test was introduced as a serological test for syphilis (STS). Although these investigators first believed that in this test, sera reacted with specific antigens derived from *Treponema pallidum,* within a year it was shown that extract of normal human or animal tissues reacted similarly with syphilitic sera [4]. The antigenic component of this test was isolated and identified from bovine heart extracts as cardiolipin by Pangborn [5] in 1941. Later, a flocculation test using suspension of liposomes containing cardiolipin, lecithin, and cholesterol was adopted as a serodiagnostic test for syphilis referred to as the VDRL (Venereal Disease Research Laboratory) test [6].

False Positive STS Using The Complement Fixation Test for Syphilis and VDRL

The presence of aPL detected as Wassermann reagin in conditions other than syphilis was reported as early as 1907 [4]. Detection of Wassermann reagin in the

---

[†] In memory of A.E. Gharavi who passed away on Oct 13, 2004.

serum of a person who did not have syphilis was called "biological false-positive serological test for syphilis" (BFP-STS) and in a retrospective study of false positive reactors, Moore and Mohr identified 2 distinct groups of patients with acute and chronic reactions [7]. Acute reactions are transient and are seen during non-syphilis infections such as viral pneumonia, viral hepatitis, measles, varicella, and scarlet fever [8]. Vaccination against smallpox may also cause BFP-STS [9]. The chronic BFP-STS reactors whose BFP test persisted for a period of 6 months or more had a high prevalence of autoimmune disorders such as systemic lupus erythematosus (SLE), Sjögren syndrome, autoimmune hemolytic anemia, Hashimoto's thyroiditis, and rheumatoid arthritis [7, 9–11]. In 1957, Laurell and Nilsson found that the so-called lupus coagulation inhibitor or "lupus anticoagulant" (LA) was frequently associated with BFP-STS [12] and Lee and Saunders [13] showed that these were aPL, and this observation was confirmed by later studies using monoclonal antibodies [14]. In clinical studies, Bowie et al reported that the LA was associated paradoxically with thrombotic episodes [15].

2.3. Solid Phase Immunoassays for Anticardiolipin Antibodies

In 1983, Harris, Gharavi, and Hughes designed a radioimmunoassay using cardiolipin as antigen [16] to detect antibodies to cardiolipin in SLE patients with a positive LA test. LA tests detect the ability of aPL to prolong phospholipid dependent clotting reactions (such as the activated partial thromboplastin time) in vitro. This assay that was later converted to an enzyme-linked immunoassay (ELISA) [17], was subsequently standardized in several international workshops [18] and gave a new dimension to the field of aPL. The anticardiolipin (aCL) ELISA was first thought to be just a more sensitive test for detecting aPL than STS. However, it was recognized soon that the 2 tests detected somewhat different antibody populations and not all sera with positive STS were always positive in solid phase assay for cardiolipin [19]. In fact, the aCL ELISA did not help diagnosing more patients with syphilis, but it resulted in the recognition of a new syndrome characterized by thrombosis, recurrent abortion, and thrombocytopenia associated with aPL, the Antiphospholipid Syndrome (APS) [20]. The aCL ELISA is now commonly used to detect autoimmune aCL present in APS.

This assay also detected aPL in patients with other infections [21], such as Lyme disease [22], mycoplasma [23], tuberculosis [24], leprosy [25], legionnaires disease [26], Q fever [27], Mediterranean spotted fever [28], etc. Furthermore, aPL in viral infections have also been reported. These include cytomegalovirus [29], Varicella Zoster virus [30], human immune-deficiency virus (HIV) [31], and hepatitis C [32]. Furthermore, transient LA activity has been reported in patients with Epstein–Barr virus infections [33].

Infection-induced aPL

Differentiation of Autoimmune and Infectious-induced aPL: β_2-glycoprotein I

The association of the aPL detected by solid phase assays with serious clinical complications such as venous and arterial thrombosis, recurrent spontaneous abortion, stroke, and myocardial infarction [20] underlined the importance of differentiating the infection-induced aPL that seemed not to be associated with these clinical complications, from aPL associated with autoimmune conditions that are closely associated with these life-threatening complications [34]. Several groups studied these 2 types of aPL with respect to the differences in binding to CL and other individual PL [35] or phospholipid mixtures [36], the differences in IgG sub-classes, in light chain distribution and in their affinity [37]. However, most of these findings remained controversial among different investigators [38].

The important observation that the autoimmune aPL required a lipid binding normal plasma protein which is an inhibitor of coagulation: β_2-glycoprotein I (β_2-GPI) by 3 groups simultaneously in 1990 [39–41] shed a new light on this issue. Matsuura et al reported that binding of aPL in sera from autoimmune diseases (SLE) to CL-coated plates is enhanced by β_2-GPI and called these autoimmune aPL β_2-GPI dependent aPL [39]. In contrast, the binding of aPL from syphilis sera (infection) is inhibited by β_2-GPI, and these infection-associated aPL were called β_2-GPI-independent aPL. It is generally believed that β_2-GPI-dependent antibodies are associated with clinical features of APS, such as thrombosis and pregnancy losses, and the β_2-GPI-independent aPL are not. Other investigators confirmed these findings. We purified IgG and IgM aPL from sera of patients with syphilis, HIV infection, SLE, and chlorpromazine-induced aPL and demonstrated that the binding of autoimmune and drug-induced aPL was enhanced by β_2-GPI, but the binding of syphilis- and HIV-induced aPL was significantly inhibited by β_2-GPI [42]. Hunt et al used purified IgG, IgA, and IgM aPL from patients with infectious or autoimmune diseases and had similar findings [43]. In an elegant study, Celli et al studied the interaction of aPL from 2 different populations (autoimmune and infectious) with CL arranged in a defined bilayer. In this system, β_2-GPI increased, the binding of autoimmune aPL to CL and induced the leakage of the fluorescent probe, carboxyfluorescein (CF), entrapped in the vesicles. In contrast, β_2-GPI inhibited the binding of syphilitic aPL to CL-containing vesicles [44]. The authors concluded that CL β_2-GPI complex is the most likely epitope for autoimmune aPL, and in syphilis β_2-GPI is not likely to be part of the epitope.

Some studies have shown that syphilis and autoimmune aPL differ not only in specificity or β_2-GPI requirement, but also in functional effects. Campbell et al studied the effects of affinity purified aCL antibodies from APS patients and syphilis on platelet activation and aggregation [45]. These investigators showed that in the presence of low concentrations of platelet activators (thrombin, ADP, or collagen), all APS samples (n = 6), but none of the syphilis (n = 5) samples induced platelet aggregation and activation [45]. In another study, affinity purified aPL from APS patients and not from syphilis were shown to inhibit the conversion of prothrombin into thrombin (prothrombinase reaction) when liposomes composed of phosphatidylserine and phosphatidylcholine were used to support the enzymatic reaction [46].

Several investigators have reported that autoimmune aPL may bind to β_2-GPI coated on irradiated, high-binding, or oxidized polystyrene plates [47, 48], and the anti–β_2-GPI antibodies that are detected by this method in the sera of APS and SLE patients would represent only the autoimmune ("pathogenic") aPL [49, 50]. In a study, Forastiero et al showed that 29 out of 35 APS samples, and only 1 out of 37 syphilis sera (that were aCL positive), bound to β_2-GPI coated on irradiated ELISA plates, concluding that performing both ELISA (aCL and anti–β_2-GPI) makes possible to distinguish between APS and syphilitic sera [51]. In another study, Leroy et al examined the prevalence of aPL, anti–β_2-GPI and anti-prothrombin antibodies in chronic hepatitis C patients. Twenty-four percent of the patients had low to moderate levels of aCL, compared with 3.5% in the control population. In contrast the prevalence of anti–β_2-GPI and anti-prothrombin antibodies was not different from the control [52]. The presence of aCL in hepatitis C patients did not correlate with thrombosis or pregnancy losses, indicating that in the absence of associated anti–β_2-GPI antibodies, aPL is not associated with the clinical complications of APS [52].

In a study involving 58 HIV positive patients, Constans et al showed that 3% to 4% of the patients were anti–β_2-GPI positive, whereas the frequency of aCL was 41% [53].

β_2-GPI-dependent aPL and anti–β_2-GPI Antibodies Associated with Infections

Recently the widely believed dogma that the infection-associated aPL are β_2-GPI-independent, do not bind β_2-GPI in the absence of phospholipids and are not associated with the clinical manifestations of APS (i.e., thrombosis and/or pregnancy losses) has been challenged by several reports. In one study, aCL antibody present in leprosy patients were shown to be heterogeneous with respect to their β_2-GPI requirement: in 10 of 31 leprosy sera, the aCL were β_2-GPI dependent and 16 of 31 did not require B_2-GPI for binding to aCL [54]. These observations were confirmed by other investigators who indicated that that these β_2-GPI-dependent aPL were associated with thrombosis. In addition anti–β_2-GPI without aPL were detected in patients with human T lymphotropic virus-1 (HTLV-1) infections associated with tropical spastic paraparesis (TSP)[55]. TSP, which is also called Jamaican neuropathy, is believed to be an autoimmune condition that complicates the HTLV-1 infection only in a small proportion of patients. In another study, parvovirus B19 associated with aCL were shown to be β_2-GPI-dependent and behaved in a similar fashion as the autoimmune aPL [56]. Furthermore, some cases of viral hepatitis C associated aPL have been reported to be complicated with thrombosis [57]. Other investigators have shown association of HCV with multiple autoimmune manifestations [58]. The immune response to HCV infection encompasses the development of autoantibodies, immune complex formation and deposition, and cryoglobulinemia complicated with vasculitis, glomerulonephritis, or neuropathy [58].

There are also several reports of LA and aPL of the "autoimmune" type associated with thrombosis in patients with Epstein–Barr virus [33], leprosy [25, 54] cytomegalovirus (CMV) [29], and HIV infection [31], hepatitis C [32], and adenovirus [59]. We have recently reported a young woman with an acute CMV infection who developed APS manifested by a common iliac vein thrombosis [60]. IgM aCL appeared with the onset of the infection, followed later by IgG aCL. Five months later, both IgM and IgG aCL levels disappeared from the serum. This was the second case of APS associated with CMV infection in the literature that we are aware of.

In 1992, Gharavi and colleagues for the first time induced high levels of aPL in rabbits and mice following immunization with heterologous (human purified) β_2-GPI [61]. These aPL were pathogenic [62, 63] and the model was easily reproduced by other investigators [64]. β_2-GPI immunized PL/J mice developed high levels of aPL and had significantly lower litter sizes compared with the ovalbumin or non-immunized groups; in addition, 3 of the 4 mice subsequently developed paraparesis and trophic changes in the tail and hind limbs resembling transverse myelopathy 8 months after the induction of APS [65, 66]. Thus, an APS-like syndrome could be induced in autoimmune "prone" mice. We hypothesize then that in susceptible humans, exposure to viral or bacterial agents with β_2-GPI-like epitopes could lead to autoimmunity to self β_2-GPI, and thus the genesis of APS, through the mechanism of molecular mimicry.

It is also possible then that certain infections may induce aPL of the "autoimmune" type that are not transient. Hence, we hypothesized that in these patients, aPL production may be induced by binding of β_2GPI-like foreign PL binding proteins (such as viral/bacterial proteins) to self PL, thus forming immunogenic complexes against which aPL are produced. The sequence similarity (molecular mimicry) of these proteins to the region (s) of $\beta2$-GPI may break tolerance to self β_2-GPI and induce anti–β_2-GPI/PL antibody production. To test this hypothesis, we first investigated whether the PL binding region of β_2-GPI alone, without the remaining of the β_2-GPI molecule, can induce pathogenic aPL production. A 15 amino acid peptide spanning the Gly^{274}-Cyc^{288} in the fifth domain of β_2-GPI, which was shown to be a major PL binding site of β_2-GPI [67], which we called GDKV, was synthesized. Binding of these peptides to CL-coated plates by ELISA confirmed its PL binding property [68]. A monoclonal antibody with aPL and anti–β_2-GPI activity was generated by fusing spleen cells from GDKV immunized mice with myeloma cell lines. We confirmed the pathogenicity of the GDKV-induced monoclonal aPL [69] using in vivo models for thrombus enhancement and microcirculation.

Do Infections Induce Autoimmune aPL? Viral Peptide–induced aPL

The next question was whether proteins other than β_2-GPI, that contain GDKV-like regions, can induce pathogenic aPL and anti–β_2-GPI production. From the Genbank database, several proteins were identified that have sequence similarity to GDKV. These proteins, much like GDKV, contain series of lysines (with positive charge) flanked at least in 1 side by hydrophobic residues. They should therefore have the potential to bind anionic PL and be suitable candidates for inducing aPL by immunization. Four of these peptides were synthesized (QBC Hopkins, MA): TADL (dnb2_ade02), TIFI (from ulbo_hcmva), VITT (us27_hcmva), and SGDF (tlpa_bacsu) that shared structural similarity with the PL binding region of β_2-GPI (GDKV). These peptides are of additional interest because they are part of human viruses (e.g., adenoviruses or CMV) to which human subjects are commonly exposed. These peptides all showed greater degrees of binding to PL compared to GDKV. Subsequently, groups of PL-J mice immunized with these peptides (conjugated to BSA in Freund's adjuvant) produced high levels of aPL and anti–β_2-GPI antibodies [70]. These findings suggest that incidental immunization during a subclinical infection with these viral and bacterial proteins may trigger aPL antibody production.

Induction of "Pathogenic" aPL with Viral and Bacterial Peptides

To determine whether aPL induced by immunization with viral peptides are pathogenic in vivo, we produced monoclonal antibodies from spleen cells of mice immunized with TIFI, the 19 amino acid CMV derived peptide. Ten monoclonal aPL were tested for finding to different PL by ELISA and for LA activity by the modified kaolin clotting test (KCT). Binding of the monoclonal antibodies to CL was inhibited by CL micelles and this inhibition was further enhanced when β_2-GPI was added to the CL micelles. Five of 10 monoclonal aPL had LA activity. Pathogenic effects of aPL induced by the CMV peptide were evaluated in vitro by incubating these monoclonal aPL with confluent monolayers of human umbilical vein endothelial cells (HUVECs) and measuring the expression of adhesion molecules ICAM-1, VCAM-1, and E-selectin by ELISA. All 10 monoclonal antibodies upregulated the expression of adhesion molecules by HUVECs [71]. The pathogenic effects of these monoclonal aPL were further evaluated using our in vivo mouse models of thrombus formation and microcirculation. Two groups of CD-1 male normal mice were injected each with 1 of the 2 monoclonal IgM aPL. The third group was injected with irrelevant control murine monoclonal IgM. The vein was pinched with standard pressure used to introduce an injury and to induce clot formation. Clot formation and dissolution in the transilluminated vein were visualized and recorded with a microscope equipped with a closed-circuit video system. Thrombus size (in square micrometers) at maximum was measured by digitizing the image and tracing its outer margin; the times (in minutes) of formation (from appearance to maximum size) and disappearance (from maximum size to disappearance) of the thrombus were also measured as described. Activation of endothelial cells was assessed by direct visualization and quantitation of adhering, "sticking" white blood cells (WBC) to endothelial cells in the microcirculation of the exposed cremaster muscle in mice [71]. The surgical procedure was performed 72 hours after the first injection with antibody preparation or with Ig control. Mice injected with monoclonal aPL had significantly larger clots that persisted longer when compared to controls. The adhesion of leukocytes to endothelial cells was significantly increased in mice injected with TIFI-induced monoclonal IgM aPL D2/AC10 or F3AA4, compared with controls [71].

The effects of TIFI-induced IgM aPL on pregnancy outcome was recently evaluated by injecting BALB/c mice on days 4, 8, and 12 of pregnancy with 50 µg of either IGM aPL or normal mouse immunoglobulin. The number of viable pups in aPL-treated groups was almost 50% of than in the control group [72].

These studies demonstrate that pathogenic aPL with properties similar to those found in APS patients can be induced by immunization with molecular structures similar to the PL binding site of β_2-GPI (GDKV), such as PL binding–CMV peptide TIFI. Because human subjects are commonly exposed to these viral products, molecular mimicry may break tolerance to itself and induce aPL and anti–β_2-GPI production in patients with APS.

Our findings were confirmed recently by Blank and Shoenfeld [73]. Those investigators employed a peptide phage display library to identify 3 hexapeptides that specifically reacted with monoclonal anti–β_2-GPI and inhibited the biological functions of the corresponding anti–β_2-GPI antibodies such as induction of APS in vivo and endothelial cell activation in vitro [73]. Using the Swiss protein database, the authors found a high homology between the hexapeptides with some bacteria and viruses. Naive mice were immunized with a panel of pathogen particles sharing the appropriate homology with the peptides. All the mice developed aPL. Affinity purified IgG anti-hexapeptide antibodies were isolated and infused IV in BALB/c mice and development of clinical manifestations of APS was then studied. Only mice infused with antibodies derived from mice immunized with *Haemophilus influenzae* or *Neisseria gonorrhoeae* directed to the hexapeptide TLRVYK had clinical manifestations resembling the experimental APS [73].

The data presented in previous paragraphs suggest that pathogenic aPL and anti–β_2-GPI can be generated with peptides of bacterial and viral origin that mimic various regions of β_2-GPI. These data strongly suggest molecular mimicry between bacterial/viral antigens and self proteins in APS.

In APS, there is evidence that additional PL binding proteins other than β_2-GPI are also involved in some APS subjects. In APS, future challenges include the possible extension of the experimental model to include other PL binding proteins. Knowledge of the causative autoantigens in APS will likely facilitate efforts to down-regulate aPL production as a method of treating APS.

Effects of Bacterial and Viral Peptides on aPL Mediated Thrombosis In Vivo

In one recent study, we examined the ability of the synthetic peptide (named peptide A, NTLKTPRVGGC) that shares similarity with common bacterial antigens, to reverse aPL mediated thrombosis in mice in vivo. Peptide A is also found in region I/II of β_2-GPI. A scrambled form of peptide A (named scA, GTKGCPNVRLT) was used as a control. Sera from 29 patients with APS bound to peptide A but not to peptide scA by ELISA in a dose-dependent fashion. Mice treated with aPL and infused with peptide scA produced significantly larger thrombi when compared to mice treated with control IgG (IgG-NHS) and peptide scA (2466 ± 462-μm^2 vs. 772.5 ± 626.4 μm^2). Treatment of mice with peptide A significantly decreased thrombus size in mice injected with aPL (1063 ± 890 μm^2 vs. 2466 ± 462 μm^2) [74].

Similarly, in another recent study we examined the ability of TIFI to affect aPL mediated thrombosis in mice. Sera from 54 patients with APS bound significantly to TIFI by ELISA [mean OD = 0.429 ± 0.078 vs. 25 control sera (mean OD = 0.228 ± 0.079)]. Cardiolipin liposomes containing TIFI inhibited completely the binding of 11 sera from APS patients to CL. Competitive studies showed that TIFI competes with β_2-GPI. Mice treated with aPL and infused with saline produced significantly larger thrombi when compared to mice treated with IgG-NHS and saline (1442 ± 162 μm^2 vs. 140 ± 26 μm^2). Treatment with TIFI significantly decreased thrombus size in mice injected with aPL (312 ± 90 μm^2 vs. 1442 ±162 μm^2). The data indicate that peptide A (from bacterial origin) and TIFI (from viral origin) inhibit thrombogenic properties of aPL in mice and this may happen by competition with β_2-GPI, hence hampering the pathogenic effects of aPL.

Altogether these findings may have important implications in designing new modalities of prevention and/or treatment of thrombosis in APS.

Drug-induced aPL

Several drugs can result in the production of aPL. These include procainamide, phenothiazines, quinine, and oral contraceptives. These compounds have been also shown to be responsible for the drug-induced lupus syndrome. Pathogenicity of drug-induced aPL is variable and is closely related to the specific drug involved. In general, phenothiazine-induced aPL are considered fairly benign [75], while procainamide and other drug-induced aPL are associated with thrombosis [76].

Chlorpromazine (CPZ) is by far the most common medication associated with drug-induced aPL. A review of over 650 LA-positive patients in 25 separate studies revealed 78 patients to have drug-induced antibodies; most were attributed to phenothiazines (n = 69) or procainamide (n = 5), but 4 patients had aPL-induced hydralazine (n = 3) and phenytoin (n = 1) [77]. Finally, drugs implicated in the series of 34 drug-induced LA from Triplett et al include quinidine (n = 7) and phenytoin (n = 4), in addition to a single case each of valproic acid, amoxicillin, hydralazine, and propranolol [76]. In this study, CPZ and procainamide accounted for a large proportion of positive tests. Procainamide accounted for 15 cases and CPZ only 4 cases. Complications such as thrombosis, abortion, and cerebrovascular accidents occurred in 10 of the 34 patients.

Susceptibility to induction of drug-induced aPL may depend on various factors: (1) acetylator status – slow acetylators develop antibodies earlier than fast acetylators; (2) HLA DR status – a high incidence of HLD DR4 has been found in hydralazine-assocaited SLE; and (3) the existence of null alleles at the C4A and CB4 loci (ir 4) inhibition of binding of C4 to activated C1S [78, 79].

The administration of procainamide for long periods of time (more than 2 months) results in the appearance of antinuclear antibodies (ANA) in 50% to 74% of asymptomatic patients [80, 81]. The presence of drug-induced aPL in the form of LA may be demonstrated in patients that have developed drug-induced lupus, and also as an isolated abnormality in the absence of features of procainamide-induced lupus or uncommonly associated with thrombotic events. In a study by Day et al, the authors found an incidence of 10% to 15% of LA among their 190 patients taking procanaimide [82]. Asherson et al, Li et al, and Schlesinger and Peterson reported several patients with thrombotic events associated with procainamide [83–85].

In one study Zarrabi et al found that 85% of their patients who had taken CPZ for more than 2–5 years had LA [86]. Subsequently Gharavi et al found that all LA-positive patients from the previous study had IgM aCL by ELISA [87]. However, none of these patients had experienced thrombotic events. Berglund et al reported that a 69-year-old woman taking CPZ suffered a kidney infarct shortly thereafter she developed BFP-STS [88]. Similarly, Mueh et al included 2 patients in their series who appeared to have aPL-related thrombosis [89]. Canoso et al studied 108 psychiatric patients receiving CPZ treatment for more than a year and only 3 of them experienced episodes of venous thrombosis [75].

One report has shown that development of lupus-like syndrome and high IgG and medium IgM aCL in a 30-year-old woman that was being treated with quinine for malaria [90]. Once quinine was withdrawn, there was a prompt release of the symptoms and the laboratory tests returned to normal shortly thereafter.

Therapy for drug-induced aPL requires prompt discontinuation of the offending drug. Duration of the therapy need not be for life, given that the antibody generally disappears over time.

Conclusions

Our observations, and those from others, give further support to our hypothesis that "autoimmune aPL" may be generated by immunization with products from bacteria or viruses after incidental exposure or infection. We also were able to generate APS-like syndrome in a strain of mice susceptible to autoimmunity, indicating that other factors are likely to be involved, such as genetic predisposition. Furthermore, not all aPL generated were pathogenic. Based on the clinical experience and on the numerous reports indicating presence of aPL in large number of infectious diseases, it may be expected that not all aPL produced during infection will be pathogenic. A limited number aPL induced by certain viral/bacterial products would be pathogenic in certain genetically predisposed individuals. Further studies to identify the agents responsible for induction the pathogenic aPL are needed. Identification of those bacterial and/or viral agents may help finding strategies for the prevention of production of aPL "pathogenic" antibodies. Alternatively, free peptides may be used to induce tolerance against aPL production or to abrogate their pathogenic effects.

Drugs such as procainamide and phenothiazines can also induce aPL. The prevalence and pathogenicity of drug-induced aPL is generally low and has been discussed in this chapter.

References

1. Wasserman A, Neisser A, Bruck C. Eine serodiagnostiche Reaction bei Syphilis. Dtsch Med Wochenschr 1906;32:745–489.
2. Gharavi AE, Wilson WA. Antiphospholipid antibodies, In: Wallace DJ, Hahn, eds. Lupus erythematosus, 5th ed. Philadelphia:Williams &Wilkins; 1996:471–491.
3. Lockshin MD, Druzin ML, Goei S, et al. Antibody to cardiolipin as a predictor of fetal distress or death in pregnant patients with systemic lupus erythematosus. N Engl J Med 1985;313:152–156.
4. Lansdteiner K, Muller R, Potzl O. Zur Frage der Komplementbindungsreaktion bei Syphilis. Wcin Klin Wochenschr 1907;20:1565–1569.
5. Pangborn MC. A new serologically active phospholipid from beef heart. Proc Soc Exp Biol Med 1941;48:484–486.
6. Harris A, Rosenberg AA, Riedel L. A microflocculation test for syphilis using cardiolipin antigen. Preliminary report. J Vener Dis Inf 1946;27:169–174.
7. Moore JE, Mohr CF. Biologically false-positive test for syphilis: type, incidence, and cause. J Am Med Assoc 1952;150:467–473.
8. Putkonen T, Jokinen EJ, Foerstroem L. Reiter protein complement fixation test in treated neurosyphilis. Acta Derm Venereol 1963;43:405–412.
9. Lynch FW, Boynton RE, Kimball AC. False positive serologic reactions for syphilis due to smallpox vaccination (vaccinia) J Am Med Assoc 1941;115:591–595.
10. Moore JE, Lutz WB. Natural history of SLE: approach to its study through chronic biologic false positive reactions. J Chron Dis 1949;1:297–316.
11. Harvey AM, Shulman LE. Systemic lupus erythematosus and chronic biological false-positive test for syphilis. In: Dubouis E, ed. Lupus, 4th ed. Los Angeles: University of California Press; 1974:196–209.
12. Laurell AB, Nilsson IM. Hypergammaglobulinemia and biological false positive Wassermann reaction: a study of two cases. J Lab Clin Med 1957;49:694–707.
13. Lee SL, Saunders M. A disorder of blood coagulation in SLE. J Clin Invest 1955;34:1814–1822.
14. Thiagarajan P, Shapiro SS, DeMarco L. Monoclonal immunoglobulin M lambda coagulation inhibitor with phospholipid specificity: mechanism of lupus anticoagulant. J Clin Invest 1980;66:397–407.
15. Bowie EJ, Thompson JH Jr, Pascuzzi CA, et al. Thrombosis in SLE despite cirulating anticoagulants. J Lab Clin Med 1963;62:416–420.
16. Harris EN, Gharavi AE, Boey M, et al. Anticardiolipin antibodies: detection by radioimmunoassay and association with thrombosis in systemic lupus erythematosus. Lancet 1983;ii:1211–1214.
17. Gharavi AE, Harris EN, Asherson RA, Hughes GRV. Antiphospholipid antibodies: isotype distribution and phospholipid specificity. Ann Rheum Dis 1987;46:1–6.

18. Harris EN, Gharavi AE, Patel BM, Hughes GRV. Evaluation of the anticardiolipin antibody test: report of an international workshop held April 4 1986. Clin Exp Immunol 1987;68:215–222.
19. Harris EN, Gharavi AE, Loizou S, et al. Cross-reactivity of antiphospholipid antibodies. J Clin Lab Immunol 1985;16:1–6.
20. Wilson WA, Gharavi AE. Hughes syndrome: perspectives on thrombosis and antiphospholipid antibody. Am J Med 1996;101:574–576.
21. Vaarala O, Kleemola M, Palosuo T, Aho K. Anticardiolipin in response in acute infections. Clin Immunol Immunopathol 1986;41:8–15.
22. Mackworth-Young CG, Harris EN, Steere AC, et al. Anticardiolipin antibodies in Lyme disease. Arthritis Rheum 1988;31:1052–1057.
23. Catteau B, Delaporte E, Hachulla E, et al. Mycoplasma infection with Stevens-Johnson syndrome and antiphospholipid antibodies: apropos of 2 cases. Rev Med Interne 1995;16:10–14.
24. Santiago MB, Cossemelli W, Tuma MF, Oliveira RM. Anticardiolipin antibodies in infectious diseases. Clin Rheumatol 1989;8:23–28.
25. Fiallo P, Ninzi. $\beta_2$glycoprotein I-dependent anticardiolipin antibodies as a risk factor for reactions in borderline leprosy patients. Int J Lepr Other Mycobact Dis 1998;66:387–388.
26. Durupt S, Rosselli S, Manchon J, Lopez M. Presence of antiphospholipid antibodies in "Legionnaires disease". Presse Med 1996;25:1649.
27. Galvez J, Martin I, Medino D, Pujol E. Thrombophlebitis in a patient with abute Q fever and anticardiolipin antibodies. Med Clin (Barc) 1997;108:396–397.
28. Chaumentin G, Zenone T, Bibollet C, et al. Malignant boutonneuse fever and polymyalgia rheumatica: a coincidental association? Infection 1997;25:320–322.
29. Labarca JA, Rabaggliatti RM, Radrigan FJ, et al. Antiphospholipid syndrome associated with cytomegalovirus infection: case report and review. Clin Infect Dis 1997;24:197–200.
30. Manco-Johnson MJ, Nuss R, Key N, Moertel C, et al. Lupus anticoagulant and protein S deficiency in children with postvaricella purpura fulminans or thrombosis. J Pediatr 1996;128:319-323.
31. Intrator L, Oksenhendler E, Desforgs L. Anticardiolipin antibodies in HIV infected patients with or without autoimmune thrombocytopenia purpura. Br J Haematol 1988;67:269–270.
32. Herzenberg Am, Telford JJ, De Luca LG, et al. Thrombotic microangiopathy associated with cryoglobulinemic membranoproliferative glomerulonephritis and hepatitis C. Am J Kidney Dis 1998;31:521–526.
33. Poux JM, Jauberteau MO, Boudet R, et al. Transient lupus anticoagulant induced by Epstein-Barr virus infections. Blood Coagul Fibrinolysis 1991;2:771–774.
34. Sammaritano LR, Gharavi AE, Lockshin MD. Antiphospholipid antibody: immunologic and clinical aspects. Semin Arthritis Rheum 1990;20:81–96.
35. Harris EN, Gharavi AE, Wasley GD, Hughes GRV. Use of an enzyme-linked immunosorbent assay and of inhibition studies to distinguish between antibodies to cardiolipin from patients with syphilis or autoimmune disorders. J Infect Dis 1988;157:23–31.
36. Harris EN, Pierangeli SS. A more specific ELISA assay for the detection of antiphospholipid antibodies. Clin Immunol 1995;15:26–28.
37. Levy RA, Gharavi AE, Sammaritano LR, et al. Characteristics of IgG antiphospholipid antibodies in patients with systemic lupus erythematosus and syphilis. J Immunol 1990;17:1036–1041.
38. Costello PB, Green FA. Reactivity patterns of human anticardiolipin and other antiphospholipid antibodies in syphilitic sera. Infect Immun 1986;51:771–775.
39. Matsuura H, Igarashi T, Fujimoto M, et al . Anticardiolipin cofactor(s) and differential diagnosis of autoimmune disease [letter]. Lancet 1990;336:177–178.
40. Galli M, Comfurius P, Hemker HC, et al. Anticardiolipin antibodies (ACA) directed not to cardiolipin but to a plasma protein cofactor. Lancet 1990;335:1544–1547.
41. McNeil HP, Simpson RJ, Chesterman CJ, Krilis SA. Antiphospholipid antibodies are directed against a complex antigen that includes lipid binding inhibitor of coagulation: β_2 glycoprotein I (apolipoprotein H). Proc Natl Acad Sci U S A 1990;87:4120–4124.
42. Gharavi AE, Sammaritano LR, Wen J, et al. Characteristics of HIV and chlorpromazine induced antiphospholipid antibodies: effect of $\beta_2$glycoprotein I on binding to phospholipid. J Rheumatol 1994;21:94–99.
43. Hunt J, Krilis S. A phospholipid-$\beta_2$glycoprotein I complex is an antigen for anticardiolipin antibodies occurring in autoimmune disease but not with infection. Lupus 1992;1:75–81.
44. Celli M, Gharavi AE, Chaimovich H. Opposite $\beta_2$glycoprotein I requirement for the binding of infectious and autoimmune antiphospholipid antibodies to cardiolipin liposomes is associated with antibody avidity. Biochim Biophys Acta 1999;12:225–238.

45. Campbell AL, Pierangeli SS, Wellhausen S, Harris EN. Comparison of the effects of anticardiolipin antibodies from patients with the antiphospholipid syndrome and with syphilis on platelet aggregation. Thromb Haemost 1995;73:529–534.

46. Pierangeli SS, Goldsmith GH, Krnic S, Harris EN. Differences in functional activity of anticardiolipin antibodies from patients with syphilis and the antiphospholipid syndrome. Infect Immun 1994;62:4081–4084.

47. Matsuura E, Igarashi M, Yasuda T, Koike T, Triplett DA. Anticardiolipin antibodies recognize $\beta_2$glycoprotein I structure altered by interacting with in oxygen modified solid phase surface. J Exp Med 1994;179:457–462.

48. Roubey RAS. Autoantibodies to phospholipid-binding plasma proteins: a new view of lupus anticoagulantas and other "antiphospholipid" autoantibodies. Blood 1994;84:2854–2867.

49. Tsutsumi A, Matsuura E, Ichikawa K, et al. Antibodies to $\beta_2$glycoprotein I and clinical manifestations in patients with systemic lupus erythematosus. Arthritis Rheum 1996;39:1466–1474.

50. Roubey RA. Comparison of an enzyme-linked immunosorbent assay for antibodies to $\beta_2$glycoprotein I and a conventional anticardiolipin immunoassay. Arthritis Rheum 1996;39:1606–1607.

51. Forastiero RR, Martinuzzo ME, Kordich LC, Carreras LO. Reactivity to $\beta_2$glycoprotein I clearly differentiates anticardiolipin antibodies from antiphospholipid syndrome and syphilis. Thromb Haemost 1996;75:717–720.

52. Leroy V, Arvieux J, Jacob MC, et al. Prevalence and significance of anticardiolipin, anti-$\beta_2$glycoprotein I and anti-prothrombin antibodies in chronic hepatitis C. Br J Haematol 1998;101:468–474.

53. Constans J, Guerin V, Couchouron A, et al. Autoantibodies directed against phospholipids or human $\beta_2$glycoprotein I in HIV-seropositive patients: relationship with endothelial activation and antimalonic dialdehyde antibodies. Eur J Clin Invest 1988;28:115–122.

54. Hojnik M, Gilburd B, Ziporen L, et al. Anticardiolipin antibodies in infections are heterogenous in their dependency on $\beta_2$glycoprotein I: analysis of anticardiolipin antibodies in leprosy. Lupus 1994;3:515–521.

55. Faghri Z, Wilson WA, Taheri F, Barton EN, Morgan OS, Gharavi AE. Antibodies to cardiolipin and $\beta_2$glycoprotein I in HTLV-1 associated myelopathy tropical spastic para paresis. Lupus 1999;8:210–214.

56. Loizou S, Cazabon JK, Walport MJ, et al. Similarities of specificity and cofactor dependence in serum antiphospholipid antibodies from patients with human parvovirus B19 infection and from those with systemic lupus erythematosus. Arthritis Rheum 1997;40:103–108.

57. Giordano P, Galli M, Del Vecchio GC, et al. Lupus anticoagulant, anticardiolipin antibodies and hepatitis C virus infection in thalassemia. Br J Haematol 1998;102:903–906.

58. Prieto J, Yuste JR, Beloqui O, et al. Anticardiolipin antibodies in chronic hepatitis C: implication of hepatitis C virus as the cause of antiphospholipid syndrome. Hepatology 1997;23:199–204.

59. Jaeger U, Kapiotis S, Pabinger I, et al. Transient lupus anticoagulant associated with hypoprothrombinemia and factor XII deficiency following adenovirus infection. Ann Hematol 1993;67:95–99.

60. Uthman I, Tabbarah Z, Gharavi AE. Hughes syndrome associated with cytomegalovirus infection. Lupus 1999;8:775–777.

61. Gharavi AE, Sammaritano LR, Wen J, Elkon KB. Induction of antiphospholipid autoantibodies by immunization with β_2 glycoprotein I (apolipoprotein H). J Clin Invest 1992;90:1105–1109.

62. Pierangeli SS, Liu XW, Anderson G, et al. Thrombogenic properties of murine anti-cardiolipin antibodies induced by β_2 glycoprotein 1 and human IgG antiphospholipid antibodies. Circulation 1996;94:1746–1751.

63. Pierangeli SS, Harris EN. Induction of phospholipid-binding antibodies in mice and rabbits by immunization with human β_2 glycoprotein I or anticardiolipin antibodies alone. Clin Exp Immunol 1993;78:233–238.

64. Blank M, Fadin D, Tincani A, et al. Immunization with anticardiolipin cofactor (β_2-glycoprotein I) induces experimental antiphospholipid antibody syndrome in naive mice. J Autoimmun 1994;7:441–455.

65. Garcia CO, Kanbour-Shakir A, Tang H, Molina JF, Espinoza LR, Gharavi AE. Induction of experimental antiphospholipid syndrome in PL/J mice following immunization with β_2 GPI. Am J Reprod Immunol 1997;37:118–124.

66. Aron AL, Cuellar ML, Brey RL, et al. Early onset of autoimmunity in MRL/++ mice following immunization with β_2-glycoprotein I. Clin Exp Immunol 1995;101:78–81.

67. Hunt J, Krilis S. The fifth domain of β_2 glycoprotein I contains a phospholipid binding site (Cys 281-Lys288) and a region recognized by anticardiolipin antibodies. J Immunol 1994;152:653–659.

68. Gharavi AE, Tang H, Gharavi E, et al. Induction of aPL by immunization with a 15 amino acid peptide. Arthritis Rheum 1995;39:S296.
69. Gharavi AE, Pierangeli SS, Colden-Stanfield M, et al. GDKV-induced antiphospholipid antibodies enhance thrombosis and activate endothelial cells in vivo and in vitro. J Immunol 1999;163:2922–2927.
70. Gharavi EE, Cucurull E, Tang H, et al. Induction of antiphospholipid antibodies by immunization with viral peptides. Lupus 1999;8:449–455.
71. Gharavi AE, Pierangeli SS, Espinola RG, et al. Antiphospholipid antibodies induced in mice by immunization with a cytomegalovirus-derived peptide cause thrombosis and activation of endothelial cells in vivo. Arthritis Rheum 2002;46:545–552.
72. Gharavi AE, Vega-Ostertag M, Espinola RG, et al. Intrauterine fetal death in mice caused by cytomegalovirus-derived peptide induced aPL. Lupus 2004;13:17–23.
73. Blank M, Krause I, Fridkin M, et al. Bacterial induction of autoantibodies to β$_2$glycoprotein I accounts for the infection etiology of antiphospholipid syndrome. J Clin Invest 2002;106:797–804.
74. Pierangeli SS, Blank M, Liu X, et al. A peptide that shares similarity with bacterial antigens reverses thrombogenic properties of antiphospholipid antibodies in vivo. J Autoimmun 2004;22:217–225.
75. Canoso RT, de Oliveira RM. Chlorpromazine-induced anticardiolipin antibodies and lupus anticoagulant: absence of thrombosis. Am J Hematol 1988;27:272–275.
76. Triplett DA, Brandt JT, Musgrave KA, Orr CA. The relationship between lupus anticoagulants and antibodies to phospholipids. JAMA 1988;259:550–554.
77. Derksen RHWM, Kator I. Lupus anticoagulant: revival of an old phenomenon. Clin Exp Rheumatol 11985;3:349–357.
78. Spiers C, Fielder AHL, Chapel H, Davey NJ, Batchelor JR. Complement system protein C4 and susceptibility to hydralazine-induced systemic lupus erythematosus. Lancet 1989;i:922–924.
79. Sim E, Gill EW, Sim RB. Drugs that induce systemic lupus erythematosus inhibit complement component C4. Lancet 1984;ii:422–424.
80. Russell AS, Ziff M. Natural antibodies to procainamide. Clin Exp Immunol 1968;3:901–909.
81. Blomgren SE, Condemi JJ, Bignall MC. Antinuclear antibody induced by procainamide. A prospective study. N Engl J Med 1969;281:61–66.
82. Day JH, Cherrey R, O'Hara D, Carabello J. Incidence of procainamide-induced lupus anticoagulants [abstract]. Thromb Haemost 1987;58:394.
83. Asherson RA, Zulman J, Hughes GRV. Pulmonary thromboembolism associated with procainamide induced lupus syndrome and anticardiolipin antibodies. Ann Rheum Dis 1989;48:232–235.
84. Schlesinger P, Peterson L. Procainamide-associated lupus anticoagulants and thrombotic events [abstract]. Arthritis Rheum 1988;31:S54.
85. Li GC, Greenberg CS, Curie MS. Procainamide induced lupus anticoagulants and thrombosis. South Med J 1988;81:262–264.
86. Zarrabi MH, Zucker S, Miller F, et al. Immunologic coagulation disorders in chlorpromazine-treated patients. Ann Intern Med 1988;81:262–264.
87. Gharavi AE, Harris EN, Asherson RA, et al. Anticardiolipin (aCL) isotypes: a study of their clinical relevance [abstract]. Clin Rheumatol 1986;5:154.
88. Berglund S, Gottfries CG, Stormby K. Chlorpromazine-induced antinuclear factors. Acta Med Scand 1970;187:67–74.
89. Mueh JR, Herbst KD, Rapaport SI. Thrombosis in patients with the lupus anticoagulant. Ann Intern Med 1980;92:156–159.
90. Rosa-Re D, Garcia F, Gascon J, et al. Quinine induced lupus-like syndrome and cardiolipin antibodies. Ann Rheum Dis 1996;55:559–560.

Section 4

Therapy

43 Management of Thrombosis in Antiphospholipid Syndrome

M.A. Khamashta and Guillermo Ruiz-Irastorza

Introduction

Among the growing variety of clinical manifestations of antiphospholipid syndrome long-term prognosis is most influenced by the risk of recurrent thrombosis in APS. Therefore, the most important aspects concerning management of patients with APS are treating thrombosis, preventing re-thrombosis (i.e., secondary prophylaxis) and, ideally, reducing the number of individuals having aPL who develop the syndrome (i.e., primary prophylaxis).

Unfortunately, the optimal therapy for each of these scenarios has not been yet defined. The paucity and relative low quality of the studies performed, mainly due to selection criteria of patients, lies behind the lack of agreement among authors. These discrepancies have been recently shown in the consensus documents published after the 10th Conference on Antiphospholipid Antibodies held at Taormina, Sicily, in September 2002 [1–3].

However, important advances have taken place during the past few years, and, specifically, since the first edition of this text was published in 2000. Therefore, this chapter deals with the task of presenting available data, discussing their strengths and limitations and defining the arguable position of these authors on conflicting issues.

Treatment of Thrombosis in APS: Acute Therapy and Secondary Prophylaxis

The description of APS by Hughes in 1983 [4] provided a new insight into vascular disease. Here, for the first time, was a common prothrombotic disorder which resulted in arterial as well as venous thrombosis. Treatment of the acute thrombotic event, if identified, is no different in APS than in the general population. Patients with venous thromboembolism are given heparin (currently low-molecular-weight in most countries) followed by warfarin. Fibrinolytic therapy has been used successfully in patients with APS [5]. Antiaggregation is commonly used in the first place in patients with arterial events as aPL status is unknown in many cases.

The risk of recurrent thrombosis in patients with APS is high. The level of this risk has been variously reported ranging between 22% to 69% [6–10]. The type of thrombosis is predictive; retrospective analysis of patients with APS and recurrent thrombosis showed that a venous thrombosis is followed by another venous thrombosis in more than 70% of cases, and an arterial thrombosis is followed by another arterial thrombosis in more than 90% of cases [6, 7]. Two recent large and prospective long-term follow-up studies of patients with venous thromboembolism have confirmed that the risk of recurrence in APS patients is significantly higher than in patients without aPL [9, 10]. The cerebral circulation appears to be particularly targeted, with strokes and transient ischemic attacks, movement disorders, epilepsy, myelopathy, and migraine being major manifestations. The rate of recurrent stroke has also been shown to be extremely high in patients with moderate-to-high titers of aCL [11, 12].

Retrospective studies published between 1992–1995 by Rosove et al [6], Derksen et al [13], and Khamashta et al [7] showed the need for prolonged anticoagulation of patients with APS presenting with thrombosis, because the risk of recurrent thrombosis in patients not having, and especially stopping anticoagulation, was unacceptably high – and consistently shown across the studies. Based on these data, indefinite anticoagulation has been accepted by most authors as the standard secondary prophylaxis for thrombosis in patients with APS [14, 15]. It is not clear, however, whether prolonged anticoagulation is necessary in APS patients whose first thrombotic episode developed in association with surgery, oral contraceptive pill, pregnancy, or other circumstantial thrombotic risk factors.

The second relevant finding of the studies by Rosove at al [6] and Khamashta et al [7] was the decreased risk of recurrent thrombosis of patients treated with oral anticoagulation targeted to an international normalized ratio (INR) higher than 3.0 as compared with those aimed to a lower intensity. In addition, low-dose aspirin alone was less effective in preventing recurrent thrombosis than high-intensity anticoagulation. The message from these studies would be to target the intensity of anticoagulation to a higher level than the standard for other conditions such as atrial fibrillation.

Criticism of these studies includes the retrospective design and thus, the non-randomized assignment of treatment, which is obviously a major limitation. Also, patients with arterial and venous events could not be analysed separately in any of these series due to sample size issues. Furthermore, a number of small subsequent series of patients with venous thromboembolism and aPL found no increased risk of thromboembolic events in patients treated with standard intensity warfarin [9, 10, 16–18]. All the above, together with the fear of increasing hemorrhage as INR rises, made some authors claim a standard 2.0–3.0 anticoagulation target for all patients with APS and thrombosis, irrespective of the vascular bed [19].

Three studies recently published aimed to shed some light on this controversy. In the first, our group analysed a series of 66 patients with definite APS according to Sapporo classification criteria [20] treated with oral anticoagulation to a target INR 3.0–4.0 [21]. The major results of our study were 3-fold: The intensity of anticoagulation was frequently lower than desired, although the INR was very rarely below 2.0; the frequency of life-threatening bleeding was not higher than in patients from other series and treated with lower intensities of anticoagulation, and several APS patients experienced recurrent thrombosis at INRs between 2.0–3.0 (5 documented cases with INRs ranging from 2.1–2.6), most of them having additional risk factors for vascular events. The main limitations of this study were the retrospective design – somewhat limited by a personal interview with each participant in the study – and the lack of a control group with a lower target INR.

In 2003, Crowther et al published the first randomized clinical trial comparing low-and high-intensity oral anticoagulation in a group of 114 patients with APS and previous thrombosis [22]. They found a similar rate of recurrent thrombosis in both groups, which, in addition, was lower than expected according to previous studies, and concluded that a usual INR range of 2.0–3.0 is enough for preventing re-thrombosis in patients with APS.

Unfortunately, and despite the optimal design of the study, including double-blindness and intention-to-treat analysis, some important issues biased this trial rendering its conclusions difficult to generalize. First, patients having recent strokes or thrombosis under anticoagulant treatment were excluded; as an expected consequence, 76% of patients had venous thrombosis only, thus conclusions regarding patients with arterial thrombosis were not possible. Second, and probably most important, patients in the high-intensity group were below the "therapeutic range" 43% of the time. Therefore, high-intensity anticoagulation was not achieved. Not surprisingly, most thrombotic episodes in both groups (6 out of 8) took place when INRs were lower than 3.0.

A second prospective study focusing on the secondary prevention of thrombosis in patients with APS was published in JAMA in 2004 [23]. Taking advantage of an on-going randomized clinical trial (the Warfarin vs. Aspirin Recurrent Stroke Study, comparing low-intensity anticoagulation with aspirin for secondary prevention of stroke), the authors aimed to define the role of aPL in predicting recurrent strokes and response to therapy (Antiphospholipid Antibodies and Stroke Study). Blood samples were stored from 1770 patients (80% of WARSS participants) and aCL (including IgG, IgM, and IgA isotypes) and LA were determined.

The results showed similar frequencies of the primary end points (death, recurrent ischemic stroke, transient ischemic attack, myocardial infarction, peripheral or visceral artery thrombosis, and venous thromboembolism) among aPL-positive and aPL-negative patients. Response to warfarin or aspirin was uniformly similar among patients with and without aPL. Thus, the conclusions of this study can be summarized as follows:

1. Testing for LA or aCL did not confer important knowledge for prognosis or treatment of patients with recently diagnosed ischemic stroke.
2. Warfarin was not associated with fewer thrombotic events than aspirin among patients with aPL and stroke.

It is our view that a potentially outstanding study has been substantially weakened by important limitations with regard to the population studied. Performing a single aPL determination and considering patients with low titers aCL only as positive, including IgA isotype, is unacceptable to sustain a classification of APS according to currently accepted criteria [20]. Not surprisingly, most patients with aCL were positive at low titers only, which explains the huge proportion of aPL-positive patients (41% of the cohort) in a population averaging 63 years old, suggesting a low specificity of aPL definitions used. In fact, the study by the APASS group found an increased risk of the main outcome (death or thrombosis at any site) among patients positive for both aCL and LA, who were only 6.7% of the whole group.

Contrary to the opinion of the authors, it is our view that the lack of a differences between aPL-positive patients treated with aspirin or warfarin in terms of recurrent thrombosis, may actually support the idea that oral anticoagulation to an INR below 3.0 (the range in the study was 1.4–2.8) is not enough for patients with APS and arterial events [21].

In conclusion, we advocate prolonged oral anticoagulation as the standard secondary prophylaxis of thrombosis in patients with APS. Intensity of anticoagulation should be individually targeted according to risk of thrombosis, thrombosis related damage and bleeding: patients with arterial events (specially stroke) and life-threatening pulmonary embolism should be maintained at INRs higher than 3.0; a lower target INR could be acceptable for patients with non-severe venous thromboembolism. Special caution must be paid to patients with leukoaraiosis and/or previous serious bleeding. It goes without saying that other risk factors for thrombosis, such as smoking, hypertension, hyperlipidemia, diabetes, and use of estrogens must be strictly corrected.

Primary Thromboprophylaxis of aPL-positive Subjects

Available data from clinical studies suggest that the thrombotic risk associated with aPL may be substantial. In a prospective study of healthy men, those with aPL suffered 5 times the risk for venous thrombosis or pulmonary embolus [24]. Women initially referred to an obstetrical group for pregnancy-related aspects of APS had 15.7 thromboses per 100 patient-years in an average of 3 years of follow up [25].

Finazzi et al [26] designed a large prospective study in 360 unselected patients with aPL and showed that high titer IgG anticardiolipin antibody (aCL) was a significant predictor for thrombosis. Vaarala et al [27] showed that patients with high levels of aCL had a higher risk of myocardial infarction and that this risk was independent of any other factors. While there have been few rigorously designed epidemiological studies, available data suggest that the stroke risk associated with aPL may be substantial, especially in young adults [28–30]. A study of lupus patients with aPL but no thrombosis showed that no less than one half (52%) had developed the syndrome over 10-year follow up [31]. Recently, Gomez-Pacheco et al [32] have suggested that the detection of antibodies directed against β_2-glycoprotein I may predict the risk of thrombosis in asymptomatic individuals with aPL.

Despite the accumulating data that aPL is a serious risk factor for thrombosis, to date, no study has attempted to address the prophylactic management of the aPL-positive individuals. In treating patients with aPL it is important to remove or reduce other risk factors for thrombosis. Patients are advised to stop smoking, and women are counselled against the use of estrogen-containing oral contraceptive pills.

Although low-dose aspirin (75 mg/day) has been considered to be a logical prophylaxis, the Physician Health Study showed that low-dose aspirin use in men with aCL did not protect against deep venous thrombosis or pulmonary embolus [24]. Hydroxychloroquine has well-documented antiplatelet effects and has been shown to reduce the risk of thrombosis in both SLE patients [33–36] and animal models of APS [37]. Low-intensity oral anticoagulation with target INR around 1.5 has been shown to be effective in other prothrombotic states including central venous catheterization [38], stage IV breast cancer [39], and ischaemic heart disease in men at increased risk [40]. A prospective randomized trial comparing low-dose aspirin with low-intensity warfarin in subjects with SLE and/or an adverse pregnancy history is currently in progress in the United Kingdom. Until these results are available, we suggest that individuals with lupus or obstetric APS with persistently positive aCL (medium-high levels) and/or LA take low-dose aspirin (75 mg/day) indefinitely. Furthermore, high-risk situations such as surgery should be covered with subcutaneous heparin prophylaxis.

Miscellanea

Some patients with APS continue to have recurrent thrombotic events despite an INR of 3.0–4.0. Whether additional therapy with low-dose aspirin is efficacious in this situation is not known, but the risk of hemorrhage is increased when aspirin is used alongside oral anticoagulant therapy [41]. As already commented, hydroxychloroquine use may aid preventing thrombosis in lupus patients [33–36]. Due to its excellent safety profile, this drug might empirically be given to patients with APS with insufficient control despite optimal oral anticoagulation.

It is increasingly evident that many patients have uncontrollable fluctuations of INR. Concerns exist over the validity of the INR in control oral anticoagulant dosing if LA is present. The inhibitor occasionally increases the prothrombin time and, in turn, the INR, which may thus not reflect the true degree of anticoagulation [42]. This phenomenon seems to be more likely when certain recombinant thromboplastin reagents are used and can usually be circumvented by careful selection of the thromboplastin to be used for the prothrombin time test [43, 44]. One of the features of APS is that some patients appear relatively resistant to warfarin, some requiring up to 25 mg daily to maintain adequate anticoagulation. In our experience, most of these patients were receiving other drugs and, notably, azathioprine at the same time as warfarin therapy. Azathioprine interacts with warfarin, reducing its efficacy by possible hepatic enzyme induction [45]. Conversely, patients on warfarin who stop azathioprine may be at risk of bleeding and should be monitored carefully.

The role of steroids and immunosuppressive drugs in the treatment of patients with aPL and thrombosis is uncertain. Such drugs have severe side effects when given for prolonged periods and aPL are not always suppressed by these agents. Furthermore, in our series of patients with APS, corticosteroids and immunosuppressive therapy, prescribed in some patients to control lupus activity, did not prevent further thrombotic events [7]. The use of these drugs is probably justified only in patients with life-threatening conditions with repeated episodes of thrombosis despite adequate anticoagulation therapy, namely catastrophic APS. In this rare but life-threatening condition, plasmapheresis has also been used [46]. It is tempting to speculate that more targeted immunosuppressive therapy may be a future option in this antibody mediated disease.

Autoimmune thrombocytopenia is an accompanying problem in 25% of individuals with APS [47]. Generally, it is mild (platelet counts between 50,000–150,000/mm^3), but occasionally severe thrombocytopenia occurs. The treatment of choice is corticosteroids. The treatment of thrombosis and thrombocytopenia in the same patient is a difficult clinical problem and requires careful management. It is worth noting that thrombocytopenia does not necessarily protect patients against thrombosis [8] and platelet counts of 50,000–100,000/mm^3 in APS should not modify the treatment policy of thrombosis with warfarin.

Oral anticoagulation therapy carries an inevitable risk of serious hemorrhage. The rate of life-threatening bleeding in subjects taking warfarin, based on an Italian prospective study, is at least 0.25% per annum [48]. This rises rapidly when the INR exceeds 4.0. In APS, serious bleeding complications may occur, but their risk is not higher than that observed in other thrombotic conditions warranting oral anticoagulation [49]. Actually, our own experience has shown that serious hemorrhagic events are unusual even in patients treated with high-intensity oral anticoagulation [21]. However, it should be kept in mind that these data have been obtained from series of young patients with primary or SLE-related APS. Age has been demonstrated to be a risk factor for severe bleeding episodes in patients placed on long-term anticoagulation [48] and Piette and Cacoub have recently reported similar experience in their elderly patients with APS [50]. The presence of leukoaraiosis has been regarded as a major risk factor for cerebral hemorrhage in patients taking oral anticoagulants [51]. As has been previously discussed, all these facts must be borne in mind when targeting INR in an individual patient with APS [21].

References

1. Brey RL, Chapman J, Levine SR, et al. Stroke and the antiphospholipid syndrome: consensus meeting Taormina 2002. Lupus 2003;12:508–513.
2. Meroni PL, Moia M, Derksen RH, et al. Venous thromboembolism in the antiphospholipid syndrome: management guidelines for secondary prophylaxis. Lupus 2003;12:504–507.
3. Khamashta MA, Shoenfeld Y. Antiphospholipid syndrome: a consensus for treatment? Lupus 2003;12:495.
4. Hughes GRV. Thrombosis, abortion, cerebral disease and the lupus anticoagulant. Br Med J 1983;287:1088–1099.
5. Julkunen H, Hedman C, Kauppi M. Thrombolysis for acute ischemic stroke in the primary antiphospholipid syndrome. J Rheumatol 1997;24:181–183.
6. Rosove MH, Brewer PMC. Antiphospholipid thrombosis: clinical course after the first thrombotic event in 70 patients. Ann Intern Med 1992;117:303–308.
7. Khamashta MA, Cuadrado MJ, Mujic F, Taub N, Hunt BJ, Hughes GRV. The management of thrombosis in the antiphospholipid antibody syndrome. N Engl J Med 1995;332:993–997.
8. Krnic-Barrie S, O'Connor CR, Looney SW, Pierangeli SS, Harris EN. A retrospective review of 61 patients with antiphospholipid syndrome. Analysis of factors influencing recurrent thrombosis. Arch Intern Med 1997;157:2101–2108.
9. Schulman S, Svenungsson E, Granqvist S, the Duration of Anticoagulation Study Group. Anticardiolipin antibodies predict early recurrence of thromboembolism and death among patients with venous thromboembolism following anticoagulant therapy. Am J Med 1998;104:332–338.
10. Kearon C, Gent M, Hirsh J, et al. A comparison of three months of anticoagulation with extended anticoagulation for a first episode of idiopathic venous thromboembolism. N Engl J Med 1999;340:901–907.
11. Levine SR, Salowich-Palm L, Sawaya KL, et al. IgG anticardiolipin titer >40 GPL and the risk of subsequent thrombo-occlusive events and death. Stroke 1997;28:1660–1665.
12. Verro P, Levine SR, Tietjen GE. Cerebrovascular ischemic events with high positive anticardiolipin antibodies. Stroke 1998;29:2245–2253.
13. Derksen RHWM, de Groot PG, Kater L, Nieuwenhuis HK. Patients with antiphospholipid antibodies and venous thrombosis should receive long term anticoagulant treatment. Ann Rheum Dis 1993;52:689–692.
14. Levine JS, Branch DW, Rauch J. The antiphospholipid syndrome. N Engl J Med 2002;346:752–763.

15. Brunner HI, Chan WS, Ginsberg JS, Feldman BM. Longterm anticoagulation is preferable for patients with antiphospholipid antibody syndrome. result of a decision analysis. J Rheumatol 2002;29:490–501.
16. Ginsberg JS, Wells PS, Brill-Edwards P, et al. Antiphospholipid antibodies and venous thromboembolism. Blood 1995;10:3685–3691.
17. Prandoni P, Simioni P, Girolami A. Antiphospholipid antibodies, recurrent thromboembolism and intensity of warfarin anticoagulation. Thromb Haemost 1996;75:859.
18. Rance A, Emmerich J, Fiessinger JN. Anticardiolipin antibodies and recurrent thromboembolism. Thromb Haemost 1997;77:221–222.
19. Greaves M, Cohen H, Machin SJ, Mackie I. Guidelines on the investigation and management of the antiphospholipid syndrome. Br J Haematol 2000;109:704–715.
20. Wilson WA, Gharavi AE, Koike T, et al. International consensus statement on preliminary classification criteria for definite antiphospholipid syndrome. Arthritis Rheum 1999;42:1309–1311.
21. Ruiz-Irastorza G, Khamashta MA, Hunt BJ, Escudero A, Cuadrado MJ, Hughes GRV. Bleeding and recurrent thrombosis in definite antiphospholipid syndrome: analysis of a series of 66 patients treated with oral anticoagulation to a target INR of 3.5. Arch Intern Med 2002;162:1164–1169.
22. Crowther MA, Ginsberg JS, Julian J, et al. A comparison of two intensities of warfarin for the prevention of recurrent thrombosis in patients with the antiphospholipid syndrome. N Engl J Med 2003;349:1133–1138.
23. Levine SR, Brey RL, Tilley BC, et al. APASS Investigators. Antiphospholipid antibodies and subsequent thrombo-occlusive events in patients with ischemic stroke. JAMA 2004;291:576–584.
24. Ginsburg KS, Liang MH, Newcomer L, et al. Anticardiolipin antibodies and the risk for ischemic stroke and venous thrombosis. Ann Intern Med 1992;177:997–1002.
25. Silver RM, Draper ML, Scott JR, Lyon JL, Reading J, Branch DW. Clinical consequences of antiphospholipid antibodies: an historic cohort study. Obstet Gynecol 1994;83:372–377.
26. Finazzi G, Brancaccio V, Moia M, et al. Natural history and risk factors for thrombosis in 360 patients with antiphospholipid antibodies: a four year prospective study from the Italian registry. Am J Med 1996;100:530–536.
27. Vaarala O, Manttari M, Manninen V, et al. Anticardiolipin antibodies and risk of myocardial infarction in a prospective cohort of middle-aged men. Circulation 1995;91:23–27.
28. Kittner S, Gorelick PB. Antiphospholipid antibodies and stroke: an epidemiological perspective. Stroke 1992;23:I19–I22.
29. Brey RL, Stallworth CL, McGlasson DL, et al. Antiphospholipid antibodies and stroke in young women. Stroke 2002;33:2396–2400.
30. Brey RL, Abbott RD, Curb JD, et al. Beta(2)-glycoprotein 1-dependent anticardiolipin antibodies and risk of ischemic stroke and myocardial infarction: the Honolulu heart program. Stroke 2001;32:1701–1706.
31. Shah N, Khamashta MA, Atsumi T, Hughes GRV. Outcome of patients with anticardiolipin antibodies: a 10 year follow-up of 52 patients. Lupus 1998;7:3–6.
32. Gomez-Pacheco L, Villa AR, Drenkard C, Cabiedes J, Cabral AR, Alarcon-Segovia D. Serum anti-β_2-glycoprotein I and anticardiolipin antibodies during thrombosis in systemic lupus erythematosus patients. Am J Med 1999;106:417–423.
33. Wallace DJ, Linker-Israeli M, Metzger AL, Stecher VJ. The relevance of antimalarial therapy with regard to thrombosis, hypercholesterolemia and cytokines in SLE. Lupus 1993;2(suppl):S13–S15.
34. Petri M. Hydroxychloroquine use in the Baltimore lupus cohort: effects on lipids, glucose and thrombosis. Lupus 1996;5(suppl):S16–S22.
35. Erkan D, Yazici Y, Peterson MG, Sammaritano L, Lockshin MD. A cross-sectional study of clinical thrombotic risk factors and preventive treatments in antiphospholipid syndrome. Rheumatology 2002;41:924–929.
36. Molad Y, Gorshtein A, Wysenbeek AJ, et al. Protective effect of hydroxychloroquine in systemic lupus erythematosus. Prospective long-term study of an Israeli cohort. Lupus 2002;11:356–361.
37. Edwards MH, Pierangeli S, Liu X, et al. Hydroxychloroquine reverses thrombogenic properties of antiphospholipid antibodies in mice. Circulation 1997;96:4380–4384.
38. Bern MM, Lokich JJ, Wallach SR, et al. Very low doses of warfarin can prevent thrombosis in central venous catheters: a randomized prospective trial. Ann Intern Med 1990;112:423–428.
39. Levine M, Hirsh J, Gent M, et al. Double-blind randomised trial of very low-dose warfarin for prevention of thromboembolism in stage IV breast cancer. Lancet 1994;343:886–889.
40. The Medical Research Council's General Practice Research Framework. Thrombosis prevention trial: randomised trial of low-intensity oral anticoagulation with warfarin and low-dose aspirin in the primary prevention of ischaemic heart disease in men at increased risk. Lancet 1998;351:233–241.

41. Meade TW, Miller CJ. Combined use of aspirin and warfarin in primary prevention of ischemic heart disease in men at risk. Am J Cardiol 1995;75:23B–26B.
42. Moll S, Ortel TL. Monitoring warfarin therapy in patients with lupus anticoagulant. Ann Intern Med 1997;127:177–185.
43. Robert A, Le Querrec A, Delahousse B, et al. Control of oral anticoagulation in patients with the antiphospholipid syndrome: influence of the lupus anticoagulant on International Normalized Ratio. Thromb Haemost 1998;80:99–103.
44. Lawrie AS, Purdy G, Mackie IJ, Machin SJ. Monitoring of oral anticoagulant therapy in lupus anticoagulant positive patients with the antiphospholipid syndrome. Br J Haematol 1997;98:887–892.
45. Rivier G, Khamashta MA, Hughes GRV. Warfarin and azathioprine: a drug interaction does exist. Am J Med 1993;95:342.
46. Asherson RA, Cervera R, Piette JC, et al. Catastrophic antiphospholipid syndrome. Clues to the Pathogenesis from a Series of 80 Patients. Medicine (Baltimore) 2001;80:355–377.
47. Cuadrado MJ, Mujic F, Munoz E, Khamashta MA, Hughes GRV. Thrombocytopenia in the antiphospholipid syndrome. Ann Rheum Dis 1997;56:194–196.
48. Palareti G, Leali N, Cocheri S, et al. Bleeding complications of oral anticoagulant treatment: an inception-cohort, prospective collaborative study (ISCOAT) Italian study on complications of oral anticoagulant therapy. Lancet 1996;348:423–428.
49. Al-Sayegh FA, Ensworth S, Huang S, Stein HB, Kinkhoff AV. Hemorrhagic complications of longterm anticoagulant therapy in 7 patients with systemic lupus erythematosus and antiphospholipid syndrome. J Rheumatol 1997;24:1716–1718.
50. Piette JC, Cacoub P. Antiphospholipid syndrome in the elderly: caution. Circulation 1998;97:2195–2196.
51. Gorter JW. Major bleeding during anticoagulation after cerebral ischemia: patterns and risk factors. Neurology 1999;53:1319–1327.

44 Management of Antiphospholipid Syndrome in Pregnancy

Lorin Lakasing, Susan Bewley, and Catherine Nelson-Piercy

Introduction

Antiphospholipid syndrome (APS) predominantly affects young women and there has been a growing awareness of this condition amongst obstetricians and gynecologists over the last 15 years. In this chapter we discuss the association between APS and adverse pregnancy outcome and present some of the dilemmas in the management of on-going pregnancies in women with APS. Although clinicians are becoming increasingly familiar with these management options, knowledge of the pathogenesis of poor pregnancy outcome in APS remains incomplete, and in the last part of this chapter we outline some of the areas of research in this rapidly evolving field.

Making the Diagnosis of APS

The criteria for the classification of APS are well described [1] and it is critical that these are applied strictly to avoid inappropriate management of patients [2]. Similarly, even in those with a robust diagnosis, all adverse pregnancy outcomes should not be entirely attributed to the syndrome as there are numerous other associations with poor outcome that may be causative or contributory, for example, cervical incompetence, "unexplained" intrauterine death. It is therefore essential to apply good clinical judgment in each individual case to avoid interventions that may be unnecessary or even harmful.

The Effect of Pregnancy on APS

Pregnancy is a hypercoagulable state and women with APS are at increased risk of thrombosis unless thromboprophylaxis or anticoagulation is adequate. Some studies have demonstrated that a significant proportion of pregnant patients still have thrombotic episodes despite thromboprophylaxis [3, 4]. These patients need long-term anticoagulation with warfarin aiming for an international normalized ratio (INR) of at least 2.0–2.9 [5]. Pregnancy can also exacerbate pre-existing thrombocytopenia, and this may be further compounded by medication because aspirin and heparin administered during pregnancy may cause thrombocytopenia. Thromboprophylaxis, full anticoagulation, and the management of thrombocytopenia in pregnant women with APS are discussed in more detail below.

The Effect of APS on Pregnancy

APS and Early Pregnancy Complications

Many cases of APS are diagnosed following investigation of recurrent miscarriage. The association between APS and recurrent miscarriage is well known [6–9], with second trimester loss being particularly common [10]. The prospective fetal loss rate in primary APS is reported to be 50% to 75% [11, 12]. In patients with systemic lupus erythematosus (SLE) and secondary APS some studies suggest this may be as high as 90% [13, 14], although this is likely to be an overestimate. It has been suggested that the risk of fetal loss is directly related to the antibody titer [15, 16], but this is certainly not true of all cases. Some studies have shown maternal IgG aCL to be a particularly reliable predictor of miscarriage [17, 18]. Although this makes theoretical sense as this subfraction of antibodies can cross into the fetoplacental circulation [19], many women with recurrent miscarriage have IgM aCL antibodies only. It is impossible to predict which women will develop complications in pregnancy, and some women with persistently elevated aPL titers and a history of thromboses and/or thrombocytopenia will have no obstetric complications at all. Previous poor pregnancy outcome remains the most important predictor of future risk [20–22].

APS and Late Pregnancy Complications

In pregnancies that do not end in miscarriage or fetal loss, there is a high incidence of early onset pre-eclampsia (PET) [23–26] and intrauterine growth restriction (IUGR) [20, 27], placental abruption [28], and premature delivery [29, 30]. Because patients with APS form a heterogeneous group, the incidence of these complications varies between units. Indeed it is now clear that the substantial differences in APS patient populations in studies of pregnancy inevitably results in large differences in reported adverse pregnancy outcomes, and whilst attempts are being made to define management in certain subgroups, many recommendations are not strictly evidence based [31, 32]. Those units which manage women with systemic manifestations of APS have a higher incidence of complications in pregnancy [33], whilst those which recruit women predominantly from recurrent miscarriage clinics have a lower incidence of these complications [34, 35]. It is essential to appreciate these differences in order to critically appraise the literature, advise women appropriately, and rationalize therapy [36]. In a recent study from our own unit, 35 pregnancies in women with primary APS resulted in a live birth in 32 cases (91%) with a mean gestation of 38.4 (27.5–42) weeks and a mean birth weight of 2895 ± 165 g. Complications included miscarriage in 3 cases (9%), fetal growth restriction in 4 cases (12%), placental abruption in 1 case (3%), pre-eclampsia in 2 cases (6%), preterm delivery in 8 cases (24%), and maternal thrombotic events in 5 cases (14%). Labor was induced in 8 (25%) cases and delivery was by Caesarean section in 19

Table 44.1. Pregnancy outcomes in different populations of women with antiphospholipid syndrome.

Study	Utah [28]	St. Thomas [1]	Liverpool [29]	St. Mary's [30]
Pregnancies (n)	82	60	53	150
Population	Predominantly systemic	Predominantly systemic	Predominantly recurrent miscarriage	All recurrent miscarriage
PET (%)	51	18	3	11
IUGR (%)	31	31	11	15
Preterm delivery (%)	37	43	8	24

Adapted from Ref. 36.

(59%) cases. Five (16%) babies required neonatal intensive care [37]. A summary of the outcomes in APS pregnancies reported in the main studies is shown in Table 44.1.

The early prediction of women with APS who are likely to develop complications in pregnancy remains a challenge. Several studies have recommended uterine artery Doppler waveform analysis in these women [38, 39]. In a study of APS pregnancies, bilateral uterine artery notches at 22–24 weeks gestation represented a likelihood ratio for prediction of pre-eclampsia of 12.8 [95% confidence interval (CI), 2.2-75] with a sensitivity of 75% and a specificity of 94% and a negative predictive value of 94%, and similar statistics were obtained for the prediction of fetal growth restriction [40]. Other studies in APS pregnancies have confirmed the reassuring nature of absence of bilateral uterine artery notches at even lower gestations [41]. Histological evidence of impaired trophoblast migration in placental bed biopsies from women showing these high resistance Doppler waveforms has been reported [42], although the extent of uteroplacental pathology does not always correlate with the severity of maternal or fetal disease.

Therapeutic Options in APS Pregnancies

Many therapeutic options have been tried in APS pregnancies and the risks and benefits of each form of therapy continue to be an active area of debate [43]. A meta-analysis of therapeutic trials in pregnant women with APS has recently been published but the conclusions need to be interpreted with caution due to the small number of patients in most studies, differences in diagnostic laboratory methods, and variable inclusion criteria [44]. The most commonly used medications are aspirin, heparin, warfarin, and steroids. A summary of the side-effects of these drugs is shown in Table 44.2. Pre-conceptual review of medication is useful as it allows clinicians to place each patient in a risk category and treat her accordingly. These individualized treatment regimes limit the problems associated with polypharmacy in pregnancy and enable resources to be invested appropriately.

Aspirin

Women with APS are advised to take low-dose aspirin (75 mg daily) in pregnancy. The rationale for this is aspirin-mediated inhibition of thromboxane, increased vasodilation, and subsequent reduced risk of thromboses in the placenta and else-

Table 44.2. Therapeutic options in antiphospholipid syndrome pregnancies.

	Maternal side effects	Fetal side effects	Breastfeeding
Aspirin	GI disturbances	Safe	Safe
Warfarin	GI disturbances Hypersensitivity Hemorrhage	Teratogenic Hemorrhage Miscarriage	Safe
Heparin	Osteoporosis Thrombocytopenia Hemorrhage/bruising Hypersensitivity	Safe	Safe
Prednisolone	Infection Diabetes Hypertension Osteoporosis Peptic ulceration Muscle wasting Cushing's syndrome Depression/psychosis	Safe	Safe ?adrenal suppression (very rare, only if > 30 mg daily)

where. However, the use of aspirin in APS pregnancies has never been subjected to a randomized trial, although several non-randomized studies suggest it is beneficial [45–47], and there are animal data to support this [48]. In low risk APS pregnancies, that is, no previous thromboses or miscarriages, a randomized controlled trial of aspirin versus no aspirin failed to show any benefit of treatment [49]. Damage to the developing trophoblast occurs early in pregnancy and therefore if aspirin is used it is likely to be of most benefit if administered from the pre-conceptual period as use of aspirin from the mid-trimester onwards has been shown to be of no benefit in reducing the incidence of adverse pregnancy outcome in high risk groups [50]. Treatment is usually continued at least until delivery if not into the puerperium. Low-dose aspirin does not affect the use of regional anesthesia during labor. Renal and hepatic impairment do not occur with this dose of aspirin and bronchospasm is exceptionally rare affecting a minority of asthmatics. There are no adverse fetal or neonatal effects from the use of low-dose aspirin.

Heparin

Women with APS and a previous history of thromboembolism are treated with heparin as thromboprophylaxis in pregnancy. For those with recurrent pregnancy loss or previous adverse pregnancy outcome but without a history of thromboembolism, there is as yet no consensus of opinion [51]. Some studies have suggested that heparin therapy in addition to aspirin may contribute to improved fetal outcome [52]. One group has shown improved fetal outcome using heparin [53] or LMWH alone [54]. Most specialist units caring for pregnant women with APS use aspirin and low-molecular-weight heparin (LMWH) together in women with a history of thrombosis or second trimester loss, and there is some evidence of improved pregnancy outcome with the use of heparin in women with recurrent first trimester loss [55, 56], although not all studies have shown a benefit in this sub-group [57]. Those women who wish to take LMWH during pregnancy for fetal indications, for example, recurrent miscarriage, previous intrauterine death, pre-eclampsia, or fetal growth restriction, usually receive once daily thromboprophylactic doses. However, those with previous thromboses are often given high dose thromboprophylaxis in the form of twice daily administration (e.g., Enoxaparin 40 mg SC b.i.d.) to minimize the risk of recurrent thromboses during pregnancy which might necessitate treatment with either therapeutic doses of LMWH or oral anticoagulation with warfarin. Whether LMWH is being administered for fetal or maternal indications or both, the potential benefits of treatment should be balanced against the risk of heparin-induced osteoporosis [58-60]. The problem of osteoporosis is compounded by concomitant use of steroid medication, and indeed by pregnancy itself [61-63]. LMWHs are commonly used in APS patients because of the convenience of once daily administration (in most cases), the improved antithrombotic (áXa) to anticoagulant (áIIa) ratio, the decreased risk of heparin-induced thrombocytopenia, and the probable decreased risk of heparin-induced osteoporosis [64]. However, there have been small case series reporting osteoporotic fractures with LMWH administered in therapeutic doses [65]. Systematic review of all studies of LMWH use in pregnancy confirms a very low (0.09%) risk of osteoporosis [66]. Although Factor Xa levels may be used to monitor LMWH [67], experience has shown that doses are virtually never altered as a result [60], and therefore it is not necessary to measure Factor Xa levels routinely [68]. LMWH administration is omitted at least 12 hours prior to elective delivery, but in case urgent delivery is necessary, reversal with protamine sulphate is possible. The molecular weight of unfractionated heparin ranges from 12–15 kDa and that of LMWH from 4–5 kDa therefore neither preparation is able to cross the placenta. Heparin is not excreted into breast milk [69].

Warfarin

When there has been a thrombotic event in the index pregnancy despite heparin thromboprophylaxis, or in women with a history of previous cerebrovascular thromboses, the risk of recurrence is sufficiently high to consider antenatal administration of warfarin [70]. In practice the use of warfarin is avoided in the first trimester unless a woman develops transient ischemic attacks or other thrombotic events at that time. This is because, unlike heparin, warfarin does cross the placenta and is potentially teratogenic producing a typical embryopathy characterized by nasal hypoplasia, stippled epiphyses, rhizomelia (short proximal limbs), digital dysplasia, eye abnormalities, and developmental delay [71]. The exact incidence of these anomalies is unknown largely due to case-reporting bias. Review of the literature suggests that it is between 2% to 4% [72], but there appears to be a dose dependent incidence of complications with a higher number of complications in pregnant women receiving more than 5 mg per day [73, 74]. Patients require close supervision and regular INR estimates maintaining values between 2.0–2.5. It must be remembered that the maternal INR does not accurately reflect the fetal coagulation status and animal studies show that the risk of fetal intravascular hemorrhage is still present despite optimum maternal control [75]. The fetus is therefore at risk throughout pregnancy during the period of warfarin administration [76]. A fortnight before planned delivery, warfarin is discontinued and either an intravenous infusion of unfractionated heparin or therapeutic doses of subcutaneous LMWH is commenced. This allows sufficient time for clearance of warfarin by both mother and fetus to occur. Every attempt should be made to avoid rapid reversal of warfarin anticoagulation with vitamin K at the time of delivery as this makes subsequent anticoagulation in the post-natal period difficult. There is no evidence to suggest that fetal outcome is improved with the use of warfarin. There is no significant excretion of warfarin into breast milk [77, 78].

Steroids

In the past, high dose steroids (greater than or equal to 60 mg daily) were used to suppress lupus anticoagulant (LA) and anticardiolipin antibodies (aCL) and some studies reported improved fetal survival [79, 80]. However, these therapeutic regimes resulted in considerable maternal morbidity including gestational diabetes, hypertension, and sepsis, and subsequent studies failed to show an improvement in pregnancy outcome [46, 81]. Cowchock et al demonstrated that aspirin and heparin gave equivalent fetal outcomes when compared with aspirin and steroids with significantly less maternal morbidity [52], and more recently there have been suggestions that steroid use may be detrimental to fetal outcome by promoting preterm delivery [82]. Therefore the use of steroids in APS pregnancies has been abandoned except for the treatment of maternal thrombocytopenia or co-existent SLE for which prednisolone is still first line therapy. Regular blood glucose monitoring is required with long-term administration of steroids. Patients requiring more than7.5 mg prednisolone daily for more than 2 weeks prior to delivery should be given intra-partum intravenous hydrocortisone 100 mg t.i.d.. Breastfeeding is rarely contraindicated, although women taking greater than 60 mg prednisolone with healthy term babies may consider bottle-feeding because of the theoretical risk of neonatal hypothalamic–pituitary adrenal suppression at these high doses.

Others

Immunosupression with azathioprine, intravenous immunoglobulin [83–85], plasma exchange [86], and interleukin-3 therapy [87] have all been tried in APS pregnancies. Due to the cost of immunoglobulin therapy, this treatment has previously been limited to salvage therapy in women who develop complications despite treatment with aspirin and heparin [88]. Initial reports using a 2 g/kg course of intravenous immunoglobulin administered in divided doses over 2–5 days in the second or early third trimester in pregnancies complicated by IUGR suggested a temporary improvement in uteroplacental Doppler waveforms [89]. More recently, a randomized controlled trial of intravenous immunoglobulin versus aspirin and heparin in 40 women with APS associated recurrent miscarriage showed a live birth rate of only 57% in the immunoglobulin group compared with 84% in the aspirin and heparin group [90]. Thus, although initially promising, immunoglobulin therapy does not appear to be beneficial in APS pregnancies.

Management of APS Pregnancies at St. Thomas' Hospital

St. Thomas Hospital is a national referral center for APS and there is a weekly antenatal clinic for pregnant women with APS. Many of these women are well known to the rheumatology and hematology services and this allows pre-conceptual counseling in most cases. At this visit women undergo a risk assessment and future therapy is planned. Many women with APS have related disorders also addressed at that time, for example, SLE or thrombocytopenia. Apart from the standard pre-pregnancy advice, for example, folic acid, women who are not already taking aspirin are advised to start from the pre-conceptual period onwards until delivery. LMWH is offered to women who are taking long-term oral anticoagulation, those with previous thrombotic events and those with 1 or more previous second trimester losses. LMWH is administered immediately after ultrasound confirmation of a viable intrauterine pregnancy, but not pre-conceptually in order to limit the time of heparin usage. Women are regularly reviewed by a multi-disciplinary team and the frequency of visits depends on the presence of any complications and practical issues such as commuting distance.

As well as routine aspects of ante-natal care offered to all pregnant women, for example, screening for chromosomal abnormalities and mid-trimester ultrasound examination of the fetus, women with APS are offered Doppler analysis of uterine artery wave forms at 20 and 24 weeks gestation. In the third trimester, "high risk" women with APS, for example, abnormal Doppler assessment of the uterine arteries or previous late pregnancy complications, are offered 4 weekly scans, whereas those at the milder end of the APS spectrum, for example, recurrent first trimester losses only, are offered scans at 28 and 34 weeks gestation. In cases with suspected fetal growth restriction, biophysical profiles are performed to further assess fetal well being. LMWH is discontinued at 20 weeks gestation in women with a history of recurrent first trimester miscarriage alone and normal uterine artery Dopplers at this time as the benefits of LMWH have not been demonstrated beyond this gestation in this sub-group of patients. In the other women, LMWH is continued up to the time of delivery and for 6 weeks afterwards [91]. Those with previous thromboses taking long-tern anticoagulant therapy are converted back to warfarin after delivery.

Women have direct access to hospital 24 hours a day and inpatients are regularly reviewed by a multi-disciplinary team. Women who develop pre-eclampsia are managed according to the standard hospital protocol. A specialist team of midwives care for these high risk pregnancies and this provides continuity of care. Obstetric anesthetists are involved when planning delivery especially in women who arc fully anti-coagulated. A bereavement counseling service is provided by consultant obstetricians, specialist midwives, and neonatologists where appropriate.

Pathogenesis of Adverse Pregnancy Outcome in APS

The safe and successful treatment of pregnant women with APS lies in understanding the etiology of this condition and the mechanism by which complications in pregnancy may arise. As yet there are many more questions than answers [92]. Most research has been in the form of drug trials and conclusions have been largely unconvincing due to small numbers, poor study design, and variable entry criteria and outcome measures. More recently there has been a shift in emphasis to more laboratory based research using models for trophoblast development and molecular biological techniques to determine various aspects of antibody–endothelial interactions [93].

Early Pregnancy Failure

Early pregnancy failure is likely to be due to impaired development of the trophoblast and failure to establish an effective fetoplacental circulation. The factors governing trophoblast invasion and early placental development are multiple and complex. Some factors specific to APS pregnancies have been well characterized, in particular β_2-glycoprotein I (β_2-GPI) [94]. In addition, aPL have been shown to directly alter trophoblastic hormone production and invasiveness in in vitro models [95], and, more interestingly, that LMWH restores trophoblast differentiation and invasiveness [96]. However, many others factors are also involved. It is likely that growth factors [97, 98], cytokines [99], integrins [100, 101], cell adhesion molecules [102, 103], and class I major histocompatibility complex antigens [104] are all instrumental. The effect of aPL on the function of these molecules has yet to be established.

Late Pregnancy Failure

Late pregnancy complications are likely to arise from damage to the uteroplacental vasculature. After 15 weeks gestation the vasculosyncitial membrane is porous enough for IgG antibodies to be able to cross into the fetal circulation. High concentrations of IgG antibodies have been eluted from placenta from women with aPL-positive sera with poor pregnancy outcomes [19]. Whether these aPL themselves are directly responsible for structural and/or functional damage to the placental vessels or whether they act indirectly via another secondary mechanism is unclear. It has been difficult to extrapolate antibody data from animal studies to clinical experience in humans [105, 106]. Some studies have suggested that aPL are involved in oxidant mediated damage to the vascular endothelium [107]. However, in order to recognize endothelial cells, aPL antibodies require the presence of certain cofactors [108, 109], the best characterized of which are β_2-GPI [110] and prothrombin [111]. Much work has been done in this area but few conclusions drawn. Histological examination of placenta from APS pregnancies often show thromboses of the uteroplacental vasculature and placental infarction [112]. There may be decidual vasculopathy characterized by fibrinoid necrosis and atherosis of decidual vessels [113]. These findings suggest thrombotic damage to the fetoplacental circulation, and whilst some groups have published data to support this [114–116], others disagree [117, 118]. Another possibility is that placental dysfunction and subsequent fetal demise in APS pregnancies are secondary to the maternal vasculopathy which is thought to also affect placental bed vessels, and not to primary antibody mediated fetoplacental events at all. In this way, APS related adverse pregnancy outcome may be similar to that which occurs in women with pre-eclampsia without an underlying vasculopathy [119], or those with hereditary thrombophilias [120, 121]. Although the mechanisms causing utero-placental dysfunction in these pregnancies has attracted much interest in the last decade, recent research in a murine model suggests that the complement system has a major role in APS-related adverse pregnancy outcome [122].

Summary

Pregnant women with APS are at risk of complications at all stages of pregnancy. They require specialist care and a team approach involving obstetricians, obstetric physicians, rheumatologists, hematologists, neonatologists, and specialist midwives. Close monitoring of the various aspects of the condition may reduce maternal morbidity and improve fetal outcome. Therapeutic options include aspirin, LMWH, and, less commonly, warfarin and steroids.

The pathogenesis of the adverse pregnancy outcome in APS has not yet been fully elucidated although there is active research in this field. Until this is ascertained, we must accept that many aspects of management are purely empirical and it is our duty to counsel women thoroughly such that they understand the risks and benefits of the treatment options they are offered.

References

1. Wilson WA, Gharavi AE, Koike T, et al. International consensus statement on preliminary classification criteria for definite antiphospholipid syndrome. Arthritis Rheum 1999;42:1309–1311.
2. Stone S, Langford K, Nelson-Piercy C, Khamashta MA, Bewley S, Hunt BJ. Antiphospholipid antibodies do not a syndrome make. Lupus 2002;11:130–133.
3. Lima F, Khamashta MA, Buchanan NMM, Kerslake S, Hunt BJ, Hughes GRV. A study of sixty pregnancies in patients with the antiphospholipid syndrome. Clin Exp Rheumatol 1996;14:131–136.
4. Ringrose DK. Anaesthesia and antiphospholipid syndrome – a review of 20 patients. Int J Obstet Anaesth 1997;6:107–111.
5. Levine JS, Branch DW, Rauch J. The antiphospholipid syndrome. N Engl J Med 2002;346:752–763.
6. Julkunen H. Pregnancy in systemic lupus erythematosus. Contraception, fetal outcome and congenital heart block. Acta Obst Gynecol Scand 1994;73:517–520.
7. MacLean M, Cumming G, McCall F, Walker I, Walker J. The prevalence of lupus anticoagulant and anticardiolipin antibodies in women with a history of first trimester miscarriages. Br J Obstet Gynaecol 1994;101:103–106.
8. Silver RM, Branch DW. Recurrent miscarriage: autoimmune considerations. Clin Obstet Gynaecol 1994;37:745–760.
9. Rai RS, Clifford K, Cohen H, Regan L. High prospective fetal loss rate in untreated pregnancies of women with recurrent miscarriage and antiphospholipid antibodies. Hum Reprod 1995;10:3301–3304.
10. Branch DW, Rodgers GM. Induction of endothelial cell tissue factor activity against sera from patients with antiphospholipid syndrome: a possible mechanism of thrombosis. Am J Obstet Gynecol 1993;168:206–210.
11. Lockwood CJ, Romero R, Feinberg RF, Clyne LP, Coster B, Hobbins JC. The prevalence and biologic significance of lupus anticoagulant and anticardiolipin in a general obstetric population. Am J Obstet Gynecol 1989;161:369–373.
12. Perez MC, Wilson WA, Brown HL, Scopelitis E. Anti-cardiolipin antibodies in unselected pregnant women in relationship to fetal outcome. J Perinatol 1991;11:33–36.
13. Branch DW, Scott JR, Kochenour NK. Obstetric complications associated with lupus anticoagulant. N Engl J Med 1985;313:1322–1326.
14. Lubbe WF, Butler WS, Palmer SJ, Liggins GC. Fetal survival after prednisolone suppression of maternal lupus anticoagulant. Lancet 1983;i:1361–1363.
15. Harris EN, Chan JK, Asherson RA, Aber VR, Gharavi AE, Hughes GRV. Thrombosis, recurrent fetal loss and thrombocytopenia. Predictive value of the anticardiolpin antibody test. Arch Intern Med 1986;146:2153–2156.
16. Reece EA, Garofalo J, Zheng XZ, Assimakopoulos E. Pregnancy outcome – influence of antiphospholipid antibody titer, prior pregnancy loss and treatment. J Reprod Med 1997;42:49–55.
17. Lockwood CJ, Reece EA, Romero R, Hobbins JC. Antiphospholipid antibody and pregnancy wastage. Lancet 1986;2:742–743.

18. Lynch A, Marlar R, Murphy J, et al. Antiphospholipid antibodies in predicting adverse pregnancy outcome. A prospective study. Ann Intern Med 1994;120:470–475.
19. Katano K, Aoki K, Ogasawara M, et al. Specific antiphospholipid antibodies (aPL) eluted from placentae of pregnant women with aPL-positive sera. Lupus 1995;4:304–308.
20. Pattison NS, Chamley LW, McKay EJ, Liggins GC, Butler WS. Antiphospholipid antibodies in pregnancy: prevalence and clinical associations. Br J Obstet Gynaecol 1993;100:909–913.
21. Buchanan NMM, Khamashta MA, Morton KE, Kerslake S, Baguley E, Hughes GRV. A study of 100 high risk lupus pregnancies. Am J Rep Immunol 1992;28:192–194.
22. Ramsey-Goldman R, Mientus JM, Kutzer JE, Mulvihill JJ, Medsger JTA. Pregnancy outcome in women with systemic lupus erythematosus treated with immunosuppressive drugs. J Rheumatol 1993;20:1152–1157.
23. Branch DW, Andres R, Digre KB, Rote NS, Scott JR. The association of antiphospholipid antibodies with severe pre-eclampsia. Obstet Gynecol 1988;73:541–545.
24. Moodley J, Bhoola V, Duursma J, Pudifin D, Byrne S, Kenoyer DG. The association of antiphospholipid antibodies with severe early-onset pre-eclampsia. South African Med J 1995;85:105–107.
25. Yasuda M, Takakuwa K, Tanaka K. Studies on the association between the anticardiolipin antibody and pre-eclampsia. Acta Med Biol 1994;42:145–149.
26. Dekker GA, de Vries JIP, Doelitzsch PM, et al. Underlying disorders associated with severe early-onset preeclampsia. Am J Obstet Gynecol 1995;173:1042–1048.
27. Yasuda M, Takakuwa K, Tokunaga A, Tanaka K. Prospective studies of the association between anticardiolipin antibody and outcome of pregnancy. Obstet Gynecol 1995;86:555–559.
28. Birdsall MA, Pattison NS, Chamley L. Antiphospholipid antibodies in pregnancy. Aust N Z J Obstet Gynecol 1992;32:328–330.
29. Kelly T, Whittle MJ, Smith DJ, Ryan G. Lupus anticoagulant and pregnancy. J Obstet Gynecol 1996;16:26–31.
30. Botet F, Romera G, Montagut P, Carmona F, Balasch J. Neonatal outcome in women treated for the antiphospholipid syndrome during pregnancy. J Perinat Med 1997;25:192–196.
31. Branch DW, Khamashta MA. Antiphospholipid syndrome: obstetric diagnosis, management and controversies. Obstet Gynecol 2003;101:1333–1344.
32. Derksen RHWM, Khamashta MA, Branch DW. Management of obstetric antiphospholipid syndrome. Arthritis Rheum 2004;50:1028–1039.
33. Branch DW, Silver RM, Blackwell JL, Reading JC, Scott JR. Outcome of treated pregnancies in women with antiphospholipid syndrome: an update of the Utah experience. Obstet Gynecol 1992;80:614–620.
34. Granger KA, Farquharson RG. Obstetric outcome in antiphospholipid syndrome. Lupus 1997;6:509–513.
35. Backos M, Rai R, Baxter N, Chilcott I T, Cohen H, Regan L. Pregnancy complications in women with recurrent miscarriage associated with antiphospholipid antibodies treated with low dose aspirin and heparin. Br J Obstet Gynaecol 1999;106:102–107.
36. Huong DLT, Wechsler B, Blerty O, Vauthier-Brouzes D, Lefebvre G, Piette JC. A study of 75 pregnancies in patients with antiphospholipid syndrome. J Rheumatol 2001;28:2025–2030.
37. Stone S, Hunt BJ, Khamashta MA, Bewley SJ, Nelson-Piercy C. Primary antiphospholipid syndrome in pregnancy: an analysis of outcome in 35 women. Thromb Haemost 2004. In press.
38. Kerslake S, Morton KE, Versi E, et al. Early Doppler studies in lupus pregnancy. Am J Reprod Immunol 1992;28:172–175.
39. Caruso A, De Carolis S, Ferrazzani S, Valesini G, Caforio L, Mancuso S. Pregnancy outcome in relation to uterine artery flow velocity waveforms and clinical characteristics in women with antiphospholipid syndrome. Obstet Gynecol 1993;82:970–976.
40. Venkat-Rahman N, Backos M, Teoh TG, Lo WT, Regan L. Uterine artery Doppler in predicting outcome in women with antiphospholipid syndrome. Obstet Gynecol 2001;98:235–242.
41. Bats AS, Lejeune V, Cynober E, et al. Antiphospholipid syndrome and second or third trimester fetal death: follow-up in the next pregnancy. Eur J Obstet Reprod Biol 2004;114:125–129.
42. Lin S, Shimizu I, Suehara N, Nakayama M, Aono T. Uterine artery velocimetry in relation to trophoblast migration into the myometrium of the placental bed. Obstet Gynecol 1995;85:760–765.
43. Cowchock FS. Autoantibodies and pregnancy loss. N Engl J Med 1997;337:197–198.
44. Empsom M, Lassere M, Craig JC, Scott JR. Recurrent pregnancy loss with antiphospholipid antibody: a systematic review of therapeutic trials. Obstet Gynecol 2002;99:135–144.
45. Elder MG, de Swiet M, Robertson A, Elder MA, Flloyd E, Hawkins DF. Low-dose aspirin in pregnancy. Lancet 1988;i:410.

46. Silver R, MacGregor SN, Sholl JS, Hobart JM, Neerhof MG, Ragin A. Comparative trial of pred-nisolone plus aspirin versus aspirin alone in the treatment of anticardiolipin antibody positive obstetric patients. Am J Obstet Gynecol 1993;169:1411–1417.
47. Balasch J, Carmona F, Lopez-Soto A, et al. Low-dose aspirin for prevention of pregnancy losses in women with antiphospholipid syndrome. Hum Reprod 1993;8:2234–2239.
48. Krause I, Blank M, Gilbrut B, Shoenfeld Y. The effect of aspirin on recurrent fetal loss in experi-mental antiphospholipid syndrome. Am J Reprod Immunol 1993;29:155–161.
49. Cowchock S, Reece EA. Do low-risk pregnant women with antiphospholipid antibodies need to be treated? Am J Obstet Gynecol 1997;176:1099–1100.
50. Yu CK, Papageorghiou AT, Parra M, Palma Dias R, Nicolaides KH. Randomized controlled trial using low-dose aspirin in the prevention of pre-eclampsia in women with abnormal uterine artery Doppler at 23 weeks' gestation. Ultrasound Obstet Gynecol 2003;22:233–239.
51. Lockshin MD. Which patients with antiphospholipid antibody should be treated and how? Rheum Dis Clin N Am 1993;19:235–247.
52. Cowchock FS, Reece EA, Balaban D, Branch DW, Plouffe L. Repeated fetal losses associated with antiphospholipid antibodies: a collaborative randomised trial comparing prednisolone with low-dose heparin treatment. Am J Obstet Gynecol 1992;166:1318–1323.
53. Ruffati A, Orsini A, Di Lenardo L, et al. A prospective study of 53 consecutive calcium heparin treated pregnancies in patients with antiphospholipid antibody-related fetal loss. Clin Exp Rheumatol 1997;15:499–505.
54. Ruffati A, Favoro M, Tonello M, et al. Efficacy and safety of nadroparin in the treatment of preg-nant women with antiphospholipid syndrome. Lupus 2004. In press.
55. Kutteh WH. Antiphospholipid antibody-associated recurrent pregnancy loss–treatment with heparin and low-dose aspirin is superior to low-dose aspirin alone. Am J Obstet Gynecol 1996;174:1584–1589.
56. Rai R, Cohen H, Dave M, Regan L. Randomised controlled trial of aspirin and aspirin plus heparin in pregnant women with recurrent miscarriage associated with phospholipid antibodies (or antiphospholipid antibodies). Br Med J 1997;314:253–257.
57. Farquharson RG, Quenby S, Greaves M. Antiphospholipid syndrome in pregnancy: a randomized, controlled trial of treatment. Obstet Gynecol 2002;100:408–413.
58. de Swiet M, Ward PD, Fidler J, et al. Prolonged heparin therapy in pregnancy causes bone deminer-alization. Br J Obstet Gynaecol 1983;90:1129–1134.
59. Dahlman TC. Osteoporotic fractures and the recurrence of thromboembolism during pregnancy and the puerperium in 184 women undergoing thromboprophylaxis with heparin. Am J Obstet Gynecol 1993;168:1265–1270.
60. Nelson-Piercy C, Letsky E, de Swiet M. Low molecular weight heparin for obstetric thrombopro-phylaxis: experience of 69 pregnancies in 61 high risk women. Am J Obstet Gynecol 1997;176:1062–1068.
61. Smith R, Stevenson JC, Winearls CG, Woods CG, Wordsworth BP. Osteoporosis of pregnancy. Lancet 1985;1:1178–1180.
62. Khastgir G, Studd J. Pregnancy-associated osteoporosis. Br J Obstet Gynaecol 1994;101:836–838.
63. Smith R, Athanasou NA, Ostlere SJ, Vipond SE. Pregnancy-associated osteoporosis. QJM 1995;88:865–878.
64. Nelson-Piercy C. Heparin-induced osteoporosis in pregnancy. Lupus 1997;6:500–504.
65. Byrd LM, Johnston TA, Shiach C, Hay CRM. Osteopenic fractures and low molecular weight heparin in pregnancy. J Obstet Gynaecol 2004;24:S11.
66. Greer IA, Nelson-Piercy C. Systematic review of safety and efficacy of LMWH in pregnancy. Br J Obstet Gynaecol 2004. In press.
67. Hunt BJ, Doughty H, Majumdar G, et al. Thromboprophylaxis with low molecular weight heparin (Fragmin) in high risk pregnancies. Thromb Haemost 1997;77:39–43.
68. Hunt BJ, Gattens M, Khamashta M, Nelson-Piercy C, Almeida A. Thromboprophylaxis with unmonitored intermediate-dose low molecular weight heparin in pregnancies with a previous arte-rial or venous thrombotic event. Blood Coagul Fibrinolysis 2003;14:735–739.
69. Nelson-Piercy C. Low molecular weight heparin for obstetric thromboprophylaxis. Br J Obstet Gynaecol 1994;101:6–8.
70. Hunt BJ, Khamashta MA, Lakasing L, Williams F, Nelson-Piercy C, Hughes GRV. Thromboprophylaxis in antiphospholipid syndrome pregnancies with previous cerebral arterial thrombotic events: is warfarin preferable? Thromb Haemost 1998;79:1060–1061.
71. Shaul WL, Hall JG. Multiple congenital anomalies associated with oral anticoagulants. Am J Obstet Gynecol 1977;127:191–198.

72. Ginsberg JS, Hirsh J, Turner DC, Levine MN, Burrows R. Risks to the fetus of anticoagulant therapy during pregnancy. Thromb Haemost 1989;61:197–203.
73. Vitale N, Feo M, De Santo LS, Pollice A, Tedesco N, Cotrufo M. Dose-dependent fetal complications of warfarin in pregnant women with mechanical heart valves. J Am Coll Cardiol 1999;33:1637–1641.
74. Cotrufo M, De Feo M, De Santo LS, et al. Risk of warfarin during pregnancy with mechanical valve prostheses. Obstet Gynecol 2002;99:35–40.
75. Howe AM, Webster WS. Exposure of the pregnant rat to warfarin and vitamin K1: an animal model of intraventricular hemorrhage in the fetus. Teratology 1990;42:413–420.
76. Wellesley D, Moore I, Heard M, Keeton B. Two cases of warfarin embryopathy: a re-emergence of this condition? Br J Obstet Gynaecol 1998;105:805–806.
77. Orme ML, Lewis PJ, de Swiet M, et al. May mothers given warfarin breast-feed their infants? Br Med J 1977;1:1564–1565.
78. McKenna R, Cole ER, Vasan U. Is warfarin sodium contraindicated in the lactating mother? J Paediatr 1983;103:325–327.
79. Kwak JYH, Barini R, Gilman-Sachs A, Beaman KD, Beer AE. Down-regulation of maternal antiphospholipid antibodies during early pregnancy and pregnancy outcome. Am J Obstet Gynecol 1994;171:239–246.
80. Lubbe WF, Butler WS, Palmer SJ, Liggins GC. Fetal survival after prednisolone suppression of maternal lupus anticoagulant. Lancet 1983;i:1361–1363.
81. Lockshin MD, Druzin ML, Qamar T. Prednisolone does not prevent recurrent fetal death in women with antiphospholipid antibody. Am J Obstet Gynecol 1989;160:439–443.
82. Laskin CA, Bombardier C, Hannah ME, et al. Prednisolone and aspirin in women with autoantibodies and unexplained recurrent fetal loss. N Engl J Med 1997;337:148–153.
83. Spinnato JA, Clark AL, Pierangeli SS, Harris EN. Intravenous immunoglobulin therapy for the antiphospholipid syndrome in pregnancy. Am J Obstet Gynecol 1995;172:690–694.
84. Kaaja R, Julkunen H, Ammala P, Palouso T, Kurki P. Intravenous immunoglobulin treatment of pregnant patients with recurrent pregnancy losses associated with antiphospholipid antibodies. Acta Obstet Gynaecol Scand 1993;72:63–66.
85. Arnout J, Spitz B, Wittevrongel C, Vanrusselt M, Van Assche A, Vermylen J. High-dose intravenous immunoglobulin in a pregnant patient with antiphospholipid syndrome: immunological changes associated with a successful outcome. Thromb Haemost 1994;71:741–747.
86. Fulcher D, Stewart G, Exne T, Trudinger B, Jeremy R. Plasma exchange and the anticardiolipin syndrome in pregnancy. Lancet 1989;ii:171.
87. Fishman P, Falach Vaknine E, Zigelman R, et al. Prevention of fetal loss in experimental antiphospholipid syndrome by in vivo administration of recombinant interleukin-3. J Clin Invest 1993;21:1834–1837.
88. Gordon C, Kilby MD. Use of intravenous immunoglobulin therapy in pregnancy in systemic lupus erythematosus and antiphospholipid antibody syndrome. Lupus 1998;7:429–433.
89. Gordon C, Raine-Fenning N, Brackley K, Bacon PA, Weaver J, Kilby M. Intravenous immunoglobulin (IVIG) therapy to salvage severely compromised pregnancies in SLE and antiphospholipid (aPL) syndrome. Lupus 1998;7:114.
90. Triolo G, Ferrante A, Ciccia F, et al. Randomized study of subcutaneous low molecular weight heparin plus aspirin versus intravenous immunoglobulin in the treatment of recurrent pregnancy loss associated with antiphospholipid antibodies. Arthritis Rheum 2003;48:728–731.
91. Royal College of Obstetricians and Gynaecologists. Thromboprophylaxis during pregnancy, labour and after vaginal delivery, 2004 Guidelines. London: Royal College of Obstetricians and Gynaecologists, 2004.
92. Branch DW. Thoughts on the mechanism of pregnancy loss associated with the antiphospholipid syndrome. Lupus 1994;3:275–280.
93. Lakasing L, Poston L. Adverse pregnancy outcome in antiphospholipid syndrome: focus for future research. Lupus 1997;6:1–4.
94. Di Simone N, Del Papa N, Raschi E, et al. Antiphospholipid antibodies affect trophoblast gonadotrophin secretion and invasiveness by binding directly and through adhered β_2-glycoprotein I. Arthritis Rheum 2000;43:140–150.
95. Di Simone N, Caliandro D, Castellani R, Ferrazzani S, Caruso A. Interleukin-3 and human trophoblast: in vitro explanations for the effect of interleukin in patients with antiphospholipid antibody syndrome. Fertil Steril 2000;73:1194–1200.
96. Di Simone N, Caliandro D, Castellani R, Ferrazzani S, De Carolis S, Caruso A. Low-molecular weight heparin restores in-vitro trophoblast invasiveness and differentiation in presence of immunoglobulin G fractions obtained from patients with antiphospholipid syndrome. Hum Reprod 1999;14:489–495.

97. Lala PK, Hamilton GS. Growth factors, proteases and protease inhibitors in the maternal-fetal dialogue. Placenta 1996;17:545–555.
98. McMaster MT, Bass KE, Fisher SJ. Human trophoblast invasion, autocrine control and paracrine modulation. Ann N Y Acad Sci 1994;734:122–131.
99. Guilbert L, Robertson SA, Wegmann TG. The trophoblast as an integral component of a macrophage-cytokine network. Immunol Cell Biol 1993;71:49–57.
100. Burrows TD, King A, Loke YW. Trophoblast migration during human placental implantation. Hum Reprod Update 1996;2:307–321.
101. Fisher SJ, Damsky CH. Human cytotrophoblast invasion. Sem Cell Biol 1993;4:183–188.
102. Vicovac L, Aplin JD. Epithelial-mesenchymal transition during trophoblast differentiation. Acta Anatomica 1996;156:202–216.
103. Aplin JD. The cell biology of human implantation. Placenta 1996;17:269–275.
104. McMaster MT, Librach CL, Zhou K, et al. Expression Is restricted to differentiated cytotrophoblasts. J Immunol 1995;154:3771–3778.
105. Vogt E, Ah-Kau N, Rote NS. A model for the antiphospholipid antibody syndrome: monoclonal antiphosphotidylserine antibody induces intrauterine growth restriction in mice. Am J Obstet Gynecol 1996;174:700–707.
106. Silver RM, Smith LA, Edwin SS, Oshiro BT, Branch DW. Variable effects on murine pregnancy of immunoglobulin G fractions from women with antiphospholipid antibodies. Am J Obstet Gynecol 1997;177:229–233.
107. Horkko S, Miller E, Dudl E, et al. Antiphospholipid antibodies are directed against epitopes of oxidized phospholipids. Recognition of cardiolipin by monoclonal antibodies to epitopes of oxidized low density lipoprotein. J Clin Invest 1996;98:815–825.
108. Roubey RAS. Autoantibodies to phospholipid-binding plasma proteins: a new view of lupus anticoagulants and other "antiphospholipid" autoantibodies. Blood 1994;84:2854–2867.
109. Lockwood CJ, Rand JH. The immunology and obstetrical consequences of antiphospholipid antibodies. Obstet Gynecol Surg 1994;49:432–441.
110. Galli M, Comfurius P, Maassen C, et al. Anticardiolipin antibodies (ACA) directed not to cardiolipin but to a plasma protein cofactor. Lancet 1990;335:1544–1547.
111. Fleck RA, Rapaport SI, Rao L. Anti-prothrombin antibodies and the lupus anticoagulant. Blood 1988;72:512–519.
112. De Wolf F, Carreras LO, Moerman P, Vermylen J, Van Assche A, Renaer M. Decidual vasculopathy and extensive placental infarction in a patient with repeated thromboembolic accidents, recurrent fetal loss, and a lupus anticoagulant. Am J Obstet Gynecol 1982;142:829–834.
113. Erlendsson K, Steinsson K, Johannsson JH, Geirsson RT. Relation of antiphospholipid antibody and placental bed inflammatory vascular changes to the outcome of pregnancy in successive pregnancies of 2 women with systemic lupus erythematosus. J Rheumatol 1993;20:1779–1785.
114. Labarrere CA, Faulk WP. Fetal stem vessel endothelial changes in placentae from normal and abnormal pregnancies. Am J Reprod Immunol 1992;27:97–100.
115. Rand JH, Wu XX, Guller S, Gil G, Scher J, Lockwood CJ. Reduction of annexin V (placental anticoagulant protein-1) on placental villi of women with antiphospholipid antibodies and recurrent spontaneous abortion. Am J Obstet Gynecol 1994;171:1566–1572.
116. Rand JH, Wu XX, Andree HAM, et al. Pregnancy loss in the antiphospholipid-antibody syndrome – a possible thrombogenic mechanism. N Engl J Med 1997;337:154–160.
117. La Rosa L, Meroni PL, Tinicani A, et al. $\beta_2$glycoprotein-I and placental anticoagulant protein I in placentae from patients with antiphospholipid syndrome. J Rheumatol 1994;21:1684–1693.
118. Lakasing L, Campa JS, Poston R, Khamashta MA, Poston L. Normal expression of tissue factor, thrombomodulin and annexin V in placentas from women with antiphospholipid syndrome, Am J Obstet Gynecol 1999;181:180–189.
119. Lyall F, Greer IA. The vascular endothelium in normal pregnancy and pre-eclampsia. Rev Reprod 1996;1:107–116.
120. Greer IA. Thrombophilia: implications for pregnancy outcome. Thromb Res 2003;109:73–81.
121. Brenner B. Clinical management of thrombophilia related placental vascular complications. Blood 2004;103:4003–4009.
122. Girardi G, Berman J, Redecha P, et al. Complement C5a receptors and neutrophils mediate fetal injury in the antiphospholipid syndrome. J Clin Invest 2003;112:1644–1654.

45 Management of Thrombocytopenia in Hughes Syndrome

Monica Galli and Tiziano Barbui

Introduction

The combination of lupus anticoagulants (LA) and anticardiolipin antibodies (aCL), which are the best known antiphospholipid antibodies (aPL), with arterial and venous thrombosis and recurrent miscarriages defines Hughes syndrome. Two forms of Hughes syndrome have been described: the "primary" syndrome [1], that occurs in the absence of any underlying disease, and the "secondary" syndrome [2], that develops in association with another pathological condition, mainly systemic lupus erythematosus (SLE). In 1999, a panel of experts defined the preliminary laboratory and clinical criteria for Hughes syndrome [3].

Thrombosis is the most frequent clinical event of Hughes syndrome, as it occurs in approximately 30% of patients [4], with an overall annual rate of 2.5% [5]. Venous thrombosis accounts for about 60% of all thromboembolic events, and is represented mainly by deep vein thrombosis of the legs and pulmonary embolism [6]. On the other hand, complete cerebral ischemic strokes and transient ischemic attacks are the most common arterial thrombosis [6]. Thrombosis may be recurrent and is often spontaneous. Obstetric complications are reported in about 15% to 20% of women with Hughes syndrome [7], and are considered secondary to thrombosis of the placental vessels [8].

A variable degree of thrombocytopenia is observed in as many as 20% to 40% of patients with aPL [9]. As uncertainty exists regarding its pathogenesis, therapy, and influence on the policy of treatment of thrombosis, the panel of experts decided not to include thrombocytopenia among the criteria for the diagnosis of Hughes syndrome.

Pathophysiology of Thrombocytopenia

Thrombocytopenia of Hughes syndrome is classified among the immune thrombocytopenias. Idiopathic thrombocytopenic purpura – the most common and better known of this group of conditions – has been pathogenetically linked to specific autoantibodies directed against glycoproteins IIb/IIIa and Ib/IX (less frequently, also glycoproteins Ia/IIa and V) [10]. Upon binding to platelet membrane, these

Table 45.1. Antigenic targets of antiphospholipid antibodies.

β_2-glycoprotein I
(Human) prothrombin
(Activated) protein C
Protein S
Tissue-type plasminogen activator
Annexin V
Thrombomodulin
Oxidized low-density lipoproteins
Factor XII
High- and low-molecular weight kininogens
Factor VII/VIIa
Complement components H and C4b

antibodies increase the peripheral destruction of opsonized platelets [11, 12]. Typically, the half-life of platelets becomes very short, and their scavenging from circulation takes place mainly in the spleen and the liver.

In the mid 1980s, aPL had been suggested to cause thrombocytopenia, based on the high prevalence of aCL in patients with idiopathic thrombocytopenic purpura [13], and on the interaction between platelet membrane phospholipids and these antibodies (see below). Even though this possibility cannot be excluded, the direct role of aPL in the pathogenesis of thrombocytopenia has been questioned. In fact, antibodies directed against glycoproteins IIb/IIIa and Ib/IX are found in about 40% of aPL-positive patients [14], a figure similar to that already known for idiopathic thrombocytopenic purpura [15]. Moreover, antibodies directed against a 50–70 kDa internal platelet protein have been specifically found in patients with aPL and thrombocytopenia but not in patients with idiopathic thrombocytopenic purpura [16]. Antibodies directed towards platelet glycoproteins Ia/IIa and IV and towards CD9 have also been detected in the serum of patients with primary Hughes syndrome [17]. Finally, it has been observed that immunosuppressive treatment of idiopathic thrombocytopenic purpura increased platelet number and reduced the titers of platelet-associated IgG but not those of aPL [18]. This data would indicate that aPL and antiplatelet antibodies comprise different specificities and suggest that platelet-specific antibodies, rather than aPL, play a role in the pathogenesis of thrombocytopenia of Hughes syndrome.

Interactions Between aPL Antibodies and Platelets: Parallelism with Heparin-induced Thrombocytopenia

aPL interact with negatively charged phospholipids by means of specific proteins (listed in Table 45.1). β_2-glycoprotein I and prothrombin are by far the 2 best known and characterized antigenic targets of aPL [19–22].

Anionic phospholipids are essential constituents of cell membranes. In platelets, they are located in the inner leaflet of the plasma membrane [reviewed in 23]; thus, they are not available for interaction with aPL. However, under physiologic conditions, this asymmetric distribution can be lost, resulting in exposure of anionic phospholipids on the outer leaflet of plasma membrane [23]. For platelets, this phenomenon occurs upon activation by different agonists and is accompanied by shedding of microvesicles. Because both activated platelets and platelet-derived microvesicles represent an important in vivo procoagulant surface, the interaction between aPL and cellular membranes may be relevant to the pathogenesis of thrombosis of Hughes syndrome.

Limited evidence is available regarding the interaction of aPL with platelets in vivo. Although impairment of the thromboxane A2/prostacyclin balance [24], and increased urinary excretion and plasma levels of the platelets-specific β-thromboglobulin [25] have been reported, pointing towards a condition of in vivo platelet activation, neither elution of aPL from platelet membrane [26], nor clear evidence for circulating activated platelets have been demonstrated by flow cytometry studies. Fanelli et al [27] found a statistically significant increase in the expression of CD62p above the normal cut-off in the platelet-rich plasma of 9 out of 16 patients with primary Hughes syndrome. No differences were observed for CD63 expression. Joseph et al [28] analyzed a cohort of 20 patients with primary Hughes syndrome for the expression of CD62p, CD63, percentage of circulating reticulated platelets, and levels of soluble P selectin, taken as indicators of platelet activation. These authors found an increased expression of CD63 and a higher median level of P selectin in the patients' group when compared to the control group. The same group [29] confirmed and extended this observation, showing an increased presence of monocyte–platelet complexes in patients with primary Hughes syndrome. Conversely, other groups failed to find signs of platelet activation both in patients with primary [30] or with SLE-related Hughes syndrome [31].

The presence of microvesicles has been investigated in aPL-positive patients [32]. By means of flow cytometry, employing specific antiplatelet glycoprotein antibodies, pathological levels of circulating microvesicles were observed in approximately half of the patients. By retrospective analysis, this finding was statistically associated with thrombosis.

The interaction of aPL with platelets has been investigated mainly by in vitro experiments. Even though binding of aPL to resting platelets has been occasionally reported [33], activation and/or damage appear a prerequisite for the binding of aPL [34–36]. Elegant studies with murine monoclonal antibodies to β_2-glycoprotein I demonstrated that the antibodies by themselves were unable to activate resting platelets, but that they greatly stimulated platelet activation and secretion induced by sub-threshold concentrations of ADP or epinephrine [37]. The effect was blocked by a specific inhibitor of the FcāRII. A similar pattern of reactivity was observed when platelets were substituted by neutrophils [38]. Again, the monoclonal anti-β_2-glycoprotein I antibodies interact with neutrophil surface via the FcāRII inducing activation, degranulation, and adherence of neutrophils to endothelial cells. Similarly, Font et al [39] showed the ability of monoclonal human aCL to promote platelet interaction with subendothelium under flow conditions, provided the presence of β_2-glycoprotein I. Experiments by Lutters et al [40] extended these observations by showing that dimers of β_2-glycoprotein I increase platelet deposition to collagen via interaction with phospholipids and the apolipoprotein E receptor 2'.

Noima et al [41] showed that plasma and IgG fractions displaying both aCL and LA activities were able to enhance CD62p expression of ADP-stimulated platelets. Conversely, plasmas and IgG immunoglobulins containing aCL only or LA activity only failed to induced such a stimulatory effect.

This in vitro behavior of aPL is remarkably similar to that already reported for heparin-induced thrombocytopenia (HIT) [42], another autoimmune thrombocytopenia characterized by a high rate of venous and arterial thromboembolic complications [43]. Upon recognition of the heparin/platelet factor 4 complex on the surface of slightly activated platelets [44, 45], the antibodies interact with FcγRII, in this way enhancing platelet activation, secretion, and shedding of microvesicles [46–48]. A single base polymorphism of the FcγRII has been reported at position 131, that changes the native arginine to histidine: the FcγRII[His131] was found to be associated with with a predisposition to HIT because its prevalence was higher than in normal controls [49]. Compared to the FcγRII[Arg131] isoform, the FcγRII[His131] allele has a higher affinity for IgG2 [50], which is the major IgG subtype of both heparin-induced antibodies [51] and aPL [52]. At variance with HIT, the prevalence of the different FcγRII genotypes in aPL patients was similar to that of controls [53].

The above reported clinical and laboratory similarities between HIT and Hughes syndrome prompted Vermylen et al [54] to put forward a hypothesis to explain both the high risk of thombosis and the development of thrombocytopenia in patients with the Hughes syndrome. Following a mild platelet activation, phospholipid binding proteins (i.e., β_2-glycoprotein I, prothrombin) would interact with anionic phospholipids exposed on the outer surface; aPL stabilize their binding via trimolecular complex formation [55, 56] (Fig. 45.1) and via additional FcγRII interactions.

The interaction results in 2 main consequences:

1. Sensitized platelets are quickly removed from circulation, leading to thrombocytopenia.

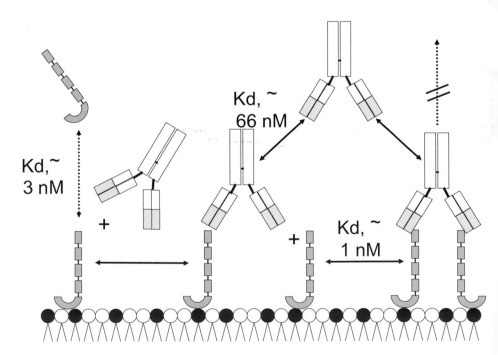

Figure 45.1. Anti–β_2-glycoprotein I antibodies form stable tri-molecular complexes with their antigen at the anionic (phospholipid) surface.

2. Platelets are further activated, leading to an increased risk of thrombosis.

Indirect support to this hypothesis comes from Nojima et al [57], who reported a high prevalence of thrombocytopenia in patients with secondary Hughes syndrome and arterial thrombosis. In a prospective study of a large cohort of thrombocytopenic patients, the presence of aPL was associated with an increased risk to develop the thrombotic complications of Hughes syndrome [58]. Finally, in an arterial thrombosis model in the hamster [59], monoclonal β_2-glycoprotein I–dependent aPL promoted thrombus formation and were immunohistochemically localized on individual platelets within the platelet-rich thrombi. Cellular activation via the Fc portion was not essential because the F(ab)2 fragments of the antibodies still promoted thrombus formation.

Prevalence, Clinical Course, and Management of Thrombocytopenia

Thrombocytopenia in the Hughes syndrome rarely requires treatment, because it is seldom associated with major bleeding [60, 61]. Among the 293 cases enrolled in the Italian Registry [6], the prevalence of thrombocytopenia was 26%, 32 patients (11%) had platelet counts below 50,000/mm^3 and only 2 of them (6%) showed severe bleeding complications. Therefore, the prevalence of major hemorrhagic events in Hughes syndrome does not appear significantly different from that reported for idiopathic thrombocytopenic purpura [62].

Thrombocytopenia has been associated with a high risk of mortality in patients suffering from SLE [63]. By univariate analysis, thrombocytopenia and arterial thrombosis were the only phospholipid-related manifestations statistically associated with mortality in 658 patients with SLE ($P < 0.001$ and $P = 0.02$, respectively). Unfortunately, the authors did not state whether and to what extent bleeding complications accounted for the death of their patients; therefore, it is possible that thrombocytopenia was simply associated with a more severe disease.

Some authors have speculated about the possibility that thrombocytopenia selects a population of patients with aPL antibodies at particular risk for the development of SLE [13], but few data exist to support this. Indeed, the first 4-year follow-up analysis of the patients enrolled in the Italian Registry of Antiphospholipid Antibodies study indicates that the rate of progression to overt SLE is low, 0.28% patients/year [5], irrespective of whether thrombocytopenia is present or not. Similar data have been reported by Stasi et al [64], who performed a long-term follow-up observation of 208 patients with idiopathic thrombocytopenic purpura. These authors identified only 4 patients who developed laboratory or clinical features consistent with SLE or other overt autoimmune diseases over a median follow up of 92 months.

Thrombocytopenia in Hughes syndrome rarely requires treatment. However, when this becomes necessary, the same policy as for idiopathic thrombocytopenic purpura should be considered [65]. Two large series of thrombocytopenic patients have been evaluated for treatment outcome according to their aPL status [18, 58]: corticosteroids, splenectomy, and intravenous immunoglobulins produced response irrespective of the presence of aCL. Most of the patients were treated with corticosteroids and splenectomy. As expected, corticosteroids produced a similar low rate of sustained response in patients with or without aCL (15% and 17%, respectively). Splenectomy was performed in 23 patients; sustained responses were obtained in approximately 60% in both groups. Therefore, the presence of aPL did not seem to affect the treatment outcome. Surgery in these cases should be considered with caution because of the risk of both bleeding and thrombosis.

The anti-CD20 monoclonal antibody Rituximab has been used to treat idiopathic thrombocytopenic purpura. Sustained increase of platelet count has been reported in 28% to 54% of thrombocytopenic patients refractory to several lines of treatments [66–69]. Little is known about its use in thrombocytopenic patients with aPL, as only 1 pediatric case has been reported so far [70]. Rituximab must be used with caution, because in occasional patients it has been associated with induction or exacerbation of autoimmune diseases, including acute agranulocytosis [71] and lupus thrombocytopenia [72].

Acquired defects of platelet function have been estimated to occur in as many as 40% of the patients with aPL [65]. Impairment of platelet aggregation has been found in the course of opportunistic infection in acquired immune deficiency syndrome patients with aPL [73] and reduced adhesion to subendothelium has been observed by Orlando et al [74]. Other defects include storage pool disease, isolated defects in response to epinephrine or collagen, and impairment of thromboxane B2 synthesis [34]. In vitro experiments performed with the immunoglobulin fractions isolated from patients' plasma led to the suggestion that aPL might be responsible for these acquired qualitative platelet defects [73, 74]. However, the evidence is inconclusive, because only in a few cases were affinity-purified aCL tested. Even though the bleeding time is generally prolonged, the defect are not associated with significant hemorrhagic complications, unless another risk factor co-exists. Therefore, defective platelet function need only be sought in case of unexplained bleeding in aPL-positive patients on antithrombotic treatment. Treatment of hemorrhagic complications not associated with thrombocytopenia remains an open question. Only a few case reports have been published: corticosteroid administration and plasma exchange have been found useful anedoctally [75, 76].

Prevalence and Treatment of Thrombosis in Relation to Thrombocytopenia

Thromboembolic events are the most common manifestation of Hughes syndrome. When their prevalence is evaluated according to the platelet number, it appears that severe, but not moderate thrombocytopenia protects, at least partly, against thrombosis. The Italian Registry [6] reported that 32% of moderately thrombocytopenic patients (platelet 50,000–100,000/mm^3) experienced at least 1 thrombotic event compared with 40% of patients with normal platelet count. Conversely, severe thrombocytopenia (platelet < 50,000/mm^3) was associated with a lower prevalence of thrombosis (9%). These retrospective data have been confirmed by the 4-year follow-up analysis of patients enrolled in the Italian Registry of Antiphospholipid Antibodies [5]. No significant differences in the incidence of thrombosis were found between patients with a normal platelet count (2.54% patients/year) and those with moderate thrombocytopenia (3.9% patients/year). Again, a lower incidence (0.95% patients/year) was observed in severely thrombocytopenic patients. This difference did not reach statistical significance, probably because of the relatively low number of patients with thrombosis (7 out of 56 patients with mild thrombocytopenia vs. 2 out of 52 severely thrombocytopenic patients).

Thrombotic complications may occur in spite of a very low platelet count, as Nojima et al [57] pointed out. This raises concern in the management of thromboembolic events when thrombocytopenia is also present.

By retrospective analysis, 2 studies [77, 78] showed that long-term high-intensity warfarin therapy [prothrombin international normalized ratio (INR) > 3.0] confers better antithrombotic protection than low-intensity warfarin and/or aspirin. Three studies analyzed the risk of recurrence of thrombosis of aPL-positive patients in relation to the intensity and duration of oral anticoagulation [79–81]. Two of them [80, 81] agreed on the benefit from a prolonged secondary prophylaxis with oral anticoagulants aimed at maintaining a PT INR range of 2.0-3-0. The third group [79], conversely, found a similar rate of recurrence of thrombosis in patients with and without aPL after discontinuation of oral anticoagulation.

The decision about the duration and intensity of oral anticoagulation must be weighted against the risk of hemorrhage. Rosove and Brewer [77] and Khamashta et al [78] reported an incidence of significant hemorrhagic complications of 3.1% and 7.1% patients/year, with an incidence of life-threatening bleeding events of 1.9% and .7 patients/year, respectively. These figures are somewhat higher than the 1% patients/year incidence of major bleeding reported in patients with prosthetic heart valve replacement, who are similarly on high intensity oral anticoagulation (PT INR 3.0–4.5) [82]. In anticoagulated patients with Hughes syndrome one cannot exclude the possibility that thrombocytopenia (or, less frequently, a platelet function defect) may play a role, at least partly, in the development of hemorrhagic complications. Unfortunately, neither study specifically addressed this problem, because no statement was made regarding platelet count at the time of bleeding events. The survey of the Italian Registry of Antiphospholipid Antibodies reported major bleeding in 3 patients under oral anticoagulation: 1 was thrombocytopenic and experienced a fatal cerebral hemorrhage [5].

Three randomized, multi-center, prospective studies have addressed the issue of the optimal intensity of oral anticoagulation to prevent recurrence of arterial and venous thrombosis in Hughes syndrome [83–85]. The study by Crowther et al [83] evaluated the rate of venous thrombosis recurrence and haemorrhage of APS patients assigned to moderate- (PT INR 2.0–3.0) or high-intensity (PT INR 3.0–4.0) warfarin treatment. Patients with platelet counts below 50,000/mm^3 were excluded from randomization. The annual risk of major bleeding was 2.2% in the moderate-intensity group, and 3.6% in the high-intensity group. Overall, 19% of patients in the former and 25% in the latter group had at least 1 episode of bleeding.

The WAPS study [85] compared moderate- (PT INR 2.0–3.3) with high-intensity (PT INR 3.0–4.5) warfarin treatment for the prevention of recurrence of venous and arterial thrombosis in APS patients. Also this study excluded patients with platelet counts below 50,000/mm^3 from randomization. Patients assigned to receive high-intensity treatment experienced more bleeding complications (27.8% vs. 14.6%, hazard ratio 2.18, 95% confidence interval, 0.92-5.15), even though the prevalence of major hemorrhagic events was similar in the 2 groups.

In both studies, the rate of thrombotic recurrence was similar in the 2 treatment arms, clearly indicating that warfarin aimed at a target PT INR of 2.3–3.0 is the treatment of choice because it has the highest efficacy and safety profile.

The APASS study [84] compared the 2-year rate of recurrence of any thrombosis in patients who – after a first documented stroke – were assigned to either moderate-intensity warfarin therapy (PT INR 1.4–2.8) or aspirin (325 mg/day). The study did not show difference in the rate of thrombotic recurrence of aPL-positive (22.2%) compared to aPL-negative (21.8%) patients. Among aPL-positive patients, aspirin and warfarin treatments were associated with similar rates of recurrence (22 and 26% after 2 years, respectively). Unfortunately, bleeding complications were not among the end points of the study, which neither provided information as to whether thrombocytopenia was an exclusion criterion.

Based on the results of these studies, moderate-intensity warfarin appears the treatment of choice to prevent recurrence of thrombosis of APS patients. Aspirin is also a good choice to prevent recurrence of non-cardiogenic stroke. The issue of the most appropriate antithrombotic treatment of thrombocytopenic APS patients (platelet count below 50,000/mm^3) still remains to be established.

Conclusions and Future Perspectives

Moderate thrombocytopenia is frequent in Hughes syndrome and, as a rule, does not modify the policy for treatment of thrombosis. Severe thrombocytopenia is relatively uncommon and it is seldom associated with bleeding events. When required, its treatment is similar to that of idiopathic thrombocytopenic purpura. Finally, much clinical and laboratory work is still required to elucidate the role of aPL antibodies and platelets in the pathogenesis of the thrombotic complications typical of Hughes syndrome.

References

1. Asherson RA, Khamashta MA, Ordi-Ros J, et al. The "primary" antiphospholipid syndrome: major clinical and serological features. Medicine (Baltimore) 1989;68:366–374.
2. Alarcon-Segovia D, Deleze M, Oria CV. Antiphospholipid antibodies and the antiphospholipid sindrome in systemic lupus erythematosus: a review of 500 consecutive cases. Medicine (Baltimore) 1989;68:353–365.
3. Wilson WA, Gharavi AE, Koike T, et al. International consensus statement on preliminary classification criteria for definite antiphospholipid syndrome. Arthritis Rheum 1999;42:1309–1311.
4. Lechner K, Pabinger-Fasching I. Lupus anticoagulant and thrombosis. Hemostasis 1985;15:252–262.
5. Finazzi G, Brancaccio V, Moia M, et al. Natural history and risk factors of thrombosis in 360 patients with antiphospholipid antibodies. A four-year prospective study from the Italian Registry. Am J Med 1996;100:530–536.
6. Italian Registry of Antiphospholipid Antibodies (IR-APA). Thrombosis and thrombocytopenia in antiphospholipid syndrome (idiopatic and secondary to SLE): first report from the Italian Registry. Haematologica 1993;78:313–318.
7. Barbui T, Cortelazzo S, Galli M, et al. Antiphospholipid antibodies in early repeated abortions: a case-control study. Fertil Steril 1988;50:589–592.
8. De Wolf F, Carreras LO, Moerman P, Vermylen J, Van Assche A, Renaer M. Decidual vasculopathy and estensive placental infarction in a patient with repeated thrombembolic accidents, recurrent fetal loss and a lupus anticoaguant. Am J Obstet Gynecol 1982;142:829–834.

9. Galli M, Finazzi G, Barbui T. Thrombocytopenia in the antiphospholipid syndrome. Br J Haematol 1996;93:1–5.
10. Kuniki TJ, Newman PJ. The molecular immunology of platelet proteins. Blood 1992;80:1386–1404.
11. Harrington WJ, Minnich W, Hollingsworth WJ, Moore CV. Demonstration of a thrombocytopenic factor in the blood of patients with thrombocytopenic purpura. J Lab Clin Med 1951;38:1–10.
12. Aster RH, Jandl JH. Platelet sequestration in man. II. Immunological and clinical studies. J Clin Invest 1962;43:856–869.
13. Harris EN, Gharavi AE, Hedge U, et al. Anticardiolipin antibodies in autoimmune thrombocytopenic purpura. Br J Haematol 1985;59:231–234.
14. Galli M, Daldossi M, Barbui T. Anti-glycoprotein Ib/IX and IIb/IIIa antibodies in patients with antiphospholipid antibodies. Thromb Haemost 1994;71:571–575.
15. He R, Reid DM, Jones CE, Shulman NR. Spectrum of IgG classes, specificities and titers of serum antiglycoproteins in chronic idiopathic thrombocytopenic purpura. Blood 1994;83:1024–1032.
16. Fabris F, Steffan A, Cordiano L, et al. Specific antiplatelet autoantibodies in patients with antiphospholipid antibodies and thrombocytopenia. Eur J Haematol 1994;53:232–236.
17. Godeau B, Piette J-C, Fromont P, Intrator L, Schaeffer A, Bierling P. Specific antiplatelet autoantibodies are associated with the thrombocytopenia of primary antiphospholipid syndrome. Br J Haematol 1997;98:873–879.
18. Stasi R, Stipa E, Masi O, et al. Prevalence and clinical significance of elevated antiphospholipid antibodies in patients with idiopathic thrombocytopenic purpura. Blood 1994;84:4203–4207.
19. McNeil HP, Simpson RJ, Chesterman CN, Krilis SA. Antiphospholipid antibodies are directed against a complex antigen that includes a lipid-binding inhibitor of coagulation: β_2-glycoprotein I (apolipoprotein H). Proc Natl Acad Sci U S A 1990;87:4120–4124.
20. Galli M, Comfurius P, Maassen C, et al. Anticardiolipin antibodies (ACA) directed not to cardiolipin but to a plasma protein cofactor. Lancet 1990;334:1544–1547.
21. Matsuura E, Igarashi Y, Fujimoto M, Ichikawa K, Koike T. Anticardiolipin cofactor(s) and differential diagnosis of autoimmune disease. Lancet 1990;335:177–178.
22. Bevers EM, Galli M, Barbui T, Comfurius P, Zwaal RFA. Lupus anticoagulant IgG's (LA) are not directed to phospholipids only, but to a complex of lipid-bound human prothrombin. Thromb Haemost 1991;66:629–632.
23. Zwaal RFA, Schroit AJ. Pathophysiologic implications of membrane phospholipid asymmetry in blood cells. Blood 1997;89:1121–1132.
24. Martinuzzo ME, Mclouf J, Carreras LO, Levy-Toledano S. Antiphospholipid antibodies enhance thrombin induced platelet activation and thromboxane formation. Thromb Haemost 1993;70:667–671.
25. Galli M, Cortelazzo S, Viero P, Finazzi G, de Gaetano G, Barbui T. Interactions between platelets and lupus anticoagulant. Eur J Haematol 1988;88–94.
26. Biasiolo A, Pengo V. Antiphospholipid antibodies are not present in the membrane of gel-filtered platelets of patients with IgG anticardiolipin antibodies, lupus anticoagulant and thrombosis. Blood Coag Fibrinolysis 1993;4:425–448.
27. Fanelli A, Bergamini C, Rapi S, et al. Flow cytometric detection of circulating activated platelets in primary antiphospholipid sindrome. Correlation with thrombocytopenia and anticardiolipin antibodies. Lupus 1997;6:261–267.
28. Joseph JE, Harrison P, Mackie IJ, Machin SJ. Platelet activation markers and the primary antiphospholipid syndrome (PAPS). Lupus 1998;7:S48–S51.
29. Joseph JE, Harrison P, Mackie IJ, Isenberg DA, Machin SJ. Increased circulating platelet-leukocyte complexes and platelet activation in patients with antiphospholipid syndrome, systemic lupus erythematosus and rheumatoid arthritis. Br J Haematol 2001;115:451–459.
30. Out HJ, de Groot P, van Vliet M, de Gast GC, Niewenhuis HK, Derksen RHWM. Antibodies to platelets in patients with antiphospholipid antibodies. Blood 1991;77:2655–2659.
31. Shechter Y, Tal Y, Greenberg A, Brenner B. Platelet activation in patients with antiphospholipid syndrome. Blood Coag Fibrinolysis 1998;9:653–657.
32. Galli M, Grassi A, Barbui T. Platelet-derived microvesicles in patients with antiphospholipid antibodies[abstract]. Thromb Haemost 1993;69:541.
33. Khamashta MA, Harris EN, Gharavi AE, et al. Immune mediated mechanism for thrombosis : antiphospholipid antibody binding to platelet membrane. Ann Rheum Dis 1988;47:849–852.
34. Hasselaar P, Derksen RHWM, Blokzijl L, de Groot P. Cross-reactivity of antibodies directed against cardiolipin, DANN, endothelial cells and blood platelets. Thromb Haemost 1990;63:169–173.
35. Mikhail MH, Szczech LAM, Shapiro SS. The binding of lupus anticoagulant (LACs) to human platelets [abstract]. Blood 1988;72:333.

36. Shi W, Chong BH, Chesterman CN. β_2-glycoprotein I is a requirement for anticardiolipin antibody binding to activated platelets: differences with lupus anticoagulants. Blood 1993;81:1255–1262.
37. Arvieux J, Roussel B, Pouzol P, Colomb MG. Platelet activating properties of murine monoclonal antibodies to beta2-glycoprotein I. Thromb Haemost 1993;70:336–341.
38. Arvieux J, Jacob MC, Roussel B, Bensa JC, Colomb MG. Neutrophil activation by anti-β_2-glycoprotein I monoclonal antibodies via Fcã receptor II. J Leukoc Biol 1995;57:387–394.
39. Font J, Espinosa G, Tassies D, et al. Etteftc of beta2-glycoprotein I and monoclonal anticardiolipin antibodies in platelet interaction with subendothelium under flow conditions. Arthritis Rheum 2002;46:3283–3289.
40. Lutters BC, Derksen RH, Tekelenburg WL, Lenting WL, Arout H, de Groot PG. Dimers of beta2-glycoprotein I increase platelet deposition to collagen via interaction with phospholipids and the apolipoprotein E receptor 2'. J Biol Chem 2003;278:33831–33838.
41. Nojima J, Suehisa E, Kuratsune H, et al. Platelet activation induced by combined effects of anticardiolipin and lupus anticoagulant IgG antibodies in patients with systemic lupus erythematosus. Thromb Haemost 1999;81:436–441.
42. Arnout J. The pathogenesis of antiphospholipid syndrome: a hypothesis based on parallelisms with heparin-induced thrombocytopenia. Thromb Haemost 1997;75:536–541.
43. George JN, Alving B, Ballem P. Immune heparin-induced thrombocytopenia and thrombosis. Nashville TN: Educational Program of the American Society of Hematology; 1994:66–68.
44. Green D, Harris K, Reynolds N, Roberts M, Patterson R. Heparin immune thrombocytopenia: evidence for a heparin-platelet complex as the antigenic determinant. J Lab Clin Med 1978;91:167–175.
45. Greinacher A, Michel I, Mueller-Eckhardt C. Heparin-associated thrombocytopenia: the antibody is not heparin specific. Thromb Haemost 1992;67:545–549.
46. Chong BH, Pitney WR, Castaldi PA. Heparin-induced thrombocytopenia: association with thrombotic complications with heparin-dependent IgG antibody that induces thromboxane synthesis and platelet aggregation. Lancet 1982;ii:1246–1249.
47. Kappa JR, Fisher CA, Addonizio VP Jr. Heparin-induced platelet activation: the role of thromboxane A2 synthesis and the extent of platelet granule release in two patients. J Vasc Surg 1989;9:574–579.
48. Warkentin TE, Hayward CP, Boshkov LK, et al. Sera from patients with heparin-induced thrombocytopenia generate thrombi-derived microparticles with procoagulant activity: an explanation for the thrombotic complications of heparin-induced thrombocytopenia. Blood 1994;84:3691–3699.
49. Burgess JK, Lindeman R, Chesterman CN, Chong BH. Single aminoacid mutation of Fcγ receptor is associated with the development of heparin-induced thrombocytoenia. Br J Haematol 1995;91:3691–3699.
50. Warderman PAM, van de Winkel JGJ, Vlug A, Esterdaal NAC, Capel PJA. A single aminoacid in the second Ig-like domain of the human Fcγ receptor II is critical for the human IgG2 binding J Immunol 1991;147:1338–1343.
51. Arepally G, Poncz M, McKanzie SE, Cines D. Charactierization of antibody subclass specificity and antigenic determinants in heparin-associated thrombocytopenia [abstract]. Blood 1994;84:181.
52. Arvieux J, Roussel B, Ponard D, Colomb MG. IgG2 subclass restriction of anti β_2-glycoprotein I antibodies in autoimmune patients. Clin Exp Immunol 1994;95:310–315.
53. Atsumi T, Caliz R, Amengual O, Khamashta MA, Hughes GRV. Fcγ receptor IIa H/R 131 polymorphism in patients with antiphospholipid antibodies. Thromb Haemost 1998;79:924–927.
54. Vermylen J, Hoylaerts MF, Arnout J. Antibody-mediated thrombosis. Thromb Haemost 1997;78:420–426.
55. Willems G, Janssen MP, Pelsers MMAL, et al. Role of divalency in the high-affinity binding of anticardiolipin antibody-β_2-glycoprotein I complexes to lipid membranes. Biochemistry 1996;35:13833–13842.
56. Willems GM, Janssen MP, Comfurius P, Galli M, Zwaal RFA, Bevers EM. Kinetics of prothrombin-mediated binding of lupus anticoagulant antibodies to phosphatidylserine-containing phospholipid membranes: an ellipsometric study. Biochemistry 2002;41:14357–14363.
57. Nojima J, Suehisa E, Kuratsune H, et al. High prevalence of thrombocytopenia in SLE patients with high levels of anticardiolipin antibodies combined with lupus anticoagulant. Am J Hematol 1998;58:55–60.
58. Diz-Kucukkaya R, Hacihanefioglu, Yenerel M, et al. Antiphospholipid antibodies and antiphospholipid syndrome in patients presenting with immune thrombocytopenic purpura: a prospective cohort study. Blood 2001;98:1760–1764.
59. Jankowski M, Vreys I, Wittevrongel C, et al. Thrombogenicity of beta2-glycoprotein I-dependent antiphospholipid antibodies in a photochemically induced thrombosis model in the hamster. Blood 2003;101:157–162.

60. Barbui T, Finazzi G. Clinical trials on antiphospholipid syndrome: what is being done and what is needed? Lupus 1994;3:303–307.
61. Machin SJ. Platelets and antiphospholipid antibodies. Lupus 1996;5:386–387.
62. Cortelazzo S, Finazzi G, Buelli M, Molteni A, Viero P, Barbui T. High risk of severe bleeding in aged patients with chronic idiopathic thrombocytopenic purpura. Blood 1991;71:31–33.
63. Drenkard C, Villa AR, Alarcon-Segovia D, Perez-Vazquez ME. Influence of the antiphospholipid sindrome in the survival of patients with systemic lupus erythematosus. J Rheumatol 1994;21:1067–1072.
64. Stasi R, Stipa E, Masi M, Cecconi M, et al. Long-term observation of 108 adults with chronic idiopathic thrombocytopenic purpura. Am J Med 1995;98:436–442.
65. Galli M, Finazzi G, Barbui T. Thrombocytopenia in the antiphospholipid sindrome. Br J Haematol 1996;93:1–5.
66. Stasi R, Pagano A, Stipa E, Amadori S. Rituximab chimeric anti-CD20 monoclonal antibody treatment for adults with chronic idiopathic thrombocytopenic purpura. Blood 2001;98:952–957.
67. Stasi R, Stipa E, Forte V, Meo P, Amadori S. Variable patterns of response to rituximab treatment in adults with chronic idiopathic thrombocytopenic purpura. Blood 2002;99:3872–3873.
68. Giagoudinis AA, Anhuf J, Schneider P, et al. Treatment of relapsed idiopathic thrombocytopenic purpura with the anti-CD20 antibody rituximab. Eur J Haematol 2002;69:95–100.
69. Zaja F, Vinelli N, Sperotto A, et al. The B-cell compartment as the selective target for the treatment of immune thrombocytopenias. Haematologica 2003;88:538–546.
70. Binstadt BA, Caldas AM, Turvey SE, et al. Rituximab therpy for multisystem autoimmune diseases in pediatric patients. J Pediatr 2003;143:598–604.
71. Voog E, Brice P, Cartron J. Acute agranulocytosis (AA) in three patients treated with rituximab for non-Hodgkin lymphoma [abstract]. Blood 2001;98:4668a.
72. Mehta AC, Mtanos GJ, Gentile TC. Exacerbation of lupus while receiving rituximab for chronic refractory thrombocytopenia [abstract]. Blood 2001;98:3862a.
73. Cohen AJ, Philip TM, Kessler CM. Circulating coagulation inhibitors in the acquired immunodeficiency syndrome. Ann Int Med 1986;104:175–180.
74. Orlando E, Cortelazzo S, Marchetti M, Sanfratello R, Barbui T. Prolonged bleeding time in patients with lupus anticoagulant. Thromb Haemost 1992;68:495–499.
75. Manoharan A, Gottlieb P. Bleeding in patients with lupus anticoagulant. Lancet 1984;ii:171.
76. Ordi J, Vilardell M, Oristell J, et al. Bleeding in patients with lupus anticoagulant. Lancet 1984;ii:868–869.
77. Rosove MH, Brewer PMC. Antiphospholipid antibodies: clinical course after the first thrombotic event in 70 patients. Ann Intern Med 1992;117:303–308.
78. Khamashta MA, Cuadrado MJ, Mujic F, Taub MA, Hunt BJ, Hughes GRV. The management of thrombocytopenia in the antiphospholipid antibody syndrome. N Engl J Med 1995;332:993–997.
79. Ginsberg JS, Wells PS, Brill-Edwards P, et al. Antiphospholipid antibodies and venous thromboembolism. Blood 1995;86:3685–3691.
80. Prandoni P, Simioni P, Girolami A. Antiphospholipid antibodies, recurrent thromboembolism, and intensity of warfarin anticoagulation [letter]. Thromb Haemost 1996;75:859.
81. Shulman S, Svegnusson E, Granqvist S, and the Duration of Anticoagulation Study Group. Anticardiolipin antibodies predict early recurrence of thrombembolism and death among patients with venous thromboembolism following anticoagulant therapy. Am J Med 1998;104:332–338.
82. Cortelazzo S, Finazzi G, Viero P, et al. Thrombotic and haemorrhagic complications in patients with mechanical heart valve prosthesis attendine an anticoagulation clinic. Thromb Haemost 1993;69:316–320.
83. Crowther MA, Ginsberg JS, Julian J, et al. A comparison of two intensities of warfarin for the prevention of recurrent thrombosis in patients with the antiphospholipid syndrome. N Engl J Med 2003;349:1133–1138.
84. The APASS Investigators. Antiphospholipid antibodies and subsequent thrombo-occlusive events in patients with ischemic stroke. JAMA 2004;291:576–584.
85. Finazzi G on behalf of the members of the Italian Registry. The Italian Registry of antiphospholipid antibodies [abstract 44]. Blood 2003;102:16a.

46 The Future of Hughes Syndrome

Michael D. Lockshin

Five years ago, in these pages, at the request of the editors, I speculated about the future of the antiphospholipid antibody (aPL) field. I argued for more precise clinical distinctions and for answers to several explicit biological questions and noted the absence of the large-scale clinical collaborations that are necessary for clinical studies to advance. Progress since then has been considerable. Table 46.1 lists the questions I raised in 2000 and compares them to the answers available in mid-2004.

What a remarkable period it has been! Many of the old questions have been answered and much new information has accrued. Major contributions have come from Asia and Europe, from the Middle East and Africa, from Australia and all the Americas. Consensus statements from the 10th International Antiphospholipid Antibody meeting in Taormina helped standardize vocabularies, clinical approaches, priorities, and more consensus documents will come from the meeting in Sydney in late 2004. Investigators in the Hughes syndrome field have learned to analyze separately, in treatment and prognosis studies, patients with arterial thromboses from those with venous thromboses or with pregnancy loss only. Most clinical

Table 46.1. Desires for the Hughes Syndrome field in 2000 and status of those desires in 2004. Those items indicated by asterisk are less close to resolution.

2000 questions	2004 status
Clinical distinctions to make	
Hughes syndrome vs. non-immunological coagulopathies	Distinct but similar causes of thrombosis are now understood
Patients with pregnancy loss vs. venous vs. arterial thrombosis	Need for separate patient groups for treatment and outcome studies now understood, but not enacted
Onset of antibody vs. onset of clinical illness	Antibody known to be present 10+ years before syndrome
Causes of thrombosis	*Trigger causes suspect, none identified
Biological questions	
Specifics of antigen and antibody	*Greater detail known, no defined pathogenesis as yet
Mechanisms of coagulation	*Greater detail known, no defined pathogenesis as yet
Mechanisms of valvulopathy, nephropathy, livedo	*Not understood
New animal models	Additional model available, more information on current models
Interpretation of discordant aCL/LAC/β_2-GP1	*Not understood
Needs	
Establishment of consortia for clinical trials	APSCORE, EuroPhospholipid Consortium, others
Clean descriptions of outcomes	Prospective studies underway

studies now carefully distinguish between patients with the primary and those with the secondary form of the syndrome. The distinctions are critical for prospective studies, especially those on treatment. Prospective studies that actually make these distinctions, however, have only just begun; definitive answers will not be available for another few years.

Thrombosis is the defining feature of Hughes syndrome. Simple thrombosis does not explain many of the syndrome's aspects, however, and it is possible that anticoagulation will prove to be an incomplete, insufficient treatment for many of its symptoms. Statins may have a therapeutic role for reasons related to their effects on endothelium or inflammatory mechanisms. We do not yet understand the pathogenesis of, and cannot assume the effectiveness of anticoagulation for livedo, valvulopathy, cognitive dysfunction (with or without hyperintense brain lesions on magnetic resonance imaging), or renal thrombotic microangiopathy. The reasons for the sudden occurrence of the catastrophic antiphospholipid syndrome (CAPS) remain a mystery, as do those for pulmonary hemorrhage. We now know that aPL arises years if not decades before clinical illness, a fact that encourages us to maintain clear distinctions between etiological agents and triggers of clinical events and between aPL and Hughes syndrome itself. How the separate parts of the concatenation of illness – genetic susceptibility, antibody acquisition, first clinical event, and long-term complications – relate to one another is unclear. We are now more aware of surgical risk and of risk of losing renal transplants to thrombosis despite prophylaxis. Systematic cross-sectional studies may have excluded one hypothesis prevalent in 2000, that aPL induces accelerated atherosclerosis; other clinical correlations remain true. Very simple facts – What is the risk in a given circumstance for a new thrombosis? What are the effects of contributing factors, such as smoking, oral contraceptive treatment, or surgery on thrombosis risk? – remain to be defined.

The basic science of this field has also advanced rapidly but has yet to yield definitive answers. We now know a great deal about the binding properties of aPL; its avidity and valence; the peptide and tertiary structure of and the effect of directed point mutations and deletions on β_2-glycoprotein I; the relationships between aPL and antibodies to other phospholipid binding proteins, such as prothrombin; and the roles in the syndrome of plasmin, tissue factor pathway inhibitor, and other effectors or markers of thrombosis and fibrinolysis. New animal models for thrombosis, knock-outs and mutated animals, and animal models for neurologic disease assist us to understand pathogenesis. Animal mutations and modulations demonstrate a requirement for complement activation in experimental pregnancy loss. Animal preparations that monitor in vivo adhesion of cells or cell particles in flowing blood may serve as tests of treatment efficacy. In humans, the roles of endothelial cell and platelet activation in clinical events have been studied in detail. Studies on microbial peptides that cross-react with β_2-glycoprotein I suggest etiologies and potential treatments. But, oddly, compared to other (rheumatic) illnesses, the science of Hughes syndrome has accrued less information about its genetics, potential roles (if any) of cytokines, functions or abnormalities of specific immunocytes, cell surface markers, and cell activation cycles. Is this because thrombosis is thought not to be immunologic or because Hughes syndrome is not thought to be a systemic autoimmune disease? Or is it that, absent evident immune attack, these sciences do not apply?

Despite thousands of papers, the clinical needs of this field remain great. Standardization of clinical definitions among studies is an absolute requirement, a process clearly aided by the Taormina consensus statements and by the creation of large consortia, such as the Euro Phospholipid Project and APSCORE (the American consortium). We have just begun to enter the era of prospective, randomized, clinical trials – dose ranging for warfarin for secondary prevention of thrombosis, dose ranging for heparin for prevention of pregnancy loss, and in-progress but not yet reported trials for asymptomatic patients with aPL: aspirin/placebo (APLASA in the United States) or aspirin/warfarin (ALIWAPAS in Britain) – which are necessarily large scale and long-term, because proof of success is absence of new thrombotic events. We lack clinical trials that test alternatives to warfarin–platelet and endothelial cell inhibitors and non-anticoagulant treatments. Patients throughout the world receive ad hoc treatments that lack an evidence base, rituximab, for instance, and antithrombins and the newer antiplatelet agents. We learn of these in anecdotes but have yet to see prospective controlled trials. New hypotheses of pathogenesis such as complement activation in pregnancy loss are beginning to be

Table 46.2. Future needs for antiphospholipid antibody and Hughes syndrome.

Clinical
Prospective studies
Seropositive clinically well patients
Withdrawal of treatment
Pathogenesis studies
    Valve disease
    Livedo
    Nephropathy
    Hyperintense brain lesions on MRI
    Renal transplant thrombosis

Treatment
    Non-warfarin inhibitors of coagulation: antiplatelet, antithrombin
    Biologics
    Peptides (particularly in prevention)
    Complement inhibitors

Etiology and mechanism
    Etiologic agent
    Trigger factors
    Mechanisms
    Endothelial activation
    Thrombosis
    Thrombocytopenia
    Relationship with other hypercoagulable states

Antibody
    Measurement
    Absolute standards
    Variability, discrepancies among LAC, aCL, anti–β_2GPI
    Molecular biology
    Function and modulation

Pathogenic vs. non-pathogenic antibody

Molecular genetics?
Cytokines?
Cell signaling?

tested; if the hypotheses prove true, treatment trial opportunities will broaden, and targeted immunodulators will be tried.

Very little information is available concerning pathogenesis or treatment of Hughes syndrome–associated valve disease, livedo, brain lesions, cognitive dysfunction, the multiple sclerosis-like syndrome, or catastrophic syndrome. We know next to nothing about identification or mechanisms of triggers or about how to measure disease activity. Though many hypercoagulable states are known, we do not truly understand the relationship among them to Hughes syndrome. If there is truly a pathogenic and a non-pathogenic version of aPL, we do not know. These are all topics ready for exploration. Cytokine profiles, genetic predisposing factors, RNA and gene activation patterns, cell surface markers and cell activation need to be explored, even though contemporary work does not suggest that exploration of these areas will be revealing. Table 46.2 lists topics likely to be valuable for future research.

The past half decade has been the most exciting period yet in the field of aPL and Hughes syndrome. As the field prepares to enter its second quarter-century, opportunities abound to explore the illness' etiology, to define the pathogeneses of its disparate elements, to describe its natural history, to perform conclusive treatment trials, and to target interventions to specific disease mechanisms. At the current rate of progress, and with the science and patient bases now in place, when the next edition of this book is printed we may be speaking of cures.

Index